STOICHIOMETRY

Fourth Edition

About the Authors

B I Bhatt is a Consultant to Chemical Industries and is based at Ahmedabad. He provides consultancy services in energy conservation, captive power generation, debottlenecking in chemical industries and other engineering services. He earlier served chemical industries for nearly 34 years. His industrial experience covered the fields of project execution, process engineering, debottlenecking, troubleshooting, production management, management reporting, etc. He spent nearly 18 years at Indian Farmers Fertiliser Cooperative Limited, Kalol Unit in various capacities. Prior to joining the industry, he served at the textile research institute (ATIRA) for nearly 5 years where he was involved in industrial research and consultation to member textile units.

Mr Bhatt carried out units conversion work from fps units to SI units of the *Introduction to Chemical Engineering Thermodynamics*, 6th Edition by Smith, Van Ness and Abbott, a publication of McGraw-Hill, USA.

Mr Bhatt graduated in Chemical Engineering from the University Institute of Chemical Technology, University of Mumbai.

S M Vora is Vice President of Technology and Chairman of Technical Review Committee with Entecgration Inc. Fogelsville, PA, USA. His responsibilities include directing technology developments and chairing technical reviews. He was earlier the Principal Engineering Associate with Air Products and Chemicals, Inc., Allentown, PA, USA where he worked for more than 27 years. His experience and responsibilities included various process improvements, debottlenecking and troubleshooting, catalyst evaluation from laboratory to commercial applications, process development and reactor scale-ups, digital simulations and modelling, atmospheric dispersion, equipment designs, standardizing and centralizing emission calculations and reporting for multi-plants, management reporting, etc. He is a graduate in Chemical Engineering from the University Institute of Chemical Technology, University of Mumbai and a Ph.D. in Chemical Engineering from the Louisiana State University, Baton Rouge, LA, USA.

STOICHIOMETRY

Fourth Edition

B I Bhatt
Consulting Engineer
Aavishkar Consultancy Services
Ahmedabad

S M Vora
Vice President of Technology and
Chairman, Technical Review Committee
Entecgration Inc.
Fogelsville, PA
USA

Tata McGraw-Hill Publishing Company Limited
NEW DELHI

McGraw-Hill Offices
New Delhi New York St Louis San Francisco Auckland Bogotá Caracas
Kuala Lumpur Lisbon London Madrid Mexico City Milan Montreal
San Juan Santiago Singapore Sydney Tokyo Toronto

Tata McGraw-Hill

© 2004, 1996, 1984, 1976 Tata McGraw-Hill Publishing Company Limited

Seventh reprint 2007
RCXDCDRYRCADX

No part of this publication can be reproduced in any form or by
any means without the prior written permission of the publishers

This edition can be exported from India only by the publishers,
Tata McGraw-Hill Publishing Company Limited

ISBN-13: 978-0-07-049494-7
ISBN-10: 0-07-049494-0

Published by Tata McGraw-Hill Publishing Company Limited,
7 West Patel Nagar, New Delhi 110 008, Typeset at Script Makers,
19, A1-B, DDA Market, Pashchim Vihar, New Delhi 110 063 and printed at
Rashtriya Printers, M-135, Panchsheel Garden, Naveen Shahdara, Delhi 110 032

Cover printer: Rashtriya Printers

Dedicated to

OUR PARENTS

Contents

Preface to the Fourth Edition

It gives us great pleasure to present the fourth edition of Stoichiometry. Use of SI units is continued in this edition. Over a period of more than 26 years the book has received overwhelming response from all the users; students and practising engineers. This edition is thoroughly revised with new problems from various industries such as water treatment, oil and fats, environmental pollution, heavy chemicals, etc. Development of a cascade steam balance with optimum energy consumption is dealt at the length that we hope will be a distinctive feature. A few innovations in the chemical industry are introduced in the form of stoichiometric problems.

Use of personal computers for solving all types of engineering problems has increased. Chemical engineering is no exception. Mathematical software has taken the place of spreadsheet programs. We have extensively used Mathcad—versatile mathematical software in solving stoichiometric problems. Simplicity of the software has enhanced the capability of an engineer in finding the optimum solution. We think that problems on optimization with Mathcad solution will be of interest to students as well as practising engineers.

We gratefully acknowledge the suggestions and comments received from various faculty members of different universities which have vastly helped us in bringing out this updated fourth edition. We are indebted to Prof. M M Sharma, Padma Vibhushan and Former Director, University Institute of Chemical Technology, University of Mumbai for his continued encouragement and support to our work. Our special thanks are due to Mr. Nishant Pandya of Nirma Institute of Diploma Studies, Ahmedabad for his supportive work in this edition. We are also grateful to various individuals, institutions and organizations for providing us copyrighted material and permitting us to reproduce them in this edition.

We are sure that all the users—students as well as our colleagues in industry and in academia—will find this edition more useful. All suggestions for further improvement are welcome.

B I Bhatt
S M Vora

Preface to the First Edition

The prime objective of this book is to present fundamentals of chemical engineering in a simple and forthright manner and provide the broad background for applying these principles to industrial and theoretical problems. The importance of stoichiometry—material and energy balances—is widely known and accepted in the chemical industry in analysing a particular process in whole or in part and also in evaluating the economics of the various processes. Basically, stoichiometry deals with the laws of conservation of mass and energy. With this, if the principles of unit operations and chemical reaction engineering are carefully bridged, the subject becomes extremely valuable to the chemical engineers who apply these principles in solving problems. This has been our main consideration in selecting and preparing the material for this book. An introduction to the topic on material and energy balances of unsteady state operations will be of special interest as the topic is gaining more and more industrial importance. In addition to these, extra care has been taken to include the most reliable thermodynamic and other useful data so that the book can serve as a standard text for students and as a reference book for practising engineers. The material has been so organised that the subject can be easily grasped by undergraduate students, nevertheless inclusion of many advanced problems makes the text quite appropriate for postgraduate students and process and design engineers.

The main advantages of the book that can be mentioned here are: a simple introduction of chemical engineering fundamentals, a careful and proper organisation of the subject that allows the student for self-progress, and a treasure of examples and exercises of advanced levels enveloping a wide range of subjects for students of all levels and practising engineers.

We are grateful to Professor M M Sharma, Head of the Department of Chemical Engineering, University Department of Chemical Technology, University of Bombay, for sparing his valuable time in reviewing the text and writing a Foreword to this book. We also thank Professor J B Cordiner and Professor P A Bryant of Louisiana State University, Baton Rouge, Louisiana, USA, and Mr J B Joshi of the Department of Chemical Technology, University of Bombay, for their valuable comments to make this book more complete. We are very grateful to various organisations and institutions for granting us permissions to reproduce their copyright material in this book. Due acknowledgements have been made at appropriate places in the book. In addition, we are thankful to all those who directly or indirectly helped us in our venture.

Special thanks are extended to the National Book Trust, India, for granting the subsidy. We are also grateful to the management and proper authorities of IFFCO, Kalol Unit, Gujarat, and Air Products and Chemicals, Inc., Allentown, Pennsylvania, USA, for granting us the permission to publish this book. Our thanks are also due to our wives, Minaxi Bhatt and Kapila Vora, whose patience and encouragement during this work were very helpful.

B I BHATT
S M VORA

Chapter 1

Dimensions and Units

1.1 INTRODUCTION

Physical theories gain their definiteness from the mathematical form in which they are expressed. The function of numbering and measuring is indispensable even in order to reproduce the raw material of facts that are to be reproduced and unified in a theory.

DR. E.A. CASSIRER[1]
German Philosopher

No better introduction can be given than the above quotes of Dr. Cassirer which clearly indicate that a thorough knowledge of dimensions and the various systems of units is not only essential but a must for a logical understanding of the subject. Mathematics and technology are international languages. Engineers converse effectively in formulae and units. To understand one another, communication is required in commonly accepted units. The expression of results of measurements and/or of calculations in a symbolic and numerical form is essential for the development of physics, chemistry and technology. The study of stoichiometry is no different than that of the other sciences and one must start with the understanding of fundamental quantities, namely, dimensions. This will facilitate appropriate and consistent units in solving stoichiometric problems. This chapter not only deals with these fundamentals but also with the methods of conversion of the units from one system to another.

1.2 DIMENSIONS AND SYSTEMS OF UNITS

According to Maxwell, every physical quantity can be expressed as a product of a pure number and an unit, where the unit is a selected reference quantity in terms of which all quantities of the same kind can be expressed. Physical entities are defined by means of certain quantities, such as mass, length, pressure, energy, etc. While defining a particular physical quantity, two questions need to be answered; (i) What would be the most convenient unit? (ii) What would be the best form and material for the standard, physically representing that unit? Physical quantities can be classified as *fundamental* quantities and *derived* quantities. The first group consist of four important quantities, namely—length, mass, time and thermodynamic temperature. These are called *dimensions* or *base units* and are represented by symbols L, M, θ and T, respectively. The second group consists of quantities derived from the fandamental quantities, such as area, force, pressure, energy etc. It follows, therefore, that *derived* quantities are represented algebraically in terms of multiplication and division of fundamental quantities.

The fundamental quantities are represented by a system of units according to the system of measurement. Basically, the *standard* physically representing the base units differs in different systems of units. In this chapter three systems of units, viz. fps, mks and SI will be discussed.

The fps system, developed in England, is based on foot, pound and second as standard measurements for length, mass and time, respectively. This is now commonly known as US Customary Units system.

In 1791, in France, a system of units entirely based on unit of length, *the metre* was created. Because of its foundation entirely based on the metre, this system got the name *Systèm Metrique* or Metric System (mks). The unit of mass in the metric system is kilogram. An important feature of this system was the decimal expression. This system was increasingly adopted in various countries, including India. In India, the mks system was introduced in 1957.

In another subsidiary system, the cgs system, the step is derived from the mks system. The base standards of the cgs system were accepted to be those of the mks system. In practice these two systems were used side by side, depending on the convenience. For example, it was common to express the density in g/cm^3 rather than in kg/m^3 (or kg/L) in mks system.

For better international understanding, in particular, in science and technology and in international and trade relations, a need for an international system of units was felt. At the 10th General Conference on Weights and Measures in 1954 at Paris, it was decided to have an international practical system of units, based on six base units, namely, metre, kilogram, second, ampere, kelvin and candela. It may be seen that first four base units are the same as those in the mks system. In 1960, the 11th General Conference on Weights and Measures in Paris gave the name *Le Système International d'Unitès* or the International System of Units and abbreviated as SI in all languages. Along with six base units, two more supplementary units, namely, *radian* and *steradian* were also defined.

Later it became evident that the quantity mass, although it may be an appropriate concept in mechanics, is entirely unsuitable for use in chemistry where the molecular structure and in particular, the number of molecules in a system are much more relevant than it total mass. For this reason, the concept *amount of substance* was introduced as a base unit by the 14th General Conference on Weights and Measures in 1971, which by definition is the amount of substance of system containing as many elementary entities as there are atoms in 0.012 kilogram of carbon-12 and this unit of quantity was called a *mole* (abbreviated as mol). The unified scale of mole thus obtained gives value of the relative atomic mass (m_u). Reference 2 give most important aspects of basic meteorology. References 2, 3, and 4 give an excellent account of SI. India adopted SI units through the Standards of Weights and Measures Act, 1976.

1.3 FUNDAMENTAL QUANTITIES

The fundamental quantities in different systems of units are given in Table 1.1.

Table 1.1 Fundamental Quantities[2, 3, 4]

Fundamental Quantity	System of Units			Symbolic Abbreviation			Dimensions
	SI	Metric	fps	SI	Metric	fps	
Length	Metre	Metre	Foot	m	m	ft	L
Mass	Kilogram	Kilogram	Pound	kg	kg	lb	M
Temperature	Kelvin	Celsius	Fahrenheit	K	°C	°F	T
Time	Second	Second	Second	s	s	s	θ
Electric current	Ampere	Ampere	Ampere	A	A	A	I
Amount of substance	Mole	—	—	mol	—	—	n
Luminous intensity	Candela	—	—	cd	—	—	

The thermodynamic temperature (kelvin), defined in SI, is accepted as the absolute temperature in the metric system. The thermodynamic temperature scale is defined by choosing the triple point of water as the fundamental fixed point, and assigning to it the exact temperature value of 273.16 degrees kelvin. In other words, kelvin, the unit of thermodynamic temperature, is 1/273.16 of the thermodynamic temperature of the triple point of water. In the fps system, the unit of absolute temperature is Rankine.

Degree Kelvin (K) = °C + 273.15*

Degree Rankine (°R) = °F + 459.67

Use of degrees Fahrenheit is not permitted in SI.

---

* The thermodynamic temperature **273.15 K** is by definition **0.01 K** below the thermodynamic temperature of the triple point of water. In the examples in the text, SI and metric units are given. While giving a conversion of K to °C or vice versa, the difference of 0.15 will be ignored for all practical purposes except for the values of high accuracy.

For expressing the temperature interval in absolute temperature scale, the same symbol is used.

$$280 \text{ K} - 235 \text{ K} = 45 \text{ K}$$
$$520°\text{R} - 480°\text{R} = 40°\text{R}$$
$$30°\text{C} = 303\text{K}$$
$$35°\text{F} = 494°\text{R}$$

The supplementary SI units, radian and steradian, are not discussed as these are not used in the book. Although, the International Organization for Standardization (ISO)[3] have recommended comma (,) as a decimal marker, the current practice of using a point (.) as the decimal marker in India will be followed in this book.

1.4 DERIVED QUANTITIES

There can be any number of derived quantities, and hence, it is difficult to list all of them. However, the commonly used quantities for stoichiometric calculations in SI, mks and cgs systems are listed in Table 1.2. The International Committee for Weights and Measures have considered that in general, cgs units should preferably not be used with SI. Considering the increasing adoption of SI in a large number of countries and also in India (particularly in science and technology), the SI will be followed in this book.

Table 1.2 Derived Quantities[2,3,4]

Derived Quantity	Units in SI/mks/cgs System	Abbreviated Units	Symbol	Dimension
Mass	Kilogram	kg	m	M
	Gram	g		M
Area	Square metres	m^2	$A(S)$	L
	Square centimetres	cm^2		L
Volume	Cubic metres	m^3	$V(v)$	L^3
	Cubic centimetres	cm^3		L^3
	Cubic decimetres	dm^3		L^3
Capacity	Litres	L	V	L^3
Linear velocity	Metres per second	m/s	u,v,w	$L\theta^{-1}$
Linear acceleration	Metres per second per second	m/s^2	a, g (free fall)	$L\theta^{-2}$
Density	Kilograms per cubic metre	kg/m^3	ρ	ML^{-3}
	Grams per millilitre	g/mL		ML^{-3}
Specific volume	Cubic metres per kilogram	m^3/kg	v	L^3M^{-1}
Force	Newtons	N	F	$ML\theta^{-2}$
	kilograms-force*	kgf	F	

* Base unit in mks system, but not used with SI.

(Contd.)

Table 1.2 Contd.

Derived Quantity	Units in SI/mks/cgs System	Abbreviated Units	Symbol	Dimension
Force	Dynes	dyn		$ML\theta^{-2}$
Pressure	Newtons per square metre (Pascals)	N/m^2 (Pa)	p (P)	$ML^{-1}\theta^{-2}$
	Kilograms-force per square centimetre	kgf/cm^2		FL^{-2}
Work/Energy	Joules	J	W	$ML^2\theta^{-2}$
	Ergs	erg		$ML^2\theta^{-2}$
	Metres kilogram force	m · kgf		MF
Heat/Enthalpy	Joules	J	q, Q, H	$ML^2\,\theta^{-2}$
	Kilocalories	kcal		$ML^2\,\theta^{-2}$
Power	Kilowatts	kW	P	$ML^2\,\theta^{-3}$
	Horsepower	HP		$MF\,\theta^{-1}$
Heat flow	Joules per second	J/s or W	ϕ	$ML^2\,\theta^{-3}$
	kilocalories per hour	kcal/h		$ML^2\,\theta^{-3}$
Specific/ Absolute humidity	Kilograms water per kilogram dry air	kg/kg	H, x	$M°L°\theta°$
Relative humidity	Nil	Nil	RH	$M°L°\theta°$
Saturation ratio	Nil	Nil	ϕ	$M°L°\theta°$
Mass flow rate	Kilograms per second	kg/s	$q_m, \dot{m}$	$M\,\theta^{-1}$
Volumetric flow rate	Cubic metres per second	m^3/s	q_v, V	$L^3\theta^{-1}$
	Litres per second	L/s		$L^3\theta^{-1}$
Heat capacity	Joules per kilogram per degree kelvin	J/(kg · K)	C	$L^2\theta^{-2}T^{-1}$
	Kilocalories per kilo-gram per degree Celsius	kcal/(kg · °C)		$L^2\,\theta^{-2}T^{-1}$
Molar heat capacity	Joules per mole per degree kelvin	J/(mol · K)	C_m	$ML^2\theta^{-2}n^{-1}T^{-1}$
	Kilocalories per kilo-gram mole per degree Celsius	kcal/(kmol · °C)		$ML^2\theta^{-2}n^{-1}T^{-1}$

Note: In general mks units are not recommended for use with SI.

1.4.1 Force

The definition of force follows from Newton's second law of motion, which states that force is proportional to the product of mass and acceleration.

$$F \propto m \times a \tag{1.1}$$

Introducing a proportionality constant K,

$$F = K\,m\,a \tag{1.2}$$

Force and acceleration are both vector quantities and hence they should act in the same direction. There are two ways of selecting the constant K. In one case, K is selected as unity (dimensionless), and with this value, the units newton (SI) and dyne are defined.

The newton (N) is the force which when applied to a body having a mass of one kilogram gives it an acceleration of one m/s^2.

The dyne (dyn) is the force which when applied to a body having a mass of one gram gives it an acceleration of one cm/s^2.

Based on these definitions,

$$1\ N = 10^5\ dyn$$

A similar unit in the fps system is the poundal which is the force, when applied to a body having a mass of one pound gives it an acceleration of one ft/s^2.

$$1\ pdl = 30.48 \times 453.5924 = 13\ 825.5\ dyn$$

Another choice of the constant K yields the technical unit of Force and is defined as a fundamental quantity. Thus, the constant K becomes a dimensional quantity. Its numerical value is not unity but fixed at $1/g_c$.

$$F = \left(\frac{1}{g_c}\right) ma \tag{1.3}$$

$$g_c = 9.806\ 65\ (kg \cdot m)/(kgf \cdot s^2) = 32.174\ (1b \cdot ft)/(1bf \cdot s^2)$$

g_c is called the Newton's law conversion factor. Its value corresponds to the acceleration due to gravity (g) at the means seal level (9.806 65 m/s^2 or 32.174 ft/s^2). It should be clearly noted that g_c does not vary even though g varies from place to place. In ordinary calculations, however, g/g_c is taken as 1.0 kgf/kg. By definition, g_c has the units of 1 (kg $\cdot$ m)/(N $\cdot$ s^2) in SI.

The technical units of force in mks and fps systems are kilogram-force and pound-force, respectively.

The kilogram-force (kgf) is the force which when applied to a body having a mass of one kilogram gives it an acceleration of 9.806 65 m/s^2.

The pound force (1bf) is the force which when applied to a body having a mass of one pound gives it an acceleration of 32.174 ft/s^2.

The force becomes weight when the body acts under gravitational acceleration (g), i.e., when $a = g$ in Eq. (1.2).

$$\text{Weight, } G = \left(\frac{1}{g_c}\right) mg \tag{1.4}$$

Since g and g_c are assumed equal for all practical purposes,

$$G = m \tag{1.5}$$

Thus, the values of weight and mass become practically equal.

In order to differentiate between the terms mass and force, their units are distinguished by writing 'f' at the end of the fundamental unit of force.

The measurement of force, pressure, mass and weight have in the past been conveniently made through the use of gravitational acceleration without taking into account the variation of this acceleration from one location to another, which was normally insignificant in the applications. However, as process industries have spread geographically and as the processes involved require more sophisticated control, the difference between the points of calibration and use of an instrument has become more significant. The practice of ignoring the difference was also fundamentally wrong. Both these reasons have necessitated the use of SI in the current practice and the term 'weight' is discarded for use with SI.

1.4.2   Volume

Volume is measured in cubic metres and litres (SI) and in gallons (fps).

A litre is the volume occupied by a mass of one kilogram of pure air free water at the temperature of its maximum density (at 277.15 K or 4°C) and under normal atmospheric pressure. The cubic decimetre and litre are unequal and differ by about 28 parts in 10^6 parts. Hence the word 'litre' can be employed as a special name of the cubic decimetre. However, the name litre should not be employed to give the results of high accuracy volume measurements.

$$1 \text{ litre} = 1.000 \ 028 \text{ cubic decimetres} \qquad \text{(exact)}$$

Approximately, 1 cubic metre = 1000 litres = 1 kilolitre

The Imperial and US gallons are different. The former is defined as the volume occupied by a quantity of distilled water, which weighs 10 lb in air at the temperature of 62°F (289.82 K or 16.67°C) and the pressure of 30 in Hg (762 torr). The US gallon is equal to 231 in^3 (3.7854 L).

1.4.3   Pressure

Pressure is defined as the force acting on unit area exposed to the pressure

$$p = \frac{F}{A} \tag{1.6}$$

The common units of pressure in SI, mks and fps units are N/m^2 (known as Pascal, Pa), kgf/cm^2 and 1bf/in^2 (commonly known as psi), respectively.

Pressure is normally measured with the help of a gauge which registers the difference between the pressure in vessel and the local atmospheric pressure. This is known as the over pressure/gauge pressure (p_e) and the letter 'g' follows the unit. The gauge pressure does not indicate the true total pressure. In order to obtain the true pressure or pressure above reference zero, it is necessary to add the local atmospheric or barometric pressure expressed in coherent units to the gauge pressure. This sum is called the absolute pressure and the letter 'a' follows the units. In general, if no letter follows the pressure units, it is taken as absolute pressure in this book.

Absolute pressure = gauge pressure + atmospheric pressure   (1.7)

Although the actual atmospheric pressure varies from one locality to another, its value at the mean sea level is 101 325 N/m^2 or Pa (1.033 kgf/cm^2) and is called the *standard* atmosphere (symbol 'atm'). In SI, the standard atmosphere and bar are accepted as the practical units.

$$1 \text{ atm} = 101\ 325 \text{ Pa (exact)}$$
$$1 \text{ bar} = 10^5 \text{ Pa} = 1.019\ 716 \text{ kgf/cm}^2 = 0.986\ 923 \text{ atm}$$

Quite often, the pressure is expressed in pressure heads.

Pressure head = absolute pressure/density   (1.8)

The more commonly used pressure heads are in terms of mercury and water columns.

$$1 \text{ atm} = 760 \text{ torr (or mm Hg)} = 10.33 \text{ m } H_2O$$

Vacuum refers to sub-atmospheric pressure.

Absolute pressure = atmospheric pressure – vacuum   (1.9)

Vacuum is usually expressed in torr (mm Hg) or Pa or mbar.

1.4.4 Work (Energy) and Power

Work (energy) is defined as the product of the force acting on a body and the distance travelled by the body.

$$W = \mathbf{F} \times d \tag{1.10}$$

The units of work (energy) in SI, mks, cgs and fps systems are joule, m·kgf, erg and ft·1bf, respectively.

Energy is a physical entity which is present in a system in different forms, e.g., mechanical (work), electromagnetic, chemical or thermal. One form of energy is convertible to another from.

One joule is the work done when the point of application of one newton force moves a distance of one metre in the direction of the applied force.

One erg is the work done when the point of application of one dyne force moves a distance of one centimetre in the direction of the applied force.

$$1 \text{ J} = 10^7 \text{ erg}$$

Power P is defined as the work W done per unit time.

$$\text{Power } P = \frac{W}{\theta} \tag{1.11}$$

$$1 \text{ Watt} = 1 \text{ J/s}$$
$$1 \text{ metric horsepower} = 75 \text{ (m·kgf)/s} = 0.7355 \text{ kW}$$
$$= 0.986\ 32 \text{ hp}$$
$$1 \text{ British horsepower} = 550 \text{ (ft·1bf)/s} = 0.7457 \text{ kW}$$

$$= 1.013\,87 \text{ metric hp}$$

Horsepower units are not recommended for use with SI.

1.4.5 Heat

Heat is one form of energy that flows from higher temperature to lower tempera-ture, i.e., enthalpy in transit. The units of heat in SI, mks, cgs and fps systems are the joule (J), kilocalorie (kcal), calorie (cal) and British thermal unit (Btu), respectively and are same as those for energy.

There are several definitions of Btu and cal. All are defined in terms of the joule. Each Btu and its corresponding cal are related by a heat capacity equa-tion.

$$1 \text{ calorie (thermochemical)} = 4.184 \text{ J} \qquad \text{(exact)}$$

$$1 \text{ calorie (International Steam Tables, called IT)} = 4.1868 \text{ J} \qquad \text{(exact)}$$

$$1 \text{ Btu (International Steam Tables, called IT)} = 1055.056 \text{ J}$$

The Celsius Heat Unit (CHU) and Therm were also used in the fps system.

$$1 \text{ CHU} = 1.8 \text{ Btu}$$

$$1 \text{ Therm} = 10^5 \text{ Btu}$$

In SI system, heat flux (i.e., heat flow) rate, ϕ, is customarily expressed in unit of power, i.e. watts (W).

1.4.6 Derived Electrical Units

Current is the undamental quantity in electricity. The volt V is the unit of electromotive force or of potential difference. Resistance (R in ohms) of the conductor is defined as

$$R = \frac{V}{I} \qquad (1.12)$$

where R is the resistance in ohms, V is the potential difference in volts and I is the current in amperes.

Coulomb is the unit of quantity of electricity and is defined as the quantity of electricity carried in one second by a current of one amperes across any cross-section

$$1 \text{ Faraday } (F) = 96\,485.309 \text{ C/mol (based on carbon-12)}$$

The quantity coulomb (C) an important quantity in electrochemistry.

1.5 CONVERSIONS

It is often required to convert units of a particular from one system to another. Table 1.3 gives a brief list of the conversions[6, 7, 8, 9, 10] in common use. Appendix I gives the conversions in a direct usable form.

The precision to which a given conversion factor is known, and its applica-tion, determine the number of significant figures which should be used. While comparing the data given in Appendix I with those given in many handbooks and standards, it may be hinted that different source disagree, in many cases, in the fifth or further figure which indicates that four or five significant figures represent the precision for these factors fairly accurately. At present, the acuracy of process instrumentation, analog or digital, needs only three significant figures. Additional accuracy is only needed in basic fundamental research and could be waste of time in the industrial practice.

Table 1.3 Condensed Table of Conversion Factors

Length:	1 m = 1.093 613 yd
	= 3.280 84 ft
	1 cm = 0.393 701 in
	1 km = 0.621 37 miles
Area:	1 m^2 = 10.763 91 ft^2
	= 1.195 99 yd^2
	1 cm^2 = 0.155 in^2
	1 km^2 = 0.386 102 mile^2
	1 ha = 100 00 m^2
	= 2.471 05 acre
	= 0.003 861 mile^2
Volume:	1 m^3 = 1000 dm^3 = 1000 L
	= 35.314 67 ft^3
	= 1.307 95 yd^3
	1 cm^3 = 0.061 024 in^3
Capacity:	1 L = 0.219 969 Imperial gal
	= 0.264 172 US gal
	= 0.035 3147 ft^3
	1 kL = 1000 L
	= 0.000 810 71 acre·ft
Mass:	1 kg = 1000 g
	= 2.204 623 lb
Mass:	1 t = 1000 kg
	= 0.984 21 T
	= 1.102 311 T (short, used in USA)
	= 2204.623 lb
	1 g = 15.4324 grain
Density:	1 kg/dm^3 = 1 kg/L
	= 70 156.8 grain/Imperial gal
	= 58 417.82 grain/US gal
	1 g/cm^3 = 62.427 95 lb/ft^3
	= 10.0224 lb/Imperial gal
	= 8.345 405 lb/US gal
	= 0.036 127 lb/in^3

(Contd.)

Table 1.3 Contd.

Specific volume:	$1\ m^3/kg$ = 16.018 48 ft^3/lb
	= 99.7765 Imperial gal/lb
	= 119.8265 US gal/lb
Force:	1 N = 0.101 972 kgf
	= 0.224 809 lbf
Pressure:	1 kPa = 0.010 197 kgf/cm^2
	= 0.145 038 lbf/in^2 or psi
	1 bar = 0.1 MPa
	= 1.019 716 kgf/cm^2
	= 14.503 77 lbf/in^2
	1 atm = 101.325 kPa (defined)
	= 1.013 25 bar
	= 1.033 227 kgf/cm^2
	= 14.695 95 lbf/in^2
	1 torr (1 mm Hg) = 133.3224 Pa
	= 1.333 224 mbar
	= 0.039 37 in Hg
	1 mbar = 0.750 06 torr
Energy:	1 J = 0.238 846 cal (IT)
	= 2.777 778 $\times$ 10^{-7} kWh
	= 9.478 172 $\times$ 10^{-4} Btu (IT)
	= 0.101 972 $kgf\cdot m$
	= 0.737 562 $lbf\cdot ft$
	= 9.869 233 $\times$ 10^{-3} $L\cdot atm$
	1 kWh = 859.8452 kcal (IT)
	= 3412.142 Btu (IT)
	1 kcal (IT) = 3.968 321 Btu (IT)
	= 4.1868 kJ
	1 $kgf\cdot m$ = 7.233 $lbf\cdot ft$
Power:	1 kW = 1.359 62 metric hp
	= 1.341 02 hp (British)
	= 859.8452 kcal (IT)/h
	= 3412.142 Btu (IT)/h
	1 $(m\cdot kgf)/s$ = 7.233 (ft.lbf)/s
Heat capacity:	1 $J/(g\cdot K)$ = 0.238 846 kcal (IT)/(kg $\cdot°C$)
	= 0.238 846 Btu (IT)/(lb $\cdot°F$)
Temperature:	$°C = 5/9\ (F° - 32)$
	$°F = (9/5)\ °C + 32$

1.6 RECOMMENDATIONS FOR USE OF UNITS

The recommendations issued by the General Conference on Weight and Measures[2], International Organization for the Standardization[3], Bureau of Indian Standards [IS : 1890 (Part 0)-1983] and American Society for Testing Materials (E – 380)[10] for the use of units are summarised as follows.

(i) SI prefixes are given in Table 1.4.

Table 1.4 SI Prefixes

Factor	Prefix	Symbol
10^{24}	yotta	Y
10^{21}	zetta	Z
10^{18}	exa	E
10^{15}	peta	P
10^{12}	tera	T
10^{9}	giga	G
10^{6}	mega	M
10^{3}	kilo	k
10^{2}	hecto	h
10^{1}	deca	da
10^{-1}	deci	d
10^{-2}	centi	c
10^{-3}	milli	m
10^{-6}	micro	μ
10^{-9}	nano	n
10^{-12}	pico	p
10^{-15}	femto	f
10^{-18}	atto	a
10^{-21}	zepto	z
10^{-24}	yocto	y

(ii) An exponent attached to compound prefix-unit implies that the exponent refers to the entire compound unit and not just to the base symbol.

1 cm³ means volume of a cube having one cm side.

(iii) The product of two or more units may be indicated in any one of the following ways.

Correct: N·m or N m   Incorrect: Nm

(iv) A solidus (oblique stroke,/), a horizontal line or negative powers may be used to express a derived unit, formed from two others dy division, e.g.,

m/s, $\dfrac{m}{s}$, m·s⁻¹ or m s⁻¹

(v) A solidus must not be repeated on the same line unless ambiguity is avoided by parentheses.

Correct: Incorrect:

m/s² or m·s⁻² or m s⁻²   m/s/s

J/(mol·K) or J·mol⁻¹·K⁻¹   J/mol.K or J/mol/K

(vi) Unit symbols do not change in the plural. For example, 5 centimetres should be abbreviated as 5 cm and not as 5 cms.

(vii) Unit symbols are not followed by a full stop (period) except at the end of a sentence.

Correct : 8 kg   Incorrect : 8 kg.

(viii) When numerical values fall outside the range of 0.1 to 1000, it is recommended that the numerals be separated into groups of three with a space replacing the traditional comma.

Recommended	Not recommended
3 600 or 3600	3,600
19 625 725	19,625,725
0.001 625	0.001,625 or 0.001625
0.046 89	0.046,89 or 0.004689

In this book, four digits or decimals are grouped.

(ix) Prefix symbols are printed without any space between the prefix symbol and unit symbol.

Correct : 10.5 kW   Incorrect : 10.5 k W

(x) Compound prefixes formed by the juxtaposition of two or more SI prefixes are not to be used.

Correct : 1 nm   Incorrect : 1 mμm

(xi) A prefix should never be used alone.

Correct : $10^6/m^3$ Incorrect : M/m^3

(xii) Although kilogram is the base unit in SI units, names of decimal multiples and sub-multiples of mass are formed by attaching prefixes to the word 'gram'.

Correct : 1 mg   Incorrect : 1 μkg

(xiii) Good practice recommends selection of a prefix which, whenever possible, provides a numerical value between 0.1 and 1000. Prefer expression 10.0 kPa over 0.01 MPa. However, when a ground of values is tabulated, they should be expressed in the same unit multiple even though their numerical value lies outside 0.1 to 1000 range.

1.2×10^4 N can be written as 12 kN.

1421 Pa can be written as 1.421 kPa.

(xiv) If the magnitude of the number is less than unity, the decimal sign should preferably be preceded by a zero, e.g.,

.125 should be written as 0.125.

(xv) The SI prefixes are not to be used with °C or K.

Example 1.1 The volumetric flow rate of kerosene in 80 mm nominal diameter pipe is 75 Imperial gallons per minute. Taking the density of kerosene as 0.8 kg/dm^3, find the mass flow in kg/s.

Solution

$$\text{Volumetric flow rate } q_v = 75 \text{ (gallon/min)} \times \left(\frac{1}{60}\right) \text{ (min/s)}$$

$$\times \left(\frac{1}{0.129\ 67}\right) \text{ (dm}^3\text{/gallon)}$$

$$= 5.683 \text{ dm}^3\text{/s}$$

$$\text{Density, } \rho = 0.8 \text{ kg/dm}^3$$

$$\text{Mass flow rate, } q_m = q_v \times \rho$$
$$= 5.683 \times 0.8 = 4.546 \text{ kg/s} \qquad Ans.$$

Example 1.2 Steam is flowing at the rate of 2000 kg/h in a 3″ NB 40 schedule pipe at 440 kPa (4.4 bar) absolute and 453 K (180°C). Calculate the velocity of the steam in the pipeline.

Solution

$$\text{Mass flow rate, } q_m = 2000 \text{ kg/h}$$

Internal diameter of 3″ NB 40 schedule pipe = 3.068 in = 77.927 mm

$$\text{Cross-sectional area of the pipe, } A = \left(\frac{\pi}{4}\right)(77.927)^2/10^6$$
$$= 47.694 \times 10^{-4} \text{ m}^2$$

Specific volume of the steam at 440 kPa a and 453 K,

$$v = 0.461\ 66 \text{ m}^3/\text{kg (ref. Steam Tables; Appendix III.3)}$$

Volumetric flow rate of

$$\text{steam, } q_v = 2000 \text{ (kg/h)} \times \left(\frac{1}{3600}\right) \text{(h/s)} \times 0.461\ 66 \text{ (m}^3/\text{kg)}$$
$$= 0.2565 \text{ m}^3/\text{s}$$

$$\text{Velocity of steam, } v_s = \frac{q_v}{A}$$
$$= 0.2565 \text{ m}^3/\text{s} \times 1/(47.694 \times 10^{-4}) \text{ 1/m}^2$$
$$= 53.77 \text{ m/s} \qquad Ans.$$

Example 1.3 A Ton of Refrigeration (TR) is classically defined as the rate of heat absorption equivalent to the latent heat in a short ton (2000 lb) of ice melted in 24 hours. Latent heat of fusion (λ_f) of ice is 144 thermochemical Btu/lb at 32°F. Calculate equivalent energy in kW equivalent to 1 TR.

Solution

$$\text{Heat absorption rate, equivalent to 1 Tr, } \phi = \left(\frac{2000}{24}\right) \text{(lb/h)} \times 144 \text{ (therm Btu/lb)}$$
$$\times 0.251\ 996 \text{ (therm kcal/therm Btu)}$$
$$\times 4.184 \text{ (kJ/therm kcal)} \times \left(\frac{1}{3600}\right) \text{(h/s)}$$
$$= 3.5145 \text{ kW} \qquad Ans.$$

Example 1.4 The conductance of a fluid-flow system is defined as the volumetric flow rate, referred to a pressure of one torr (133.322 Pa). For an orifice, the conductance C can be computed[11] from

$$C = 89.2\ A\ \sqrt{\frac{T}{M}} \text{ ft}^3/\text{s}$$

where A = area of opening, ft^2

T = temperature, °R

M = Molar mass

Convert the empirical equation into SI units.

Solution

Let C', A' and T' be the conductance, area of opening and temperature in m^3/s, m^2 and K respectively. Molar mass is unaffected by change of units.

$$C = 35.314\ 67\ C'$$

$$T = 1.8\ T'$$

$$A = 10.763\ 91\ A'$$

$$35.341\ 67\ C' = 89.2 \times 10.763\ 91\ A' \sqrt{1.8\frac{T'}{M}}$$

$$C' = 36.447\ A' \sqrt{\frac{T'}{M}}\ \text{m}^3/\text{s} \qquad\qquad Ans.$$

EXERCISES

1.1 Make following conversions:

(a)   Wavelength 5500 Å to nm.   [*Ans.* 550 nm]

(b)   175 grain moisture/lb dry air to g moisture/kg dry air.

[*Ans.* 25 g moisture/kg dry air]

1.2 In a double effect evaporator plant, the second effect is maintained under vacuum of 475 torr (mm Hg). Find the absolute pressure in kPa, bar and psi.

[*Ans.* 38 kPa, 0.38 bar, 5.51 psi]

1.3 A force equal to 192.6 kgf is applied on a piston with a diameter of 5 cm. Find the pressure exerted on the piston in kPa, bar and psi.

[*Ans.* 98.066 kPa, 0.981 bar, 14.227 psi]

1.4 Iron metal weighing 500 lb occupies a volume of 29.25 L. Calculate the density of Fe in kg/dm^3.

[*Ans.* 7.754 kg/dm^3]

1.5 The diameter and height of a vertical cylindrical tank are 5 ft and 6 ft 6 in respectively. It is full up to 75% height with carbon tetrachloride (CCl_4), the density of which is 1.6 kg/L. Find the mass in kilograms.

[*Ans.* 4336 kg]

1.6 A bag filter of 5 micron rating is designed for a pressure drop of 0.05 lbf/in^2 per US gallon per minute of water solution in clean conditions. Calculate pressure drop in kPa from the filter for water flow rate of 10 m^3/h.

[*Ans.* 15.178 kPa]

1.7 Corrosion rates are normally reported in mills per year (mpy) in the chemical process industry. For the measurement of the rates, a corrosion test coupon is inserted in the process stream for a definite period. The loss of weight is measured during the period of insertion.

In a particular test, a coupon of carbon steel was kept in a cooling water circuit. The dimensions of the coupon were measured to be 7.595 cm × 1.276 cm × 0.1535 cm. Mass of the coupon before insertion in the circuit and after exposure for 50 days were measured to be 14.9412 g and 14.6254 g, respectively. Calculate the rate of corrosion. Take the density of carbon steel to be the same as the one calculated in Exercise 1.4.

Note: 1 mil per year = 1/1000 in per year

[*Ans.* 5.3 mpy]

1.8 Vapour pressure of benzene in the temperature range of 280.65 K (7.5°C) to 377.15 K (104°C) can be calculated using the following Antoine equation.

$$\log_{10} p = 6.9057 - \frac{1211.0}{(t + 220.8)}$$

where p = Vapour pressure in torr (mm Hg), and

           t = Temperature in °C

Convert the above equation in SI units.

1.9 Heat capacity of gaseous n-butane is given by

$$C_{mp}^{o} = 4.429 + 40.159 \times 10^{-3}\, T - 68.562 \times 10^{-7}\, T^2$$

where C_{mp}^{o} = Heat capacity in Btu/(lb mole · °R) and

           T = Temperature in °R

Convert the equation in SI units.

1.10 Pressure drop across a venturi scrubber can be calculated using following Calvert equation[12].

$$\Delta p = (5 \times 10^{-5})\, v^2\, L$$

where Δp = pressure drop, in WC

           L = liquid flow rate, US gal/1000 ft^3 gas

           v = gas velocity in the venturi throat, ft/s

Convert the equation in SI units.

1.11 In the case of fluids, the local heat-transfer coefficient for long tubes and using bulk-temperature properties is expressed by the empirical equation[13].

$$h = 0.023\, G^{0.8} \times k^{0.67} \times C_p^{0.33}/(D^{0.2} \times \mu^{0.47})$$

where h = heat-transfer coefficient, Btu/(h · ft^2 · °F)

$$G = \text{mass velocity of fluids, lb/(ft}^2 \cdot \text{s})$$
$$C_p = \text{heat capacity of fluid at constant pressure, Btu/(lb} \cdot {}^\circ\text{F})$$
$$k = \text{thermal conductivity, Btu/(h} \cdot \text{ft} \cdot {}^\circ\text{F})$$
$$D = \text{diameter of tube, ft and}$$
$$\mu = \text{viscosity of liquid, lb/(ft} \cdot \text{s})$$

Convert the empirical equation into SI units.

Note: Will the above equation change when consistent SI units are used? Why?

REFERENCES

1. Cassirer, E., *Substance and Function*, Dover Publication, USA, 1953, p. 115.
2. *The International System of Units (SI)*, National Institute of Standards and Technology Publication No. 330, USA, 1991.
3. ISO 1000 : 1992/Amd. 1 : 1998 (E), *SI Units and Recommendations for the Use of their Multiples and Certain other Units (Amendment 1)*, International Organization for Standards, Switzerland.
4. Mills, I., T. Cvitas, K. Homann, N. Kallay and K. Kuchitsu, *Quantities, Units and Symbols in Physical Chemistry*, 2nd Ed., IUPAC Chemical Data Series, Blackwell Science Ltd., UK, 1993.
5. IS : 10 005-1985, *SI Units and Recommendations for the Use of their Multiples and of Certain other Units (First Revision)*, Bureau of Indian Standards, New Delhi.
6. *SI for AIChE*, American Institute of Chemical Engineers, USA, 1979.
7. *The International System of Units—Physical Constants and Conversion Factors*, Second Revision, National Aeronautics and Space Administration Document No. SP-7012, USA, 1973.
8. IS : 786-1967 *Conversion Factors and Conversion Tables (First Revision)*, Bureau of Indian Standards, New Delhi.
9. *Introduction to the TRC Thermodynamic Tables: Non-Hydrocarbons*, Thermodynamic Research Centre, USA, 1991.
10. ASTM Standard for Metric Practice E-380, American Society for Testing and Materials, USA, October 1985.
11. Green, D. W. and Malony, J. O., Perry's *Chemical Engineers' Handbook*, 6th Ed. McGraw-Hill, New York, 1984, pp. 5–33.
12. Doolittle, C., Woodhull, J. and Venkatesh, M., *Chemical Engineering*, **109** (13), Dec. 2002, p. 50.
13. McCabe, W. L., J. C. Smith and P. Harriott, *Unit Operations of Chemical Engineering*, 6th Ed. McGraw-Hill, New York, 2001, p. 348.

Chapter 2

Basic Chemical Calculations

2.1 INTRODUCTION

In Chapter 1, an attempt was made to present various systems of units and their conversions from one system of units to another. Before discussing material and energy balances, it is important to understand basic chemical principles.

Matter exist in three different forms, viz., solids, liquids and gases. Most of the elements and compounds can be had in all the three forms except a few, e.g., iodine and ammonium chloride, for which the liquid state is not visible and the solid state is sublimated into gaseous state. The easiest way of expressing the quantity of matter is mass. For solids and liquids, this can be done by weighing on a balance. However, a gas occupies the entire volume available to it, and hence it is customary to specify the volume along with its temperature and pressure. Very often, liquid volumes are also specified, in which case, additional information regarding its density is required to compute the mass of the liquid.

2.2 MOLE, ATOMIC MASS AND MOLAR MASS

Although measurement in terms of mass is of direct interest to the engineers, matter is basically made up of atoms and molecules. However, since the discovery of the fundamental laws of chemistry, chemists considered it significant to express quantity of matter in atoms and molecules rather than in terms of auxiliary properties, such as mass and volume. For instance, 'gram atom' and 'gram mole' have been used to specify amounts of chemical elements or compounds. These units have a direct relationship with 'atomic weights' 'molecular weights' which are, in fact, relative masses.

Originally, the atomic mass of oxygen was taken as a reference base and its numerical value was fixed at 16. However, the physicists discovered different isotopes of oxygen which created a conflict between the physicists and the chemists. In 1959-60, this controversy came to an end and both the groups of scientists finally agreed on a standard based on carbon-12. The table of elements based on this scale was formulated in which atomic masses (m) were listed. Appendix-II at the end of this book gives values of atomic masses and atomic numbers of naturally-occurring isotopes. The amount of substance of a system which contains as many elementary entities as there are atoms in 0.012 kilograms of carbon-12 is defined as a mole. As noted in Chapter 1, a mole is the *base unit* in SI units.

Some elements are monoatomic while others are diatomic. Potassium and sodium are examples of monoatomic elements while chlorine, oxygen, nitrogen, etc. are diatomic elements. In this book, gram mole and kilogram mole will be specified as mol and kmol, respectively.

For chemical compounds, a mole is defined as the amount of substance equal to its formula weight. The formula weight is called the molar mass (M). Based on this understanding, the molecular mass of a monoatomic element is its atomic mass while that of a diatomic element is double that of its atomic mass.

$$1 \text{ atom Al} = 27^* \text{ g Al}$$
$$1 \text{ katom Na} = 23^* \text{ kg Na}$$
$$1 \text{ mol O}_2 = 2 \text{ g atom O}_2 = 32^* \text{ g O}_2$$
$$1 \text{ kmol H}_2 = 2 \text{ kg atom H}_2 = 2^* \text{ kg H}_2$$
$$1 \text{ mol NaCl} = 23 + 35.5 = 58.5^* \text{ g NaCl}$$
$$1 \text{ mol CuSO}_4 = 63.5 + 32 + (4 \times 16) = 159.5^* \text{ kg CuSO}_4$$

From the above discussion, it follows that

$$\frac{(1 \text{ mole of compound X})}{(1 \text{ mole of compound Y})} = \frac{(\text{molar mass of X})}{(\text{molar mass of Y})} \qquad (2.1)$$

This expression is of considerable importance in the following Chapters where the material and heat balances of chemical reactions are presented. In addition, it is also invaluable in converting the mole composition into mass composition.

Example 2.1 How many grams of NH_4Cl are there in 5 mol?

Solution

$$\text{Molar mass of } NH_4Cl = 14 + 4 + 35.5 = 53.5 \text{ g}$$
$$5 \text{ mol of } NH_4Cl = 5 \times 53.5 = 267.5 \text{ g } NH_4Cl \qquad \textit{Ans.}$$

Example 2.2 Convert 499 g $CuSO_4.5H_2O$ into mol. Find equivalent mol of $Cu\,SO_4$ in the crystals.

---

* Rounded-off value

Solution

$$\text{Molar mass of CuSO}_4 = 159.5 \text{ g}$$
$$\text{Molar mass of CuSO}_4.5H_2O = 159.5 + 5\,(1 \times 2 + 16) = 249.5 \text{ g}$$
$$\text{Moles of CuSO}_4.5H_2O = \frac{499}{249.5} = 2 \text{ mol} \qquad \textit{Ans.}$$

In the formula of $CuSO_4.5H_2O$, the moles of $CuSO_4$ are equal (one in each) and hence, the equivalent moles of $CuSO_4$ in the crystals are also 2.0 mol.

Example 2.3 How many moles of K_2CO_3 will contain 117 kg K?

Solution

$$\text{Atomic mass of K, } m_K = 39$$
$$\text{Atoms of K} = \frac{117}{39} = 3 \text{ kg atom}$$

Each mole of K_2CO_3 contains 2 atoms 2 atoms of K.
$$2 \text{ atoms of K} \equiv 1 \text{ mole of } K_2CO_3$$
(The sign $\equiv$ refers to 'equivalent to' and not 'equal to')
$$\text{Moles of } K_2CO_3 = \frac{3}{2} = 1.5 \text{ kmol} \qquad \textit{Ans.}$$

The number of atoms present in a mole can be obtained from Avogadro's number.

$$1 \text{ mol} = 6.022\,1367 \times 10^{23} \text{ atom/mol}$$

From this relation it is once again clear that the number of atoms present in a matter is directly proportional to the number of moles and not the mass.

Example 2.4 How many atoms are present in 416.6 go barium chloride?

Solution

$$\text{Molar mass of BaCl}_2 = 137.3 + 2 \times 35.5 = 208.3$$
$$\text{Moles of BaCl}_2 = 416.6/208.3 = 2 \text{ mol}$$
$$\text{Atoms present in the mass of 416.6 g BaCl}_2 = 2 \times 6.022 \times 10^{23}$$
$$= 12.044 \times 10^{23} \qquad \textit{Ans.}$$

2.3 EQUIVALENT MASS

In chemical reactions, one *equivalent mass* of an element or compound has precisely the same power for chemical combination as one equivalent mass of any other element or compound. It depends strictly upon the reaction in which the molecule participates. Consider the reaction:

$$H_2 + \frac{1}{2} O_2 \rightarrow H_2O \qquad (2.2)$$

In this reaction, hydrogen is monovalent whereas oxygen is divalent. Two atoms of hydrogen combine with one atom of oxygen to form water.

Again $\qquad KOH + HNO_3 \rightarrow KNO_3 + H_2O \qquad (2.3)$

In this reaction, one equivalent mass of KOH combines with one equivalent mass of HNO_3 to produce one equivalent mass of KNO_3 and one equivalent mass of H_2O. Thus, it is clear that the reactivity of a molecule in a chemical reaction determines the equivalent mass of the molecule.

In simple terms, the equivalent mass of an element or a compound is equal to the atomic mass or molecular mass divided by the valence. The *valence* of an element or a compound depends on the number of hydrogen ions accepted or the hydroxyl ions donated for each atomic mass or molecular mass.

$$\text{Equivalent mass} = \frac{\text{molar mass}}{\text{valence}} \quad (2.4)$$

$$1 \text{ g equivalent of hydrogen} = \frac{1}{1} = 1 \text{ g of hydrogen}$$

$$1 \text{ g equivalent of oxygen} = \frac{16}{2} = 8 \text{ g of oxygen}$$

$$1 \text{ g equivalent of Cu} = \frac{63.5}{2} = 31.75 \text{ g Cu}$$

$$1 \text{ g equivalent of } H_3PO_4 = \frac{98.1}{3} = 32.7 \text{ g } H_3PO_4$$

Example 2.5 Find the equivalent mass of (a) PO_4 radical, and (b) Na_3PO_4.

Solution

$$\text{Molar mass } PO_4 \text{ radical} = 31 + 4 \times 16 = 95$$
$$\text{Valence of } PO_4 \text{ radical} = 3$$
$$\text{Equivalent mass of } PO_4 \text{ radical} = \frac{95}{3} = 31.67 \qquad \textit{Ans. (a)}$$
$$\text{Molar mass of } Na_3PO_4 = 3 \times 23 + 95 = 164$$
$$\text{Valence of } Na_3PO_4 = 3,$$

i.e., $\quad\quad\quad$ Equivalent mass of Na/mole = 3

$$\text{Equivalent mass of } Na_3PO_4 = \frac{164}{3} = 54.67 \qquad \textit{Ans. (b)}$$

Example 2.6 Find the equivalents of 3 kmol of $AlCl_3$.

Solution Aluminium ion will accept three hydroxyl ions.

$$\text{Equivalents} = (\text{moles}) \times 3 = 3 \times 3 = 9 \text{ keq} \qquad \textit{Ans.}$$

2.4 SOLIDS

The composition of solids is chiefly expressed in mass percentages.
In a mixture of two compounds A and B,

$$\text{Mass \% of A} = \left[\frac{\text{mass of A}}{(\text{mass of A} + \text{mass of B})}\right] \times 100 \qquad (2.5)$$

$$\text{Mass \% of B} = \left[\frac{\text{mass of B}}{(\text{mass of A} + \text{mass of B})}\right] \times 100$$

$$= 100 - \text{mass \% A} \qquad (2.6)$$

Another way of expressing the composition is in mole %

$$\text{Moles of A} = \frac{\text{mass of A}}{\text{molar mass of A}} \qquad (2.7)$$

$$\text{Moles of B} = \frac{\text{mass of B}}{\text{molar mass of B}} \qquad (2.8)$$

$$\text{Moles \% A} = \left[\frac{\text{moles of A}}{(\text{moles of A} + \text{moles of B})}\right] \times 100 \qquad (2.9)$$

$$\text{Moles \% B} = \left[\frac{\text{moles of B}}{(\text{moles of A} + \text{moles of B})}\right] \times 100$$

$$= 100 - \text{mole \% A} \qquad (2.10)$$

With the help of Eqs. (2.7) to (2.10), the mass % can be converted mole %. Whenever no specific mention is made about the composition, i.e., whether it is mass % or mole %, it is taken as mass % for solids.

When the mass % and mole % are expressed as fractions, they are known as mass fraction and mole fraction, respectively. Equations (2.5) to (2.10) are entirely general and can be applied to mixtures of any number of components with appropriate denominators.

Example 2.7 Sodium chloride weighing 600 kg is mixed with 200 kg potassium chloride. Find the composition of the mixture in (a) mass % (b) mole %.
Solution Basis[*]: 600 kg NaCl and 200 kg KCl

Mass of NaCl in the mixture = 600 kg

Mass of KCl in the mixture = 200 kg

Total mass of the mixture = 600 + 200 = 800 kg

$$\text{Mass \% of NaCl}, w_A = \left(\frac{600}{800}\right) \times 100 = 75$$

$$\text{Mass \% of KCl}, w_B = 100 - 75 = 25 \qquad \textit{Ans. (a)}$$

Molar mass of NaCl, $M_A = 23 + 35.5 = 58.5$

$$\text{Moles of NaCl} = \frac{600}{58.5}$$

$$= 10.26 \text{ kmol}$$

Molar mass of KCl, $M_B = 39 + 35.5 = 74.5$

---

[*] It is always desirable to start by writing a definite basis which will be used in the example.

$$\text{Moles of KCl} = \frac{200}{74.5}$$

$$= 2.68 \text{ kmol}$$

Total moles in the mixture = 10.26 + 2.68 = 12.94 kmol

$$\text{Mole \% NaCl, } x_A = \left(\frac{10.26}{12.94} \right) \times 100 = 79.23$$

Mole % KCl, x_B = 100 – 79.23 = 20.77   *Ans.* (b)

In material balance calculations involving chemical reactions, mole % is a logical expression of the composition. However, mass % is more practical and convenient in the laboratory calculations. Therefore, conversion of mass fraction to mole fraction and vice versa is frequently encountered in stoichiometric calculations. A simple graphical method, presented by Atallah[1], using rectangular graph paper is quite handy for the binary system.

Figure 2.1 is the graphical solution of Example 2.7. On the Y-axis, points representing molar masses of two components are marked as P and Q. Draw lines RP and RQ. Mass fraction $w_A = 0.75$ is marked on X-axis. Draw a vertical line to intersect RQ (*i.e.*, line representing molar mass of B component) at C. Join CE. This intersects RP at D. Draw a vertical line passing from D which gives mole fraction of component A (x_A) on X-axis. Similar is the case with component B. It may be noted that results tally with the calculated values. For conversion of mole fraction to mass fraction, the procedure is to be reversed.

In many instances, indirect reference is made to the composition and/or purity. Examples are, available nitrogen in urea, calcium oxide content of limestone, available phosphorus pentoxide in phosphatic fertilisers, etc. Example 2.8 will be useful in understanding such compositions.

Example 2.8 The available nitrogen in an urea sample is found to be 45% (by mass). Find the actual urea content in the sample.

Solution Since in the problem, the basis is not defined, a suitable basis will have to be assumed.
Basis: 100 kg urea
45 kg nitrogen is present in the sample.

Molar mass of urea (NH_2CONH_2), $MU = 60$

Nitrogen content in 1 kmol of urea = 28 kg

$$\text{Actual urea present in the sample} = \left(\frac{60}{28} \right) \times 45 = 96.43 \text{ kg}$$

Thus, the sample contains 96.43% urea.   *Ans.*

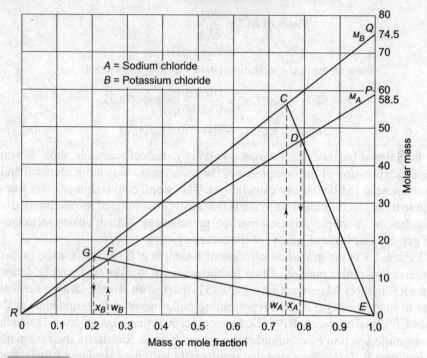

Fig. 2.1 Conversion of Mass Fraction to Mole Fraction

Very often, the impurities present in solid or liquid compounds are expressed in ppm, i.e., parts per mega (million*) (10^6) parts. This is generally expressed on a mass basis for solids and on volume basis for liquids.

Example 2.9 Caustic soda flakes obtained from a manufacturer are found to contain 60 ppm silica (SiO_2). Convert this impurity into mass %.

Solution

$$\text{Impurity} = 60 \text{ ppm}$$

$$= \frac{60 \text{ g SiO}_2}{1000\,000 \text{ g total solids}}$$

$$\text{Mass \% of SiO}_2 = \left(\frac{60}{1000\,000}\right) \times 100$$

$$= 0.006 \qquad\qquad\qquad \textit{Ans.}$$

Example 2.10 A sample of light diesel oil (LDO) from a refinery is found to contain 0.68 mass% sulphur (as S). Its density is 0.85 kg/L at 303.15 K (30°C). Convert this impurity into ppm.

---

* term used in US.

Solution

Sulphur content = 0.68%

$$= \frac{0.68 \text{ g S}}{100 \text{ g LDO}}$$

$$= \frac{0.68 \text{ g}}{100 \text{ g}} \times \frac{1000 \text{ mg}}{1 \text{ g}} \times \frac{1000 \text{ g}}{1 \text{ kg}} \times 0.85 \frac{\text{kg}}{\text{L}}$$

$$= 5780 \text{ mg/L or ppm} \qquad \qquad Ans.$$

2.5 LIQUIDS AND SOLUTIONS

As mentioned in Sec. 2.1, the volumes of pure liquids are usually specified. Along with the volume, the density and temperature of the liquids are also specified.

Regarding the solutions, there are various ways in which they can be expressed. A solution means a solute is dissolved in the solvent. The solute can be a solid, a liquid or a gas. In the case of solids, the solubility is expressed in g/100 g solvent at a definite temperature. This means that the maximum amount of solid which can be dissolved in the solvent will be equal to its solubility at that particular temperature. Solubility data can be found from various sources [2,3]. The mass % and mole% of components are expressed for liquids and solutions, the former being more common. In addition to these two, the volume % of a component is sometimes given, e.g., the alcohol content in wine. Very often, the mass % of the key component or the useful component of the solute present is also expressed, e.g., Na_2O content in caustic soda lye, P_2O_5 content of phosphoric acid, etc.

The trace impurities are either expressed in mg/L or ppm. When the solution is 'watery' (i.e., its density nearly equals 1.0 kg/L),

$$1 \text{ mg/L} = 1 \text{ ppm}$$

In water treatment and effluent treatment problems, the analysis is given in ppm or mg/L, which are both taken as being similar.

Example 2.11 A saturated solution of salicylic acid in methanol contains 64 kg salicylic acid per 100 kg methanol[3] at 298.15 K (25°C). Find (a) the mass %, and (b) mole % composition of the solution.

Solution Basis: 100 kg methanol
Solution contains 64 kg salicylic acid.

$$\text{Mass of the solution} = 100 + 64 = 164 \text{ kg}$$

$$\text{Mass \% salicylic acid} = \left(\frac{64}{164}\right) \times 100 = 39.02$$

$$\text{Mass \% methanol} = 100 - 39.02 = 60.98 \qquad \qquad Ans. \text{ (a)}$$

Molar mass methanol (CH_3OH) = 32

Molar mass of salicylic acid (HOC_6H_4COOH) = 138

$$\text{Moles of methanol} = \frac{100}{32} = 3.125 \text{ kmol}$$

$$\text{Moles of salicylic acid} = \frac{64}{138} = 0.464 \text{ kmol}$$

$$\text{Total amount} = 3.125 + 0.464 = 3.589 \text{ kmol}$$

$$\text{Mole \% methanol} = \left(\frac{3.125}{3.589}\right) \times 100 = 87.07$$

$$\text{Mole \% salicylic acid} = 100 - 87.07 = 12.93 \qquad \textit{Ans. (b)}$$

Example 2.12   What will be the % Na_2O content of lye containing 73% caustic soda?

Solution   Basis: 100 kg lye

$$\text{Caustic soda content of the lye} = 73 \text{ kg}$$

$$2 \text{ NaOH} \rightarrow Na_2O + H_2O$$

$$\text{Molar mass of NaOH} = 40$$

$$\text{Molar mass of } Na_2O = 62$$

$$\text{\% } Na_2O \text{ in the solution} = \frac{62 \times 73}{(2 \times 40)} = 56.58 \qquad \textit{Ans.}$$

In water analysis, impurities such as alkalinity, hardness, etc. are expressed in mg/L. In effluent analysis, BOD, COD, TOC, TOD, and ThOD are expressed in mg/L. For definitions of these terms, a standard book on wastewater engineering[4] or on pollution control may be referred. Among these parameters, TOC and ThOD can be theoretically calculated. TOC refers to the total organic carbon present in the solution, while ThOD refers to the theoretical oxygen demand of organic compounds present in the solution.

Example 2.13   Glycerin, weighing 600 mg, is dissolved in pure water to make a final solution of 1 litre. Find the TOC and ThOD of the solution.

Solution   Basis: 1 litre of solution

The structure of glycerin is

$$\begin{array}{l} CH_2OH \\ | \\ CHOH \\ | \\ CH_2OH \end{array}$$

1 kmol of glycering contains 3 atom (or kmol) of carbon.

$$\text{Molar mass of glycerin} = 92$$

$$\text{Glycerin concentration in the solution} = 600 \text{ mg/L}$$

$$\text{Total carbon present in the solution (TOC)} = \left(\frac{3 \times 12}{92}\right) \times 600 = 234.8 \text{ mg/L} \qquad \textit{Ans.}$$

The oxygen requirement of the compound (for complete combustion) can be determined by writing the combustion reaction as:

$$C_3H_8O_3 + 3.5 \ O_2 = 3 \ CO_2 + 4 \ H_2O$$

The O_2 requirement of glycerin present in the solution,

$$\text{ThOD} = \frac{(3.5 \times 32 \times 600)}{92} = 730.4 \text{ mg/L} \qquad Ans.$$

In the case of water analysis, the alkalinity or hardness is expressed in equivalent ppm of $CaCO_3$ although the actual values of alkalinity and hardness in terms of the compounds present will be different.

Example 2.14 By titration, it was found that a sample of water contains hardness equivalent to 500 mg/L (ppm) $CaCO_3$. Assuming that the water contains temporary hardness in 60% $Ca(HCO_3)_2$ form, and 40% $Mg(HCO_3)_2$ form. Find the concentrations of both in water.

Solution

$$\text{Molar mass of } CaCO_3 = 100$$
$$\text{Valence of } CaCO_3 = 2$$
$$\text{Equivalent mass of } CaCO_3 = \frac{100}{2} = 50$$
$$\text{Molar mass of } Ca(HCO_3)_2 = 162$$
$$\text{Valence of } Ca(HCO_3)_2 = 2$$
$$\text{Equivalent mass of } Ca(HCO_3)_2 = \frac{162}{2} = 81$$

Actual content of $Ca(HCO_3)_2$ in the

$$\text{sample of water} = \left(\frac{81}{50}\right) \times 500 \times 0.6 = 486 \text{ mg/L}$$

$$\text{Molar mass of } Mg(HCO_3)_2 = 146.3$$
$$\text{Valence of } Mg(HCO_3)_2 = 2$$
$$\text{Equivalent mass of } Mg(HCO_3)_2 = \frac{146.3}{2} = 73.15$$

Actual content of $Mg(HCO_3)_2$ in the

$$\text{sample of water} = \left(\frac{73.15}{50}\right) \times 500 \times 0.4$$
$$= 292.6 \text{ mg/L}$$

In addition to the concentration units described above, there are three other ways of expressing the concentraion of a solution containing either a solid or a liquid solute, namely, molarity (M), normality (N) and molality.

Molarity (M) is defined as the number of mol of solute dissolved in 1 litre or dm^3 of solution.

Normality (N) is defined as the number of geq dissolved in 1 litre of solution.

Molality (mol/kg) is defined as the number of mol of solute dissolved in 1 kilogram of solvent.

From the definition of normality, it is thus possible to find the concentration of solute in g/L (a modified expression of the density).

Concentration in g/L = normality $(N) \times$ equivalent mass $\qquad$ (2.11)

Example 2.15 A solution of sodium chloride in water contains 20% NaCl (by mass) at 333 K (60°C). The density of the solution is 1.127 kg/L. Find the molarity, normality and molality of the solution.

Solution Basis: 100 kg solution of sodium chloride
The solution contains 20 kg NaCl.

$$\text{Density of the solution} = 1.127 \text{ kg/L}$$

$$\text{Volume of the solution} = \frac{100}{1.127} = 88.73 \text{ L}$$

$$\text{Moles of NaCl in the solution} \frac{20}{58.5} = 0.342 \text{ kmol} \equiv 342 \text{ mol}$$

$$\text{Molarity, M} = \frac{\text{moles of solute}}{\text{volume of solution}}$$

$$= \frac{342}{88.73} = 3.85$$

For NaCl, since it is univalent,

$$\text{Molar mass} = \text{equivalent mass}$$

Therefore,

$$\text{Normality } (N) = \text{molarity (M)} = 3.85$$

$$\text{Molality} = \frac{\text{Moles of solute}}{\text{mass of solvent}}$$

$$= \frac{342}{80} = 4.275 \text{ mol/kg} \qquad\qquad Ans.$$

Example 2.16 Aqueous solution of triethanolmine (TEA), i.e., $N(CH_2CH_2OH)_3$, contains 50% TEA by mass. Find the molarity of the solution if the density of the solution is 1.05 kg/L.

Solution Basis: 100 kg TEA solution
The solution contains 50 kg TEA.

$$\text{Molar mass of TEA} = 149$$

$$\text{Moles of TEA present in the solution} = \frac{50}{149} = 0.3356 \text{ kmol}$$

$$\text{Volume of the solution} = \frac{100}{1.05} = 95.24 \text{ L}$$

$$\text{Molarity of the solution} = \left(\frac{0.3356}{95.24}\right) \times 1000 = 3.524 \text{ M} \qquad Ans.$$

The solubility of a gas in a liquid or solution is expressed in different ways. Some common ways of expression are mass %, mole %, amount of volume dissolved at specific conditions and mole ratio. Any one of them can be converted into another easily.

Example 2.17 The concentration of CO_2 is measured to be 0.206 kmol per kmol monoethanolamine (MEA) in a 20% (by mass) aqueous MEA solution. Assuming the density of the solution to be nearly 1.0 kg/L, find the concentration of CO_2 as mass % and mol % in the solution.

Solution   Basis: 100 kg aqueous MEA solution
The solution contains 20 kg MEA.

$$\text{Chemical formula of MEA} = NH_2CH_2CH_2OH$$

$$\text{Molar mass of MEA} = 61$$

$$\text{Moles of MEA in the solution} = \frac{20}{61} = 0.3279 \text{ kmol}$$

$$CO_2 \text{ dissolved in the solution} = 0.206 \times 0.3279 = 0.0675 \text{ kmol}$$

$$\text{Mass of } CO_2 = 0.0675 \times 44 = 2.97 \text{ kg}$$

$$\text{Moles of water} = \frac{(100 - 22.97)}{18} = 4.2794 \text{ kmol}$$

Table 2.1   Composition of Lean MEA

Component	kmol n_i	Mole %	Molar mass M_i	Mass kg $(n_i M_i)$	Mass %
Water	4.2794	91.54	18	77.027	77.03
MEA	0.3279	7.02	61	20	20.00
CO_2	0.0675	1.44	44	2.973	2.97
Total	4.6748	100.00	123	100.00	100.00

Ans.

Quite often, the specific gravities are used for indirect measurements of concentrations of aqueous solutions.

$$\text{Specific gravity (SG)}_{T_1/T_2} = \frac{\left(\text{Density of solution at } T_1 \text{ K}\right)}{\left(\text{Density of water at } T_2 \text{ K}\right)} \quad (2.12)$$

Various hydrometers are use in the industries to measure the specific gravity of a solution. Among them the following scales are commonly used.

(i) °Twaddell (°Tw) $= 200(SG_{288.7/288.7} - 1.000)$ $\qquad (2.13)$
(ii) For liquids heavier than water,

$$\text{°Baumè (°Bè)} = 145 - \left(\frac{145}{SG_{288.7/288.7}}\right) \quad (2.14.1)$$

For liquids lighter than water,

$$°\text{Baumè (°Bè)} = \left(\frac{140}{SG_{288.7/288.7}} \right) - 130 \qquad (2.14.2)$$

(iii) For petroleum products, American Petroleum Institute (API), USA has developed the following scale.

$$°\text{API} = \left(\frac{141.5}{SG_{288.7/288.7}} \right) - 131.5 \qquad (2.15)$$

(iv) For the sugar industry, an arbitrary scale of °Brix is developed.

$$°\text{Brix} = \left(\frac{400}{SG_{288.7/288.7}} \right) - 400 \qquad (2.16)$$

The last scale is graduated in such a way that $1°\text{Brix} = 1\%$ (mass) sugar in solution. Hydrometers of the types (i) and (ii) are used to measure the concentration of caustic lye, sulphuric acid strength, hydrochloric acid strength, etc. Table 2.2 gives the relations of °Bè/°Tw with concentrations of aqueous sulphuric acid solutions.

Table 2.2 Relationship of Degree Baumè and Degrees Twaddell with the Concentration of Sulphuric Acid[5]

°Bè	°Tw	Specific gravity $SG_{288.7/288.7}$	Mass% H_2SO_4
1	1.38	1.0069	1.02
2	2.80	1.0140	2.08
3	4.20	1.0211	3.13
4	5.68	1.0284	4.21
5	7.14	1.0357	5.28
6	8.64	1.0432	6.37
7	10.14	1.0507	7.45
8	11.68	1.0584	8.55
9	13.24	1.0662	9.66
10	14.82	1.0741	10.77
15	23.08	1.1154	16.38
20	32.00	1.1600	22.25
25	41.66	1.2083	28.28
30	52.18	1.2609	34.63
35	63.64	1.3182	41.27
40	76.20	1.3810	48.10
45	90.00	1.4500	55.07
50	105.26	1.5263	62.18
55	122.22	1.6111	69.65
60	141.18	1.7059	77.67
65	162.50	1.8125	88.65
66	167.08	1.8354	93.19

(Reproduced with the permission of Lurgi GmbH, Germany).

An important point to note about the use of these hydrometers is that the measurement of specific gravity should be made at 288.7 K (15.6°C or 60°F). If the hydrometers are used at temperatures other than 288.7 K (15.6°C), a correction should be applied. In India, the Twaddell meters in use are calibrated at 303/303 K (30/30°C). °API is very useful in knowing the nature of a petroleum product, i.e., its properties such as molar mass, viscosity, heating value, etc.

2.6 IMPORTANT PHYSICAL PROPERTIES OF SOLUTIONS

The physical properties of a pure solvent and a solution differ depending upon the amount of solute present in it. A commonly known property is pH of the solution.

It is defined as

$$pH = - \log (H^+) \tag{2.17}$$

where H^+ = hydrogen ion concentration in geq/L

The property pH is used to express acidity or alkalinity of a solution. A pH of 7 is neutral, decreasing figures below 7 indicate increasing acidity while increasing figures above 7 show increasing alkalinity. The pH of alkaline solutions[6] are plotted in Fig. 2.2.

A known property of the solvent is the vapour pressure (p_v) of the solvent. The vapour pressure of a liquid is defined as the absolute pressure at which the liquid and its vapour are in equilibrium at a given temperature. Consider the example of pure air-free water. It exerts the vapour pressure of 101.325 kPa (760 torr) at 373.15 K (100°C). The complete vapour pressure table of water is given in Chapter 6 (refer Table 6.8).

Normally, a solute dissolved in a solvent depresses the vapour pressure of the solvent. For example, the dissolution of caustic soda, sugar, salt, etc. in water reduces the vapour pressure of water. In Fig. 2.3 the vapour pressure of caustic soda solutions is plotted against temperature[7].

From Fig. 2.3, it is evident that 30% (by mass) caustic soda lye exerts a vapour pressure of 10.666 kPa (80 torr) at 333 K (60°C). While at the same temperature, the vapour pressure of water is 19.916 kPa (149.38 torr) (refer Table 6.8). Data on lowering of vapour pressures by a number of inorganic compounds in aqueous solutions is given in the CRC Handbook of Chemistry and Physics[8].

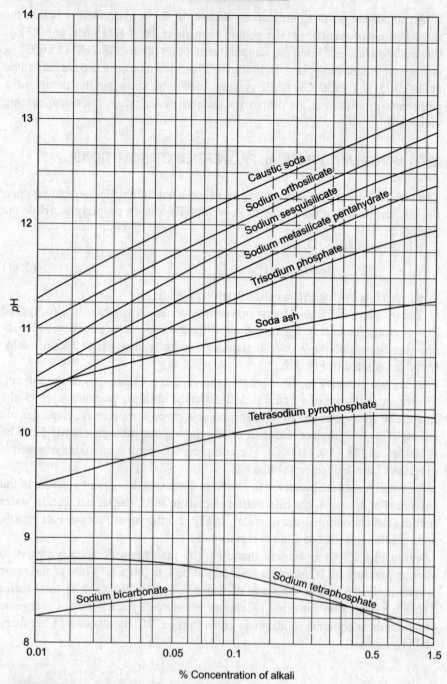

Fig. 2.2 pH of Alkaline Solutions[6]

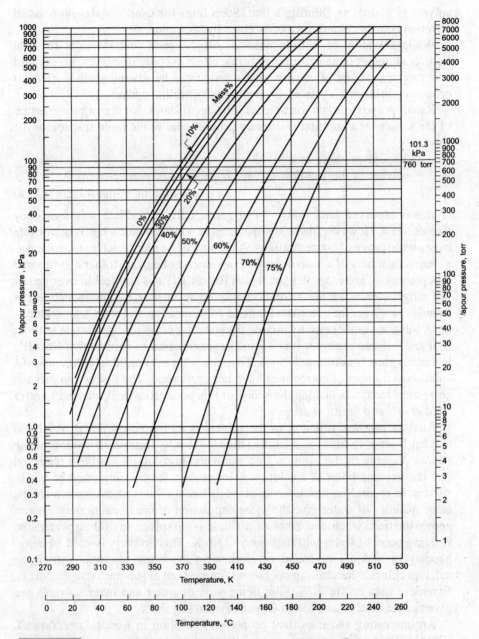

Fig. 2.3 Vapour Pressure of Caustic Soda Solutions[7]

From the above discussion, it is clear that the boiling point of a solution is higher than the boiling point of the solvent. When the temperature of a liquid is plotted against the temperature of the known reference liquid (e.g., water in case of aqueous solution), at equal vapour pressure, it is called a Dühring plot. Also a line plotting the boiling point of a solution against the boiling point of the solvent is known as Dühring's line. Such lines for caustic soda solutions of different concentrations have been given by McCabe [9].

While elevation of boiling point of caustic soda solution calls for heat transfer at higher temperature in multiple effect evaporator system, property of low vapour pressure of caustic soda solution can be advantageously used for producing brine at 5°C, using absorption refrigeration cycle.

Raoult proposed a law for an ideal solution. It states that the vapour pressure of the solvent is a solution is directly proportional to the mole fraction of the solvent.

Vapour pressure of a
solvent in the solution = (vapour pressure of pure solvent)
$$\times \text{(mole fraction of the solvent) (2.18)}$$

It was observed later that in most cases, only very dilute solutions obey Raoult's law. However, there are instances in which Raoult's law is applicable over a wide range of concentrations. A mixture of isomers, such as o-, m- and p-xylenes, members of a homologous series, such as benzene-toluene, n-hexane/n-heptane, etc. are examples for which Raoult's law is applicable over nearly full range. Hence, an ideal solution may be defined as the one which obeys Raoult's law over the complete range of concentration and at all temperatures. Such solutions are formed by mixing the constituents in the liquid state without heat and volume changes. It is a good approximation to assume that Raoult's law holds good for dilute solutions. To account for the non-ideal behaviour of a solution, a number of corrections have been proposed. The discussion on such correction factors is outside the scope of this book. Reader is advised to refer Reid *et al*[10] and Smith *et al*[11].

Another physical property of the solvent is its freezing point at which the solvent freezes to become a solid. This also results from the lowering of the vapour pressure of the solution by a non-volatile solute. It has been observed that the freezing point of a solution is lower than the freezing point of a pure solvent. In general, equimolar amounts of different solutes when dissolved in the same quantity of water give the same depression of the freezing point. As an approximation, when one kmol of a solute is dissolved in 100 kg water, the freezing point of water will depress by 18.6 K. This property is used advanta-geously in making ice-cream or circulating the brine solutions containing calcium chloride for chilling operations (carried out at sub-zero temperatures). Extensive data on freezing point depression of water and other solvents are given in the CRC Handbook of Chemistry and Physics[8].

An interesting and important property of solution in *osmotic pressure Π*. When a dilute and a concentrated solution are separated from each other by a suitable membrane, the spontaneous flow of water takes place from the dilute solution to the concentrated solution. The essential property of these membranes is that they allow the free passage of water but not of the dissolved substance. A common permeable membrane in industrial use is polyamide. In the real sense the solute cannot pass through the membrane and as a result, it will exert pressure against the wall of the membrane. The above process is called osmosis and the pressure is known as osmotic pressure which can be determined by the ideal gas as given in Eq. (2.21). The osmotic pressure is the excess pressure which must be applied to the solution to prevent the passage of solvent into the solution when they are separated by a perfectly semipermeable membrane. Rougly, osmotic pressure is equal to 6.86 kPa (51 torr) for each 100 mg/L of dissolved solids.

Reverse osmosis is a process in which the work is done against the osmotic pressure by applying pressure on the side containing the more concentrated solution. As a result the solution enclosed in the membrane gets concentrated. This technique finds application in desalination, effluent disposal, bulk drug manufacturing, dyes manufacturing, etc.

2.7 GASES

As discussed in Sec. 2.1, the direct weighing of gases is ruled out in practice. The volume of a gas can be conveniently measured and converted into mass from the density of the gas. In order to know the density of a gas, both pressure and temperature should be known. Various equations of state (also known as pVT relations) can be employed for this purpose.

2.7.1 Ideal Gas Law

According to Boyle, for a given mass of an ideal gas the product of the pressure and volume is constant at a constant temperature, i.e.,

$$p \times V = \text{constant} \tag{2.19}$$

where, p is the absolute pressure and V is the volume occupied by 1 kmol gas.

Charles proposed the law that for a given mass of an ideal gas, the ratio of the volume to temperature is constant at a given pressure.

$$\frac{V}{T} = \text{constant} \tag{2.20}$$

where, T is the absolute temperature.

Combining the above two law, an ideal gas law can be formulated as

$$\frac{(p \times V)}{T} = \text{constant} \tag{2.21}$$

The constant of Eq. (2.21 is designated by the symbol R, known as *Universal Gas Constant*.

Therefore $$pV = RT \tag{2.22}$$

Eq. (2.22) is called Ideal Gas Law.

When V' is the volume of gas in cubic metres of n kmol, Eq. (2.22) gets modified as

$$pV' = nRT \tag{2.23}$$

The value of R is listed in different units in Table 2.3.

Table 2.3 Value of Universal Gas Constant (R) in Different Units

Numerical Value of R	Units
0.083 14	$m^3 \cdot bar/(kmol \cdot K)$
8.314 51	$m^3 \cdot kPa/(kmol \cdot K)$
8.314 51	$J/(mol \cdot K)$
1.987 216	$kcal/(kmol \cdot K)$ or $Btu/(lb\ mol \cdot {}^\circ R)$
0.082 058	$L \cdot atm/(mol \cdot K)$ or $m^3 \cdot atm/kmol \cdot K)$
62 363.95	$cm^3 \cdot torr/(mol \cdot K)$
10.731 64	$ft^3 \cdot psia/(lb\ mol \cdot {}^\circ R)$

In Eq. (2.21), V is called the molar volume. At 273. 15 K (0°C or 32°F) and 101.325 kPa a (1 atm a or 14.696 psia or 760 torr), $V = 22.4136$ m³/kmol or L/mol. These conditions are said to be normal temperature and pressure (NTP). In the fps system, the molar volume at NTP equals 359.03 ft³/lb mol.

Local conditions vary from place to place and, therefore, if standard temperature and pressure (STP) are considered, the molar volume will differ at different places. In the USA, 101.325 kPa a (1 atm a) and 288.7 K (15.6°C or 60°F) are consideref to be STP.

Knowing the values of p and T, it is easy to calculate the molar volume ussing Eq. (2.22).

If p_1, V_1 and T_1 are the conditions of an ideal gas under one situation, and if p_2, V_2, T_2 are the conditions of the gas under another situation, from Eq.(2.21), it follows that

$$\frac{p_1 V_1}{T_1} = \frac{p_2 V_2}{T_2} \qquad (2.24)$$

If Eq. (2.24) is utilised instead of Eq. (2.22) one situation may be taken as NTP, i.e., $p_1 = 101.325$ kPa, $V_1 = 22.4136$ m³/kmol and $T_1 = 273.15$ K (0°C) or $p_1 = 100$ kPa, $V_1 = 22.7111$ m³/kmol and $T_1 = 273.15$ K (0°C).

2.7.2 Other Equations of State

According to Boyle's law, the volume occupied by a gas is inversely proportional to its pressure. However, real gases exhibit considerable deviation from ideal behaviour. For every gas, the ratio pV/RT is constant over only a definite range of pressure. Within this range, Boyle's law is obeyed. In general, the extent of the deviation from Boyle's law is small at low pressures, expecially when the temperature is relatively high.

In order to account for non-ideal behaviour of the gases, J.D. van der Waals proposed another equation of state in 1873 as follows:

$$\left(p + \frac{a}{V^2}\right)(V - b) = RT \qquad (2.25)$$

In eq. (2.25), a and b are constants depending on the gas. The values of a and b can be evaluated using the following equations.

$$a = 27\,\frac{R^2\,T_c^2}{64\,p_c}\ \text{L}^2\cdot\text{MPa/mol}^2\ \text{or}\ (\text{m}^3)^2\cdot\text{MPa/(kmol)}^2 \qquad (2.26)$$

$$\text{or} \qquad\qquad \text{J}\cdot\text{m}^3/\text{mol}^2$$

$$\text{and} \qquad b = \frac{RT_c}{8p_c}\ \text{L/mol or m}^3/\text{kmol} \qquad\qquad (2.27)$$

where, p_c and T_c are the critical pressure and the critical temperature of the gas, respectively.

The critical temperature is the maximum temperature at which a gas can be liquefied. The critical pressure is the saturation pressure corresponding to the critial temperature. Above the critical temperature a gas cannot be liquefied regardless of the pressure. The volume occupied by a gas under critical conditions is called the critical volume (V_c). At the critical point, the densities of coexisting liquid and gaseous phases are identical. Table 2.4 gives the critical constants of various gases[12].

Table 2.4 Critical Constants of Various Compounds[12]

Chemical	Formula	Molar mass M kg/kmol	Critical temperature T_c K	Critical pressure p_c bar	Critical Volume V_c dm³/kmol
A. Inorganic Compounds:					
Air (R*–729)	–	28.9679	132.45	37.72	88.3
Ammonia (R*–717)	NH_3	17.0305	405.50	113.50	72.0
Argon (R*–740)	Ar	39.948	150.69	48.63	75.2
Bromine	Br_2	159.808	588.00	103.00	127.0
Carbon dioxide (R*–744)	CO_2	44.0095	304.12	73.74	94.0
Carbon disulphide	CS_2	76.141	552.00	79.00	173.0
Carbon monoxide	CO	28.0101	132.85	34.94	92.2
Chlorine	Cl_2	70.9060	416.90	79.77	124.0
Deuterium (normal)	D_2	4.0282	38.40	16.60	60.0
Fluorine	F_2	37.9968	144.30	52.15	66.0
Helium-3	He	3.016	3.31	1.14	72.0
Helium-4 (R*–704)	He	4.0026	5.30	2.29	57.8
Hydrazine	N_2H_4	32.0452	653.00	14.70	103.8
Hydrogen (normal) (R*–702n)	H_2	2.0159	33.20	12.97	65.0
Hydrogen bromide	HBr	80.9119	363.20	85.50	103.2
Hydrogen chloride	HCl	36.4609	324.70	83.10	81.0
Hydrogen cyanide	HCN	27.0253	456.79	53.90	139.0
Hydrogen fluoride	HF	20.0063	461.00	64.80	69.0

(Contd.)

Table 2.4 Contd.

Chemical	Formula	Molar mass M kg/kmol	Critical temperature T_c K	Critical pressure p_c bar	Critical Volume V_c dm³/kmol
Hydrogen iodide	HI	127.9124	424.00	83.10	129.1
Hydrogen sulphide	H_2S	34.0809	373.54	90.08	98.0
Krypton	Kr	83.798	209.40	55.01	92.2
Neon (R^*-720)	Ne	20.1797	44.50	27.25	41.7
Nitric oxide	NO	30.0061	180.00	64.80	58.0
Nitrogen (R^*-728)	N_2	28.0134	126.09	33.94	89.5
Nitrogen dioxide	NO_2	46.0055	431.00	101.00	167.0
(Di) Nitrogen teroxide	N_2O_4	92.011	431.00	101.00	167.0
Nitrous oxide	N_2O (R^*-744A)	44.0128	309.60	72.40	97.0
Oxygen (R^*-732)	O_2	31.9988	154.58	50.42	73.0
Ozone	O_3	47.9982	261.00	55.70	89.4
Sulphur dioxide	SO_2 (R^*-764)	64.0638	430.80	78.84	122.0
Sulphur trioxide	SO_3	80.0632	491.00	82.10	127.0
Water (R^*-718)	H_2O	18.0153	647.11	220.76	55.9
Xenon	Xe	131.293	289.75	58.68	118.8
B. *Organic Compounds*					
Acetaldehyde	CH_3CHO	44.0526	461.00	61.33	113.0
Acetic acid	CH_3COOH	60.052	592.71	57.86	171.0
Acetone (2-propanone)	C_3H_6O	58.0791	508.10	47.00	209.0
Acetylene (ethyne)	C_2H_2	26.0373	308.33	61.39	113.0
Aniline (phenylamine)	$C_6H_5NH_2$	93.1265	699.00	53.10	274.0
Benzene	C_6H_6	78.1118	562.16	48.98	259.0
Biphenyl (diphenyl)	$C_{12}H_{10}$	154.2078	789.00	38.50	502.0
n–Butane (R^*-600)	C_4H_{10}	58.1222	425.18	37.97	255.0
i-Butane (2-methylpropane) (R^*-600a)	C_4H_{10}	58.1222	408.15	36.48	263.0
1-Butene	C_4H_8	56.1063	419.57	40.23	240.0
cis-2-Butene	C_4H_8	56.1063	435.58	42.43	234.0
trans-2-Butene	C_4H_8	56.1063	428.63	49.85	238.0
n-Butyl alcohol (1-butanol)	C_4H_9OH	74.1216	563.05	44.23	275.0
Carbon tetrachloride (R^*-10)	CCl_4	153.8227	556.40	45.60	276.0
Chlorobenzene	C_6H_5Cl	112.5569	632.40	45.20	308.0

(Contd.)

Table 2.4   Contd.

Chemical	Formula	Molar mass M kg/kmol	Critical temper- ature T_c K	Critical pressure p_c bar	Critical Volume V_c dm^3/kmol
Chlorodi- fluromethane (R^* −22)	$CCIF_2H$	86.4684	369.30	49.71	166.0
Chloroform (trichloromethane) (R^* −20)	CCl_3H	119.3776	536.50	54.00	240.0
Chloromethane (methyl chloride) (R^* −40)	$CCIH_3$	50.4875	416.25	66.79	139.0
Chlorotrifluoro ethylene	C_2CIF_3	116.4699	379.00	40.50	212.0
Chlorotrifluoro methane (R^* −13)	$CCIF_3$	104.4589	302.00	38.70	180.0
Cyclohexane	C_6H_{12}	84.1595	553.50	40.70	308.0
Dichlorodifluro methane (R^* − 12)	CCl_2F_2	120.9135	384.95	41.36	217.0
1,1 Dichloro- ethane	$C_2H_4Cl_2$	98.9592	523.00	50.70	236.0
1,2 Dichloro- ethane	$C_2H_4Cl_2$	98.9592	561.00	53.70	225.0
Dichlorofluoro- methane (R^* −21)	CCl_2FH	102.9227	451.58	51.84	196.0
Dichloromethane (R^*−30)	CH_2Cl_2	84.9326	510.00	60.80	185.2
(Di) ethyl ether (methylene chloride) (R^* −610)	$C_4H_{10}O$	74.1216	466.74	36.38	280.0
Ethane (R^* − 170)	C_2H_6	30.069	305.42	48.80	147.0
Ethanol (ethyl alcohol)	C_2H_5OH	46.0684	513.92	61.37	167.0
Ethylbenzene	C_8H_{10}	106.165	617.20	36.00	374.0
Ethylene (ethene) (R^* −1150)	C_2H_4	28.0538	282.34	50.39	130.0
Ethylene oxide (epoxyethane)	C_2H_4O	44.0526	469.00	71.90	140.0
n-Heptane	C_7H_{16}	100.2019	540.30	27.36	425.0
n-Hexane	C_6H_{14}	86.1754	507.50	30.12	370.0
Methane (R^* −50)	CH_4	16.0425	190.50	46.04	98.9
Methanol (methyl alcohol)	CH_3OH	32.0419	512.64	80.92	118.0
(Di) Methyl ether	C_2H_6O	46.0684	400.00	53.70	190.0
Methyl ethyl ether	C_3H_8O	60.095	437.80	44.30	221.0
Methyl ethyl ketone (2-butanone)	C_4H_8O	72.1057	536.78	42.07	267.0
Naphthalene	$C_{10}H_8$	128.1705	748.40	40.51	413.0
n-Octane	C_8H_{18}	114.2285	568.83	24.87	492.0

(Contd.)

Table 2.4 Contd.

Chemical	Formula	Molar mass M kg/kmol	Critical temperature T_c K	Critical pressure p_c bar	Critical Volume V_c dm³/kmol
n-Pentane	C_5H_{12}	72.1488	469.70	33.69	304.0
iso-Pentane (2-methylbutane)	C_5H_{12}	72.1488	460.43	33.81	306.0
neo-pentane (2,2-dimethylpropane)	C_5H_{12}	72.1488	433.78	31.99	303.0
Propane (R* – 290)	C_3H_8	44.0956	369.82	42.47	200.0
n-Propyl alcohol (2-propanol)	C_3H_7OH	60.095	536.78	51.70	219.0
Propylene (propene) (R* – 1270)	C_3H_6	42.0797	364.85	46.01	181.0
Pyridine	C_5H_5N	79.0999	620.00	56.30	254.0
Styrene	C_8H_8	104.1491	647.00	39.91	–
Tetrafluoro ethane (R* – 134a)	$C_2H_2F_4$**	102.0309	374.25	40.67	201.0
Toluene (methylbenzene)	C_7H_8	92.1384	591.79	41.04	316.0
Trichlorofluoro-methane (R* – 11)	CCl_3F	137.3681	471.20	44.10	248.0
m-Xylene (1,3–dimethyl-benzene)	C_8H_{10}	106.165	617.05	35.35	376.0
o-Xylene (1,2-dimethyl-benzene)	C_8H_{10}	106.165	630.30	37.30	369.0
p-Xylene (1,4–dimethyl-benzene)	C_8H_{10}	106.165	616.20	35.11	371.7

(*Reproduced with the permission of Dr G.R. Somayajulu[12]*)
*Refrigerant designation system, based on ASHRAE Standard 34-1992.
** Extracted from Technical Bulletin No. 645, 1993 of AlliedSingal Inc.[13], USA.

There are other equations of state, e.g., Beattie Bridgeman equation, Berthelot equation, Benedict Webb and Rubin equation, three parameter corresponding states prinicple of Pitzer and co-workers, etc. The discussion of these equations is beyond the scope of this book. For further study of these equations reference 11 can be consulted.

In various equations of state, the constants for different compounds are required to be calculated from other properties. Calculations of the constants involve quite complex formulae and may require use of a programmable calculator or a computer. The advantage of the complex equations is the accuracy of the results. However, for quick estimations, non-ideality of a gas can be expressed by the *compressibility factor Z* where,

$$Z = \frac{pV}{RT}$$

(2.28)

For an ideal gas $Z = 1.0$. For real gases, values of Z can be obtained from the Nelson-Obert generalised compressibility charts and acentric factor (ω) [10,11].

In order to convert the molar volume into density, molar mass (M) should be employed.

$$\text{Density of gas} = \frac{\text{molar mass } (M)}{\text{molar volume}} \qquad (2.29)$$

Another important parameter, used in gas industry, is *specific gravity* of a gas. Unlike liquids, it is defined as

$$\text{Specific gravity of a gas} = \frac{\text{molar mass of the gas}}{\text{molar mass of the air}} \qquad (2.30)$$

2.7.3 Gas Mixtures

In industries, very ofter, mixtures of various gases are handled. The analysis of the components present in the mixture is usually given on a volume basis. Take an example of air in which the oxygen and nitrogen are present nearly in 21% and 79% proportion on a volume basis respectively.

If V_i is the volume of pure component i, present in the mixture, the total volume of gas

$$V = \Sigma \, V_i \qquad (2.31)$$

This is known as Amagat's laws.

Actually, all the components of a gas mixture occupy the total volume, and hence V_i is truly speaking that volume which would be occupied by the component i, if it alone is present at pressure p and temperature T of the mixture

$$V_i = \frac{n_i RT}{p} \qquad (2.32)$$

where, n_i is the number of moles of component i.

From Eq. (2.32), it is clear that V_i is proportional to n_i. In other words, the volume % of a component in a gas mixture equals to mole % of it. This is strictly true for ideal gases. For non-ideal gases, the compressibility factor Z of the component should be considered for each gas, present in the mixture. In the Chapters that follow, volume % would be considered to be equal to mole % which is an accepted practice for stoichiometric calculations.

In the foregoing discussions, the volume V_i occupied by a component i in the gas mixture seemed to be a hypothetical proposition. However, it is logical to follow that in a gas mixture, each component exerts a different pressure, depending on the mole fraction of that component. This pressure exerted by each component is called *partial pressure or pure-component pressure*, the former term being more commonly used. It is defined as

$$p_i = p \cdot y_i \qquad (2.33)$$

where, p_i is the partial pressure of the ith component, p is the total pressure and y_i is the mole fraction of the ith component in the gas mixture.

Equation (2.33) is strictly valid for an ideal gas mixture.

$$\Sigma p_i = p \cdot \Sigma y_i \tag{2.34}$$

Since $\Sigma y_i = 1.0$,

$$p = \Sigma p_i \tag{2.35}$$

Equation (2.35) is the mathematical form of Dalton's law, which states that in an ideal gas mixture, the total pressure is the sum of the partial pressures exerted by each component. In this definition, it is assumed that the component i fills up the entire volume available to it. In other words,

$$p_i = \frac{n_i RT}{V} \tag{2.36}$$

Equation (2.36) is again valid only for an ideal gas mixture. For a non-ideal gas mixture, the compressibility factor Z for each gas, present in the mixture should be considered [10,11].

From Eq (2.32) and (2.36), it is clear that **for an ideal gas mixture**,

volume % = mole % = pressure % (2.37)

Equation (2.37) is a very important relationship in stoichiometry. The density and specific gravity of a gas mixture can be evaluated using Eq. (2.29) and Eq. (2.30) in which the average molar mass should be taken into account. Mathematically, the average molar mass M is defined as

$$M = \Sigma (M_i \cdot y_i) \tag{2.38}$$

where, M_i is the molar mass of the i th component.

From eq. (2.38), it can be deduced that the mass of a gas mixture equivalent to its average molar mass will occupy molar volume.

When trace quantities of a particular component are present in a gaseous mixture, it is expressed either as ppm (v/v) or mg/m^3, e.g., traces of SO_2 in flue gases, traces of NO_x in tail gas from nitric acid plant, etc.

2.7.4 Joule-Thomson Effect

Throttling of gases is often encountered in the industry. In such a process when a gas is passed through an orifice, a nozzle or a throttling valve, its pressure is reduced. This process essentially takes place at constant enthalpy; also called *isenthalp*. For an ideal gas, throttling should not change the temperature of the gas. However, for most real gases, throttling results in a decrease in temperature. This is known as Joule-Thomson effect. Ratio of the change in temperature to respective pressure reduction is defined as Joule-Thomson coefficient (μ).

Throttling of compressed air, refrigerant gases, steam, etc. are experienced in industry. In cryogenic separation of gases, Joule-Thomson effect has an important role. It is advantageously used in supplying relatively cold air in air breathing apparatus, commonly known as pressure suits, worn by a person, working in an hazardous environment.

2.7.5 Gas-Liquid Mixtures

It has been seen in Sec. 2.6 than an ideal liquid-liquid mixture obeys Raoult's law. The same law also applies to a gas-liquid mixture, i.e., the partial pressure of a pure component in a gas mixture at equilibrium at a given temperature equals the mole fraction of the component in liquid mixture multiplied by the vapour pressure of pure liquid at the same temperature.
Mathematically,

$$y_i \cdot p = x_i \cdot p_v \qquad (2.39)$$

Left term of the equation is the partial pressure as defined in Eq. (2.33).

At low concentrations of a gas in the liquid, Raoult's law does not hold good. For such non-ideal behaviour, Henry's law is found to be useful. If p_i is the partial pressure of the solute gas i,

$$p_i = H_i \cdot x_i \qquad (2.40)$$

where, x_i is the mole fraction of the ith component in the solution and H_i is the Henry's law constant. Note that according to Raoult's law, H_i should be equal to the vapour pressure p_v for an ideal solution. Although Henery's law was proposed for low concentraions of gas in the liquid, it is one of the most used principles of physical chemistry because of its simplicity. Henry's law may lead to erroneous results if appropriate assumptions are not made.

Example 2.18 Calculate the average molar mass and composition by mass of air.
Solution An average composition of air at sea level by volume is given below.

Table 2.5 Composition of Air at Mean Seal Level

Gas	Mole%
Nitrogen	78.084
Oxygen	20.946
Argon	0.934
Carbon dioxide	0.033
Neon	18×10^{-4}
Helium	5.2×10^{-4}
Krypton	1.1×10^{-4}
Hydrogen	0.5×10^{-4}
Xenon	0.08×10^{-4}

In general, it can be taken that oxygen, nitrogen and argon are present to the extent of 21%, 78% and 1%, respectively (on volume basis). For combustion calculations in Chapter-7, air with average composition of 21% oxygen and 79% nitrogen (by volume) is considered.
Basis: 100 kmol air

Table 2.6 Composition of Air Without Trace/Noble Gases

Gas	Formula	Molar mass	kmol	Mass kg	Mass %
Oxygen	O_2	31.9988	21	671.786	23.19
Nitrogen	N_2	28.0135	78	2185.051	75.43
Argon	Ar	39.948	1	39.948	1.38
Total			100	2896.785	100.00

Average molar mass of air = $\dfrac{2897}{100}$ = 28.97   *Ans.*

> **Note:** Molar mass of each gas component is calculated using atomic masses, given in Appendix-II. The average molar mass of air, used at various places in later Chapters, will be taken approximately as 29.

Example 2.19 Cracked gas from a petroleum refinery has the following composition by volume: methane 45%, ethane 10%, ethylene 25%, propane 7%, propylene 8%, *n*-butane 5%.

Find (a) the average molar mass of the gas mixture, (b) the composition by mass, and (c) specific gravity of the gas mixture.

Solution In this type of problem, it is convenient to assume the basis of 100 kmol of cracked gas.

Since volume % equals mole %, methane present in the mixture is equal to 45 kmol.

$$\text{Molar mass of methane} = 12 + 4 = 16$$
$$\text{Mass of methane} = 45 \times 16 = 720 \text{ kg}$$

In a similar way, for all the components of the mixture, weights can be calculated. These calculations are summarized in Table 2.7.

Table 2.7 Composition of Refinery Gas

Gas	Formula	Molar mass	kmol	Mass kg	Mass %
Methane	CH_4	16	45	720	27.13
Ethane	C_2H_6	30	10	300	11.30
Ethylene	C_2H_4	28	25	700	26.37
Propane	C_3H_8	44	7	308	11.61
Propylene	C_3H_6	42	8	336	12.66
n-Butane	C_4H_{10}	58	5	290	10.93
Total	–	–	100	2654	100.00

$$\text{Average molar mass of gas mixture} = \frac{2654}{100} = 26.54$$

$$\text{Specific gravity of gas mixture} = \frac{26.54}{28.97} = 0.9161 \qquad Ans.$$

Example 2.20 Calculate the specific volume of superheated steam at 100 bar a and 623.15 K (350°C) using (a) the ideal gas law, and (b) the van der Waals equation.

If the actual specific volume* of steam at the above conditions is 0.022 42 m³/kg, find the percentage error in the above cases.

---

* From 1980 JSME Steam Tables

Solution

Molar mass of steam (water) = 18.0153

Ideal gas law states
$$pV = RT$$
$$p = 100 \text{ bar a}, \quad T = 623.15 \text{ K}$$

Molar volume $V = \dfrac{RT}{p}$

$$= \frac{0.083\,14 \times 623.15}{100} = 0.5180 \text{ m}^3/\text{kmol}$$

Specific volume $v = \dfrac{V}{M}$

$$= 0.518/18.0153 \text{ (m}^3/\text{kmol)} \text{ (kmol/kg)}$$
$$= 0.0288 \text{ m}^3/\text{kg} \qquad\qquad Ans. \text{ (a)}$$

Evaluation of van der Waals constants:

$$\left(p + \frac{a}{V^2}\right)(V - b) = RT$$

where
$$a = \frac{27\,R^2\,T_c^2}{64\,p_c} \text{ (m}^3)^2. \text{ bar/(kmol)}^2$$

and
$$b = \frac{RT_c}{8p_c} \text{ m}^3/\text{kmol}$$

$p_c = 220.76$ bar, $T_c = 647.11$ K for water,

$$a = \frac{\left[27 \times (0.083\,14)^2 \times (647.11)^2\right]}{(64 \times 220.76)}$$

$$a = 5.5315 \text{ m}^6. \text{ bar/(kmol)}^2$$

$$b = \frac{(0.083\,14 \times 647.11)}{(8 \times 220.76)}$$

$$= 0.030\,46 \text{ m}^3/\text{kmol}$$

Substituting the value of a and b in van der Waals equation.

$$\left(\frac{100 + 5.5315}{V^2}\right)(V - 0.030\,46) = 0.083\,14 \times 623$$

Simplifying
$$10\,V^3 - 5.4836\,V^2 + 0.5526\,V - 0.0168 = 0$$

Such equations can be solved by using a numerical method such as Newton-Raphson method. According to this method, if $F(V) = 0$ then

$$V_{n+1} = V_n - \frac{F(V_n)}{F'(V_n)} \qquad\qquad (2.41)$$

where, V_n is the starting root and V_{n+1} is the corrected root. To start with, V_1 may be taken as 0.5180 m^3/kmol which is the value obtained with the help of the ideal gas law. Using V_1, calculate V_2. Compare V_1 and V_2. If they are close enough, V_2 is the final root. If they are quite different evaluate V_3 and so on. Within four or five iterations, it is possible to get the exact root. Using this method,

$$V = 0.4285 \text{ m}^3/\text{kmol}$$

$$\text{Specific volume, } v = \frac{0.4285}{18.0153} = 0.0238 \text{ m}^3/\text{kg} \qquad \qquad Ans. (b)$$

Such equations can be readily solved by specialised mathematical software like Mathcad®.

$$\text{Define } f(V): = 100V^3 - 54.8422V^2 + 5.5315V - 0.168$$

or

$$f(V): = \left[100 + \frac{5.5315}{V^2}\right] (V - 0.03046) - 51.7962$$

Guess

$$V: = 0.518$$

$$\text{soln}: = \text{root} \, (f(V), V)$$

$$\text{soln}: = 0.429 \text{ m}^3/\text{kmol}$$

or

$$v = \frac{0.429}{18.0153} = 0.2381 \text{ m}^3/\text{kg}$$

$$\text{Correct value} = 0.022\,42 \text{ m}^3/\text{kg}$$

$$\% \text{ Error by using ideal gas law} = \left[\frac{(0.0288 - 0.022\,42)}{0.022\,42}\right] \times 100 = 28.01$$

$$\% \text{ Error by using van der Waals equation} = \left[\frac{(0.0238 - 0.022\,42)}{0.022\,42}\right] \times 100 = 6.16$$

Example 2.21 Carburetted water gas has the following composition by volume: Hydrogen 35.2%, Methane 14.8% Ethylene 12.8%, Carbon dioxide 1.5%, Carbon monoxide 33.9% and Nitrogen 1.8%.

The gas is available at 773.15 K (500°C) and 4 bar a. Find the molar volume of the mixture using (a) the ideal gas law, and (b) the van der Waals equation.

Solution Ideal gas law: $pV = RT$

$$p = 4 \text{ bar } a$$

$$T = 773.15 \text{ K}$$

$$V = \frac{RT}{p}$$

$$= 0.08314 \times \frac{773}{4} = 16.067 \text{ L/mol}$$

Evaluation of van der Waals constants:

For a gas mixture, a single value of the critical pressure or critical temperature cannot be used, and hence, *pseudo*-critical properties are evaluated using Kay's additive rule as shown in Table 2.8. However, this rule leads to significant errors, particularly when widely boiling components are present in the mixture. Lee and Kesler[14] have presented a set of mixing rules to find the critical properties of the mixtures based on a three parameter corresponding states principle that are claimed to give the best results. The discussion on the complex rules is outside the scope of this book. According to Kay's rule,

Psuedo critical property of

a component in the mixture = (mole fraction of the component)

$$\times \text{(critical property of the component)} \qquad (2.42)$$

Table 2.8 Composition of Carburetted Water Gas

Component	Formula	Mole Fraction	Critical temp., K		Critical pressure, bar a	
		y_i	T_c	$y_i \cdot T_c$	p_c	$y \cdot p_c$
Hydrogen	H_2	0.352	32.20	11.334	12.97	4.57
Methane	CH_4	0.148	190.50	28.194	46.04	6.81
Ethylene	C_2H_4	0.128	282.34	36.140	50.39	6.45
Carbon monoxide	CO	0.339	132.85	45.036	34.94	11.84
Carbon dioxide	CO_2	0.015	304.12	4.562	73.74	1.11
Nitrogen	N_2	0.018	126.09	2.270	33.94	0.61
Total		1.000		127.536		31.39

$$a = \frac{27 R^2 T_c^2}{64 p_c}$$

$$= \frac{\left[27 (0.083\,14)^2 \times (127.536)^2\right]}{(64 \times 31.39)} = 1.511 \ \text{L}^2 \cdot \text{bar/(mol)}^2$$

$$b = \frac{R T_c}{8 p_c}$$

$$= 0.083\,14 \times \frac{127.536}{(8 \times 31.390)} = 0.042\,32 \ \text{L/mol}$$

substituting these values,

$$\left(4 + \frac{1.511}{V^2}\right)(V - 0.042\,32) = 0.083\,14 \times 773.15$$

$$= 64.267\,22$$

Solving the equation by the Newton-Raphson method,

$$V = 15.74 \ \text{L/mol} \qquad \qquad \textit{Ans.}$$

Mathcad solution:

Define $\qquad f(V): = \left[4 + \dfrac{1.511}{V^2}\right](V - 0.04232) - 64.267\,22$

$\qquad$ Guess $V: = 16.067$

$\qquad \qquad$ soln: $= \text{root}\,(f(V), V)$

$\qquad \qquad$ soln $= 16.086 \ \text{L/mol} \qquad \qquad \textit{Ans.}$

Example 2.22 A ternary mixture of n-butane, 1-butene and furfural is analysed to find the content of each in it[15]. The mixture is stripped off with the help of carbon dioxide without appreciable entrainment of furfural due to its very low vapour pressure. The stripped gases are passed through an absorber column in which CO_2 is absorbed in 25% (by mass) KOH solution. The mixture of hydrocarbons, saturated with water vapour is collected in a measuring burette.

The test data are as follows:

> Sample mass = 6.5065 g
>
> Volume of saturated gases collected at 296.4 K (23.25°C) and
>
> > 102.5 kPa (769 torr) = 415.1 ml

n-Butane present in the hydrocarbons (dry)

> > in the burette = 43.1 mol %

Find the analysis of the liquid mixture (both on mole and mass basis).

Data: Vapour pressure of water over

> 25% KOH solution at 296.4 K = 2.175 kPa

Solution Basis: 6.5065 g furfural-n butane-1-butene mixture

> > Partical pressure of water
> >
> > vapour in the saturated
> >
> > hydrocarbon gas mixture = Vapour pressure of water
> >
> > > over KOH solution
> > >
> > > = 2.175 kPa

Partial pressure of n-butane and 1-butene (p) = 102.5 − 2.175

> > > > = 100.325 kPa

If n is the total number of mol of n-butane and 1-butene, then according to Eq. (2.23),

$$n = \frac{pV}{RT}$$

$$= \frac{100.325 \times 415.1}{8.314 \times 296.4 \times 1000}$$

$$= 0.0169 \text{ mol}$$

n-Butane in the hydrocarbon mixture = 0.0169 × 0.431 = 0.007 284 mol

Mass of n-butane in the mixture = 0.007 284 × 58 = 0.422 g

1-Butene in the hydrocarbon mixture = 0.0169 − 0.007 284 = 0.009 616 mol

Mass of 1-butene in the mixture = 0.009 616 × 56 = 0.5379 g

Mass of furfural in the liquid mixture = 6.5065 − 0.422 − 0.5379 = 5.5466 g

Moles of furfural in the liquid mixture = $\dfrac{5.5466}{96}$ 0.057 78 mol

The result are summarized in Table 2.9.

Table 2.9 Composition of Ternary Mixture

Component	Formula	Molar mass	mol	Mole %	Mass g	Mass %
n-Butane	C_4H_{10}	58	0.007 284	9.75	0.4225	6.49
1-Butene	C_4H_8	56	0.009 616	12.87	0.5379	8.27
Furfural	$C_5H_4O_2$	96	0.057 780	77.38	5.5469	85.24
Total			0.074 680	100.00	6.5073	100.00

Ans.

Example 2.23 The liquid mixture cited in the above example is boiled at 338.15 K (65°C) and 5.7 bar g. The mole fraction of n-butane in the ternary vapour mixture in equilibrium with the liquid is found to be 49.1 volume%. Assuming ideal behaviour of the liquid and vapour mixture, find the composition of the vapour mixture.

Data: Vapour pressure of furtural at 338.15 K = 3.293 kPa = 24.7 torr

Solution

Absolute total pressure 5.7 + 1.01 = 6.71 bar

According to Raoult's law,

Actual vapour pressure of

the furtural = (vapour pressure of pure furtural at 338.15 K) × (mol fraction of furfural in the liquid mixture)

= 3.293 × 0.7738 = 2.548 kPa

According to Dalton's law of partial pressures,

Molar fraction of furfural in the vapour mixture $= \dfrac{2.548}{6.71 \times 100}$

$= 0.0038$

Mole fraction of 1-butene

in the vapour mixture = 1.0000 − 0.0038 − 0.491 = 0.5052 *Ans.*

Example 2.24 Ambient air on a particular day in Ahmedabad has the following condition

Total pressure = 100 kPa (750 torr)

Dry bulb temperature = 308.15 K (35°C)

Dew point = 294.45 K (21.3°C)

Find the absolute humidity of the air

Data: Vapour pressure of water at 294.45 K = 2.5326 kPa = 19 torr

Solution

Partial pressure of water

vapour in the air, p_w = vapour pressure for water at dew point

= 2.5326 kPa

Now, according to Dalton's law),

$$\frac{(\text{Moles of water vapour})}{(\text{Moles of dry air})} = \frac{(\text{Partial pressure of water vapour})}{(\text{Partial pressure of air})}$$

$$= \frac{2.5326}{100 - 2.5326} = \frac{2.5326}{97.4674}$$

$$\frac{(\text{Mass of water vapour})}{(\text{Mass of dry air})} = \frac{2.5326}{97.4674} \times \frac{(\text{Molar mass of water})}{(\text{Molar mass of air})}$$

$$= \frac{2.5326}{97.4674} \times \frac{18.0153}{28.9679}$$

$$= 0.016\ 16 \text{ kg/kg}$$

$$\equiv 16.16 \ \frac{\text{g water vapour}}{\text{kg dry air}} \qquad Ans.$$

Example 2.25 Refrigerant 12 is expanded through a nozzle from 20.7 bar a and 355.15 K(82°C) to 8.7 bar a. If the average Joule-Thomson coefficient (μ) for R-12 is 1.616 K/bar, calculate the outlet temperature of the gas from the nozzle.
Solution

$$T_i - T_f = \mu\,(p_i - p_f)$$

p_f = final pressure, 8.7 bar a

p_i = initial pressure, 20.7 bar a

μ = 1.616 K/bar

T_i = 355.15 K

$T_f = T_i - \mu\,(p_i - p_f)$

$\quad = 355.15 - 1.616(20.7 - 8.7)$

$\quad = 335.76$ K or 62.61°C $\qquad Ans.$

Note: From enthalpy-pressure-temperature data of R-12[16], the outlet temperature of the gas is interpolated to be 333.35 K(60.4°C).

2.8 CONCLUSION

The chapters that follow will require the use of the principles outlined in this chapter. Hence, it is needless to stress upon the importance of understanding these fundamentals. The discussion on the principles is limited to the extent that it is useful in the later chapters. For greater knowledge of chemical principles, standard textbooks should be referred [11, 17].

EXERCISES

2.1 Find the moles of oxygen present in 500 g.

[*Ans.* 15.625 mol]

2.2 How many grams of carbon are present in 600 g $CaCO_3$?

[*Ans.* 72 g]

2.3 Find the molar mass of $KMnO_4$.

[*Ans.* 158]

2.4 A mass of 100 g each of HNO_3 and H_2SO_4 is filled in two separate bottles. Which bottle contains more atoms? How many more?

[*Ans.* Bottle containing HNO_3 will have 0.567 mol or 3.415×10^{23} atoms more than the other bottle.]

2.5 How many kilogram of carbon disulphide will contain 3.5 kmol carbon?

[*Ans.* 266 kg]

2.6 What is the equivalent mass of $Al_2(SO_4)_3$?

[*Ans.* 57]

2.7 How many equivalents are there in 500 g $KMnO_4$?

[*Ans.* 15.82 g eq]

2.8 The analysis magnesite ore obtained from Chalk Hill area, Salem district, yields 81% $MgCO_3$. 14% SiO_2 and 5% H_2O (by mass), Convert the analysis into mole %.

[*Ans.* 65.3% $MgCO_3$, 15.8% SiO_2, 18.9% H_2O (mole basis)]

2.9 The analysis of a sample of glass yields 7.8% Na_2O, 7.0% MgO, 9.7% ZnO, 2.0% Al_2O_3, 8.5% B_2O_3 and 65.0% SiO_2 (by mass). Convert this composition into mole%

[*Ans.* 7.65% Na_2O, 10.57% MgO, 7.25% ZnO, 1.19% Al_2O_3, 7.43% B_2O_3 and 65.91% SiO_2 (mole basis)]

2.10 A sample of sea water contains 35 000 ppm solids. Express the concentration of the solids as mass percentage.

[*Ans.* 3.5% (mass)]

2.11 A sample of milliolite limestone, obtained from Porbandar, Gujarat, is found to contain 54.5% CaO (by mass). If this CaO is present as $CaCO_3$ in the limestone, find the content of $CaCO_3$ in the limestone.

[*Ans.* 97.32 mass %]

2.12 Calculate the available nitrogen in the following:
  (a) Commercial ammonium sulphate (96% pure)
  (b) Pure sodium nitrate (100%)

[*Ans.* (a) 20.36%; (b) 16.47% (mass basis)]

2.13 A sample of caustic soda flakes contains 74.6% Na_2O (by mass). Find the purity of the flakes.

[*Ans.* 96.26% NaOH]

2.14 Nitric acid and water forms a maximum boiling azeotrope containing 62.2 mole % water [boiling temperature = 403.6 K (130.6°C).]. Find the composition of the azeotrope by mass.

[*Ans.* 68.02% HNO_3 (mass)]

2.15 An aqueous solution of common salt (NaCl) contains 25% salt (by mass) at 298.15 K (25°C). Find the mole % of NaCl in the solution.

[*Ans.* 9.3 mol% NaCl]

2.16 An aqueous solution contains 19.0% NH_3, 65.6% NH_4NO_3 and 6.0% urea (by mass). Calculate the available nitrogen content solution.

[*Ans.* 41.41% Nitrogen]

2.17 Ethanol is present in the aqueous solution to the extent of 1000 mg/L. Find TOC and ThOD of the solution in mg/L.

[*Ans.* TOC = 522 mg/L; ThOD = 2087 mg/L]

2.18 The strength of a phosphoric acid sample is found to be 35% P_2O_5 (by mass). Find out the actual concentration of H_3PO_4 (by mass) in the acid

[*Ans.* 48.31% H_3PO_4 (by mass)]

2.19 Spent acid from a fertiliser unit has the following composition by mass; H_2SO_4: 20%, $NH_4 HSO_4$: 45%, H_2O: 30% and organic compounds: 5% Calculated the total acid content of the spent acid in terms of H_2SO_4 after adding the acid content, chemically bound in ammonium hydrogen sulphate.

[*Ans.* 58.35% (mass)]

2.20 A sample of aqueous triethanolamine (TEA) solution contains 47% TEA (on volume basis). If the density of pure TEA is 1125 kg/m³, find the mass % of TEA in the solution.

[*Ans.* 49.94% (mass)]

2.21 A sample of wine contains 20% alcohol (ethanol) on volume basis. Find the mass % of a alcohol in the wine. Assume the densities of alcohol and alcohol free liquid (essentially water) to be 0.79 kg/L and 1.0 kg/L, respectively.

[*Ans.* 16.49% alcohol]

2.22 Convert the following into equivalent ppm $CaCO_3$:

(a) 800 ppm Na_2CO_3 in water

(b) 85 ppm $MgSO_4$ in water

[*Ans.* (a) 754.7 ppm $CaCO_3$; (b) 70.7 ppm $CaCO_3$]

2.23 Make the following conversions:

(a) 294 g/L H_2SO_4 to normality (N)

(b) 4.8 mg/mL $CaCl_2$ to normality (N)

(c) 5 N H_3PO_4 to g/L

(d) 54.75 g/L HCl to molarity (M)

(e) 3 M K_2SO_4 to g/L

[*Ans.* (a) 6 N; (b) 0.0865 N; (c) 163.35 g/L (d) 1.5 M (e) 522 g/L]

2.24 An aqueous solution of acetic acid of 35% concentration (by mass) has density 1.04 kg/L at 298.15 K (25°C). Find the molarity, normality and molality of the solution.

[*Ans.* 6.066 M; 6.066 N; 8.974 Molality]

2.25 An aqueous solution of monoethanolamine contains 20% MEA (by mass). It is utilised for the absorption of CO_2. Rich solution from the absorber contains 40 volume CO_2. Calculate CO_2 loading in term of moles CO_2 dissolved per mole MEA assuming that the density of the solution is 1.011 kg/L. [*Hint*: 40 volumes CO_2 concentration means that a litre solution will liberate 40 L CO_2 at 101.325 kPa a and 273.15 K (0°C)]

[*Ans.* 0.5385 mol CO_2/mol MEA]

2.26 The strength of an aqueous hydrogen peroxide solution is 60 volumes. Its density is measured to be 1.075 kg/L at 293 K (20°C). Find the mass % of H_2O_2 in the solution [*Hint*: A quantity of 1 L of 60 volume hydrogen peroxide will liberate 60 L oxygen at 101.325 kPa a and 288.75 K(15.6°C)].

[*Ans.* 16.02 mass %]

2.27 Calculate the elevation in the boiling point of a 40% (by mass) caustic soda solution over pure water (at standard atmospheric pressure) using Fig. 2.3.

[*Ans.* 29 K(29°C)]

2.28 A gas mixture has the following composition by volume:

Ethylene	30.6%
Benzene	24.5%
Oxygen	1.3%
Methane	15.5%
Ethane	25.0%
Nitrogen	3.1%

Find (a) the average molar mass of the gas mixture, (b) the composition by mass and (c) the density of the mixture in kg/m^3 at NTP.

[*Ans.* (a) 38.94; (b) ethylene 22.0%, benzene 49.07%, oxygen 1.07%, methane 6.37%, ethane 19.26%, nitrogen 2.23% (by mass); (c) 1.737 kg/m^3]

2.29 The analysis of a sewage gas sample from a municipal sewage treatment plant is given below on a volume basis:

Methane	68%
Carbon dioxide	30%
Ammonia	2%
H_2S, SO_2, etc.	Traces

Find (a) the average molar mass of the gas; and (b) the density of the gas at NTP.

[*Ans.* (a) 24.42; (b) 1.09 kg/m^3]

2.30 A weight of 1.10 kg of carbon dioxide occupies a volume of 33 L at 300.15 K(27°C). Using the van der Waals equation of state, calculate the pressure.

Data: For CO_2, take $a = 3.60$ [(m^3)^2.kPa]/(kmol)^2 and $b = 4.3 \times 10^{-2}$ m^3/kmol

[*Ans.* 19.52 bar a]

2.31 Calculate the density of chlorine gas 503.15 K(230°C) and 152 bar a using (a) the ideal gas law, and (b) the van der Waals eauation.

[*Ans.* (a) 258.1 kg/m^3; (b) 464.05 kg/m^3]

2.32 Ethane gas is processed at 73 bar a and 423.15 K(150°C). It follows the following Beattie-Bridgeman equation of state, i.e.

$$p = \left[\frac{RT\,(1-\varepsilon)}{V^2}\right](V + B) - \frac{A}{V^2}$$

where,

$$A = A_0\left(1 - \frac{a}{V}\right)$$

$$B = B_0\left(1 - \frac{b}{V}\right)$$

$$\varepsilon = \frac{c}{VT^3}$$

For ethane[18], $A_0 = 5.88$ bar $(m^3)^2/(kmol)^2$, $B_0 = 0.094$ m^3/kmol, $a = 0.058\,61$ m^3/kmol, $b = 0.019\,15$ m^3/kmol and $c = 90 \times 10^4$ $m^3 \cdot (K)^2$/kmol.

Find the density of ethane gas at the given conditions using the above equation.

[*Ans.* 75.176 kg/m^3]

2.33 Second order virial equation of state for dimethyl ether (DME) is given by following equation[19].

$$pV = ZRT$$

where $Z = 1 - \frac{Bp}{RT}$

$$B = \frac{RT_c}{p_c}(f^0 + \omega \cdot f^1)$$

$$\omega = 0.192 \text{ for DME}^{19}$$

$$f^0 = 0.1445 - 0.330/T_r - 0.1385/T_r^2$$
$$\quad - 0.0121/T_r^3 - 0.607 \times 10^{-3}/T_r^8.$$
$$f^1 = 0.0637 + 0.331/T_r^2 - 0.423/T_r^3 - 0.8 \times 10^{-2}/T_r^8$$
$$T_r = T/T_c$$

Calculate molar volume of DME at 15 bar a and 353.15 K(80°C).

[*Ans.* 2.239 m^3/kmol]

2.34 In the manufacture of nitric acid, initially ammonia and air are mixed at 7.09 bar g and 923 K (650°C). The composition of the gas mixture (by volume) is as follows:

Nitrogen	70.5%
Oxygen	18.8%
Water	1.2%
Ammonia	9.5%

Find (i) the density of the gas mixture using (a) ideal gas law, and (b) the van der Waals equation and (ii) the specific gravity of the gas mixture.

[*Ans.* (i) (a) 2.912 kg/m^3; (b) 2.907 kg/m^3; (ii) 0.952]

2.35 In Exercise 2.34 water vapour is considered as an impurity. Assuming that the gas mixture behaves ideally, find the concentration of water vapour in (a) mg/m^3 and (b) ppm.

[*Ans.* (a) 22 761 mg/m^3, (b) 7816 ppm (or mg/kg)]

2.36 A binary mixture of *n*-butane and furfural is analysed to find the butane content in it [20]. First, the *n*-butane present in the mixture is stripped off with the help of carbon dioxide with negligible entrainment of furfural. The mixture of carbon dioxide and *n*-butane is then passed through the solution containing 25% NaOH (by (mass) in which carbon dioxide is absorbed. The saturated hydrocarbon is collected over the solution in a burette. The test data on a specific run are given below:

Weight of sample *n*-butane and furfural) = 9.082 g

Volume of saturated *n*-butane stripped off at 295.35 K (22.2°C) and

101.75 kPa (763.2 torr) = 105.7 mL

Find the amount of *n*-butane present in the liquid mixture on mole and weight basis.

Data: Vapour pressure of water over 25% NaOH solution at 295.35 K (22.2°C) = 1.666 kPa (12.5 torr)

[*Ans.* 4.48 mole % and 2.75 mass % *n*-butane]

2.37 The Orsat (dry) analysis of the flue gas from a boiler house is given as (volume basis); CO_2: 10.0%, O_2: 7.96%, N_2: 82.0% and SO_2: 0.04%. The temperature and pressure of flue gases are 463 K (190°C) and 100 kPa (750 torr), respectively. The dew point of the gas is found to be 320 K (20°C). Find the absolute humidity of the flue gases

[*Ans.* 8.6 g/kg dry flue gas]

2.38 In Exercise 2.37, SO_2 is undesirable from the point of view of occupational hazards (environmental pollution). Express the concentration of SO_2 in ppm and mg/m^3 on dry basis.

[*Ans.* 855.2 ppm (or mg/kg); 665 mg/m^3]

2.39 In the Monsanto process for the manufacture of formaldehyde, air, methanol and steam are mixed in the proportion 4:2:1.33 (by weight) at 373 K (100°C). The total pressure is 68.6 kPa g. Calculate the partial pressure of each of the components present in the mixture.

[*Ans.* methanol 38.71; steam 45.78; oxygen 17.94; nitrogen 67.49 (kPa)]

2.40 A domestic liquefied petroleum gas (LPG) cylinder, conforming to IS:4576, is stored at 313.15 K (40°C). It is a mixture of 30% propane, 45% *n*-butane, and 25% *i*-butane by volume. Calculate (a) average molar mass of LPG, (b) specific gravity of LPG, and (c) pressure in the cylinder.

Date: Vapour pressures of propane, *n*-butane and *i*-butane are 1350, 383 and 535 kPa, respectively at 313.15 K(40°C). [Ref. : Table 5.4]

[*Ans.* : (a) 53.916, (b) 2.25 and (c) 7.11 bar a]

2.41 An absorber is utilised to scrub ammonia from the purge gas of an ammonia synthesis loop. The composition of purge gas is H_2: 62.0%, N_2: 20.6%, Ar: 4.1%, CH_4: 11.1% and NH_3: 2.2% (by volume). Ammonia is absorbed in demineralised water and a solution of 3% NH_3 (by mass) strength is produced. The absorber operates at 6.77 MPa g and the solution leaves the absorber at 305.75 K (32.6°C).

Calculate the quantity of the gas mixture dissolved in 5 m³ solution. Use the data given in Table 2.10.

Table 2.10 Solubility of Gases in Aqueous Ammonia

Gas	Solubility at 101.325 kPa a and 305.75 K (32.6°C), Nm³/100 m³ 3% NH_3 soln.
Nitrogen	1.35
Hydrogen	1.60
Argon	2.75
Methane	2.80

(*Hint:* At higher pressure, solubilities can be taken proportional to partial pressures.)

[*Ans.* 5.873 Nm³/5 m³ solution]

2.42 A breathing apparatus (pressure suit) is supplied with compressed air at 7 bar g and 313.15 K(40°C). Its pressure is reduced to near atmospheric in the apparatus. If the overall Joule-Thomson coefficient[2] in this pressure range is 0.21 K/bar, calculate the air temperature after the letdown.

[*Ans.* 311.68 K(38.53°C)]

2.43 A capacity test is conducted of a reciprocating air compressor in which air receiver, located at the downstream of aftercooler, is pressurised from 1 bar g to 7.5 bar g at 313.15 K(40°C) in 4 min. Geometric volume of the air receiver is 2 m³. Neglect the volume of interconnecting piping. Calculate the capacity of the air compressor.

[*Ans.* 167.9 Nm³/h]

REFERENCES

1. Atallah, S. I., *Chem Engg.*, **68**(8), April 17, 1961, p. 200.
2. Green, D. W. and J. O. Malony, *Perry's Chemical Engineers' Handbook,* 6th Ed., McGraw-Hill, New York, 1984.
3. Technical Bulletin on *Dow Products and Services*, Dow Chemical Co., USA, 1972.

4. Tchobanoglous, G. and F. L. Burton, *Wastewater Engineering; Treatment, Disposal and Reuse,* 3rd Ed., McGraw-Hill, Singapore, 1991.

5. *H_2SO_4 Atlas,* Lurgi GmbH, Germany, 1984.

6. Technical Bulletin on *Soda Ash,* Wyandotte Chemicals Corporation, USA, 1955.

7. Technical Bulletin on *Caustic Soda,* Hooker Chemical Corporation, USA, 1966.

8. Weast, R. C., *CRC Handbook of Chemistry and Physics,* 64th Ed., CRC Press Inc., USA, 1983, p. E-1.

9. McCabe, W.L., J.C. Smith and P. Harriott, *Unit Operations of Chemical Engineering,* 6th Ed., McGraw-Hill, New York, 2001, p. 481.

10. Reid, R. C., J. M. Prausnitz and B. E. Poling, *The Properties of Gases and Liquids,* 4th Ed., McGraw-Hill, USA, 1987.

11. Smith, J. M., H. C. Van Ness, M. M. Abbott and B. I. Bhatt, *Introduction to Chem. Engg. Thermodynamics,* 6th Ed., Tata McGraw-Hill, New Delhi, 2003.

12. Somayajulu, G. R., *J. Chem. Engg. Data,* **34**, 1989, p. 107

13. *Technical Bulletin No. 645,* AlliedSignal Inc., USA, 1993.

14. Lee, B. I. and M. G. Kesler, *AIChE J.,* **21**(3), May 1975, p. 510.

15. Gerster, J. A., T. S. Martes and A. P. Colbern. *Ind. Engg. Chem.,* **39**(6), 1947, p. 797.

16. GENETRON, *a* WINDOWS based Computer Programme by Allied-Signal Inc., USA for the refrigerants, 1999.

17. Himmelblau, D. V., *Basic Principles and Calculations in Chemical Engineering,* 5th Ed., Prentice-Hall, USA, 1989.

18. Beattie, J. A., C. Hadlock, and N. Poffenberger, *J. Chem. Phys.,* **3**(2), 1935, p. 93.

19. Teng. H., J. C. McCandless, and J. B. Schneyer, ; *Thermolchemical Characteristics of Dimethyl Ether,* a paper presented at SAE World Congress, Detroit, Michigan USA, March 2001.

20. Martes, T. S. and A. P. Colburn, *Ind. Engg. Chem.,* **39**(60), 1947, p. 787.

Chapter 3

Material Balances without Chemical Reaction

3.1 INTRODUCTION

A process design starts with the development of a *process flow sheet* or *process flow diagram*. For the development of such a diagram, material and energy balance calculations are necessary. These balances follow the *laws of conservation of mass and energy*. Fundamental quantity mass remains constant regardless of the changes which occur in a physical process or a chemical reaction. According to the *law of conservation of mass*, the total mass of various compounds remains unchanged during an unit operation or a chemical reaction. Before attempting the study of mass or energy balance, it is necessary to understand the salient aspects of a process flow sheet.

3.2 PROCESS FLOW SHEET

A process flow sheet is one in which all incoming and outgoing materials and utilities are shown. It should be clearly understood that such a diagram is different from the piping and instrumentation (P & I) diagram. The latter diagram is not intended to give quantitative picture but is intended to specify the flow sequence, all relevant instrumentation and controls, pipes and fittings, material specifications of pipes and any other specific information for carrying out detailed engineering design. On the other hand, a process flow sheet includes.

  (i)   Flow rate or quantity of each stream.
  (ii) Operating conditions of each stream, such as pressure and temperature.
  (iii) Heat added/removed in a particular equipment.
  (iv) Any specific information which is useful in understanding the process.

For example, symbolic presentation of a hazard, safety precautions, sequence of flow if it is a batch process, corrosive nature of materials, etc.

From the above discussion, it is clear that the process flow diagram is a very useful diagram in the chemical process industry. It presents information in readily understandable form. It helps the operator in adjusting his parameters, the supervisor in checking/controlling the plant operation, the management in discussions across the table and the project engineers in the comparison and evaluation of different processes. If the basic process is simple and involves only a few steps, the P & I diagram and the process flow sheet can be combined into one sheet.

Chemical processes and reactions can be basically divided into two categories, batch and continuous. Batch distillation and extraction, adsorption of solvent on activated carbon and regeneration, and so on are batch unit operations. Continuous distillation, drying of cloth, and so on are common examples of unit operations that are continuous in nature. Water treatment by ion exchangers, bulking of effluents and batch production of organic chemicals are examples of batch-type chemical reactions. The manufacture of ammonia, urea, methanol, petrochemicals, and so on fall under the category of continuous chemical reactions. Continuous ion exchange columns have also been developed. Batch as well as continuous deodorizers are common in refining edible oils. Thus, it may be seen that whether a particular process is batch or continuous purely depends on the scale of economics. Practically any batch process can be converted to a continuous one.

Figures 3.1 to 3.6 give typical flow sheets of batch and continuous processes. Figure 3.1 gives a flow sheet of the bench-scale production of phenylethyl alcohol as developed by Prug[1]. This alcohol is produced by a typical Friedel-Crafts reaction. Ethylene oxide is reacted with excess benzene in the presence of anhydrous aluminum chloride. The alcohol yield is increased by diluting the ethylene oxide with air and methylamine is added to neutralise the hydrogen chloride generated during the reaction. The product is washed with sodium carbonate solution and is distilled to recover excess benzene and remove the byproduct biphenyl. It may be seen that the diagram provides nearly complete information on the process. Each of the streams is numbered, illustrating the sequence in batch operations and the stream details are given in a tabular form. To highlight the hazards of the reactants, small diamond markers are shown on the flow sheet and the numbers in the diamonds refer to the health, flammability and reactivity hazards as defined in the Standard 704 of the National Fire Protection Association, USA. The seriousness of hazards is shown by numbers on a scale from 0 to 4, with number 4 indicating 'most serious'.

Figure 3.2 gives the process details of a softening process using ion-exchange technology (see Exercise 4.18). This is a cyclic process in which the service cycle and regeneration cycle are repeated alternatively. It may be noted that tabular data on regeneration steps help in understanding the process. Since this is nearly an isothermal process, temperatures are not indicated on the diagram.

Figures 3.3 to 3.5 give process flow diagrams of continuous processes. Acid gas removal has great importance in the process industry and variety of processes have been developed by a number of companies. Figure 3.3 represents acid gas removal in a SNG plant (see Example 8.5). Dealkylation of toluene to benzene (Fig. 3.4) is an important unit process in organic industry (see Exercise 8.13). Figure 3.5 represents hydrogenation of benzene to cyclohexane[2] (Exercise 4.33). The reaction taken place in a fixed bed catalytic reactor. Exothermic heat of reaction is removed by boiling water outside the tubes which contain catalyst. It is desired that the mole ratio of hydrogen to benzene be maintained 3.3 kmol/kmol at the reactor inlet. In all these diagrams, operating conditions change during each process step. Material balance at each point can be given in a separate table as can be seen in Tables 8.18 and 8.30 or can be given at the bottom of the diagram as shown in Figs 3.1 and 3.5.

Figure 3.6 depicts continuous atmospheric distillation of crude oil. It is designed for a throughput of Indonesian crude at the rate of 0.226 m^3/s (120 000 US barrels per day). Product summary of Fig. 3.6 is an useful table for discussions across the table for product planning.

It is interesting to note that each flow sheet is presented in a different form. One process engineer may wish to give the component balance on the flow diagram while another may prefer to give it in a tabular form at the bottom. Some flow sheets may include safety aspects, such as explosibility, flammability, toxicity, corrosivity, radioactivity hazards and so on. while others may have the sequence of flow of a batch process in a tabular form. The extent to which information is required to be given in a process flowsheet also depends on the type of flowsheet. For example, a process flow sheet prepared on the basis of laboratory or pilot plant studies (Fig. 3.1) may include more information on safety aspects for safe scale-up and for speedy transition of a bench-scale process. However, ultimately the person who prepares the flowsheet is the best judge to decide the extent of information to be covered by his flow sheet. At times, one does not wish to give patented information on the flow sheet. Also, many vendors do not give complete information at the quotation stage but would like to give adequate information at the contract stage. In summary, process flow sheet can be an important aid between the process design engineer and the contractor. In fact process design starts with the preparation of a process flowsheet.

Flowsheets can also be block diagram. Boxes in such diagrams represent various stages of the process while lines represent the streams that go between the boxes. Such flowsheets can include as much information as one desires. In this book large number of block diagrams are presented in the various examples that are solved or in the exercises. Such block diagrams can easily be prepared with the help of a spreadsheet programme on a personal computer. Such electronic flowsheets are very useful in process development or in answering *what if* questions relations relating to the material and energy balances. Mathematical software such as Mathcad® also permits development of a process flow sheet. Discussion on the use of a spreadsheet software and Mathcad for stoichiometric calculations is detailed in Chapter 9.

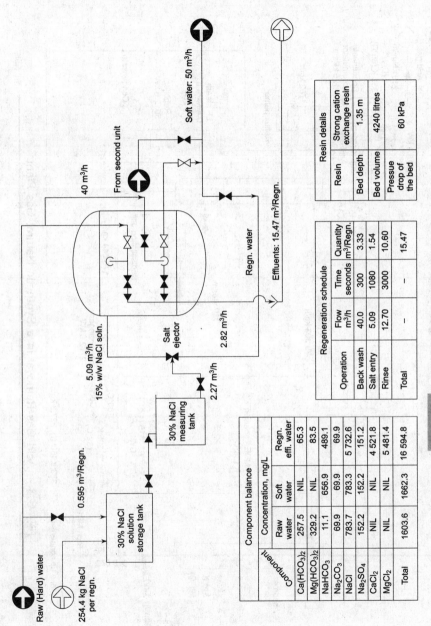

Fig. 3.2 Water Softening by Ion-exchange

Raw (Hard) water

254.4 kg NaCl per regn.

30% NaCl solution storage tank

0.595 m³/Regn.

30% NaCl measuring tank

2.27 m³/h

Salt ejector

40 m³/h

5.09 m³/h 15% w/w NaCl soln.

From second unit

Soft water: 50 m³/h

Regn. water

2.82 m³/h

Effluents: 15.47 m³/Regn.

Regeneration schedule			
Operation	Flow m³/h	Time seconds	Quantity m³/Regn.
Back wash	40.0	300	3.33
Salt entry	5.09	1080	1.54
Rinse	12.70	3000	10.60
Total	–	–	15.47

Resin details		
Resin	Strong cation exchange resin	
Bed depth	1.35 m	
Bed volume	4240 litres	
Pressure drop of the bed	60 kPa	

Component balance

Component	Concentration, mg/L			
	Raw water	Soft water	Regn. effl. water	
Ca(HCO₃)₂	257.5	NIL	65.3	
Mg(HCO₃)₂	329.2	NIL	83.5	
NaHCO₃	11.1	656.9	489.1	
Na₂CO₃	69.9	69.9	69.9	
NaCl	783.7	783.3	5 732.6	
Na₂SO₄	152.2	152.2	151.2	
CaCl₂	NIL	NIL	4 521.8	
MgCl₂	NIL	NIL	5 481.4	
Total	1603.6	1662.3	16 594.8	

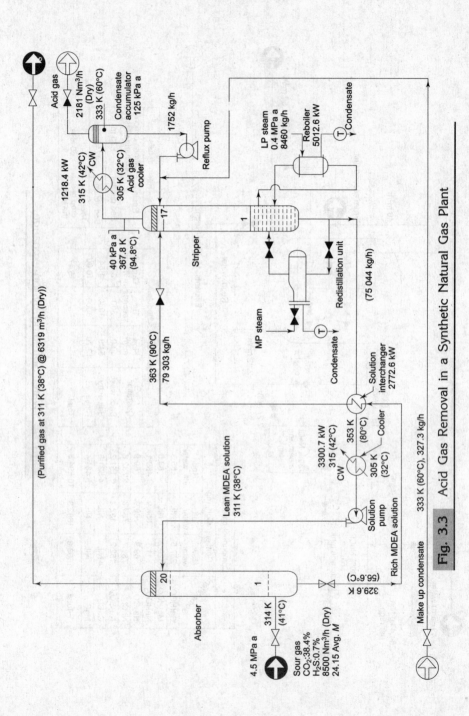

Fig. 3.3 Acid Gas Removal in a Synthetic Natural Gas Plant

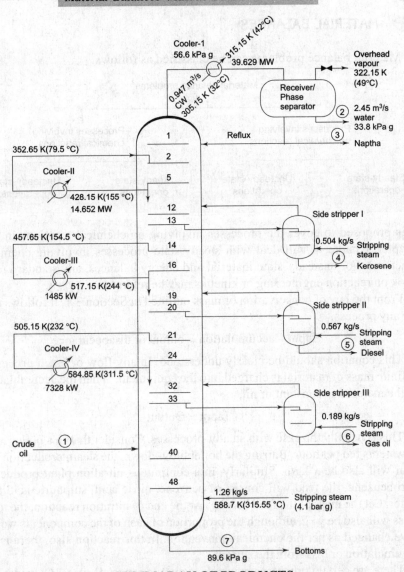

SUMMARAY OF PRODUCTS

Stream No.	Product	Flowrate		°API	Temperature
		kmol/s	m³/s		K(°C)
1.	Crude oil	0.825	0.221	29.4	505.15 K(232°C)
2.	Water	0.136	0.0025	–	322.15 K(49°C)
3.	Naphtha	0.362	0.048	61.5	322.15 K(49°C)
4.	Kerosene	0.127	0.027	40.7	353.75 K(80.6°C)
5.	Diesel	0.081	0.023	31.2	533.35 K(262.2°C)
6.	Gas oil	0.087	0.031	25.2	607.15 K(334°C)
7.	Bottoms	0.171	0.091	14.1	635.65 K(362.5°C)

Fig 3.6 Atmospheric Distillation of Indonesian Crude Oil

3.3 MATERIAL BALANCES

Material balance problems can be classified as follows.

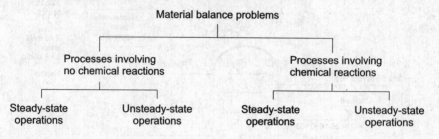

It is proposed to cover the processes involving no chemical reactions in this chapter. Chapter 4 will deal with steady-state processes involving chemical reactions. For unsteady-state material and energy balances, any standard textbook on reaction engineering or kinetics may be referred[3].

From the law of conservation of mass outlined in Section 3.1, it follows that for any process.

$$\text{Input} - \text{accumulation} = \text{output or disappearance}$$

This equation should be clearly understood. In any flow or batch process, a definite mass of material is charged into the equipment. When the accumulation of the material is constant or nil,

$$\text{Input} = \text{Output}$$

This is usually the case with steady-processes. Consider that in a boiler, x kg of water is fed per hour. Barring the boiler blow-down, the steam production per hour will also be x kg/h. Similarly, in a continuous nitration plant producing nitrobenzene, the feed will consist of benzene, nitric acid, sulphuric acid and water. Let the mass of the feed be y kg. At the end of nitration reaction, the total mass will also be y kg, although the proportion of each of the components would have changed as per the chemical conversion. In this reaction also, there is no accumulation or loss from the system.

There are certain processes in which accumulation takes place. Consider the example of a storage tank of drinking water. The input into the tank may be a m³/h, while the draw from the tank may be b m³/h ($a > b$). Under these circumstances, the input does not equal to the output, and the accumulation in the tank amounts to $(a - b)$ m³/h.

In a kiln treating magnesium hydroxide, the feed is moist magnesium hydroxide. The heat is supplied directly to the kiln. As a result, the magnesium hydroxide decomposes into magnesium oxide and water. From the stack, water escapes. In such a system, input equals the output plus the evaporated moisture.

3.3.1 Material Balances Without Chemical Reactions

There are three general methods of solving material balance problems for systems involving no chemical reactions.

(i) Make the balance of a *tie* material, the quantity of which does not change during the particular operation. The examples falling under this category include concentration of a solution in an evaporator in which the dissolved solids do not change, which is a *tie* material for the material balance. While drying the material, bone dry material is unchanged and only the solvent is evaporated.

(ii) Very often one or several *inert* chemical species which do not take part in the operation are involved in the system. By making balance of this *inert* portion, the material balance calculations can be simplified. Examples of this type of problems include leaching of solids, ash present in coal, nitrogen in combustion air entering a furnace, and so on. While leaching copper from the ore, the gangue is unaffected and acts as an inert material. During the combustion of coal, ash is left out on the grate and it does not take part in the combustion process. Extraction of oils from various seed is carried out using supercritical carbon dioxide.

(iii) When two or more compounds are present in the system and if all the compounds are affected simultaneously, it is required that the material balance equations be solved by satisfying simultaneous equations. Fortifying spent acids with strong acids (Example 3.8) and material balances of distillation and extraction of liquids (Examples 3.5, 6.1 and 6.4), establishing a cascade type steam balance (Example 8.6), solving a material balance problem of competitive chemical reactions in series, and so on fall under this category.

3.3.2 Degrees of Freedom

Concept of *Degrees of Freedom* is well known to chemical engineers. This concept is useful in physical chemistry to defined a system in equilibrium having more than one phase. The same concept is also useful in stoichiometry in solving the problems of a multi-variable system. This is an index which fixes the number of independent equations that are required to be solved for finding the specified number of unknowns. If the number of independent equations are less than the number of unknowns, the system is considered under-defined. In such a case, an optimum solution can be found by fixing some unknowns based on a judgment. In Chapter 8, steam balance calculations (Example 8.6) are given in which certain assumptions are made to arrive at an optimum steam balance. In simulation studies (Chapter 9), a specific parameter is varied and other parameters are calculated and thereby a trend analysis is generated. For such systems the degree of freedom is positive.

In certain systems, the degree of freedom is negative which indicates that the system is over-defined. For such calculations, redundant information should be discarded to obtain an unique solution. For example, when a quadratic equation is solved, two values of a parameter—usually positive and negative figures—are obtained. Negative value is discarded thereby increasing the degree of freedom. In another case, there may be contradictory demands of the variables. Consider the dilution of a hazardous gas by an inert gas. If the limiting concentration of the hazardous gas and available quantum of the inert gas are specified, it may not be possible to match them. Under such circumstances, inconsistency has to be removed by fixing one of the variables.

For a balanced system the degree of freedom is zero.

3.3.3 Solving Material Balance Problems

In any given problem, one has to first determine the particular class under which the problem falls. Then a definite basis is assumed. Often, the basis is defined in the statement of the problem itself. If this basis is convenient, it may be adopted, otherwise, a new, more convenient basis can be selected. Using this basis, the problem must be solved with consistent units.

In the case of gaseous systems, the temperature and pressure are often specified in the statement of the problem. As discussed in Chapter 2, these two parameters are needed to evaluate the density of the gas. With the help of density calculations the conversion of volume to mass or *vice versa* is possible.

The following illustrative examples will give an idea of the different types of problems.

Example 3.1 A Lancashire boiler is fed with soft water containing 1200 mg/L dissolved solids. IS: 10 392-1982 specifies that the maximum dissolved solids in the boiler water should not exceed 3500 mg/L for boilers, operating up to 20 bar g. In order to maintain the specified level, a continuous blow-down system is adopted. Find the percentage of the feed water which will be blown down, assuming that no carryover is observed.

Solution In this example, the basis is not defined. Therefore, assume a basis of 1 kg feed water. During evaporation of water in the boiler, the dissolved solids are unaffected and hence the balance of dissolved solids (a tie material) in the feed water and boiler water will provide the clue to the problem. Thus, the example is of type (i).

1 kg feed water will contain 1200 mg dissolved solids. Let x kg be the amount of feed water that will be blown down. This blow-down will contain dissolved solids to the extent of 3500 mg (same as boiler water).

Therefore $x \times 3500 = 1200 \times 1$ or $x = 0.343$ kg

% Blow-down = $(0.343/1) \times 100 = 34.3$ *Ans.*

Note: Density of feed water and boiler water is assumed to be 1.0 kg/L.

Example 3.2 In a textile mill, a double-effect evaporator system concentrates weak liquor containing 4% (by mass) caustic soda to produce a lye containing 25% solids (by mass). Calculate the evaporation of water per 100 kg feed in the evaporator.

Solution In this problem, the basis is defined.

Basis : 100 kg weak liquor (feed)

It contains 4 kg caustic soda.

Let the quantity of the lye be x kg.

Caustic soda in the lye = 0.25 x

However, the caustic soda does not take part in the evaporation.

$$0.25 \ x = 4$$
$$x = 4/0.25 = 16 \text{ kg}$$
$$\text{Evaporation} = 100 - 16 = 84 \text{ kg} \qquad \textit{Ans.}$$

Example 3.3 The analysis of a sample of Babul bark (of northern India) yield 5.8% moisture, 12.6% tannin, 8.3% soluble non-tannin organic matter and the rest lignin. In order to extract tannin out of the bark, a counter-current extraction process is employed. The residue from the extraction process is analysed and found to contain 0.92% tannin and 0.65% solute non-tannin organic matter on a dry basis. Find the percentage of tannin recovered on the basis of the original tannin present in the bark. All analyses are given on mass basis.

Solution Basis: 100 kg Babul bark

It contains 5.8 kg moisture, 12.6 kg tannin and 8.3 kg soluble non-tannin organic material.

$$\text{Lignin in the bark} = 100 - 5.8 - 12.6 - 8.3 = 73.3 \text{ kg}$$

In this leaching process it is evident that lignin is unaffected. Therefore, it will be considered inert. Thus, the example is of type (ii).

Since the analysis of residue is given on dry basis, its lignin content will be given by

$$\text{Lignin content} = 100 - 0.92 - 0.65 = 98.43 \text{ kg}/100 \text{ kg dry residue}$$

If the final weight of the dry residue is x kg,

$$x \times 0.9843 = 73.3$$
$$x = \frac{73.3}{0.9843} = 74.47 \text{ kg}$$
$$\text{Tannin present in the residue} = 74.47 \times 0.0092 = 0.685 \text{ kg}$$
$$\text{Tannin recovered} = [12.6 - 0.685)/12.6] \times 100 = 94.56 \ \% \qquad \textit{Ans.}$$

Example 3.4 Dry neem leaves were subjected to extraction with super critical carbon dioxide at 200 bar and 333 K (60°C). Dry leaves are analysed to contain 0.46% α-tocopherol and 0.0% β-carotene[4]. Extract is found to contain 15.5% α-tocopherol and 0.41% β-carotene. All percentages are by mass. If β-carotene content of the leached residue is nil, calculate (a) the mass of extra phase per kg of dry leaves, and (b)% recovery of α-tocopherol.

Solution

Basis: 1 kg dry neem leaves

β-carotene content of the leaves = 0.01/100 = 0.0001 kg

Extract contains 0.41% β-carotene.

$$\text{Extract quantity} = \frac{0.0001}{0.41} \times 100$$
$$= 0.0244 \text{ kg}$$

α-tocopherol in the extract $= 0.0244 \times 0.155$
$$= 0.003\ 782 \text{ kg}$$

α-tocopherol in the neem leaves $= 0.46/100 = 0.0046 \text{ kg}$

$$\text{Recovery of } \alpha\text{-tocopherol} = \frac{0.003\ 782}{0.0046} \times 100$$

$$= 82.2\% \qquad\qquad \textit{Ans. (b)}$$

Example 3.5 A 100 kg mixture of 27.8% of acetone (A) and 72.2% of chloroform (B) by mass is to be batch- extracted with a mixed solvent at 298 K(25°C). The mixed solvent of an unknown composition is known to contain water (S_1) and acetic acid (S_2). The mixture of the original mixture and the mixed solvent is shaken well, allowed to attain equilibrium, and separated into two layers. The compositions of the two layers are given below[5].

Table 3.1 Composition of Immiscible Layers

Layer	Composition, mass %			
	A	B	S_1	S_2
Upper layer	7.5	3.5	57.4	3.16
Lower layer	20.3	67.3	2.8	9.6

Find (a) the quantities of the two layers, (b) the mass-ratio of the mixed solvent to the original mixture, and (c) the composition of the mixed solvent (mass basis).

Solution B
asis: 100 kg original mixture

The mixture contains 27.8 kg of A and 72.2 kg of B.

This problem is of type (iii) because here the system contains more than one component, and the balance of each of the components will yield the complete material balance.

Let x and y be the amount of upper and lower layers respectively. According to the principle of Degrees of Freedom, two equations are required to find the unknowns

$$\text{Total mixture} = (x + y) \text{ kg}$$

$$\text{Balance of A: } 0.075x + 0.203y = 27.8 \qquad\qquad (1)$$

$$\text{Balance of B: } 0.035x + 0.673y = 72.2 \qquad\qquad (2)$$

Solving Eqs. (1) and (2) by elimination,

$$x = 93.42 \text{ kg and } y = 102.42 \text{ kg} \qquad \textit{Ans. (a)}$$

For two unknowns, it is relatively easy to solve the simultaneous equations   ially by elimination or by determinants. However, when number of unknowns are more, it is somewhat laborious to solve. Mathcad® (a mathematical software) can be conveniently used to solve simultaneous equations.

Mathcad solution:

Matrix

$$\text{M:} = \begin{bmatrix} 0.075 & 0.203 \\ 0.035 & 0.673 \end{bmatrix}$$

$$\text{V:} = \begin{bmatrix} 27.8 \\ 72.2 \end{bmatrix}$$

$$\text{soln:} = \text{M}^{-1} \cdot \text{v}$$

$$\text{soln} = \begin{bmatrix} 93.447 \\ 102.421 \end{bmatrix}$$

$x = 93.45$ kg and $y = 102.42$ kg   *Ans.* (a)

Total mixture = 93.45 + 102.42 = 195.87 kg

Mixed solvent = 195.87 – 100 = 95.87 kg

Mass-ratio of mixed solvent

to the original mixture = 95.87/100 = 0.9587   *Ans.* (b)

Balance of water (S_1):

Total S_1 in the system = 93.47 × 0.574 + 102.42 × 0.028 = 56.51 kg

Balance of acetic acid (S_2):

Total S_2 in the system = 93.47 × 0.316 + 102.42 × 0.096 = 39.35 kg

Quantity of the solvent = 56.51 + 39.35 = 95.86 kg

% S_1 in the mixed solvent = (56.51/95.84) × 100 = 58.95

% S_2 in the mixed solvent = 100 – 58.95 = 41.05   *Ans.* (c)

Example 3.6   A pressure swing adsorption (PSA) unit produces nitrogen for inerting purpose. It is fed with compressed air at 7 bar g and 313 K(40°C) at the rate of 170 Nm^3/h. Unit consists of carbon molecular sieves which adsorbs nitrogen under pressure. Nitrogen is produced from the unit at the rate of 50 Nm^3/h having 99% purity (by volume). Calculate the average composition of the reject stream.

Solution

Basis: 170 Nm^3/h air having 79% N_2 and 21% O_2 by volume

Nitrogen stream has 99% N_2 and 1% O_2 by volume.

Nitrogen content of the nitrogen stream = 50 × 0.99 = 49.5 Nm^3/h

Oxygen content of the nitrogen stream = 50 × 0.01 = 0.5 Nm^3/h

Table 3.2	Reject Stream Composition	
Component	Flow, Nm^3/h	Vol. %
Nitrogen	170 × 0.79 – 49.5 = 84.8	70.67
Oxygen	170 × 0.21 – 0.5 = 35.2	29.33
Total	120.0	100.00

Ans.

Example 3.7   A sample of mixed acid contains 55% HNO_3 and 48% H_2SO_4 with 3% negative water (mass) basis[6]. Find the actual constituents present in it.

The above mixed acids is prepared by mixing 100% HNO_3 and oleum. Find the required strength of oleum and the proportions of the two acids in which they should be mixed.

Solution   The mixed acid contains 55% HNO_3 and 48% H_2SO_4 which is theoretically impossible as the total of the percentages comes to 103. The real meaning of the expression is that SO_3 dissolved in 100 kg mixed acid of composition 55% HNO_3 + 45% H_2SO_4 which requires 3 kg water to convert SO_3 into H_2SO_4.

Basis: 100 kg SO_3-free mixed acid

It contains 55kg HNO_3 and 45 kg H_2SO_4.

The basic reaction with SO_3 and water is

$$SO_3 + H_2O \rightarrow H_2SO_4$$

Thus, 1 kmol $H_2O \equiv 1$ kmol SO_3

SO_3 equivalent to 3 kg water $= (80/18) \times 3 = 13.33$ kg

Thus, 1113.33 kg mixed acid contains 55 kg HNO_3, 45 kg H_2SO_4 and 13.33 kg SO_3. Since the available HNO_3 for mixing is of 100% strength, 55 kg of it will be required.

Quantity of oleum required to be mixed $= 45 + 13.33 = 58.33$ kg

$$\text{Strength of oleum} = \left(\frac{13.33}{58.33} \right) \times 100 = 22.85\% \text{ free } SO_3$$

$$\text{Ratio of } HNO_3/\text{oleum} = \frac{55}{58.33} = 0.943$$

Hence, HNO_3 and oleum are required to be mixed in the proportion of 0.943:1 (by mass) *Ans.*

───

Example 3.8 It required to make 1000 kg mixed acid containing 60% H_2SO_4, 32% HNO_3 and 8% water by blending (i) the spent acid containing 11.3% HNO_3, 44.4% H_2SO_4 and 44.3% H_2O, (ii) aqueous 90% HNO_3, and (iii) aqueous 98% H_2SO_4. All percentages are by mass. Calculate the quantities of each of the three acids required for blending.

Solution Basis: 1000 kg mixed acid

It contains 600 kg H_2SO_4, 320 kg HNO_3 and 80 kg water. Let x, y and z be the quantities of spent, aqueous nitric and aqueous sulphuric acids respectively, required for blending

Overall material balance:

$$x + y + z = 1000 \tag{1}$$

Balance of sulphuric acid:

$$0.444\,x + 0.98\,z = 600 \tag{2}$$

Balance of nitric acid:

$$0.113\,x + 0.9\,y = 320 \tag{3}$$

Solving Eqs. (1), (2) and (3), by elimanation,

$$x = 76.3 \text{ kg} \quad y = 346.0 \text{ kg} \quad z = 577.7 \text{ kg} \qquad Ans.$$

Mathcad solution:

$$M: = \begin{bmatrix} 1 & 1 & 1 \\ 0.444 & 0 & 0.98 \\ 0.113 & 0.9 & 0 \end{bmatrix}$$

$$V: = \begin{bmatrix} 1000 \\ 600 \\ 320 \end{bmatrix}$$

$$\text{soln: } = M^{-1}.v$$

$$\text{soln} = \begin{bmatrix} 76.414 \\ 345.961 \\ 577.625 \end{bmatrix}$$

or $\qquad x = 76.4 \text{ kg}, \quad y = 346.0 \text{ kg} \quad \text{and } z = 577.6 \text{ kg}$ $\qquad$ *Ans.*

Example 3.9 An analysis of a sample of borewell near Ahmedabad is given in Table 3.3.

Table 3.3 Analysis of Raw Water Sample

1. Solids, mg/L	
$\quad$ Total solids	1845
$\quad$ Dissolved solids	1625
$\quad$ Supended solids (by difference)	220
2. Alkalinity, expressed as $CaCO_3$, mg/L	
$\quad$ Total alkalinity	456.5
$\quad$ Total carbonates	65.9
$\quad$ Total bicarbonates	390.6
3. Hardness, expressed as $CaCO_3$ mg/L	
$\quad$ Temporary hardness	384.0
$\quad$ Permanent hardness	Nil
$\quad$ Total hardness	384.0
$\quad$ Magnesium hardness	225.0
4. pH	8.7
5. Chlorides as Cl, mg/L	475.6
6. Sulphates as SO_4, mg/L	102.9

Find the actual analysis of the water and check whether the reported analysis is correct.

Solution Basis: 1 litre water

$\qquad$ The water contains only temporary hardness and hence it is due to bicarbonates of calcium and magnesium (alkaline hardness). Thus, chlorides and sulphates present in the water are of sodium (neglecting potassium).

$$\text{Chlorides as Cl} = 475.6 \text{ mg}$$
$$58.5 \text{ mg NaCl} \equiv 23 \text{ mg Na} \equiv 35.5 \text{ mg Cl}$$
$$\text{NaCl present in the water} = (58.5/35.5) \times 475.6 = 783.7 \text{ mg}$$
$$\text{Sulphates as } SO_4 = 102.9 \text{ mg}$$
$$142 \text{ mg } Na_2SO_4 \equiv 46 \text{ mg Na} \equiv 96 \text{ mg } SO_4$$

$$Na_2SO_4 \text{ present in the water} = \left(\frac{142}{96}\right) \times 102.9 = 152.2 \text{ mg}$$

Carbonates presents in the Water can be only due to Na_2CO_3.

$$\text{Equivalent mass of } CaCO_3 = \frac{100}{2} = 50$$

$$\text{Equivalent mass of } Na_2CO_3 = \frac{106}{2} = 53$$

$$\text{Na}_2\text{CO}_3 \text{ present in the water} = \left(\frac{53}{50}\right) \times 65.9$$
$$= 69.9 \text{ mg}$$

$$\text{NaHCO}_3 \text{ present in the water} = \text{total bicarbonates}$$
$$- \text{temporary hardness}$$
$$= 390.6 - 384 = 6.6 \text{ mg as CaCO}_3$$

$$\text{Equivalent mass of NaHCO}_3 = 84$$

$$\text{NaHCO}_3 \text{ present in the water} = \left(\frac{84}{50}\right) \times 6.6 = 11.1 \text{ mg}$$

$$\text{Equivalent mass of Mg(HCO}_3)_2 = \frac{146.3}{2} = 73.15$$

$$\text{Mg(HCO}_3)_2 \text{ present in the water} = \left(\frac{73.15}{50}\right) \times 225 = 329.2 \text{ mg}$$

$$\text{Hardness due to Ca(HCO}_3)_2 = 384 - 225 = 159 \text{ mg as CaCO}_3$$

$$\text{Equivalent mass of Ca(HCO}_3)_2 = \frac{162}{2} = 81$$

$$\text{Ca(HCO}_3)_2 \text{ present in the water} = \left(\frac{81}{50}\right) \times 159 = 257.6 \text{ mg}$$

Thus, the water sample contains the compounds given in Table 3.4.

Table 3.4 Component Analysis of Raw Water

Compound	mg/L
Ca(HCO$_3$)$_2$	257.6
Mg(HCO$_3$)$_2$	329.2
NaHCO$_3$	11.1
Na$_2$CO$_3$	69.9
NaCl	783.7
Na$_2$SO$_4$	152.2
Total	1603.7

This total corresponds to dissolved solids. To this add 220 mg/L suspended solids, which brings the total solids to 1823.6 mg/L. By actual test, total solids were found to be 1845 mg/L. The calculated and experimental values are not very different and hence, the reported analysis is correct. The difference between the two values can be attributed to experimental errors.

3.4 GRAPHICAL SOLUTION OF PROBLEMS

In a number of cases, graphical methods offer the solution to the problems. An attempt is made here to review two such methods of solving material balance problems involving chemical reactions. A well-known method of solving simultaneous equations with the coordinate plots can be used for solving Examples 3.6 and 3.8.

Example 3.10 Solve Example 3.5 with the help of geometric plots.

Solution Balance of acetone (A) and chloroform (B) yielded the following two simultaneous equations.

$$0.075\,x + 0.203\,y = 27.8 \tag{1}$$
$$0.035\,x + 0.673\,y = 72.2 \tag{2}$$

It is necessary to tabulate values of y for different values of x.

Table 3.5 Coordinate Values of Linear Equation

$x =$	Value of y				
	70	80	90	100	110
Equation (1)	111.1	107.4	103.7	100	96.3
Equation (2)	103.6	103.1	102.6	102.1	101.6

Based on the values tabulated above, straight lines are plotted for both the equations in Fig 3.7.

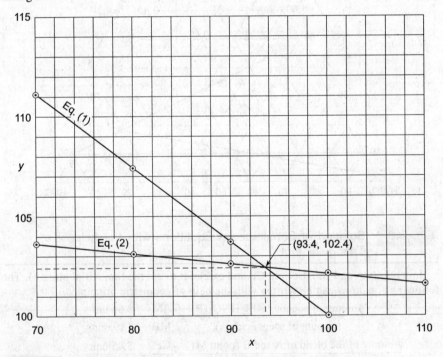

Fig. 3.7 Solution of Simultaneous Equations with the Help of a Coordinate Plot

The intersection point of these two lines represents coordinates $x = 93.4$ kg and $y = 102.4$ kg.

Ans.

In Example 3.8, three unknowns are to be evaluated. It is therefore necessary to reduce three equations to two equations by substituting the values of z from Eq. (1) in terms of x and y in Eq. (2) and then a graph, similar to Fig. 3.7, can be plotted to evaluate x and y. Alternatively, a triangular chart may be used for solving the three equations.

Example 3.11 Solve Example 3.8 with the help of a triangular plot.

Solution Figure 3.8 is a triangular chart in which spent acid, aqueous 90% HNO_3 and aqueous 98% H_2SO_4 are represented by points A, B and C respectively. Point F represents the mixed acid to be obtained by blending the three acids.

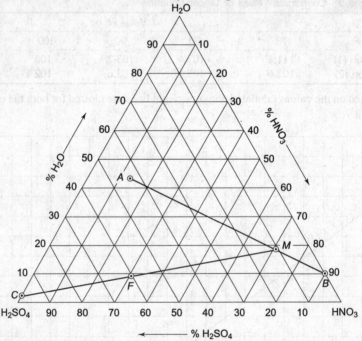

Fig. 3.8 Solution of Simultaneous Equations with the help of a Triangular Plot

---

Join points A and B. Also join CF and extend it to cut the line AB at point M. The following equations can be written with the help of geometric principles.

$$\frac{\text{Amount of aqueous } 90\% \text{ HNO}_3\text{(B)}}{\text{Amount of spent acid (A)}} = \frac{\text{AM}}{\text{MB}} = \frac{8.64 \text{ units}}{1.19 \text{ units}}$$

$$\frac{\text{Amount of the blend of A and B (point M)}}{\text{Amount of aqueous } 98\% \text{ H}_2\text{SO}_4\text{(C)}} = \frac{\text{CF}}{\text{FM}} = \frac{5.45 \text{ units}}{7.45 \text{ units}}$$

Thus, 12.90 kg of the final blend (F) will consist of 7.45 kg of 98% H_2SO_4 and 5.45 of the blend M.

$$90\% \text{ HNO}_3 \text{ required} = \frac{8.64 \times 5.45}{(8.64 + 1.19)} = 4.46 \text{ kg}$$

Spent acid required = 5.45 − 4.46 = 0.99 kg

Basis : 1000 kg final mixed acid (F)

$$\text{Amount of spent acid} = \left(\frac{0.99}{12.90}\right) \times 1000 = 76.7 \text{ kg}$$

$$\text{Amount of 90\% } HNO_3 = \left(\frac{4.45}{12.90}\right) \times 1000 = 345.7 \text{ kg}$$

$$\text{Amount of 98\% } H_2SO_4 = \left(\frac{7.45}{12.90}\right) \times 1000 = 577.6 \text{ kg} \qquad \textit{Ans.}$$

In certain cases, experimental data are to be processed for making material balance calculations. It may not be possible to fit these data in a simple equation such as those obtained in Examples 3.5 and 3.8. For such cases, graphical plots are quite handly and permit easy evaluations. In particular, where cyclic or curved plots obtained, this method is very useful. Ion exchange and adsorption/desorption operations are examples which fall under this category This method is well illustrated by the following example.

Example 3.12 The ion exclusion process is an unit operation which utilises ion exchange resins to separates solutes without the use of chemical reagents. It permits separation of ionised materials from non-ionised or slightly ionised or inorganic substances. In this process, when an aqueous solutions of two or more solutes is percolated through an ion-exchange column, a separation of solutes occurs and they appear in separate fractions in the effluent. Crude glycerine, obtained by saponification of vegetable oils or animal fats can be commercially purified by this technique [7,8,9]. Sodium chloride is the chief solute which can be separated based on the distribution coefficient.

In a pilot plant, a column is first filled to the depth with the ion exchange resin and flooded with water. A volume of the feed solution considerably less than the bulk resin volume is then added with proper distribution at the top of the resin bed. After the feed solution has passed down the column at a constant flow rate and approximately all of the feed has entered the top of the resin bed, a gradual separation of the solutes occurs and they are eluted from the column with the help of water (as a regenerant), they appear in separate fractions.

In a batch recycle technique, concentration and volume data were collected during elution. These data are presented in Table 3.6 where

C_e = concentration of solute in effluent

C_f = concentration of solute in feed solution

V_e = effluent volume

V_T = bulk volume of resin bed

Data of Table 3.6 are also plotted in Fig. 3.9.

Table 3.6   Elution Data during Ion Exclusion Process

Time from start, min	C_e/C_f of NaCl	C_e/C_f of Glycerine	$\dfrac{V_e}{V_T}$
2	0.0	0.0	0.325
5	0.105	0.0	0.35
10	0.465	0.0	0.40
15.	0.865	0.0	0.45
20	0.93	0.0	0.50
25	0.94	0.09	0.55
30	0.925	0.335	0.60
35	0.140	0.655	0.65
40	0.0	0.945	0.68
45	0.0	0.850	0.75
50	0.0	0.655	0.80
55	0.0	0.495	0.85
60	0.0	0.340	0.90
65	0.0	0.210	0.95
70	0.0	0.110	1.0
75	0.0	0.045	1.05
80	0.0	0.000	1.10

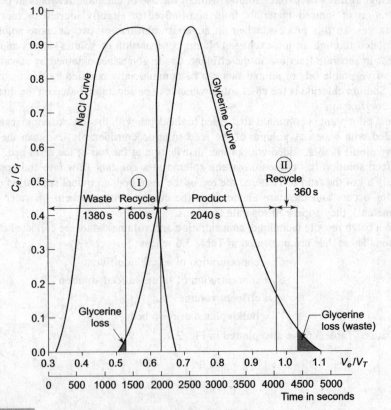

Fig. 3.9   Plot of an Ion Exclusion Process

The effluent, represented by the area of cross-contamination under the elution curves and a portion of the area under the trailing edge of the non-ionic curve is recycled to a recycle tank. A quantity of crude glycerine is then added to the recycled material. This mixture in turn becomes the feed for the second cycle. A complete cycle would then consist of feeding crude glycerine, followed by a water rinse. The effluent would contain cuts designated as waste, Recycle I or the cross-contaminated area, product, Recycle II or the dilute proportion of the trailing edge and waste (glycerine loss).

Table 3.7 Areas under the Curve

Effluent cut	Area under salt curve, square units	Area under glycerine curve, square units
Waste	4942	16
Recycle I	3436	959
Product	238	8124
Recycle II	Nil	266
Waste	Nil	83
Total	8616	9448

Assuming that C_f (glycering) = $12C_f$ (salt), Calculate: (a) % recovery of glycerine based on the mixed feed, (b)% loss of glycerine based on the mixed feed, and (c) product contamination with respect of salt content.

Soultion This type of problem can be conveniently solved by calculating the area under the curves.

$$\text{Recovery of glycerine} = \frac{8124}{9448} \times 100 = 85.99\% \qquad Ans. (a)$$

$$\text{Loss of glycerine in waste} = \frac{(16+83)}{9448} \times 100 = 1.05\% \qquad Ans. (b)$$

$$\text{Recycle of glycerine} = 100 - 85.99 - 1.05 = 12.96\%$$

$$\text{NaCl recycled} = \frac{3436}{8616} \times 100 = 39.88\%$$

NaCl in product as contaminant

$$\text{of total NaCl fed} = \frac{238}{8124} \times 100 = 2.93\%$$

Let $\quad C_f$ (salt) concentration = x

C_f (glycerine) concentration = $12\,x$

NaCl in the product = $0.0293\,x$

Glycerine in the product = $0.8599 \times 12\,x = 10.3188\,x$

Total solute = $(0.0293 + 10.3188)\,x = 10.3481x$

$$\text{NaCl of total solutes in product} = \frac{0.0293\,x}{10.3481x} \times 100$$

$$= 0.28\% \qquad Ans.$$

> **Note:** It may be interesting to note that the NaCl recycled is substantial (in Recycle I) as compared to the glycerine recycle. For example, if fresh crude glycerine contains 30% glycerine and 2.5% salt (by mass) after five batches of recycle, glycerine and salt concentrations will be 55.3% and 13.5%, respectively, based on the above recoveries. Hence, a stage will come when Recycle I will be required to be discarded to maintain low salt concentration in the mixed feed.

3.5 RECYCLING AND BYPASSING OPERATIONS

Recycling and bypassing operations are commonly encountered in unit operations as well as in chemical reactions. These operations are performed for a variety of reasons. A few important ones are listed below.

   (i) To utilise the valuable component reactant to their maximum and avoid wastage, for example, chemical reactions. For example, CO_2 sublimed during manufacture of dry ice is recycled for reprocessing. Hydrogen and nitrogen are recycled in ammonia synthesis for maximizing ammonia production.

  (ii) To utilise the heat being lost in the outgoing stream, for example, hot-air dryers, calcining the lime in the kiln, and so on.

 (iii) To improve the performance of the equipment. For example, SO_3 cannot be easily dissolved in oleum.

  (iv) To control the operating variable in a reaction, namely, pressure, temperature, and so on. For example, in ammonia synthesis, quenching (bypass) is carried out to control the reactor-bed temperature. While demineralizing water with high dissolved solids, a portion of raw water is bypassed through reverse osmosis plant to reduce salinity of the effluents.

   (v) To improve the selectivity of a product, for example, the manufacture of chlormethanes.

  (vi) To improve the safety of the chemical process. For example, in manufacture of formaldehyde, tail gas is recycled to reduce oxygen concentration below flammability limit.

 (vii) To minimize waste generation. For example, reverse osmosis technology is widely used for treatment of aqueous effluents thereby good quality permeate (a major portion of effluents) is recycled for reprocessing.

In almost all recycling operations, a definite stream has to be remove/purged to control the concentration of a particular component. In this chapter only unit operations with recycling operations will be considered. In Chapter 4, chemical reactions with recycling will be discussed. In Example 3.12 it was noted that Recycle I will have to discarded at some stage to maintain low salt concentration in the mixed feed to the ion-exchange column. This can be considered intermittent purging to control the mixed feed composition.

Example 3.13 An air-conditioning plant is employed to maintain 300 K(27°C) dry bulb (*DB*) temperature and 50% relative humidity (*RH*) in an auditorium. the air flow rate to the auditorium is measured to be 5.806 m³/s at 290 K(17°C) *DB* and 83.5% *RH*. The effluent air from the auditorium is partially recycled and mixed with the incoming fresh air due to economic reasons. The fresh ambient air is fed at the rate of 1.25 m³/s at 308 K (35°C) *DB* and 70% *RH*. The mixed air is found to have 302.5 K (29.5°) *DB* and 54% *RH* and is passed through the air-conditioning plant to make it suitable for feeding to the auditorium. For all practical purposes, the total pressure can be assumed to be 101.3 kPa a (760 torr). Table 3.8 gives the molar humidity. (Refer Fig. 6.11 for data on absolute humidity values for various air conditions.)

Table 3.8	Data on Molal Humidity		
Stream	Dry bulb temperature K (°C)	Absolute molar Humidity, kmol/ kmol dry air	Relative humidity, %
Fresh ambient air	308 (27)	0.0405	70
Mixed air	302.5 (29.5)	0.0225	54
Air entering the auditorium	290 (17)	0.0163	83.5
Air leaving the auditorium	300 (27)	0.0181	50

Figure 3.10 shows the flow diagram of the above air-conditioning plant plant.

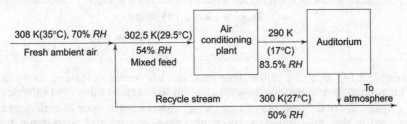

Fig. 3.10 Air-Conditioning System of an Auditorium

(a) Calculate the moisture removed in the air-conditioning plant.
(b) Calculate the moisture added in the auditorium.
(c) Calculate the recycle ratio as moles of air recycled per mole of fresh ambient air input.

Solution Basis: 1.25 m³/s of fresh ambient air feed and 5.806 m³/s of air entering into the auditorium

Specific volume of moist air

at 290 K and 101.3 kPa $a = 8.314 \times 290/101.3 = 23.80$ m³/kmol

$$\text{Molal flow rate of air entering the auditorium} = \left(\frac{5.806}{23.8}\right)1000 = 243.95 \text{ mol/s}$$

$$\text{Moisture accompanying the air} = \frac{243.95 \times 0.0163}{1.0163} = 3.91 \text{ mol/s}$$

Dry air flow = 243.95 – 3.91 = 240.04 mol/s

In the air-conditioning plant, the moisture is removed as is evident from Table 3.9. However, the flow rate of dry air remains unchanged.

Moisture removed in the air-conditioning plant = 5.4 – 3.91 = 1.94 mol/s

$$\equiv 26.82 \text{ g/s} \equiv 96.55 \text{ kg/h}$$

Ans. (a)

In the auditorium, the air picks up moisture. Here also the flow rate of dry air is unchanged.

Moisture in the air leaving the auditorium = 240.04 × 0.0181

$$= 4.345 \text{ mol/s}$$

Moisture added inthe auditorium = 4.345 – 3.91 = 0.435 mol/s

$$\equiv 7.83 \text{ g/s} \equiv 28.19 \text{ kg/h} \qquad \textit{Ans. (b)}$$

Spefific volume of the fresh air = 8.314 × 308/101.3 = 25.28 m^3/kmol

Molal flow rate of the fresh air = (1.25/25.28) 1000 = 49.45 mol/s

Moisture in the fresh air = (0.0405/1.0405) × 49.45 = 1.925 mol/s

Dry air flow in the fresh air = 49.45 – 1.925 = 47.525 mol/s

Moisture in the recycle stream = moisture in the mixed feed

– moisture in the fresh ambient air

$$= 5.40 – 1.925 = 3.475 \text{ mol/s}$$

Dry air flow in the recycled stream = 240.04 – 47.525 = 192.515 mol/s

Molal flow rate of the recycled stream = 192.515 + 3.475 = 195.99 mol/s

Recycle ratio = 195.99/49.45

$$= 3.96 \text{ kmol of recycle stream/}$$
kmol of fresh feed *Ans.* (c)

Example 3.14 In a pulp mill a three-stage cascade screening system, shown in Fig. 3.11, is employed to remove the over-size foreign particles from dilute slurries[10]. If E_1, E_2 and E_3 are the fractions of foreign particles (i.e., efficiency of each screen100) removed in the three screens respectively, develop a general relationship for the overall efficiency of the system.

Definition: Efficiency of a screen = (foreign material rejected/foreign material entering) × 100

Solution

Basis: Let N kg be the amount of foreign material entering the screen 1.

Material balance of foreign materials:

Screen 1: Feed = N kg

Oversize particles = NE_1 kg

Undersize particles = $N – NE_1$

$$= N(1 – E_1) \text{ kg}$$

Screen 2: In this screen, the feed is the mixture of oversize particles form screen 1 and the recycled undersize particles from screen 3. Let the recycled under-sized particles from the screen 3 be X kg.

Feed = $NE_1 + X$ kg

Oversize particles = $(NE_1 + X) E_2$ kg

Undersize particles = $(NE_1 + X) (1 – E_2)$ kg

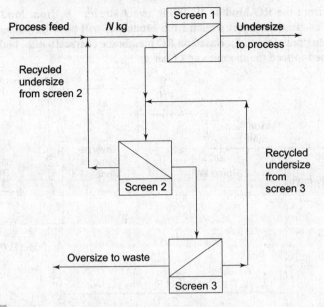

Fig. 3.11   Three-stage Cascade Screening System

The undersize particles from screen 2 are recycled and mixed with process feed to give N kg particles in the mixed feed to screen 1.

$$\text{Foreign particles in the process feed} = N - (NE_1 + X)(1 - E_2) \text{ kg}$$

Screen 3: The feed to the screen 3 consists of oversized particles from screen 2.

$$\text{Feed} = (NE_1 + X) E_2 \text{ kg}$$
$$\text{Oversize particles} = (NE_1 + X) E_2 E_3 \text{ kg}$$
$$\text{Undersize particles} = (NE_1 + X) E_2 (1 - E_3) \text{ kg}$$

However, it is assumed that undersize particles from screen 3 are X kg.

$$(NE_1 + X) E_2 (1 - E_3) = X \quad \text{or} \quad X = NE_1 E_2 \frac{(1 - E_3)}{\left[1 - E_2 (1 - E_3)\right]}$$

$$\text{Overall efficiency of the system} = \left(\frac{\text{Oversize particles from screen 3}}{\text{Particles in process feed}} \right) \times 100$$

$$= \frac{(NE_1 + X) E_2 E_3}{\left[N - (NE_1 + X)(1 - E_2) \right]} \times 100$$

Substituting for X and simplifying,

$$\text{Overall efficiency} = \frac{E_1 E_2 E_3}{\left[(1 - E_1)(1 - E_2) + E_2 E_3 \right]} \times 100 \qquad Ans.$$

Example 3.15   Production of treated water is required at the rate of 5 m^3/h with 5 mg/L (max.) dissolved solids (i.e. < 10 µS/cm conductivity) in a bulk drug plant. Raw water with 4200 mg/L dissolved solids (DS) is available for the purpose.

For the treatment of raw water, two-stage reverse osmosis (RO) plant is designed as shown in Fig. 3.12. RO Module I is designed for 66% recovery of the feed to the module while RO Module II is designed for 80% recovery. Rejection of 98.5% salts is achieved from the RO Module II. While reject stream R_1 from Module I will be discarded as effuents, reject stream from Module II will be recycled and mixed with the incoming raw water (F). Based on RO membrane characteristics, both feed pumps are designed to feed the modules at 12 bar g.

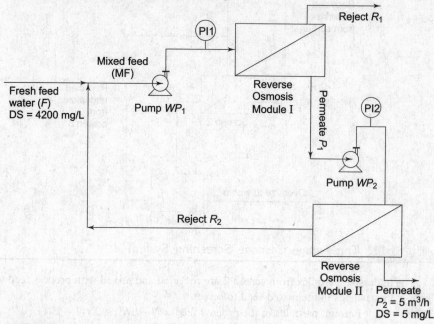

Fig. 3.12 Two Stage Reverse Osmosis Plant

Make complete material balance of the system and calculate F, R_1, P, R_2, recycle ratio, defined as R_2/F, and rejection of salt from Module I.

Solution

Overall Balance:
$$F = R_1 + P_2 \tag{1}$$
Balance across Module I:
$$F + R_2 = R_1 + P_1 \tag{2}$$
Substitute value of F from Eqn. (1).
$$R_1 + P_2 + R_2 = R_1 + P_1$$

or $P_1 = P_2 + R_2$ which represents material balance across Module II.

$$P_2 = 5 \text{ m}^3/\text{h}, \quad P_2/P_1 = 0.08 \quad \text{or} \quad P_1 = 5/0.8 = 6.25 \text{ m}^3/\text{h}$$

$$R_2 = P_1 - P_2 = 6.25 - 5 = 1.25 \text{ m}^3/\text{h}$$

$$\frac{P_1}{F + R_2} = 0.66$$

$$P_1 = 0.66 \, (F + R_2)$$

$$6.25 = 0.66(F + 1.25)$$

or
$$F = 8.22 \text{ m}^3/\text{h}$$

$$R_1 = F - P_2 = 8.22 - 5 = 3.22 \text{ m}^3/\text{h}$$

Balance of DS:

Let x represent concentration of DS in water in mg/L (i.e. same as g/m^3).

$$F x_f = R_1 \, x_{R_1} + P_2 \, x_{P_1}$$

$$8.22 \times 4200 = 3.22 \times x_{R_1} + 5 \times 5$$

or $\qquad\qquad x_{R_1} = 10\,714$ mg/L   or g/m^3

Since rejection in Module II is 98.5% DS in P_2 will be 1.5% of that in P_1

$$\text{DS in } P_1, \; x_{P_1} = \frac{5 \times 5}{0.015 \times 6.25} = 267 \text{ g/m}^3 \text{ or mg/L}$$

$$P_1 \, x_{P_1} = P_2 \, x_{P_2} + R_2 \, x_{R_2}$$

$$6.25 \times 267 = 5 \times 5 + 1.25 \times x_{R_2}$$

or $\qquad\qquad x_{R_2} = 1315$ g/m^3 or mg/L

$$\text{DS in mixed feed (MF)} = Fx_F + R_2 \, x_{R_2}$$
$$= 8.22 \times 4200 + 1.25 \times 1315$$
$$= 36\,168 \text{ g}$$

$$\text{Concentration of DS in MF} = \frac{36\,168}{(8.22 + 1.25)} = 3819 \text{ g/m}^3 \text{ or mg/L}$$

$$\text{DS in } R_1 = 3.22 \times 10\,714 = 34\,499 \text{ g}$$

$$\text{Rejection in Module I} = \frac{34\,499}{36\,168} \times 100$$
$$= 95.4\%$$

$$\text{DS in } P_1 = 36\,168 - 34\,499 = 1669 \text{ g}$$

$$\text{Concentration of DS in } P_1 = \frac{1669}{6.25} = 267 \text{ g/m}^3 \text{ or mg/L} \quad \text{Check!}$$

$$\text{Recycle ratio } \frac{R_2}{F} = \frac{1.25}{8.22} = 0.152 \text{ m}^3 \text{ reject recycle/m}^3 \text{ fresh feed}$$

Ans.

Example 3.16 An activated sludge process has been developed as a continuous operation by recycling biological sludge. This process uses microorganisms in suspension to oxidise soluble (and colloidal) organics, also known as volatile solids, to CO_2 and H_2O in the presence of molecular oxygen. In the process, an industrial waste water stream is treated with air to convert BOD into suspended solids which is subsequently removed in the clarifier[11]. The process is illustrated in Fig. 3.13. Waste water (stream 1) enters the process having a soluble BOD content S_F. The purpose of the treatment is to reduce this value to S_e (final effluent BOD content i.e., that of stream 4) by oxidation through aerobic biological degradation. Usually BOD removal efficiency of such a process varies from 90 to 95%. Fresh feed is combined with recycled sludge (stream 7) and enters the aeration tank. Biological sludge is continuously formed in the aeration tank which is usually operated under steady-state conditions with complete mixing. The reaction kinetics of such processes is normally represented by a first order reaction. The concentration of soluble BOD in stream 3 and stream 5 is the same as that of stream 4. The secondary clarifier underflow (stream 5) is split into two streams—waste sludge and recycle studge.

The kinetic model of the process can be established by setting up relation between the BOD concentration and the suspended solids that enter the aeration tank. This relation can be varied by varying the recycle ratio.

Establish a mathematical mode for such a process. For calculating the recycle ratio, assume that the overflow from the secondary clarifier does not contain any solids and the quantity of air absorbed in the tank is negligible as compared to the feed steam.

Solution   Basis: Feed flow rate of Q_F L/s having no suspended solids (i.e., $X_F = 0$) and BOD concentration equal to S_F kg/L

$$X_e = 0$$

$$Q_F = Q' + Q'' \tag{1}$$

$$Q = Q_F + Q_r$$

$$\text{Recycle ratio, } r = \frac{Q_R}{Q_F}$$

$$Q = Q_F (1 + r) \tag{2}$$

BOD balance across the aeration tank:

$$Q_F S_F - Q (S_O - S_e) = Q_F S_e$$

$$Q_F (S_F - S_e) = Q(S_O - S_e)$$

$$S_F - S_e = (1 + r) (S_O - S_e)$$

simplifying,
$$r = \frac{S_F - S_O}{S_O - S_C} \tag{3}$$

Suspended solids balance across the aeration tank:

$$Q_F X_F + (X_a - X_O) Q = Q' X_e + Q'' X_u$$

$$\text{But } X_F = X_e = 0$$

Using Eqs. (1) and (2)

$$(X_a - X_O)(Q_r + Q_F) = (Q_F - Q')X_u$$

$$(1 + r) (X_a - X_O) = \left(1 - \frac{Q'}{Q_F}\right) X_u \tag{4}$$

Suspended solids balance across secondary clarifier:

$$QX_a = Q' X_e + Q'' X_u + Q_R X_u$$

Since
$$X_e = 0$$

$$QX_a = (Q'' + Q_R) X_u$$

Using Eq. (2),

$$(1 + r) = (1 + r) X_u - \frac{Q'}{Q_F} X_u \tag{5}$$

Eliminating Q'/Q_F from Eqs. (4) and (5),

$$(X_u - X_o) = \frac{X_u}{(1 + r)}$$

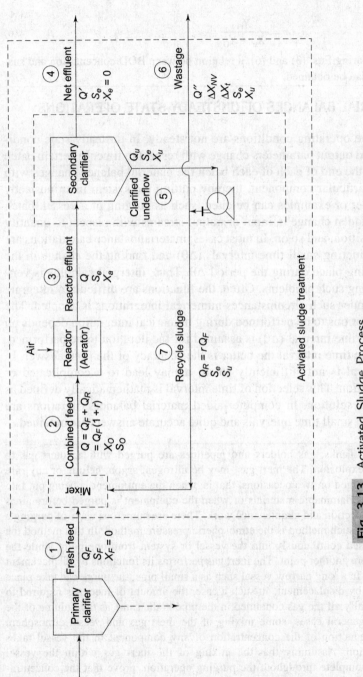

Fig. 3.13 Activated Sludge Process

Solving for r,

$$r = \frac{X_O}{X_u - X_O} \qquad (6)$$

By comparing Eqs. (3) and (6), a relation between BOD concentraion and suspended solids can be obtained. *Ans.*

3.6 MATERIAL BALANCES OF UNSTEADY-STATE OPERATIONS

Very often, the operating conditions are not steady. In unsteady-state conditions, input and output parameters change with respect to time. In certain batch operations, at the end of each of each batch the material balance changes with respect to a particular component, thereby putting the system in an unsteady state. A number of examples can be cited, such as purging of a vessel, batch distillation, sudden change in input or output streams with respect to quantity and/or composition, and so on. In most cases, material balance calculations are made by considering small time intervals ($\Delta\theta$) and finding the change in the parameter taking place during the period $\Delta\theta$. Thus, intergral calculus is very useful in solving such problems. Often, the functions are difficult to integrate directly and under such circumstances numerical integrations is adopted. The number of iterations to be performed during numerical integration depends on how small the time interval ($\Delta\theta$) is assumed for the iteration to be performed. The smaller the time interval the better is the accuracy of the final answer. In case the interval is not sufficiently small, it may lead to a complicated or erroneous solution. This selection of time interval is mathematically defined as stability of the solution. In computer-aided material balances, iterations are performed with small time intervals and quite accurate answers are obtained.

Example 3.17 Tanks, gas holders and pipelines are purged with an inert gas to prevent fire or explosion. The inert gas may be nitrogen, argon, helium or any rare gas. They are purged on two occasions, that is, when the equipment is being put into operation with inflammable materials or when the equipment is purged before air is admitted for inspection and maintenance work. There are numerous ways of purging a system[12, 13]. One such method is the atmospheric pressure method. In this method the inert gas is passed continuously into the vessel or system from one point while the purge leaves from another point. The inert gas performs its functions by displacement and/or dilution. In a long narrow vessel such as a small pipe, the purge can take place almost entirely by displacement. In such a case, the amount of inert gas required to sweep out virtually all the gas contained in the pipe is the same as the volume of the pipe. In more general cases, some mixing of the inert gas and vessel atmosphere occurs and a reduction of the concentration of any component in the vessel takes places by dilution. Assuming that the mixing of the inert gas within the vessel atmosphere is complete throughout the purging operation, prove that the concentration of any component of the original vessel atmosphere will be $1/e$ times the original concentraion after passing one vessel volume of the inert gas for purging.

Solution Let the initial concentration of a component in the vessel atmosphere by X_o kmol/L at atmospheric pressure and the vessel volume be V L. Introduce a small volume v L of inert gas into the vessel and allow it to mix well. As a result of the introduction of a small volume of inert gas, pressure will be slightly increased, which will be released.

Concentration of the component after introduction of v volume of iner gas,

$$X_1 = \frac{VX_0}{V+v} = \frac{X_0}{\left(1+\dfrac{v}{V}\right)}$$

After the introduction of an additional v volume of inert gas, concentration

$$X_2 = \frac{X_1}{\left(1+\dfrac{v}{V}\right)} = \frac{X_0}{\left(1+\dfrac{v}{V}\right)^2}$$

Similarly,
$$X_n = \frac{X_0}{\left(1+\dfrac{v}{V}\right)^n}$$

When the volume of the inert gas used for purging reaches the V, i.e., $n = V/v$ and the concentration of the component after purging by one vessel volume,

$$X_V = \frac{X_0}{\left(1+\dfrac{1}{n}\right)^n}$$

Continuous purging operation will mean that the volume v is very small. Mathematically,

$$\lim_{n \to \infty} \left(1+\frac{1}{n}\right)^n = e$$

Therefore,
$$X_V = \frac{X_0}{e}$$

If two vessel volumes of inert gas is used for purging,

$$X_{2V} = \frac{X_0}{e^2} \text{, and so on.}$$

Example 3.18 A storage tank of a deminearlised (DM) water has a holding capacity of 1500 m³ upto an overflow point. The inflow of DM water to the tank is 25 L/s having silica (as SiO_2) content of 0.005 mg/L. The supply of DM water to the high pressure boilers from the tank amount to 25 dm³/s. With time the DM water quality deteriorates and the silica content in the feed DM water increases to 0.02 mg/L. Assume that the inflow into and the outflow from the tank remains constant at 25 L/s. Calculate the time for the silica content in the storage tank to increase to 0.01 mg/L.

Solution Basis: Inflow of DM water to the tank = 25 L/s

When the inflow DM water and the outflow DM water contain the same silica level (0.005 mg/L), the system is defined as steady, which is shown is Fig. 3.14. The upset in the inflow of DM water creates the unsteady-state conditions. Figure 3.15 represents the upsets in silica concentration

Total water in the tank = 1500 m³ = 1500 000 L

Let c be the concentration of silica in the tank in mg/L at any time θ, $\Delta\theta$ be the time interval during which the change in the concentration is observed, and Δc be the change in the concentration during the time interval $\Delta\theta$. Consider $\theta = 0$ when the silica level in the incoming DM water increases to 0.02 mg/L.

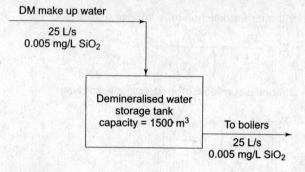

Fig. 3.14   Steady-state Conditions of Demineralised Water Storage Tank

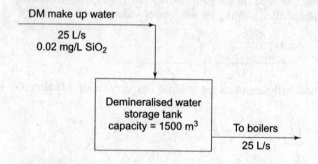

Fig. 3.15   Unsteady-state Conditions of a Demineralised Water Storage Tank

Silica Balance:

$$\text{Input into the tank in } \Delta\theta \text{ s} = 25 \times 0.02 \times \Delta\theta$$
$$= 0.5\ \Delta\theta \text{ mg/s}$$
$$\text{Output from the tank in } \Delta\theta \text{ s} = 25 \times c \times \Delta\theta \text{ mg/s}$$
$$\text{Accumulation of silica in the tank in } \Delta\theta \text{ s} = 1\,500\,000\ \Delta c \text{ mg/s}$$
$$\text{Input} - \text{Output} = \text{Accumulation}$$
$$0.5\ \Delta\theta - 25\ c\ \Delta\theta = 1\,500\,000\ \Delta c$$
$$\Delta\theta\ (1-50c) = 3\,000\,000\ \Delta c$$

Converting into the differential form and integrating,

$$d\theta = 3\,000\,000 \times \left[\frac{dc}{1 - 50c} \right]$$

$$= 3\,000\,000 \int_{c_1}^{c_2} \frac{dc}{(1 - 50c)}$$

$$\theta = \frac{-3000\,000}{50}\left[\ln\frac{(1-50c_2)}{(1-50c_1)}\right]$$

Now when $\qquad \theta = 0, \quad c_1 = 0.005$ mg/L

$\qquad\qquad\qquad \theta = \theta, \quad c_2 = 0.01$ mg/L

$$\theta = \frac{(60\,000)}{\ln\left[(1-50c_1)/(1-50c_2)\right]}$$

$\qquad\qquad \theta = (60\,000) \times 0.4055 = 24\,330$ s $\equiv 6.76$ h $\qquad\qquad$ *Ans.*

Example 3.19 In Example 3.18 assume that the inflow to the tank was reduced to 14 L/s as soon as the silica concentration was noticed to be 0.02 mg/L. The outflow from the tank remains constant at 25 L/s. Calculate the time required to increase the silica content in the storage tank to 0.008 mg/L. Also calculate the hold-up of the tank at the time when the silica concentration is 0.008 mg/L.

Solution The unsteady-state flow process is shown in Fig. 3.16. Using the same nomenclature as in Example 3.18 the silica balance may be considered.

$\qquad\qquad$ Input to the tank = $14 \times 0.02 \times \Delta\theta = 0.28\,\Delta\theta$ mg/s

$\qquad\qquad$ Output from the tank = $25\,c\,\Delta\theta$ mg/s

$\qquad\qquad$ Accumulation in the tank = $[1500\,000 - (25 - 14)\,\Delta\theta]\Delta c$

$\qquad\qquad\qquad\qquad\qquad = (1500\,000 - 11\,\Delta\theta)\,\Delta c$ mg/s

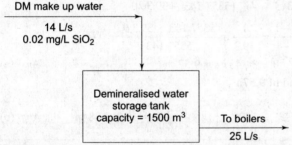

DM make up water

14 L/s
0.02 mg/L SiO₂

Demineralised water
storage tank
capacity = 1500 m³

To boilers
25 L/s

Fig. 3.16 Unsteady-state Conditions of the Demineralised Water Storage Tank with Reduced Inflow

$\qquad\qquad$ Input – Output = accumulation

$\qquad\qquad 0.28\,\Delta\theta - 25\,c\,\Delta\theta = (1500\,000 - 11\,\Delta\theta)\,\Delta c$

$\qquad\qquad \Delta\theta\,(1 - 89.3c) = (5357\,143 - 39.3\,\Delta\theta)\,\Delta c \qquad\qquad\qquad$ (1)

The above equation requires double integration. It can be solved it by numerical integration, performing the iterations.

Let $\qquad\qquad \theta = 1000$ s

$\qquad\qquad c = c_1$, i.e., the concentration of silica in the tank at the start
$\qquad\qquad\qquad\qquad\qquad\qquad\qquad$ of the period

$\qquad\qquad \Delta c = c_2 - c_1$

Iteration 1:

$\qquad\qquad 1000\,(1 - 89.3\,c_1) = (5357\,149 - 39.3 \times 1000)\,(c_2 - c_1)$

Simplifying $\qquad\qquad 10\,000\,c_2 = 9832\,c_1 + 1.88$

$$c_1 = 0.005 \text{ mg/L to start with}$$
$$c_2 = 0.005\ 104 \text{ mg/L at the end}$$

Iteration 2:

In this case
$$c_1 = 0.005\ 104 \text{ mg/L}$$
$$c_2 = 0.005\ 206 \text{ mg/L}$$

Similar iterations can be performed. At the end of 36th iteration,
$$c_2 = 0.00\ 799 \text{ mg/L} \approx 0.008 \text{ mg/L}$$
$$\text{Total time} = \Sigma\ \Delta\theta_i$$
$$= 36 \times 1000 = 36\ 000 \text{ s} \approx 10 \text{ h} \qquad Ans.(a)$$

Hold-up of the tank

at the end of 10h $= 1500 - \left(\dfrac{14 \times 36\ 000}{1000}\right) = 996 \text{ m}^3$ \qquad Ans.(b)

Alternate integral method:

Equation (1) can be converted to differential form,

$$\frac{dc}{(1 - 89.3\ c)} = \frac{d\theta}{(5357\ 143 - 39.3\theta)}$$

Integrating the above differential between $c = 0.\ 005$, and $c = 0.008$,

$$\int_{0.005}^{0.008} \frac{dc}{(1 - 89.3\ c)} = \int_0^\theta \frac{d\theta}{(5357\ 143 - 39.3\theta)}$$

$$\frac{1}{89.3} \ln \frac{89.3 \times 0\ .008 - 1}{89.3 \times 0.005 - 1} = \frac{1}{39.3} \ln \frac{5357\ 143 - 39.3\ \theta}{5357\ 143}$$

$$\theta = 34\ 437 \text{ s} \equiv 9.57 \text{ h} \qquad Ans.\ (a)$$

Hold-up of the tank at the end of 9.57h

$$= 1500 - \left(14 \times \frac{34\ 437}{1000}\right) = 1017.88 \text{ m}^3 \qquad Ans.\ (b)$$

Example 3.20 In a batch process, the reaction takes place in the presence of an acid medium. The process is illustrated in Fig. 3.17. The acid is drained from the reaction vessel at the rate of 15 mL/s as a result of the density difference of the acid from the reacting component. To avoid wastage of acid, it is recycled to an acid tank which has 1000 L capacity. The acid, drained from the reaction vessel, picks up 50 g/L of solids from the reactor. Acid is fed once again to the process from the acid tank. When the batch is started, the acid is almost pure in the tank as a result of filtration. As the reaction proceeds, acid in the tank gets more and more contaminated with the solids. The concentration of the solids should not exceed 100 g/L from the process point of view. The batch time is 16 h. Check whether the concentration of the solids will exceed 100 g/L during the batch reaction.

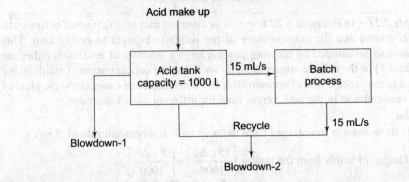

Fig. 3.17 Batch Reaction in an Acid Medium

Solution Consider the material balance of the solids across the acid tank. Let the acid concentration of the solids be c in the tank at any time θ. Consider a time interval of $\Delta\theta$ during which concentraion of the solids changes by Δc.

$$\text{Input of solids to the tank} = 15\,(c + 50)\,\frac{\Delta\theta}{1000}\;\text{g}$$

$$\text{Output of solids from the tank} = 15\,c\,\Delta\theta\;\text{g}$$

$$\text{Accumulation in the tank} = 1000\,(c + \Delta c) - 1000c$$

$$= 1000\,\Delta c\;\text{g}$$

$$\text{Input} - \text{output} = \text{accumulation}$$

$$\frac{1}{1000}\,[15\,(c + 50)\,\Delta\theta - 15\,c\,\Delta\theta] = 1000\,\Delta c$$

$$750\,\Delta\theta = 1\,000\,000\,\Delta c$$

Converting into differential from, $d\theta = 1333.33\,dc$, when

$\theta = 0$ and $c = 0$. Integration therefore yields

$\theta = 1333.33\,c$

$c = 100$ g/L is the limit

$\theta = 100 \times 1333.33$

$= 133\,333$ s

$\equiv 37.04$ h

Since this period is higher than batch period, solids concentration will not exceed 100 g/L during the batch. *Ans.*

The above answer can be also obtained by simple material balance.

$$\text{Total solids pick-up permitted} = 1000 \times 100$$

$$= 100\,000\;\text{g}$$

$$\text{Total solids pick-up} = 15 \times \frac{50}{1000} = 0.75\;\text{g/s}$$

Time reqired to attain 100 g/L solids concentration,

$$\theta = \frac{1000}{0.75}$$

$$= 133\,333\;\text{s}$$

$$\equiv 37.04\;\text{h}$$ *Ans.*

Example 3.21 In Example 3.20 above, it is assumed that acid is filtered before each batch is started and the concentration of the solids is brought to nearly zero. This filtration can be avoided by blowing down a known quantity of acid from either the tank (case 1) or the recycle stream (case 2) such that the concentration of solids in the acid fed to the process vessel is controlled. For both the above cases, draw the plots of solids concentraion in the tank versus time for different blowdown rates.

Solution

Case 1: Blowdown is maintained from the acid tank at a constant rate of B m/Ls.

$$\text{Output of solids from the tank} = \left[\frac{15\,c\,\Delta\theta}{1000}\right] + \left[\frac{B\,c\,\Delta\theta}{1000}\right] g$$
$$= (15\,c\,\Delta\theta + B\,c\,\Delta\theta)\,10^{-3}g$$

Material balance therefore yields,

$$\frac{[15\,(c+50)\,\Delta\theta]}{1000} - \frac{(15\,c\,\Delta\theta + B\,c\,\Delta\theta)}{1000} = 1000\,\Delta c$$
$$75\,\Delta\theta - B\,c\Delta\theta = 1000\,000\,\Delta c$$

Converting into differential form,

$$d\theta = 10^6\left(\frac{dc}{750 - Bc}\right)$$

when $\theta = 0$, $c = 0$. Therefore integration yields

$$\theta = \frac{10^6}{B}\ln\left(\frac{750}{750 - Bc}\right) \text{ or } c = \frac{750}{B}\left(1 - e^{-B\theta/10^6}\right)$$

The above equation permits computation of c by assuming values of B and θ. Therse data are presented in Table 3.9 and Fig. 3.18.

Table 3.9 Concentration of Solids with Blowdown from Acid Tank, g/L

B, mL/s	Time (θ) in seconds				
	18×10^3	36×10^3	90×10^3	180×10^3	360×10^3
1	13.379	26.520	64.552	123.547	226.743
3	13.142	25.593	59.155	104.313	165.101
5	12.910	24.709	54.356	89.015	125.205
7	12.684	23.867	50.079	76.751	98.522

It can be seen from Fig. 3.18 that for each blowdown rate the graph converges as the time elapses. Therefore at infinite time, the concentration of solids will become constant for each of the blowdown rate.

$$\text{When } \theta \to \infty, e^{-B\theta/10^6} \to \theta, c = \frac{750}{B}$$

For a limited concentration of $c = 100$ g/L,

$$B = \frac{750}{100} = 7.5 \text{ mL/s}$$

Case 2: Blowdown is maintained from the recycle stream at a constant rate of B ml/s

$$\text{Input of solids to the tank} = \frac{(15 - B)(c + 50)\Delta\theta}{1000} g$$

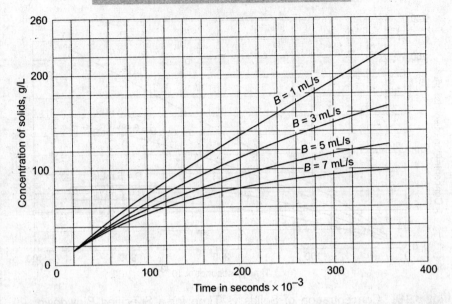

Fig. 3.18 Concentration of Solids vs Time for a Specified Blowdown Rate from the Acid Tank

Material balance therefore yields,

$$\left(\frac{(15-B)(c+50)\,\Delta\theta}{1000}\right)-\left(\frac{15\,c\,\Delta\theta}{1000}\right)=1000\,\Delta c$$

Converting into differential form,

$$\frac{10^6\,dc}{750-50B-Bc}=d\theta$$

Integration yields,

$$\frac{10^6}{B}\,\ln\left(\frac{50B-750}{Bc+50B-750}\right)=\theta$$

Simplifying,

$$\frac{Bc}{750-50B}=1-e^{-B\theta/10^6}$$

or

$$c=\left(\frac{750-50B}{B}\right)\left(1-e^{-B\theta/10^6}\right)$$

Based on the above equation, Table 3.10 is prepared and the same data are plotted in Fig. 3.19.

Table 3.10 Concentration of Solids with Blowdown from Recycle Stream, g/L

B, mL/s	18×10^3	36×10^3	90×10^3	180×10^3	360×10^3
1	12.487	24.752	60.248	115.311	211.627
3	10.514	20.474	47.324	83.450	132.081
5	8.607	16.473	36.237	59.343	66.040
7	6.765	12.729	26.709	40.934	52.545

Time (θ) in seconds

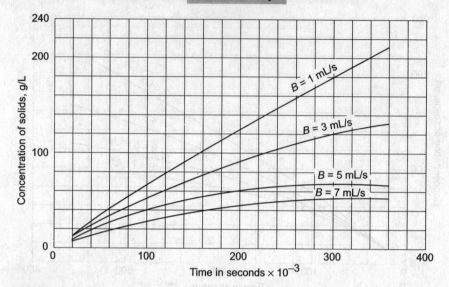

Fig. 3.19 Concentration of Solids vs Time for a Specified Blowdown Rate from the Recycle Stream

When $\theta \rightarrow \infty$, $e^{-B\theta/10^6} \rightarrow 0$, $c = \dfrac{750}{B} - 50$

For $\qquad c = 100$ g/L

$$B = \frac{750}{150} = 5 \text{ mL/s}$$

Note: It can be observed that blowdwon from recycle stream results in a lower concentration of solids in the acid fed to the process vessel.

EXERCISES

3.1 The feed water to the reverse osmosis plant has dissoved solids to the extent of 5000 mg/L[14]. The feed-to-product ration (on mass basis) is 4:3. The treated water (product) from the plant contains 600 mg/L of solids. Find the dissolved solids in the reject stream.

[*Ans.*18 200 mg/L]

3.2 A multiple-effect evaporator system has a capacity of processing one tonne per day of solid caustic soda when it concentrates weak liquor from 4 to 25% (both on mass basis). When the plant is fed with 5% weak liquor and if it is concentrated to 50% (both on mass basis), find the capacity of the plant in terms of solid caustic soda, assuming the water evaporating capacity to be the same in both cases.

[*Ans.* 1.167 t/d]

3.3 A sample of coal from Andrew Yules colliery, West Bengal, is found to contain 67.2% carbon and 22.3% ash (mass basis). The refuse obtained at the end of combustion is analysed to contain 7.1% carbon and the rest ash. Compute the % of the original carbon remaining unbrunt in the refuse.

[Ans. 2.53%]

3.4 Soybean seeds are extracted with n-hexane in batch extractors. The flaked seeds contain 18.6% oil, 69.0% solids and 12.4% moisture. At the end of the extraction process, de-oiled cake (DOC) is separated from the n-hexane-oil mixture. DOC analysis yields 0.8% oil, 87.7% solids and 11.5% moisture. Find the percentage recovery of oil. All percentage are by mass.

[Ans. 96.6% recovery]

3.5 A vent stream from an ethylbenzene plant has a composition: 66% H_2, 33% CH_4 and 1% other components (CO + C_2H_6 + C_2H_4 etc.). It is passed through a PSA Unit where hydrogen is recovered as 98% pure stream with 2% CH_4 as an impurity. Recovery of hydrogen is 85% at feed pressure of 50 bar. Calculate the composition of reject stream.

[Ans. Composition of reject stream: 23.15% H_2, 74.51% CH_4 and 2.34% other components (on mole basis)]

3.6 Composition of soybean oil deodorizer distillate[4] is C_{16}-fatty acids 19.8%, C_{18}-fatty acids 56.1%, monoglycerides 9.2%, squalene 12.0%, mixed tocopherols 11.5%, sterols 14.8%, diglycerides 1.7%, and triglycerides 1.7%. High vacuum distillation in a short path distillation unit is carried out at 5 mbar a and 463 K(190°C) to recover a stream consisting of 95% fatty acids, 0.25% mixed tocopherols and balance other components. Bottom residue is found to contain 10% fatty acids. All percentages are by mass. Calculate the ratio of overhead product to bottom residue.

[Ans. 3.45:1]

3.7 Crystals of $MgCl_2.6H_2O$ have a solubility[15] of 190 g per 100 g ethanol at 298.15 K(25°C). It is desired to make 1000 kg of saturated solution. Calculate the quantities of the crystals and ethanol required to make the above solution. Also, find the composition of the saturated solution by mass.

[Ans. Crystals = 655.5 kg, ethanol = 344.5 kg, composition: $MgCl_2$ = 30.73%, H_2O = 34.82%, C_2H_5OH = 34.45% (mass basis)]

3.8 A spent solution of chloroacetic acid in ether contains 20 mole % chloroacetic acid. It is desired to make 500 kg of a saturated solution at 298.15 K(25°C). Find the quantities of spent solution and chloroacetic acid required to make the above solution.

Data:The solubility of chloroacetic acid in ether[15] is 190 g/100 g ether at 298.15 K(25°C).

[Ans. 227.4 kg of chloroacetic acid and 272.6 kg of spent solution]

3.9 A mixture of $CuSO_4.5H_2O$ and $FeSO_4.7H_2O$ weighs 100 g. It is heated in an oven at 378 K (105°C) to evaporate the water of hydration. The mass of mixture after removal of water is 59.78 g. Calculate the mass ratio of $CuSO_4$ to $FeSO_4$ in the mixture.

[*Ans.* 1.23:1]

3.10 The average molar mass of a flue gas sample is calculated by two different engineers. One engineer uses the correct molar mass of 28 for N_2 and determines the average molar mass to be 30.08, the other engineer, using an incorrect value of 14, calculates the average molar mass to be 18.74.

(a) Calculate the volume % of N_2 in the flue gases.

(b) If the remaining components of the flue gases are CO_2 and O_2, calculate the volume % of each of them.

[*Ans.* (a) N_2 = 81%; (b) CO_2 = 11.0% and O_2 = 8% (by volume)]

3.11 In refining mineral oils, a technique of mixed solvent extraction is employed. In a particular method, acetic acid is used as principal solvent and chloroform as an auxiliary solvent. A particular oil having a viscosity graviy constant (VGC) of 0.8553 is first treated with acetic acid. The acetic acid-oil mixture (a complex) has a composition 63.4% acetic acid and 36.6% oil. At 298.15 K(25°C) the complex separated into two coexisting liquid phases having the compositions shown in Table 3.11.

Table 3.11 Composition of an Acetic Acid-Oil Mixture

	Composition, mass %		VGC of solvent free oil
	acetic acid	oil	
Complex	63.4	36.6	0.8553
Upper layer	9.62	90.38	0.8418
Lower layer	93.03	6.97	0.9532

To the above complex, chloroform is added. The resultant mixture (a new complex) is separated again in two at 298.15 K (25°C), having the compositions given in Table 3.12.

Table 3.12 Composition of the Complex (See Table 3.11) plus Chloroform

	Composition, mass %			VGC of solvent free oil
	acetic acid	chloroform	oil	
New complex	57.8	9.7	Balance	0.8553
Upper layer	14.5	18.93	Balance	0.8424
Lower layer	87.5	3.62	Balance	0.9210

Calculate: (a) the mass ratio of two layers given in Table 3.11, (b) the mass ratio of two layers given in Table 3.12 and (c) the amount of chloroform added to the original complex. Also solve the problem by graphical method.

[*Ans.* (a) 0.55:1, (b) 0.686:1 and (c) 9.7 kg chloroform
per 100 kg original complex]

3.12 A spent lye sample obtained from a soap-making unit contains 9.6% glycerol and 10.3% salt (NaCl). It is concentrated at the rate of 50 000 kg/h in a double-effect evaporator until the final solution contains 80% glycerol and 6% salt. Assume that about 4.5% glycerol is lost by entrainment. All percentages are by mass.
Find: (a) The evaporation taken place in the system; and (b) the amount of salt crystallised out in the salt box of the evaporator.

[*Ans.* (a) 3946.5 kg/h, (b) 480.5 kg/h]

3.13 A mixed fertiliser, having the NPK composition 10:26:26 as % N, % P_2O_5 and % K_2O by mass respectively, is to be formulated by mixing ammonia, phosphoric acid, potassium chloride and/or urea.
 (a) If anhydrous ammonia, anhydrous phosphoric acid and 100% pure potassium chloride are used for mixing, calculate the amount of each of them required for formulating 100 kg mixed fertiliser. Assume that the filler will make-up the balance.
 (b) If 100% pure urea is used in place of anhydrous ammonia calculate the ammount of urea required for formulating 100 kg mixed fertiliser.
 (c) If anhydrous ammonia and 98% potassium chloride (mass %) are available, calculate the strength of H_3PO_4 required for making the required mixed fertiliser.

Note: This example can be worked out with the help of simple nomograph such as the one proposed by Sisson[16].

[*Ans.* (a) 12.14 kg NH_3, 35.89 kg H_3PO_4 and 41.18 kg KCl;
(b) 21.43 kg urea; (c) 78.29% H_3PO_4 (mass)]

3.14 For carrying out nitration reaction, it is desired to have a mixed acid containing 39% HNO_3, 42% H_2SO_4 (mass). Nitric acid of 68.3% (mass) is readily available (azeotropic composition). Calculate: (a) the required strength of sulphuric acid to obtain the above mixed. Also solve the problem using a triangular chart.

[*Ans.* (a) 97.9% (mass) (b) 1.33:1]

3.15 In Example 3.8 aqueous 98% H_2SO_4 is used for blending. If, instead of this, 10% oleum is used, find the quantities of each of the three acids required to be blended. Which blending should be preferred? How can a triangular chart be used for this problem?

[*Ans.* 128.6 kg spent acid, 339.4 kg 90% HNO_3 and
532.0 kg 10% oleum]

3.16 A mixed acid is to be prepared from spent acid, 99% H_2SO_4, 95% HNO_3 and water, if necessary. Determine the following graphically.
 (a) The mass of sulphuric acid, nitric acid and water necessary to convert 1000 kg of spent acid containing 40% H_2SO_4, 20% HNO_3 40% H_2O to a mixed acid containing 50% H_2SO_4, 40% HNO_3 and 10% H_2O.

(b) The mass of water that must be evaporated from 1000 kg of spent acid to produce a mixed acid containing 66% H_2SO_4, 33% HNO_3; and 1% H_2O.

All percentages are on mass basis.

[*Ans.* (a) 1000 kg spent acid, 2267.0 kg 99% H_2SO_4 and 2013.0 kg 95% HNO_3; (b) 393.4 kg water to be evaporated]

3.17 Benzene and cyclohexane form a positive azeotrope which boils at 350.4 K(77.4°C) containing 54 mole% benzene. Acetone is used as an entrainer for separation of the azeotrope. Acetone forms an azeotrope only with cyclohexane that boils at 326.1 K(53.1°C) containing 74.6 mole % acetone. Assume that a mixture of benzene and cyclohexane containing male 38.2 mass% benzene is to be azeotropically distilled with the addition of acetone. Calculate the mass of acetone required per 100 kg of feed using a triangular plot such that the distillate is the acetone-cyclohexane azeotrope and the bottom product is pure benzene. Also read the composition of the ternary mixture.

[*Ans.* 127.9 kg acetone]

3.18 Slabs of building boards contain 16% moisture. They are dried to a water content of 0.5% by circulating hot air over them. The outgoing air contains 0.09 kg water vapour per kg dry air. Calculate the quantity of fresh air required per 1000 kg/h net dry board, if the fesh air is supplied at 301 K(28°C) and 101.325 kPa containing 0.2 kg/kg dry air humidity.

[*Ans.* 2337.3 m³/h]

3.19 The component tri-glycerides present in lard [17] are given in Table 3.13.

Table 3.13 Composition of Lard[17]

No.	Tri-glyceride	Formula		Mass %
1.	Palmitodistearin	C_3H_5	$(OOCH_{31}C_{15})$ $(OOCH_{35}C_{17})_2$	3
2.	Stearodipalmitin	C_3H_5	$(OOCH_{31}C_{15})_2$ $(OOCH_{35}C_{17})$	2
3.	Oleopalmitostearin	C_3H_5	$(OOCH_{31}C_{15})$ $(OOCH_{35}C_{17})$ $(OOCH_{33}C_{17})$	11
4.	Oleodistearin	C_3H_5	$(OOCH_{35}C_{17})_2$ $(OOCH_{33}C_{17})$	2
5.	Palmitodiolein	C_3H_5	$(OOCH_{31}C_{15})$ $(OOCH_{33}C_{17})_2$	82

Compute the composition of lard in terms of fatty acids.

[*Ans.* Palmitic acid: 31.24%; stearic acid: 7.92%; and oleic acid: 60.84% (mass basis)]

3.20 The analysis of the water obtained from an underground source is given in Table 3.14.

Table 3.14 Analysis of Raw Water Sample

a. Solids, mg/L.		
	Total solids	2688.0
	Dissolved solids	2510.0
	Suspended solids (by difference)	178.0
b. Alkalinity, expressed as $CaCO_3$, mg/L		
	Total alkalinity	572.6
	Total carbonates	80.5
	Total bicarbonates	492.1
c. Hardness, expressed as $CaCO_3$, mg/L		
	Temporary hardness	284.0
	Permanent hardness	Nil
	Total hardness	284.0
	Magnesium hardness	194.0
d. pH		8.5
e. Chlorides as Cl, mg/L		775.6
f. Sulphates as SO_4, mg/L		230.4

Find (a) the actual analysis of water, and (b) % Na of total cations (based on milliequivalents).

[*Ans.* (a) Analysis in mg/L; $Ca(HCO_3)_2$ 145.8; $Mg(HCO_3)_2$ 283.8; $NaHCO_3$ 349.6; Na_2CO_3 85.3; $NaCl$ 1278.1; Na_2SO_4 340.8 Dissolved solids 2483.3 (b) 85% Na of total cations]

3.21 A dyehouse effluent is found to contain sodium (as Na) and calcium (as Ca) to the extent of 245.7 mg/L and 37.6 mg/L respectively. This effluent is to be discharged on the land used for irrigation purposes. According to IS: 2490 the tolerance limit for % Na of total cations (on equivalent basis) is 60. In order to bring the sodium level down to 60%, how much gypsum (essentially $CaSO_4$) is to be dissolved in the effluent. Also, calculate the % Na of total cations as such in the effluents.

[*Ans.* % Na in the effluent = 85.04; Dosage of $CaSO_4$ required = 356.3 mg/L]

3.22 Coking of catalyst is common phenomenon in the process industry. Masking of active pores by coke results in reduction of catalytic activity, therfore decoking of catalyst is carried out periodically.

Decoking with air from the beginning means supply of excess oxygen; thereby combustion reaction can 'run away' which can result in hot spots in the catalyst bed. Such a phenomenon can destroy catalyst and may result in explosion if temperature control is not exercised.

To control the catalyst bed temperature effectively, oxygen concentration in the feed stream is to be regulated. This will impart heat, generated by combustion, to the flowing gaseous stream as fast as generated. Laboratory experimentation for fixing various parameters proves useful.

In one experiment[18], 0.1 kg coked catalyst is charged in the laboratory reactor. Ultimate analysis of the coke suggests its average composition to be $CH_{0.6}$. Temperature sensing element is provided in the catalyst bed. Analyzers for oxygen at inlet and outlet are also provided.

Initially, the reactor is purged with pure nitrogen for about 900 s at a flowrate of 0.025 L/s at NTP to achieve bed temperature of 723 K (450°C). Keeping N_2 flow rate constant, air is introduced in it so that feed stream contains 5% oxygen (by vol.). Decoking (combustion) reaction consumes oxygen from the strem. Bed temperature is controlled around 723 K (450°C). After 1800 s, flow of nitrogen is stopped and only air is allowed to flow at 0.025 L/s at NTP. Oxygen concentration was measured at the exit of reactor at different time intervals. Results are as under.

Table 3.15 Oxygen Concentration Data

Time from start, s	Oxygen concentration at the exit of reactor, vol. %
300	0
600	0
775	0
900	0.17
1200	0.86
1500	1.46
1800	2.15
1950	2.59
2000	2.75
2100	10.34
2250	17.24
2400	20.30
2550	20.52
2700	21.0 – same as air

After 3600 s, air stream is stopped. Reactor is then purged with pure nitrogen for about 600 s and cooled.

Calculate total oxygen consumption during the experiment.

[*Ans.* 0.128 mol or 4.096×10^{-3} kg]

3.23 In particular drying operation, it is necessary to hold the moisture content of feed to a calciner to 15% (mass) to prevent lumping and sticking. This is accomplished by mixing the feed having 30% moisture (mass) with a recycle stream of dried material having 3% moisture (mass). The drying operation is shown in Fig. 3.20. What fraction of the dried product must be recycled? [*Ans.* 63.4%]

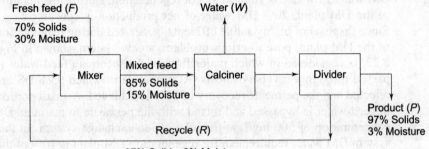

Fig. 3.20 Drying of Solids

3.24 Cloth is dried in a stenter (hot-air dryer) in a texile mill. In this machine, fresh air first mixes with recirculated air. The mixture then passes through a heater. Hot air as jetted over the cloth to evaporate the mixture. A major portion of the jetted air is recirculated while the remaining small portion is exhausted out. The operation is shown schematically in Fig. 3.21.

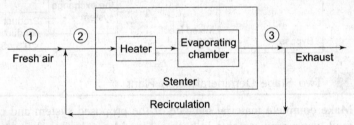

Fig. 3.21 Cloth Drying in Stenter

Test data on particular run of a stenter are given below:
Cloth details: Width = 90 cm; Density = 90 g/m^2; Speed = 1 m/s;
Inlet moisture regain = 80% and Outlet moisture regain = 8%

     Air conditions:

     Moisture of air at point (1) = 0.015 kg/kg dry air

     Moisture of air at point (2) = 0.095 kg/kg dry air

     Moisture of air at point (3) = 0.10 kg/kg dry air

Calculate: (a) the rate of evaporation in the stenter, (b) the mass flow rate of fresh air, (c) the volumetric flow rate of fresh air, if it is supplied at 303 K (30°C) and 100 kPa (755 torr), and (d) the mass flow rate of recirculating dry air.

Note: (i) Moisture regain of cloth = (kg moisture in cloth/kg dry cloth) × 100 (ii) Use the ideal gas law.

[*Ans.* (a) 210 kg/h; (b) 2470.6 kg/h; (c) 2146.2 m^3/h; (d) 39 530 kg/h]

3.25 A demineralisation (DM) plant employs ion exchange system for production of high purity water with conductivity of 0.5 μS/cm (max.). Feed water to the plant contains 2500 mg/L dissolved solids (DS) and DM water flow rate is 10 m³/h, net of regeneration. During regeneration of the DM plant, 20% DM water of net production is consumed.

Since disposal of highly saline effluents, generated during regeneration of the DM plant, pose a serious problem, a new system, shown in Fig. 3.22, is considered in which major flow of the incoming feed water is passed through a reverse osmosis (RO) module in which 95% DS are rejected and the permeate recovery of 80% is achieved. A small portion of feed water is bypassed and mixed with the permeate to maintain DS concentration of 500 mg/L at the inlet of ion exchange system. In this system DM water requirement for regeneration DM plant is 10% of the net production.

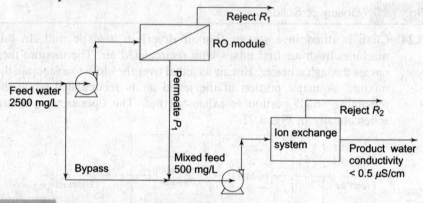

Fig. 3.22 Two Stage Demineralization Plant

Make complete material balance of the proposed system and compare feed water requirements in both cases. Also calculate the ratio of the permeate to bypass feed water flow rate and concentration of DS in the reject water.

[*Ans.* Feed water to ion exchange = 12 m³/h
Feed water to new system = 13.347 m³/h
Ratio of permeate to bypass = 5.82 m³/m³
Concentration of DS in reject = 11 875 mg/L]

3.26 In Example 3.15, recovery of permeate in RO Module I is taken as 66%. Rework material balance with recoveries of 60% and 70% of RO Module I.

[*Ans.* Table 3.16 Material balance with different recoveries]

Table 3.16 Material Balance with Different Recoveries

Recovery, %	Reject R_1 flow rate m³/h	Recycle ratio, R_2/F, m³/m³	DS concentration in R_1, mg/L	Rejection of DS in RO module I, %
60	4.17	0.136	9 230	95.84
70	2.68	0.163	12 026	95.07

3.27 In a textile industry, it is desired to make a 24% solution (by mass) of caustic soda for a mercerisation process. Due to the very high heat of dissolution of caustic soda in water, the above solution is prepared by two-step process.

First, in a dissolution tank, caustic soda is dissolved in the correct quantity of water to produce 50% (by mass) solution. After complete dissolution and cooling, the solution is taken to dilution tank where some more water is added to produce 24% solution. The two-step process is shown in Fig. 3.23.

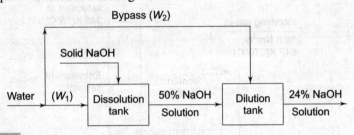

Fig. 3.23 Dissolution of Caustic Soda in Water

Assuming no evaporation loss in the dissolution tank, calculate the mass ration W_1/W_2.

[*Ans.* $W_1/W_2 = 0.462$]

3.28 In the preparation of cooking liquor for a sulphite pulp mill, an absorption column is used to absorb SO_2 in a weak liquor[19]. The weak liquor enters the top of the column at the rate of 20 L/s with SO_2 concentration of 0.5% (by mass) and leaves with SO_2 concentration of 1.0% (by mass). The gas steam entering the bottom of the column passing in the counter-current direction to the liquor stream contains 17.0% (by volume) SO_2. When the gas leaves the top of the column, 75% of SO_2 gets absorbed. The pressure in the column becomes 50 kPa g and operates isothermally at 308 K (35°C). Assuming that the liquor has a specific gravity of 1.0, calculate: (a) the molar flow rate of enterings gas, and (b) the volumetric flow rate of entering gas.

[*Ans.* (a) 12.26×10^{-3} kmol/s (b) 207.4 dm³/s]

3.29 An effluent sample from a formaldehyde plant is found to contain methanol and formaldehyde. The analysis of the solution indicated that TOC and ThOD are 258.3 mg/L and 956.5 mg/L, respectively. Find the concentration of each of the compounds in the sample.

[*Ans.* Methanol: 535 mg/L formaldehyde: 144 mg/L]

3.30 Hot acid gases from a calciner are fed to a venturi scrubber[20] at 643 K(370°C) as shown in Fig. 3.24. The volumetric flow rate of the moist gases is 16.5 Nm³/s which contain 4.2 Nm³/s of water vapours, 1600 mg SO_3/Nm³ of dry gas and 9000 mg solids/Nm³ dry gas of which chlorides (as Cl) amount to 1.5 g/s. After scrubbing the gases in the venturi scrubber, the exit gases from the separator are saturated at 348 K(75°C).

Eighty percent SO_3, entering the scrubber, is scrubbed in the circulating liquor. Solids concentration in the exit gas mixture is found to be 120 mg/Nm³ dry gas. Practically all chlorides in the incoming gases are scrubbed. The make-up water which is added to the circulating liquor contains 50 mg/L chlorides (as Cl). The scrubber, separator and other parts of the system are made of stainless steel. At the low pH (because of SO_3 dissolution), the concentration of chlorides is limited to 200 mg/L in the circulating liquor to prevent corrosive attack.

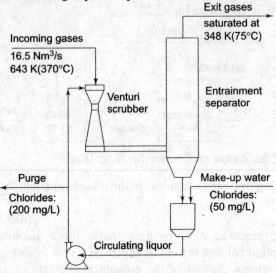

Fig. 3.24 Scrubbing of Acid Gases in a Venturi Scrubber

For this purpose a continuous bled is maintained from the circulating system. Calculate the purge rate, concentration of solids and sulphuric acid in it and make-up water requirement.

Note: Humidity of exit gases from separator = 0.614 kmol/kmol dry gas.

[*Ans.* Purge rate = 10.9 kg/s bleed; Solid concn. = 1.00%, H_2SO_4 concn. = 0.18 % (by mass); Make-up water rate = 13.6 kg/s]

3.31 Wastewaters from rice-processing industry is required to be treated in an activated sludge plant before being discharged in public sewer owing to high BOD loading (~12 500 mg/L). Waste steam contains 485 mg/L suspended solids which are non-bacterial in nature. The process flow diagram is similar to the one shown in Fig. 3.13, except that a primary clarifier is not employed. After aeration in the aeration tank, all the suspended solids are separated in the secondary clarifier. The sludge (underflow) from the clarifier is partially recycled. From kinetic considerations of the aeration tank and design considerations of the clarifier, the minimum recycle ratio leading to minimum sludge waste can be achieved when the bacterial suspended solids concentration in the recycle stream is five times[21] higher than that in the total combined feed entering the aeration tank. Prove that the minimum recycle ratio $r (= Q_r/Q_F)$ is exactly 1/4 assuming that suspended solids concentration in the total combined feed is 2% (mass). The wastage amount can be neglected for calculation purposes.

Note: It may be noted that $X_F = 485$ mg/L in this problem which was assumed to be zero in Example 3.16 as the effluents passed through a primary clarifier.

3.32 In Example 3.17, the atmospheric pressure method of purging is described. There are two more methods of purging.
  (a) Pressure Cycle Method: In this method, the equipment to be purged is pressurised with inert gas and on complete mixing of the inert gas with vessel atmosphere, the pressure is released to the initial pressure. Assume that the initial pressure is p_1 kPa a in the vessel. It is pressurised with inert gas to p_2 kPa a and then depressurised to p_1. Prove that the concentration of the component will be p_1/p_2 times the initial concentration (c_0) after one cycle of pressurisation/depressurisation. Also prove that the number of vessel volumes of inert gas required per cycle will be $(p_2 - p_1)/p_1$.
  (b) Vacuum Cycle Method: This method is similar to the pressure cycle method except that sub-atmospheric pressure is used. In this method, the vessel is evacuated to p kPa a and then it is refilled with inert gas to the normal atmospheric pressure (i.e. 101.3 kPa a). Prove that the concentration of the component will reduce to $c_0 (p/101.3)$ after one cycle and $c_0(p/101.3)^n$ after n cycles of evacuation/refilling. Also prove that the amount of inert gas required for purging per cycle will be $(1 - p/101.3)$ vessel volumes.

Note: It is assumed in all the cases that temperature changes taking place in the system are negligible.

3.33 An isotank is used for long distance transportation of oxygen sensitive liquid organic product. It is a horizontal pressure vessel having 2.5 m diameter and 6 m length. It is normally filled upto 85% height. Empty volume above the liquid has to have inert atmosphere with oxygen concentration less than 1% (v/v).
Initially the empty space is occupied by atmospheric air (ref. Example 2.18). It is pressure purged with pure nitrogen (containing less than 0.1% O_2) at 308.15 K(35°C). from cylinders. Considering design limitations of the isotank, it is pressurised up to 2 bar g each time with nitrogen and depressurised to atmospheric (1.0197 bar a) pressure.
Neglecting oxygen in nitrogen, and negligible solubility of nitrogen in organic liquid, calculate
  (a) number of cycles required to achieve desire oxygen concentration in the empty space,
  (b) final concentration of oxygen in the empty space, and

(c) total requirement of pure nitrogen for purging.

[*Ans.* (a) 3 cycles; (b) 0.8% (v/v); (c) 14.54 Nm^3]

3.34 Gas mixture leaving high temperature shift converter in a typical natural gas based ammonia plant, has the following compositions on dry basis: H_2: 56%, CO: 15%, CO_2: 7%, N_2: 21.7% and Ar: 0.3%. Steam (essentially in the gas form) to dry gas ratio in the feed is 1.2 kmol/kmol (ref. Exercise 5.35). Converter is normally operated under pressure (around 25 bar g) and 618.15 K(345°C). Shift reaction is exothermic in nature.

Reaction: $CO + H_2O \rightarrow CO_2 + H_2$

During a shutdown of the ammonia plant, the converter must be pressure purged after isolation to limit the concentration of steam in it so that the reaction is practically stopped and chances of hot spot formation in the catalytic bed are eliminated. Pure nitrogen (< 1% O_2 by vol.) is available at 308.15 K (35°C) at 6 bar g. At first the converter is depressurised to low pressure (to 0.25 bar g). Subsequently it is pressurised with pure nitrogen to 5 bag g and depressurised again to 0.25 bar g.

(a) Assuming converter's void and empty volume of 40 m^3, calculate the number of cycles required to achieve steam concentration below 1% (by vol.) on wet basis.

(b) Calculate final concentration of steam and carbon monoxide at the end of purging on wet basis.

(c) Calculate total requirement of nitrogen at NTP.

[*Ans.* (a) 3 cycles; (b) H_2O: 0.5%, CO: 0.06%; (c) 498.6 Nm^3]

3.35 Combustion can occur when a flammable vapour is mixed with oxygen (or air) within certain concentration ranges. This concentration range is known as flammability envelope (limit). The minimum fuel content requirement to support combustion is called the lower flammability limit and the maximum is called the upper flammability limit. An ignition source is required to cause combustion of the mixture within the flammability limit which is also a function of pressure and temperature.

In a number of gas (vapour) phase oxidation processes, the mixture of gases may be within the flammability limits. To ensure the intrinsic safety of the process, operating conditions must be established in such a way that the process vapours remain outside the flammability envelope at all times or oxygen content does not exceed a certain percentage. Often, it is not possible to operate the process with altered composition of the flammable material and oxygen (or air) to be away from the flammable limits due to desired process conditions. For such a case, two alternatives are available[22].

In one alternative, addition of an inert gas (such as nitrogen, argon, carbon dioxide, superheated steam, etc.) is practiced such that oxygen content can be brought down to a safe level. In the second alternative, addition of another flammable gas can be considered, the amount of which can be calculated using the Le Chatelier's relationship:

$$\frac{n_1}{N_1} + \frac{n_2}{N_2} + \frac{n_3}{N_3} \dots = 1$$

where n_i = mole % of ith flammable gas

and N_i = lower or upper flammability limit of ith gas

In reactor, 100 kmol of hydrogen and 100 kmol of air are available at 101.325 kPa a and 293.15 K(20°C). As such this mixture is to be made non-flammable by addition of (a) nitrogen, and (b) methane. Calculate the minimum requirements of nitrogen and methane in the two cases. Data:

(i) Hydrogen-air mixture is non-flammable when oxygen is less than 5 mole %.

(ii) Flammability data:

Table 3.17 Flammability Data

| Gas | Flammability limits (vol.%) in air at 101.325 kPa and 293.15 K(20°C) | |
	Upper limit	Lower limit
Hydrogen	75 %	4 %
Methane	14 %	5 %

[*Ans.* (a) 219 kmol nitrogen; (b) 10.85 kmol methane]

Note: It is interesting to note that a flammable gas mixture can be readily made non-flammable by a small amount of another flammable gas than a substantial amount of an inert gas.

3.36 An average astronaut inhale 123 kg of air and exhales 112 kg air, 1.8 kg water vapour and 8.8 kg carbon dioxide every day. He can safely breath gases containing 100% to 20% oxygen (v/v). The cabin of a spaceship has free volume of 4500 L and is filled with pure oxygen at a pressure 154.6 kPa a and a temperature of 293.15 K(20°C). In flight. the temperature is held at 293.15 K(20°C) and the water is absorbed by a desiccant.

(a) How long can a mission astronaut sustain, without an external oxygen supply?

(b) What will be the total pressure and partial pressures of carbon dioxide and oxygen at the end of the mission?

[*Ans.* (a) 26 h 16 min; (i.e. 94 560s), (b) Total pressure = 147.5 kPa a
p_{O_2} = 29.5 kPa; p_{CO_2} = 118 kPa]

3.37 In a continuous kraft pulp bleaching, caustic soda is required at a concentration of 10% NaOH (by mass) and a flow rate of 1.65 kg/s. This solution is prepared by introducing 50% caustic lye (by mass) and diluted with water continuously in a 1900 L tank, equipped with an agitator, and withdrawing the 10% solution continuously at the desired rate. During the operation, the inflow of 50% caustic lye suddenly fails while the dilution water continues to enter the tank. Assuming that a perfect mixing takes place in the tank and the volume is constant (1900 L), calculate the time required for the effluent concentration to fall to 8% NaOH by mass[10].

Data: Take the specific gravity of NaOH solution in the range of 10% to 8% concentration to be constant at 1.10.

[*Ans.* 2827 s]

3.38 Compressed air at 710 kPa g and 318.15 K(45°C) (fully saturated) is dried in a silica gel column. It is desired to dry air at the rate of 150 Sm^3/h [(measured at 101.325 kPa and 288.15 K (15°C)] to use it in pneumatic instruments. The maximum permissible moisture content of the instrument air is 25 mg/m^3 [(approximate atmospheric dew point = 241.15 K(−32°C)]. The air passes through a column in which 220 kg bone-dry silica gel is packed. The regenerated silica contains 2.5 kg moisture per 100 kg bone-dry desiccant. The laboratory experiment reveal the following performance of the silica gel.

Table 3.18 Dehydration of Air with Silica Gel[23]

Moisture in silica gel kg moisture/100 kg dry desiccant	Residual water in mg/Sm^3 in air
2.500	5.0
3.750	10.0
5.625	15.0
6.563	20.0
7.344	25.0

Calculate the expected service time of the bed, after which it is required to be regenerated.

Data: Moisture of fully-saturated air at 710 kPa g and 318.15 K (45°C) = 0.011 95 kmol/kmol dry air.

[*Ans.* 7.935 h (i.e. 28 566 s)]

3.39 A cooling water system comprises of a cooling tower and a cooling water circuit through various heat exchangers. It has a total hold up of 3000 m^3. On a particular day, the suspended solids were measured to be 50 mg/L. A side-stream sand filter is installed to reduce the turbidity in the cooling water. The filter is fed with cooling water at the rate of 100 m^3/h. The performance of the filter is expected to be as given in Table 3.19.

Table 3.19 Performance of a Side Stream Filter

Suspended solids in the ingoing cooling water, mg/L	Suspended solids in the outcoming cooling water, mg/L
50-40	10
40-30	9
30-27.5	8
27.5-25	7
25-20	6
20-10	5

Assuming that there is no addition of suspended solids from the surroundings, calculate the time required to bring down the suspended solids in the cooling water to 10 mg/L. Refer Fig. 3.25 for the flow diagram.

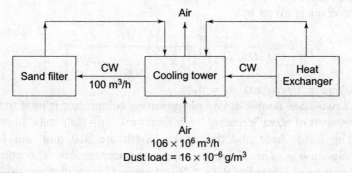

Fig. 3.25 Performance of a Side Stream Filter in Cooling Water System

[*Ans.* 68 h]

3.40 In Exercise 3.39, it was assumed that there is no addition of dust from the atmosphere. However, in actual practice, the dust amounts to a sizable turbidity in the cooling water. Assume that incoming air @ 106×10^6 m^3/h brings in the dust at a rate of 16×10^{-6} g/m^3. Calculate the time required to bring down the suspended solids of the cooling water to 25 mg/L based on the filter performance outlined in Table 3.20.

3.41 In the exponential dilution technique for preparation of calibration gas mixture, a bottle fitted with a magnetic stirrer, is filled with a gas mixture, having the concentration of component A as C_{A_0}. The volume of the bottle is V mL. Inert gas, free from A, is introduced at a rate of F mL/s into the bottle, thoroughly mixed with the contents and the dilute gas mixture is drawn from the bottle at the rate of F mL/s. Prove that the concentration of A in the bottle at time θ (in s) from the start of introducing gas is given by

$$C_A = C_{A_0} \cdot e^{-(F\theta/V)}$$

Note: This is basically a mixing model in which the dependency of the concentration of the component A in the exit stream with time θ is expressed. Fowler[24] has presented a mixing model for dilution of a solution or purging a vessel on the same principle.

3.42 A single-stage single acting reciprocating compressor is used to fill a receiver having the volume V m^3. The compressor operates as s strokes/s, has the geometric volume v_0 m^3 of the cylinder and the clearance c. It is required to increase the absolute pressure in the receiver from p_0 to p_1. The volumetric efficiency of the compressor is defined as

$$\eta_v = 1 + c - \frac{p}{100\, p_0} - c\left(\frac{p}{p_0}\right)^{1/\gamma}$$

where p = discharge pressure after time θ (in s) and γ = ratio of heat capacities of the gas = C_p/C_v. Prove that the time required to fill the receiver is given by

$$\theta = \frac{V}{(3600\, s\, v_0)} \int_0^{R_1} \frac{dr}{\left[1 + c - \dfrac{r}{100} - c(r)^{1/\gamma}\right]}$$

where $r = p/p_0$ and $R_1 = p_1/p_0$.

3.43 A two-stage double-acting reciprocating compressor is used to fill up a receiver of 60 m^3 capacity with air for use with pneumatic instruments. The inside bore and the stroke length are 310 mm and 150 mm respectively. The clearance in the cylinder is 7%. The compressor operates at a speed of 9.2 s^{-1}. It is designed for equal compression ratio in each stage. Calculate the time required to pressurise the receiver from normal atmospheric conditions to 7 bar g.

Data: γ for air = 1.4.

[*Ans.* 1562 s]

REFERENCES

1. Prugh, R. W., *Chem. Engg. Prog.*, **70**(11): 1974, p. 72.
2. Private Communication with Aspen Technology, Inc., USA.
3. Levenspiel, O., *Chemical Reaction Engineering*, 2nd Ed., John Wiley & Sons, Inc., USA, 1972, p. 972.
4. Mukhopadhyay, M., *Natural Extracts using Supercritical Carbon Dioxide*, CRC Press LLC, USA, 2000, p. 238
5. Hunter, T. G., *Ind. Engg. Chem.*, **34**(8): 1942, p. 963.
6. Kirk, R. E. and D. F. Othmer, *Encyclopedia of Chemical Technology*, 1st Ed., Vol. 9, The Interscience Encyclopedia, Inc., USA, 1952, p. 315.
7. Prielipp, G. E. and H. W. Keller. *J. of the American Oil Chemists' Soc.*, **XXXIII** (3): 1956, p. 103.
8. US Patent No. 3078 140, 1963.
9. *Chemical processing by Ion Exchange*, Dow Chemical Co., USA.
10. *Chemical Engineering Problems in Pulp and Paper Industry*, Technical Association of the Pulp and Paper Industry (TAPPI), USA, 1965.
11. Ramalho, R. S. *Hydrocarbon Processing*, **57**(10): 1978, p. 112.
12. Saigal, R. S., *Gas News*, **1**(12): 1978, p. 3.
13. Kinsley, G. R., *Chemical Engineering Progress*, **97**(2), 2001, p. 57.

14. Chandodkar, M. V. and D. J. Mehta, *Chemical Age of India*, **24**(5): 1973, p. 302.
15. *Technical Bulletin on Dow Products and Services* Dow Chemical Co., USA, 1972.
16. Sisson, B., *Chem Engg.*, **84**(6): March 14, 1977, p. 156.
17. Guillaudan, A., *Ind. Engg. Chem.*, **29**(7): 1937, p. 729.
18. Fulton, J. W., *Chem. Engg.*, **95**(1), Jan. 18, 1988, p. 111.
19. *Tappi*, **47**(8): 1964, p. 114a.
20. Gleason, T. G., *Chem Engg.*, **84**(23): Oct. 24, p. 146.
21. *AIChE Student Contest Problem*, 1972.
22. Talmage W. P., *Chemtech*, Feb. 1971, p. 117.
23. Davis, K. G. and K. D. Manchanda, *Chem. Engg.*, **81**(19): Sept. 16, 1974, p. 102.
24. Flowler, W. B., *Chem. Engg.*, **88**(25): Dec. 14, 1981, p. 110.

Chapter 4

Material Balances Involving Chemical Reactions

4.1 INTRODUCTION

Chemical reactions play a vital role in the manufacturing processes. For the design of a chemical reaction equipment, the operating conditions, such as pressure, temperature, composition and flow rates of the streams should be known. The material and energy balance calculations come to the rescue of the designer and allow him to calculate the various flow rates and temperatures of the streams. Although the rates of reaction, reactor design and other kinetic aspects of reaction engineering do not fall within the scope of this book, a few terms such as limiting component, excess reactant, degree of conversion, selectivity and yield will be defined in order to have a clear understanding of the subject. Assuming that the kinetic data of a reaction are available, the overall material balance of the steady-state conditions will be discussed in this chapter.

4.2 EQUATIONS FOR CHEMICAL REACTIONS

International Union for Pure and Applied Chemistry (IUPAC) recommend following symbols, connecting the reactants and products in a chemical equation.

$$C_6H_6 + HNO_3 = C_6H_5NO_2 + H_2O \qquad \text{Stoichiometric relation} \qquad (4.1)$$

$$HCl + NaOH \longrightarrow NaCl + H_2O \qquad \text{Net forward reaction} \qquad (4.2)$$

$$CO + H_2O \rightleftharpoons CO_2 + H_2 \qquad \text{Reactions in both directions} \qquad (4.3)$$

$$NH_3 + HCl \rightleftharpoons NH_4Cl \qquad \text{Equilibrium} \qquad (4.4)$$

4.3 MATERIAL BALANCES INVOLVING CHEMICAL REACTIONS

The law of conservation of mass stated in Chapter 3 holds good for the material balances involving chemical reactions also.

The general mathematical statement can be written as:

Total mass entering the chemical reactor = total mass of products leaving the chemical reactor.

Very often, it is convenient to work with moles rather than with mass, particularly in gaseous systems. It should be noted that in chemical reactions, the total mass of the input remains constant, but the total moles may or may not remain constant. This fact can be understood by studying the following two reactions. Consider the shift reaction:

$$CO + H_2O = CO_2 + H_2 \qquad (4.5)$$
$$\text{1 mole} \quad \text{1 mole} \quad \text{1 mole} \quad \text{1 mole}$$

In this, it can be observed that two moles react with each other and produce also two moles. Thus, the number of moles of the reactants entering the reactor equals the number of moles of the products leaving the reactor. The ammonia synthesis reaction can be written as

$$N_2 + 3H_2 \rightleftharpoons 2NH_3 \qquad (4.6)$$
$$\text{1 mole} \quad \text{3 moles} \quad \text{2 moles}$$

It can be observed that four moles (of reactants) produce two moles of ammonia in forward direction. Thus, the number of moles have been reduced, although the total mass of the reactants entering and of the products leaving the reactor are equal. For reaction (4.5), one can write

$$\text{1 mole } CO \equiv \text{1 mole } H_2O \equiv \text{1 mole } H_2 \equiv \text{1 mole } CO_2$$

Similarly, for reaction (4.6), 1 mole $N_2 \equiv$ 3 moles $H_2 \equiv$ 2 moles NH_3

The above equalities decide the stoichiometric requirements of the components. (The sign $\equiv$ represents *equivalent to* from the point of view of the chemical equilibrium, and not *equal to* from the mathematical point of view.)

4.4 DEFINITION OF TERMS

Some of the terms used in chemical reaction engineering will now be defined.

In most chemical reactions, two or more components reacting together are not in stoichiometric proportions due to technical, economic or safety considerations. In such cases, a *limiting component* is defined as one which decides the conversion in the reactions. An *excess reactant* is the one which is in excess amount over the stoichiometric requirement of the reactant as determined by the desired chemical reaction.

Consider the reforming reactions between methane and steam.

$$CH_4 + H_2O \longrightarrow CO + 3H_2 \qquad (4.7)$$

$$CH_4 + 2H_2O \longrightarrow CO_2 + 4H_2 \qquad (4.8)$$

In actual practice, the steam that is fed to the reformer is usually much in excess of the stoichiometric requirement. Therefore, methane is the limiting component while steam is the excess reactant.

Urea is produced by the reaction of carbon dioxide and ammonia as per the following reaction:

$$CO_2 + 2NH_3 \longrightarrow NH_2CONH_2 + H_2O \qquad (4.9)$$

Normally, NH_3 is the excess reactant and CO_2 is the limiting component in the above synthesis. The feed may consist of CO_2 and NH_3 in $1:4.5$ molar ratio in a typical process.

Consider the ammonia synthesis [reaction (4.6)]. The synthesis gas normally enters the reactor in stoichiometric proportions, i.e. $1:3$ molar ratio of $N_2:H_2$. In this reaction, none is in excess (unlike most chemical reactions).

Chlorination of methane presents an interesting example. The following four reactions take place simultaneously.

$$CH_4 + Cl_2 \longrightarrow CH_3Cl + HCl \qquad (4.10)$$

$$CH_3Cl + Cl_2 \longrightarrow CH_2Cl_2 + HCl \qquad (4.11)$$

$$CH_2Cl_2 + Cl_2 \longrightarrow CHCl_3 + HCl \qquad (4.12)$$

$$CHCl_3 + Cl_2 \longrightarrow CCl_4 + HCl \qquad (4.13)$$

In a typical vapour phase chlorination reaction, normally chlorine is completely consumed while a portion of methane may escape unreacted. Since all the reactions take place simultaneously, it is difficult to specify the stoichiometric requirement of chlorine. In fact, the amount of chlorine determines the products pattern. Therefore, in this type of reaction, conversion of chlorine is 100% and it can be termed as a limiting component. However, conversion of methane need not be 100%.

Distinction between *conversion*, *selectivity* and *yield* should be clear before attempting to solve any problem involving chemical reaction. These terms, however, are not uniformly employed in various scientific publications. Definitions, accepted in most publications, are presented here.

Conversion is defined as the ratio of the reacting amount of a component to its initial amount. The amounts can be expressed in moles, masses or volumes. Accordingly, the conversion is also expressed as mole %, mass % or volume %.

In reforming reactions, (4.7) and (4.8), two parallel reactions are taking place. CO and CO_2 are co-products. In both reactions H_2 is the common product.

Let a be the kmol of CH_4 fed of which b kmol of CH_4 are reacted by reaction (4.7) and c kmol of CH_4 are reacted by reaction (4.8)

$$\text{Total moles of } CH_4 \text{ reacted} = b + c \text{ kmol}$$

$$\text{Percentage conversion of } CH_4 = \left\{ \frac{b+c}{a} \right\} 100$$

$$\text{Unreacted CH}_4 = a - (b + c) \text{ kmol}$$

Since steam is the excess reactant, conversion is normally not defined on the basis of consumption of steam.

In the manufacture of nitrobenzene, benzene and nitric acid are reacted.

$$C_6H_6 + HNO_3 \longrightarrow C_6H_5NO_2 + H_2O \qquad (4.14)$$

The chief product is nitrobenzene but in practice, it is observed that some of the nitrobenzene reacts with additional quantity of nitric acid to produce dinitrobenzene.

$$C_6H_5NO_2 + HNO_3 \longrightarrow C_6H_4(NO_2)_2 + H_2O \qquad (4.15)$$

Thus, it can be seen that the final product mixture will contain nitrobenzene as well as dinitrobenzene, the amount of latter depends on the excess quantity of HNO_3, present in the mixture. Reaction (4.15) can also be written as

$$C_6H_5 + 2 HNO_3 \longrightarrow C_6H_5(NO_3)_2 + 2 H_2O \qquad (4.16)$$

Yield is defined as under:

$$\text{Yield} = \frac{\text{moles of desired product formed} \times \text{stoichiometric factor}}{\text{moles of specific reactant consumed}}$$

where, stoichiometric factor = Stoichiometric requirement of the
specific reactant (in moles) per
mole of the desired product

For the production of nitrobenzene,
stoichiometric factor = 1

$$\text{Percentage yield of nitrobenzene} = \frac{\text{moles of nitrobenzene produced}}{\text{moles of benzene consumed}} \times 100$$

Consider the reactions (4.7) and (4.8). The aim of reforming reactions is to maximise the yield of hydrogen. Calculation of yield of hydrogen is complex. Stoichiometric factor for reaction (4.7) for hydrogen production is 1/3 and that for reaction (4.8) is 1/4 based on methane consumption.

Percentage yield of hydrogen = [moles of hydrogen produced by reaction
(4.7)/3 + moles of hydrogen produced by
reaction (4.8)/4]/[moles of methane con-
sumed] × 100

Formation of chloroform [reaction (4.12)] can be written as

$$CH_4 + 3 Cl_2 \longrightarrow CHCl_3 + 3 HCl \qquad (4.17)$$

$$\text{Percentage yield of chloroform} = \frac{[\text{moles of chloroform formed}]}{[\text{moles of chlorine consumed} \times 3]}$$

In all the above cases, it is seen that the competitive reactions take place and hence the yield of desired product is worked out by finding the moles of specific reactant consumed for the formation of the desired product. Competitive reactions can either be secondary reactions [(4.14) and (4.15)] or parallel reactions [(4.7) and (4.8)]. When there are no competitive reactions, yield is 100% at any conversion.

Selectivity in another term which measures the proportion of the total reaction which produces the desired product. Different conventions are used for assigning a numerical value to the selectivity in literature. One definition of selectivity would be the ratio of amount of limiting reactant that reacts to give the desired product to the amount that reacts to give undesirable product(s). The term selectivity is more often used in catalysis where a catalyst is judged by its selectivity. If yield is 100%, then selectivity is 1.

4.5   GENERALIZED APPROACH FOR SOLVING PROBLEMS

Material Balance Involving Chemical Reactions

In Sec. 3.3, it was seen that Law of Conservation of Mass can be applied to solve material balance problems of any system. Having understood the definitions of various terms of reaction engineering in the previous section, a generalized approach to solve material balance problems involving chemical reactions can now be studied.

At first it is important to note that in chemical reactions, moles are important rather than mass. Therefore for material balance calculations mass (m) of reactants or products are converted to moles using molar mass (M) values. Data on conversion of a chemical reaction and yield are then used to arrive at moles of products. When consecutive reactions are taking place, conversion of each reaction will have to be considered for finding the quantity of products.

Consider dehydrogenation of methanol to produce formaldehyde using silver catalyst. In this reaction, a mixture of methanol vapours, steam and small quantity of air are fed to a reactor packed with a catalyst. Following stoichiometric reactions are known to take place; the first one is the chief one.

$$CH_3OH = HCHO + H_2 \tag{4.18}$$

$$CH_3OH = CO + 2 H_2 \tag{4.19}$$

$$CH_3OH + \frac{1}{2} O_2 = HCHO + H_2O \tag{4.20}$$

$$CH_3OH = CH_4 + 1/2 O_2 \tag{4.21}$$

Conversion of methanol will mean total methanol reacted by all four reactions. Yield will determine product quantities.

Reaction (4.20) can also be written as

$$2 CH_3OH + O_2 = 2 HCHO + 2 H_2O \tag{4.20a}$$

Since mathematically both sides of the reaction are multiplied by a common multiplier, material balance (and heat balance) calculations are unaffected.

Consider reforming reactions (4.7) and (4.8). Actually production of CO_2 is the result of shift reaction of CO by the following reaction.

$$CO + H_2O = CO_2 + H_2 \tag{4.5}$$

Thus there are two consecutive reactions and conversion of each reaction is determined by kinetic considerations at the operating pressure and temperature.

In many cases compositions of reaction mixture and product mixture are given. Reforming reactions and combustion reactions are examples where such compositions are specified. This type of problem is normally solved by taking 100 mol of outgoing product gas mixture as a basis and back calculating the reactant requirements.

Multiplier of a reactant or a product in a chemical reaction is called *Stoichiometric Number* (v_i) when expressed with proper sign. Normal convention is a positive sign for the stoichiometric number of a product and negative sign for the reactant. Sum of all stoichiometric numbers gives change in total number of moles in the reaction. Any change in total number of moles of a gaseous reaction will mean change in extensive property, i.e. volume and/or pressure, but will not mean change in total mass. In case of liquids, change in volume is relatively small.

Many a times inert material (such as nitrogen, steam, etc.) is present in the reaction mixture. It is deliberately introduced to either reduce the concentration of the reactant (to reduce the rate of reaction) and/or to keep the temperature under control of an exothermic reaction. When air is used for combustion, nitrogen does enter with oxygen. Inert component has zero stoichiometric number. Although it increases total number of moles of the reaction mass, it does not take part in the reaction. Stoichiometric equations remain unchanged. Again total mass of reaction mixture remains constant.

For reaction (4.18), $\Sigma v_i = + 1$, for reaction (4.19), $\Sigma v_i = + 2$, for reaction (4.9), $\Sigma v_i = - 1$ and for reaction (4.5), $\Sigma v_i = 0$.

Following examples illustrate steady material balance calculations involving chemical reactions. Steady state means equilibrium state at given pressure and temperature in which no further changes occur.

Example 4.1 Monochloroacetic acid (MCA) is manufactured in a semibatch reactor by the action of glacial acetic acid with chlorine gas at 373 K (100°C) in the presence of PCl_3 catalyst. MCA thus formed will further react with chlorine to form dichloroacetic acid (DCA). To prevent the formation of DCA, excess acetic acid is used. A small-scale unit which produces 5000 kg/d MCA, requires 4536 kg/d of chlorine gas. Also, 263 kg/d of DCA is separated in the crystalliser to get almost pure MCA product. Find the % conversion, % yield of MCA and selectivity.

Solution Basis: One-day operation
Reactions:

CH_3COOH	+	Cl_2	=	$CH_2ClCOOH$	+	HCl
Acetic Acid		Chlorine		MCA		Hydrogen Chloride
$CH_2ClCOOH$	+	Cl_2	=	$CHCl_2COOH$	+	HCl
MCA		Chlorine		DCA		Hydrogen Chloride

In this example, the amount of chlorine determines the product distribution while acetic acid is in excess. Hence, chlorine becomes the limiting component.

$$\text{Chlorine charged} = \frac{4536}{71} = 63.89 \text{ kmol}$$

For each mole of MCA production, one mole of chlorine is consumed.

$$\text{Chlorine utilised for MCA production} = \frac{5000}{94.5} = 52.91 \text{ kmol}$$

Similarly, for each mole of DCA production, two moles of chlorine are consumed.

$$\text{Chlorine utilised for DCA production} = \frac{263 \times 2}{129} = 4.08 \text{ kmol}$$

$$\text{Total chlorine utilised} = 52.91 + 4.08 = 56.99 \text{ kmol}$$

$$\text{Conversion} = \frac{(56.99 \times 100)}{63.89} = 89.2\% \qquad \textit{Ans. (a)}$$

$$\text{Yield of MCA} = \frac{(52.91 \times 100)}{56.99} \; 92.84\% \qquad \textit{Ans. (b)}$$

$$\text{Selectivity of MCA} = \frac{52.91}{4.08} = 12.97 \qquad \textit{Ans. (c)}$$

Example 4.2 Bechamp process is classically known for reduction of nitro compounds to corresponding primary amino compounds using iron in an acidic medium. Orthotoluidine (OT) is manufactured from ortho-nitro toluene (ONT) by Bechamp process.

In a batch of 700 kg ONT, 800 kg iron turnings (containing 90% Fe) and 400 kg water are added. Reaction mixture is heated to 333 K (60°C) and formic acid is added (approx. 6 kg) as a catalyst in batches. The mixture is stirred for about 18 hours and then total mass is allowed to settle in two layers. Upper layer of OT is sucked out by vacuum in a distillation unit where it is purified by vacuum distillation.

Reactions:

$$
\begin{array}{ccc}
4 \times 137 & 9 \times 56 \quad 16 \times 18 & 4 \times 107 \qquad 3 \times 90 \qquad 6 \times 107
\end{array}
$$

$$3 \, Fe(OH)_2 \; + \; 6 \, Fe(OH)_3 \; = \; 3 \, Fe_3O_4 \; + \; 12 \, H_2O$$

$$
\begin{array}{cccc}
3 \times 90 & 3 \times 107 & 3 \times 232 & 12 \times 18
\end{array}
$$

At the end of the batch, 505 kg 99% pure OT is obtained. Assuming 98% completion of reduction, calculate (a) the yield of OT, and (b) excess quantity of iron powder.

Solution Basis: 700 kg ONT charged to reactor

$$\text{OT produced} = 505 \times 0.99 = 500 \text{ kg}$$

$$\text{ONT required} = \frac{4 \times 137 \times 500}{4 \times 107} = 640.2 \text{ kg}$$

$$\text{ONT reacted} = 700 \times 0.98 = 686 \text{ kg}$$

$$\text{Yield of OT} = \frac{640.2 \times 100}{686} = 93.32\% \qquad \textit{Ans. (a)}$$

$$\text{Theoretical iron requirement} = \frac{9 \times 56 \times 700}{4 \times 137} = 643.8 \text{ kg}$$

$$\text{Iron charged} = 800 \times 0.9 = 720 \text{ kg}$$

$$\text{Excess iron} = \frac{(720 - 643.8)\,100}{643.8}$$

$$= 11.84\% \qquad\qquad \textit{Ans. (b)}$$

Note: Many small scale industries use Bechamp process for reduction of nitrocompounds. Recent trend is to use hydrogen for reduction which is available from chlor-alkali plants.

Example 4.3 Chlorobenzene is nitrated using a mixture of nitric acid and sulphuric acid[1]. During the pilot plant studies, a charge consisted of 100 kg chlorobenzene (CB), 106.5 kg 65.5% (by mass) nitric acid, and 108.0 kg 93.6% (by mass) sulphuric acid. After two hours of operaion, the final mixture was analysed. It was found that the final product contained 2% unreacted chlorobenzene. Also, the product distribution was found to be 66% p-nitrochlorobenzene (p-NCB) and 34% o-nitrochlorobenzene (o-NCB).

Calculate: (a) the analysis of charge, (b) the percentage conversion of chlorobenzene, and (c) the composition of the product mixture.

Solution Basis: 100 kg chlorobenzene

The charge consists of chlorobenzene and mixed acid.

$$HNO_3 \text{ in the charge} = 106.5 \times 0.655 = 69.758 \text{ kg}$$

$$H_2SO_4 \text{ in the charge} = 108 \times 0.936 = 101.088 \text{ kg}$$

$$\text{Water in the charge} = 106.5 \times 0.345 + 108.0 \times 0.064 = 43.654 \text{ kg}$$

The analysis of the reactants can be tabulated as shown in Table 4.1.

Table 4.1 Composition of Feed

Component	Molar mass	Charge, kg	Mass %
Chlorobenzene	112.5	100.000	31.80
HNO_3	63.0	69.758	22.18
H_2SO_4	98.0	101.088	32.14
H_2O	18.0	43.654	13.88
Total		314.500	100.00

Ans. (a)

The reactions taking place in the reactor are:

chlorobenzene + HNO₃ (nitric acid) = o-nitrochlorobenzene + H₂O (water)

chlorobenzene + HNO₃ (nitric acid) = p-nitrochlorobenzene + H₂O (water)

As given in the problem, the yield of *p*-NCB is 66%. Since the total charge (mass) remains constant.

$$\text{Unreacted CB in the product} = 314.5 \times 0.02 = 6.29 \text{ kg}$$

$$\text{Amount of CB that has reacted} = 100 - 6.29 = 93.71 \text{ kg}$$

$$\text{Conversion of CB} = \left(\frac{93.71}{100}\right) \times 100 = 93.71\% \qquad \textit{Ans.}(b)$$

Sulphuric acid remain unreacted.

From the reactions, it is clear that,

$$1 \text{ kmol CB} \equiv 1 \text{ kmol HNO}_3$$

$$\equiv 1 \text{ kmol NCB}$$

$$\equiv 1 \text{ kmol H}_2\text{O}$$

Thus, 63 kg HNO_3 will be consumed for converting 112.5 kg CB into NCB (See Table 4.1).

$$\text{Total HNO}_3 \text{ consumed} = \left(\frac{63}{112.5}\right) \times 93.71 = 52.478 \text{ kg}$$

$$\text{Unreacted HNO}_3 = 69.758 - 52.478 = 17.28 \text{ kg}$$

$$\text{Total NCB produced} = \left(\frac{157.5}{112.5}\right) \times 93.71 = 131.194 \text{ kg}$$

$$p\text{-NCB} = 0.66 \times 131.194 = 86.588 \text{ kg}$$

$$o\text{-NCB} = 0.34 \times 131.194 = 44.606 \text{ kg}$$

$$\text{Water produced} = \left(\frac{18}{112.5}\right) \times 93.71 = 14.994 \text{ kg}$$

Total water in the product mixture = 43.654 + 14.994 = 58.648 kg
The final analysis of the products is given in Table 4.2.

Table 4.2   Composition of Product Stream

Component	Mass, kg	Mass %
CB	6.290	2.00
p-NCB	86.588	27.53
o-NCB	44.606	14.18
HNO$_3$	17.280	5.49
H$_2$SO$_4$	101.088	32.15
H$_2$O	58.648	18.65
Total	314.500	100.00

Ans. (c)

Example 4.4 Dehydrogenation of ethanol is a commercial process of manufacturing acetaldehyde[2,3]. Ethyl alcohol vapours are preheated and mixed with air in such a proportion that the exothermic heat of oxidation will just exceed the heat of dehydrogenation. This facilitates the reaction to proceed to dehydrogenation without any external application of heat. The reaction temperature is usually around 720 K (447°C).

Pre-mixed ethanol-air mixture was passed over a silver catalyst. The content of ethanol in the mixture was found to be 2.0 kg ethanol per kg air. The different reactions taking place in the reactor are as follows:

$$CH_3CH_2OH = CH_3CHO + H_2 \qquad (1)$$

$$2\,CH_3CH_2OH + O_2 = 4\,CO + 6\,H_2 \qquad (2)$$

$$2\,CH_3CH_2OH + 3\,O_2 = 4\,CO_2 + 6\,H_2 \qquad (3)$$

$$2\,CH_3CH_2OH + 2\,H_2 = 4\,CH_4 + O_2 \qquad (4)$$

$$2\,H_2 + O_2 = 2\,H_2O \qquad (5)$$

The exit gases from the converter were passed through a scrubber where cold dilute alcohol cools the gases and dissolves both alcohol and acetaldehyde. The stripped gases leaving the scrubber were scrubbed again with water in the second scrubber and released from the system. The dilute alcohol-acetaldehyde solution from the bottom of the first scrubber was sent to a distillation tower to produce 99% pure acetaldehyde as the overhead product. The gases leaving the second scrubber were analysed to contain 0.7% CO_2, 2.1% O_2, 2.3% CO, 7.1% H_2, 2.6% CH_4 and 85.2% N_2 on dry basis (by volume). Find (a) the conversion of ethanol in the converter, and (b) the yield of acetaldehyde.

Solution Basis: 100 kmol of outgoing gases (from second scrubber)

N_2 present in the gases = $100 \times 0.852 = 85.2$ kmol

Nitrogen comes from which remains unchanged during the reactions. For every 79 kmol of N_2, O_2 entering the converter is 21 kmol.

$$O_2 \text{ supplied through air} = \left(\frac{21}{79}\right) \times 85.2 = 22.65 \text{ kmol}$$

The outgoing gases contain 2.1 kmol of O_2.

$$\text{Reacted } O_2 = 22.65 - 2.1 = 20.55 \text{ kmol}$$

Oxygen balance:

[Oxygen consumed by reactions (2), (3) and (5)] –

[Oxygen produced by reaction (4)] = 20.55 kmol

Let a, b and c be the kmol of ethanol reacted by reactions (2), (3) and (4) respectively, Also, let d be the kmol of H_2 reacted by reaction (5). Therefore, oxygen balance will yield:

$$\left(\frac{a}{2}\right) + 1.5b + \left(\frac{d}{2}\right) - \left(\frac{c}{2}\right) = 20.55$$

or $\qquad\qquad\qquad a + 3b - c + d = 41.10 \qquad\qquad (6)$

Balance of carbon monoxide:

$$2a = 2.3 \text{ [reaction (2)] or } a = 1.15 \text{ kmol}$$

Balance of carbon dioxide:

$$2b = 0.7 \text{ [reaction (3)] or b} = 0.35 \text{ kmol}$$

Balance of methane:

$$2c = 2.6 \text{ [reaction (4)] or } c = 1.3 \text{ kmol}$$

Substiuting the values of a, b and c in Eq. (6),

$$d = 41.1 - 1.15 - 1.05 + 1.3 = 40.2 \text{ kmol}$$

Balance of hydrogen:

Total hydrogen produced = Hydrogen is outgoing gases

+ hydrogen reacted by reaction (5)

+ hydrogen reacted by reaction (4)

$$= 7.1 + c + d$$

$$= 7.1 + 1.3 + 40.2$$

$$= 48.6 \text{ kmol}$$

The above hydrogen is produced by reaction (1), (2) and (3).

Therefore, hydrogen produced by reaction (1) = $48.6 - (3 \times 0.35 + 3 \times 1.15)$

$$= 44.1 \text{ kmol}$$

Ethanol reacted by reaction (1) = 44.1 kmol

Total ethanol reacted = $44.1 + 1.15 + 0.35 + 1.3$

$$= 46.9 \text{ kmol} \equiv 2157.4 \text{ kg}$$

Total dry air entering the converter = $85.2 + 22.65$

$$= 107.85 \text{ kmol} \equiv 3127.7 \text{ kg}$$

Total ethanol entering the converter = 2×3127.7

$$= 6255.4 \text{ kg} \equiv 135.99 \text{ kmol}$$

$$\text{Conversion of ethanol} = \left(\frac{\text{total ethanol consumed}}{\text{total ethanol charged}} \right) \times 100$$

$$= \left(\frac{2157.4}{6255.5} \right) \times 100 = 34.49\% \qquad \textit{Ans. (a)}$$

Yield of acetaldehyde =

$$\left(\frac{\text{moles of acetaldehyde produced} \times \text{stoichiometric factor}}{\text{moles of ethanol reacted}} \right) \times 100$$

$$= \left(44.1 \times \frac{1}{46.9} \right) \times 100 = 94.03\%$$

Selectivity of acetaldehyde = $44.1/2.8 = 15.75$ *Ans. (b)*

Example 4.5   The analysis of water (Table 3.3) has been given in Example 3.9. The same water is treated by the lime-soda process. Calculate the theoretical (stoichiometric) amounts of chemicals required for the treatment.

Solution   Basis: 1 L of water

Since the water contains only temporary hardness, only lime addition is required. The reactions of lime with bicarbonates are:

$$Ca(HCO_3)_2 + CaO = 2\ CaCO_3 + H_2O \qquad (1)$$

$$Mg(HCO_3)_2 + CaO = MgCO_3 + CaCO_3 + H_2O \qquad (2)$$

$$2\ NaHCO_3 + CaO = CaCO_3 + Na_2CO_3 + H_2O \qquad (3)$$

From these equations, it is clear that 1 mole of lime is required for each mole of $Ca(HCO_3)_2$ or $Mg(MCO_3)_2$ and for every 2 moles of $NaHCO_3$.

$$56 \text{ mg } CaO \equiv 162 \text{ mg } Ca(HCO_3)_2$$

$$\equiv 146.3 \text{ mg } Mg(HCO_3)_2$$

$$\equiv 2 \times 84 \text{ mg } NaHCO_3$$

$$\text{Total lime required} = \left(\frac{56}{162} \right) \times 257.6 + \left(\frac{56}{146.3} \right) \times 329.2$$

$$+ \left(\frac{56}{168} \right) \times 11.1 = 218.7 \text{ mg}$$

Thus, theoretically, the lime dosage of the order of 218.7 mg/L is required to treat the water. The dosage can be calculated by knowing te bicarbonate alkalinity in terms of equivalent $CaCO_3$.

$$1 \text{ mole } CaCO_3 \equiv 1 \text{ mole } CaO$$

$$100 \text{ mg } CaCO_3 \equiv 56 \text{ mg } CaO$$

$$\text{Lime required} = \left(\frac{56}{100}\right) \times 390.6 = 218.7 \text{ mg/L} \qquad Ans.$$

Note: From the above calculations, it may be seen that the lime requirement can be readily calculated by knowing the total bicarbonate alkalinity (taken to be entirely as $CaCO_3$) alone. Thus, one reason for expressing alkalinity in terms of $CaCO_3$ is the ease in calculations. In actual practice, lime is added in excess by 10 to 50%, depending on the process (hot or cold).

Example 4.6 A fertiliser plant manufactures ammonia using water gas and producer gas as raw materials[4]. The compositions of the gases are given in Table 4.3.

Table 4.3 Analysis of Gases

Component	Analysis, % of by volume	
	Water gas	Producer gas
N_2	2	63
H_2	51	5
CO	43	25
CO_2	4	5
Ar	Nil	2
Total	100	100

Both the gases are mixed in proper proportions to provide a stoichiometric mixture of nitrogen and hydrogen after converting carbon monoxide to carbon dioxide using steam. Calculate: (a) the kmol of water gas and producer gas required to obtain 100 kmol of dry mixed gas, (b) the analysis of dry mixed gas, and (c) the theoretical amount (in kg) of steam required to convert CO to CO_2 per 100 kmol of dry mixed gas.

Solution Basis: 100 kmol dry mixed gas

Let x be the kmol of water gas and y the kmol of producer gas, mixed to obtain 100 kmol of dry mixed gas.

Overall material balance:

$$x + y = 100 \qquad (1)$$

Total carbon monoxide present in the mixed gas = $0.43x + 0.25y$ kmol

The shift reaction is

$$CO + H_2O = CO_2 + H_2$$

Thus, each kmol of CO will give 1 kmol of CO_2 and H_2 each, when it combines with 1 kmol of steam.

Total H_2 formed due to shift reaction = $0.43x + 0.25y$ kmol

Amount of H_2 entering with

$$\text{Water gas and producer gas} = 0.51x + 0.05y \text{ kmol}$$

$$\text{Total } H_2 \text{ after shift reaction} = 0.43x + 0.51x + 0.25y + 0.05y$$

$$= 0.94x + 0.30y \text{ kmol}$$

Amount of N_2 coming with both

$$\text{the gases} = 0.02x + 0.63y \text{ kmol}$$

For ammonia synthesis, the stoichiometric N_2 to H_2 ratio requirement is 1:3. Thus, stoichiometrically, 3(moles of N_2) = moles of H_2, obtained after the shift reaction.

$$3.(0.02x + 0.63y) = 0.94x + 0.30y$$

Simplifying,

$$x = 1.807\, y \tag{2}$$

Solving Eqs. (1) and (2),

$$x = 64.46 \text{ kmol of water gas}$$

$$y = 35.54 \text{ kmol of producer gas} \qquad \textit{Ans. (a)}$$

Using the values of x and y, the analysis of the dry mixed gas can be calculated as shown in Table 4.4.

Table 4.4 Analyses of Gases

Component	Water gas vol.%	Water gas kmol	Producer gas vol.%	Producer gas kmol	Mixed gas kmol	Mixed gas vol.%
N_2	2	1.29	63	22.39	23.68	23.68
H_2	51	32.87	5	1.78	34.65	34.65
CO	43	27.72	25	8.88	36.60	36.60
CO_2	4	2.58	5	1.78	4.36	4.36
Ar	—	—	2	0.71	0.71	0.71
Total	100	64.46	100	35.54	100.00	100.00

Ans. (b)

$$\text{Amount of steam required} = \text{amount of CO converted}$$

$$= 0.43x + 0.25y = 0.43 \times 64.46 + 0.25 \times 35.54$$

$$= 36.6 \text{ kmol or } 658.9 \text{ kg} \qquad \textit{Ans. (c)}$$

As there is no competitive reaction to the shift reaction, yield of hydrogen is 100%. Also the conversion of CO is assumed to be 100%.

Example 4.7 Tallow is essentially glyceryltristearate[5]. It is desired to saponify the tallow with caustic soda. For 100 kg tallow, calculate: (a) the theoretical requirement of caustic soda, and (b) the amount of glycerine liberated.
Solution Basis: 100 kg tallow
The saponification reaction is

$$
\begin{array}{ccccc}
CH_2OOCH_{35}C_{17} & & & & CH_2OH \\
| & & & & | \\
CHOOCH_{35}C_{17} & + & 3\,NaOH & = & 3\,C_{17}CH_{35}COONa & + & CHOH \\
| & & & & | \\
CH_2OOCH_{35}C_{17} & & & & CH_2OH
\end{array}
$$

Glyceryltristearate	Caustic soda	Sodium stearate	Glycerine
890	3×40	3×306	92

$$\text{Caustic soda required} = \left[\frac{3 \times 40}{890}\right] \times 100 = 13.48 \text{ kg} \qquad \textit{Ans. (a)}$$

$$\text{Glycerine liberated} = \left(\frac{92}{890}\right) \times 100 = 10.34 \text{ kg} \qquad \textit{Ans. (b)}$$

Example 4.8 Pure sulphur is burnt in a burner[6] at the rate of 0.3 kg/s. Fresh dry air is supplied at 303 K (30°C) and 100 kPa a (750 torr). The gases from the burner contain 16.5% SO_2, 3% O_2 and rest N_2 on SO_3-free volume basis. The gases leave the burner at 1073 K (800°C) and 101.325 kPa a (760 torr). Calculate: (a) the fraction of sulphur burnt into SO_3, (b) the percentage excess air over the amount required to oxidise the sulphur to SO_2, (c) the volume of dry air in m^3/s, and (d) the volume of burner gases in m^3/s.

Notes: (i)The analysis of sulphur burner gases is always given on SO_3 free basis as SO_3 creates interference in the analysis of the gases. Usually, an Orsat apparatus, with mercury as the working fluid, is used in analysing the gases. (ii) In this example, although a basis of 0.3 kg/s sulphur is given, it would be easier to start solving the problem using a basis of 100 kmol of SO_3 free burner gases

Solution Basis: 100 kmol SO_3 free gases
The gases contain 16.5 kmol SO_2, 3.0 kmol O_2 and 80.5 kmol N_2. The reactions taking place in the burner are:

$$S + O_2 = SO_2 \qquad (1)$$

$$S + \frac{3}{2} O_2 = SO_3 \qquad (2)$$

Based on Eq. (1),

O_2 required to form 16.5 kmol SO_2 = 16.5 kmol

$$\text{Total } O_2 \text{ supplied to the burner} = \left(\frac{21}{79}\right) \times 80.2 = 21.32 \text{ kmol}$$

$$\text{Unaccounted } O_2 = 21.32 - (16.5 + 3.0) = 1.82 \text{ kmol}$$

Thus 1.82 kmol O_2 have been consumed as per Eq. (2).

$$SO_3 \text{ produced} = \left(\frac{2}{3}\right) \times 1.82 = 1.21 \text{ kmol}$$

Sulphur burnt into SO_2 = 16.5 kmol

Sulphur burnt into SO_3 = 1.21 kmol

Total sulphur burnt in the burner = 16.5 + 1.21 = 17.71 kmol

$$\text{Mass of sulphur burnt} = 17.71 \times 32 = 566.7 \text{ kg}$$

$$\text{Fraction of S burnt to } SO_3 = \frac{1.21}{17.71} = 0.0683 \qquad \textit{Ans. (a)}$$

Now, if all sulphur would have been burnt into SO_2, O_2 requirement would have been 17.71 kmol [Eq. (1)].

$$\text{Excess } O_2 = 21.32 - 17.71 = 3.61 \text{ kmol}$$

$$\text{Percentage excess air} = \left(\frac{3.61}{17.71}\right) \times 100 = 20.38 \qquad \textit{Ans. (b)}$$

$$\text{Air supplied to the burner} = 21.32 + 80.5 = 101.82 \text{ kmol}$$

However, the actual charge to the burner is 0.3 kg/s.

$$\text{Air supply rate} = \left(\frac{101.82}{566.7}\right) \times 0.3 = 0.054 \text{ kmol/s}$$

$$\text{Specific volume of incoming fresh air} = 22.414 \times \left(\frac{303}{273}\right) \times \left(\frac{100}{101.325}\right)$$

$$= 24.55 \text{ m}^3/\text{kmol}$$

Volumetric flow rate of fresh air = $0.054 \times 24.55 = 1.326$ m³/s   *Ans.* (c)

For a basis of 100 kmol SO₃-free gases,

$$\text{Total gases from burner} = 100 + 1.21 = 101.21 \text{ kmol}$$

For 0.3 kg/s sulphur charge, Total gas = $\left(\frac{101.21 \times 0.3}{566.7}\right) = 0.0536$ kmol/s

$$\text{Specific volume of burner gases} = 22.414 \times \left(\frac{1073}{273}\right) = 88.1 \text{ m}^3/\text{kmol}$$

Volumetric flow rate of burner gases = $88.1 \times 0.0536 = 4.722$ m³/s   *Ans.* (d)

Example 4.9 Refined soybean oil is hydrogenated at 2 bar g and 453 K (180°C) in an autoclave to produce 'Vanaspati' (hydrogenated fat) in presence of nickel catalyst. Reaction was considered complete when product's slip melting point was recorded 312 K (39°C). Samples of refined soybean oil and hardened (hydrogenated) fat were chromatographically analysed and found to contain following fatty acids.

Table 4.5 Composition of Edible Oil and Fat

Fatty acid	Refined Soybean oil mass %	Hardened fat mass%
Palmitic acid	11.1	11.0
Stearic acid	3.8	14.6
Oleic acid	27.3	71.8
Linoleic acid	51.1	2.6
Linolenic acid	6.7	Nil

Calculate: (a) theoretical hydrogen requirement for complete saturation, (b) actual hydrogen requirement, and (c) Iodine values (IV) of refined oil and hardened fat.

Note: Iodine value is defined as kg of iodine absorbed by 100 kg oil or fat.

Solution:
Basis: 100 kg soya fatty acids

Table 4.6 Composition of Soybean Fatty Acids

Fatty acid	kg	Molar mass	kmol
Plamitic acid	11.1	256.42	0.0433
Stearic acid	3.8	284.48	0.0134
Oleic acid	27.3	282.46	0.0967
Linoleic acid	51.1	280.45	0.1822
Linolenic acid	6.7	278.43	0.0241
Total	100.0		0.3597

Average molar mass of fatty acids $= \dfrac{100}{0.3597}$

$$= 278.00$$

All the fatty acids are in triglyceride form which is known as oil. When 3 moles of fatty acids react with 1 mole of glycerol (molar mass $= 92.09$), one mole of triglyceride and three moles of water are produced.

Average molar mass of Soybean oil $= 278.0 \times 3 + 92.09 - 3 \times 18.02$

$$= 872.03$$

Quantity of soybean oil $= \dfrac{872.03 \times 100}{278.00 \times 3}$

$$= 104.56 \text{ kg}$$

In other words if 104.56 kg soybean oil is split, 100 kg fatty acids (of analysis given in Table 4.5) and 11.04 kg glycerol will be obtained. When oil is hydrogenated, unsaturated fatty acids (oleic, linoleic and linolenic) will be saturated.

Reactions are as follows.

$$CH_3 (CH_2)_7 \; CH{:}CH(CH_2)_7 \; COOH + H_2 = CH_3(CH_2)_{16} \; COOH$$

Oleic acid   Stearic acid

(9- octadecenoic acid)   (octadecanoic acid)

$$CH_3(CH_2)_4 \; CH : CHCH_2 \; CH : CH \; (CH_2)_7 COOH + 2\,H_2 = CH_3(CH_2)_{16} \; COOH$$

Linoleic acid   Stearic acid

(9,12- octadecadienoic acid)   (octadecanoic acid)

$$CH_3CH_2CH : CHCH_2 \; CH : CHCH_2 \; CH : CH \; (CH_2)_7 \; COOH + 3\,H_2$$

$$= CH_3(CH_2)_{16} \; COOH$$

Linolenic acid   Stearic acid

(9,12,15- octadecatrienoic acid)   (octadecanoic acid)

Based on above reactions.

theoretical H_2 requirement $= 0.0967 + 0.1822 \times 2 + 0.241 \times 3$

$$= 0.5334 \text{ kmol/100 kg soy fatty acid}$$

$$\equiv 0.5101 \text{ kmol/ 100 kg soybean oil}$$

$$\equiv 11.434 \text{ Nm}^3/100 \text{ kg soybean oil} \qquad \textit{Ans.} \text{ (a)}$$

In actual practice, refined oil is partially hydrogenated for edible purpose. Hardened fat does not contain any linolenic acid and hence assume its full conversion to oleic acid. Let x kg linoleic acid gets converted to oleic acid and y kg oleic acid gets converted to stearic acid.

Oleic acid production due to conversion of linolenic acid

$$= \dfrac{282.46}{278.43} \times 6.7 = 6.797 \text{ kg}$$

Oleic acid production due to conversion of linoleic acid

$$= \dfrac{282.46}{280.45} \times x = 1.007\,17\,x \text{ kg}$$

Stearic acid production due to conversion of oleic acid

$$= \dfrac{284.48}{282.46} \times y$$

$$= 1.007\,15\,y \text{ kg}$$

Oleic acid remaining after partial hydrogenation

$$= 27.3 + 6.797 + 1.007\,17x - y$$

$$= 34.097 + 1.007\,17x - y \text{ kg}$$

Fatty acids after partial hydrogenation:

         Palmitic acid   11.1 kg

           Stearic acid $3.8 + 1.007\ 15\ y$ kg

            Oleic acid $34.097 + 1.007\ 17x - y$ kg

           Linoleic acid $51.1 - x$ kg

                 Total $100.097 + 0.007\ 17x + 0.007\ 15\ y$

Based on analysis given in Table 4.5;

Stearic acid balance:

$$\frac{3.8 + 1.007\ 15y}{100.097 + 0.007\ 17x + 0.007\ 15y} = 0.146$$

or $-0.001\ 05x + 1.006\ 11y = 10.8142$ (1)

Linoleic acid balance:

$$\frac{51.1 - x}{100.097 + 0.007\ 17x + 0.007\ 15y} = 0.026$$

or $1.000\ 19x + 0.000\ 19\ y = 48.4975$ (2)

Solving Eqs. (1) and (2).

                       $x = 48.5$ kg, $y = 10.8$ kg

Table 4.7   Composition of Hardened Fat

Fatty acid	kg	mass %	kmol	H_2 requirement kmol
Palmitic acid	11.10	10.94	0.0433	–
Stearic acid	14.68	14.60	0.0516	–
Oleic acid	72.14	71.77	0.2554	0.2554
Linoleic acid	2.60	2.59	0.0093	0.0186
Total	100.52	100.00	0.3596	0.2740

Average molar mass of fatty acids in hardened fat $= \dfrac{100.52}{0.3596} = 279.53$

Average molar mass of hardened fat $= 279.53 \times 3 + 92.09 - 3 \times 18.02$

                                     $= 876.62$

          Quantity of hardened fat $= \dfrac{876.62 \times 100.52}{279.53 \times 3}$

                                $= 105.08$ kg/100 kg soya fatty acids

                                $\equiv 100.5$ kg/100 kg soybean oil

H_2 requirement of hardened fat $= 0.274$ kmol for full saturation

Net hydrogen requirement for partial hydrogenation

                         $= 0.5334 - 0.274$

                         $= 0.2594$ kmol/ 100 kg soya fatty acids

                         $\equiv 0.248$ kmol/100 kg soybean oil

                         $\equiv 5.561$ Nm^3/100 kg soybean oil

                         $\equiv 55.61$ Nm^3/t soybean oil   *Ans.* (b)

Iodine reacts with unsaturated fatty acids in the same locations as shown for hydrogenation reactions. Molar mass of iodine = 253.81

For soybean oil:

$$\text{Iodine consumption} = 0.5334 \text{ kmol } I_2/100 \text{ kg soya fatty acids}$$
$$\equiv 0.5101 \text{ kmol } I_2/100 \text{ kg soybean oil}$$
$$\text{Iodine value (IV)} \equiv 129.5 \text{ kg } I_2/100 \text{ kg soybean oil}$$

Ans. (c-i)

For hardened fat,

$$\text{Iodine consumption} = 0.274 \text{ kmol}/100.52 \text{ kg fat}$$
$$\equiv 0.2726 \text{ kmol}/100 \text{ kg fat}$$
$$\text{Iodine value (IV)} \equiv 69.2 \text{ kg } I_2/100 \text{ kg fat} \qquad \textit{Ans.} \text{ (c-ii)}$$

Note: Iodine value (IV) is a good indication of unsaturation of fatty acids / oils. It can be determined experimentally easily and hence offers a quick quality check of fatty acids/oils. For the same slip melting point of 312 K (39°C), there can be variation in IV, indicating quality of hydrogenation. For instance, if for the above example, experimentally IV is found higher than 69.2, it indicates presence of more of linoleic or linolenic acid which may not be desirable.

Example 4.10 In the Formox process, a mixture of metal oxides, consisting of Fe, Mo and V, is used as a catalyst for partial oxidation of methanol to formaldehyde[7]. Different reactions taking place in the reactor are as follows.

$$CH_3OH + \frac{1}{2} O_2 = HCHO + H_2O \qquad (1)$$

$$CH_3OH + \frac{3}{2} O_2 = CO_2 + 2 H_2O \qquad (2)$$

$$CH_3OH = CO + 2 H_2 \qquad (3)$$

$$CH_3OH = CH_4 + \frac{1}{2} O_2 \qquad (4)$$

$$2 CH_3OH = (CH_3)_2O + H_2O \qquad (5)$$

Methanol feed is passed through a steam heated evaporator. Ambient air, containing 0.011 kg moisture/kg dry air, is heated by product gas stream, leaving the reactor, and mixed with methanol vapours in a static mixer.

The gaseous feed, containing 8.4% methanol (by volume on wet basis), employs excess air and is a flammable mixture. It is passed at 170 kPa through catalyst-filled tubes in a heat exchanging type reactor. Dowtherm - A circulates outside the tubes and removes the heat of reaction. Reactions take place isothermally at 613 K (340°C). Steam is generated at 6 bar a in a waste heat boiler (WHB) by condensing Dowtherm-A vapours. Gas mixture from the reactor is cooled to 383 K (110°C) in a heat exchanger by heating incoming air.

The gas mixture then enters the bottom of the absorber. Formaldehyde concentration at the bottom of the absorber is controlled at 37% (by mass) by fresh water, entering at the top at 303 K (30°C.) A forced circulation cooler for the bottom solution maintains formaldehyde solution to 323 K (50°C). Tail gas leaves the absorber at 120 kPa a and 323 K (50°C) at the top.

Assume 99% conversion of methanol with 90% yield to formalehyde. Based on kinetic considerations, reactions (2) to (5) consume 71%, 8%, 5% and 16% respectively of 10% methanol yield.

Make complete material balance of the plant for a methanol feed rate of 4000 kg/h.

Solution

Basis: Methanol feed rate of 4000 kg/h

$$\text{Molar feed rate of methanol} = \frac{4000}{32} = 125 \text{ kmol/h}$$

Concentration of methanol in the gaseous mixture to reactor is 8.4% by volume.

$$\text{Gaseous mixture flow rate} = \frac{125}{0.084}$$
$$= 1488.1 \text{ kmol/h}$$

$$\text{Flow of ambient (wet) air} = 1488.1 - 125$$
$$= 1363.1 \text{ kmol/h.}$$

Moisture content of ambient air = 0.011 kg/kg dry air

$$\equiv 0.011 \times \frac{29}{18}$$
$$\equiv 0.017\ 72 \text{ kmol/kmol dry ar.}$$

$$\text{Dry air flow rate} = \frac{1363.1}{(1 + 0.017\ 72)}$$
$$= 1339.37 \text{ kmol/h}$$

$$O_2 \text{ supply rate} = 1339.37 \times 0.21 = 281.27 \text{ kmol/h}$$

$$N_2 \text{ supply rate} = 1339.37 - 281.27 = 1058.10 \text{ kmol/h}$$

$$\text{Moisture, entering with air} = 1363.1 - 1339.37 = 23.73 \text{ kmol/h}$$

Table 4.8 Composition of Gaseous Mixture Entering Reactor

Component	n_i kmol/h	Mole %
CH_3OH	125.00	8.40
O_2	281.27	18.90
N_2	1058.10	71.10
H_2O	23.73	1.60
Total	1488.10	100.00

$$\text{Conversion of methanol} = 99\%$$
$$\text{Total methanol reacted} = 125 \times 0.99$$
$$= 123.75 \text{ kmol/h}$$
$$\text{Unreacted methanol} = 125.00 - 123.75$$
$$= 1.25 \text{ kmol/h}$$

Reaction (1):

$$\text{Methanol reacted} = 123.75 \times 0.9 = 111.375 \text{ kmol/h}$$
$$\text{HCHO produced} = 111.375 \text{ kmol/h}$$
$$O_2 \text{ consumed} = 111.375/2 = 55.688 \text{ kmol/h}$$
$$H_2O \text{ produced} = 111.375 \text{ kmol/h.}$$

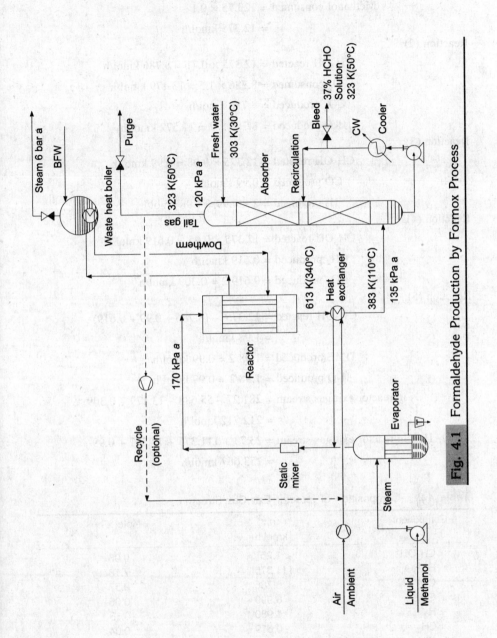

Fig. 4.1 Formaldehyde Production by Formox Process

Reaction (2) to (5):

$$\text{Methanol consumed} = 123.75 \times 0.1$$
$$= 12.375 \text{ kmol/h}$$

Reaction (2):

$$\text{CH}_3\text{OH reacted} = 12.375 \times 0.71 = 8.786 \text{ kmol/h}$$
$$\text{O}_2 \text{ consumed} = 8.786 \times 1.5 = 13.179 \text{ kmol/h}$$
$$\text{CO}_2 \text{ produced} = 8.786 \text{ kmol/h}$$
$$\text{H}_2\text{O produced} = 8.786 \times 2 = 17.572 \text{ kmol/h}$$

Reaction (3):

$$\text{CH}_3\text{OH reacted} = 12.375 \times 0.08 = 0.99 \text{ kmol/h}$$
$$\text{CO produced} = 0.99 \text{ kmol/h}$$
$$\text{H}_2 \text{ produced} = 2 \times 0.99 = 1.98 \text{ kmol/h}$$

Reaction (4):

$$\text{CH}_3\text{OH reacted} = 12.375 \times 0.05 = 0.619 \text{ kmol/h}$$
$$\text{CH}_4 \text{ produced} = 0.619 \text{ kmol/h}$$
$$\text{O}_2 \text{ produced} = 0.619/2 = 0.309 \text{ kmol/h}$$

Reaction (5):

$$\text{CH}_3\text{OH reacted} = 12.375 - (8.786 + 0.99 + 0.619)$$
$$= 1.98 \text{ kmol/h}$$
$$\text{DME produced} = 1.98/2 = 0.99 \text{ kmol/h}$$
$$\text{H}_2\text{O produced} = 1.98/2 = 0.99 \text{ kmol/h}$$
$$\text{O}_2 \text{ in reactor exit gas stream} = 281.27 - 55.688 - 13.179 + 0.309$$
$$= 212.712 \text{ kmol/h}$$
$$\text{H}_2\text{O in reactor exit gas stream} = 23.73 + 111.375 + 17.572 + 0.99$$
$$= 153.667 \text{ kmol/h}$$

Table 4.9 Composition of Reactor Exit Gas Stream

Component	n_i kmol/h	Mole %
CH_3OH	1.25	0.08
HCHO	111.375	7.18
CO_2	8.786	0.57
CO	0.990	0.06
H_2	1.980	0.13
CH_4	0.619	0.04
$(CH_3)_2O$	0.990	0.06
O_2	212.712	13.72
N_2	1058.100	68.25
H_2O	153.667	9.91
Total	1550.469	100.00

In the exit gas stream, CO_2 CO, H_2, CH_4 and $(CH_3)_2O$ are undesired components (UC).

$$UC \text{ in exit gas stream} = 8.786 + 0.99 + 1.98 + 0.619 + 0.99.$$

$$= 13.365 \text{ kmol/h}$$

At the top of the absorber, fresh water is introduced and hence it is safe to assume that negligible quantities of methanol and formaldehyde will escape.

$$p_w \text{ at } 323.15 \text{ K } (50°C) = 12.335 \text{ kPa (Refer Table 6.8)}$$

$$\text{Moisture content of tail gas} = \frac{12.335}{(120 - 12.335)}$$

$$= 0.1146 \frac{\text{kmol}}{\text{kmol dry gas}}$$

$$\text{Dry tail gas mixture} = 1550.469 - (1.25 + 111.375 + 153.667)$$
$$= 1284.177 \text{ kmol}$$

$$\text{Moisture in tail gas} = 1284.177 \times 0.1146 = 147.167 \text{ kmol/h}$$

$$\equiv 2649 \text{ kg/h}$$

Table 4.10 Composition of Tail Gas

Component	n_i kmol		Mole%	
	Dry	Wet	Dry	Wet
UC	13.365	13.365	1.04	0.93
O_2	212.712	212.712	16.56	14.86
N_2	1058.100	1058.100	82.40	73.92
H_2O	–	147.167	–	10.29
Total	1284.177	1431.344	100.00	100.00

Material balance across absorber:
Bottom solution contains formaldehydehyde and water.

$$\text{HCHO in bottom solution} = 111.375 \times 30 = 3341.25 \text{ kg/h}$$

$$\text{Concentration of HCHO} = 37\% \text{ by mass}$$

$$\text{Solution withdrawl rate} = \frac{3341.25}{0.37}$$

$$= 9030.4 \text{ kg/h}$$

$$CH_3OH \text{ in bottom solution} = 1.25 \times 32 = 40 \text{ kg/h}$$

$$\text{Water in bottom solution} = 9030.4 - (3341.25 + 40)$$

$$= 5649.15 \text{ kg/h}$$

Gases enter the absorber at 135 kPa a and 110°C.

$$\text{Moisture entering the absorber} = 153.667 \times 18$$

$$= 2766.0 \text{ kg/h}$$

Fresh water added at the top of the absorber

$$= 2649 + 5649.15 - 2766.0$$

$$= 5532.15 \text{ kg/h} \qquad \textit{Ans.}$$

Example 4.11 Pyrites fines are roasted in a chamber plant for making sulphuric acid. The reaction taking place in the burner is

$$4\,FeS_2 + 11\,O_2 = 2\,Fe_2O_3 + 8\,SO_2$$

The gases leaving the roaster have the composition 7.12% SO_2, 10.6% O_2 and rest N_2 on SO_3-free volume basis. The temperature and pressure of the gases are 798 K (525°C) and 100 kPa a (750 torr) respectively. Pyrites contain 42% sulphur and rest inerts (majority Fe and rest gangue). The refuse in the roaster (cinder) carried 2.3% S in the form of SO_3. Dry air is supplied for roasting the pyrites at 300 K (27°C) and 100 kPa a (750 torr).

The gases pass through a catalytic converter where 96% of SO_2 gets converted to SO_3. Gases from the converter are passed through an absorber where 98% SO_3 is absorbed. Based on the charge of 4 kg/s of pyrites, calculate: (a) percentage of sulphur that remained in the cinder based on the original charge, (b) percentage of burnt-up sulphur leaving the roaster as SO_3 in the gases, (c) volumetric flow rate of air in m^3/s, (d) volumetirc flow rate of roaster gases in m^3/s, (e) analysis of the gases leaving the SO_3 converter, and (f) amount of sulphuric acid produced per day assuming 98% strength for the acid from the absorber.

Solution Basis: 100 kg pyrites
The pyrites contain 42 kg sulphur and 58 inerts.
It may be noted from the problem statement that during roasting not only SO_2 is formed but some pyrites get converted to SO_3 also. The reactions are:

$$4\,FeS_2 + 11\,O_2 = 2\,Fe_2O_3 + 8\,SO_2 \tag{1}$$

$$4\,FeS_2 + 15\,O_2 = 2\,Fe_2O_3 + 8\,SO_3 \tag{2}$$

Some SO_3 is absorbed in the form of basic sulphur in the cinder and the rest escapes through the roaster exhaust. From the above two reactions, it is clear that:

$$8 \text{ moles of } SO_2 \text{ or } SO_3 \equiv 2 \text{ moles of } Fe_2O_3$$

$$8 \text{ moles of } S \equiv 3 \text{ moles of } O_2 \text{ in } Fe_2O_3$$

Thus, the amount of O_2

$$\text{combined to form } Fe_2O_3 = \left[\frac{3\times32}{8\times32}\right] \times 42 = 15.75 \text{ kg}$$

This O_2 and other inerts will be in the cinder.

$$\text{Mass of } SO_3\text{- free cinder} = 58 + 15.75 = 73.75 \text{ kg}$$

Now, 100 kg cinder contains 2.3 kg sulphur.

$$\text{Equivalent } SO_3 = \left(\frac{2.3}{32}\right) \times 80 = 5.75 \text{ kg}$$

$$SO_3\text{- free cinder} = 100 - 5.75 = 94.25 \text{ kg}$$

Thus, for 94.25 kg SO_3-free cinder, 100 kg is the actual amount of cinder. Therefore, for 73.75 kg SO_3-free cinder,

$$\text{Actual amount of cinder} = \left(\frac{100}{94.25}\right) \times 73.75 = 78.25 \text{ kg}$$

$$\text{Sulphur in the cinder} = 78.25 \times 0.023 = 1.8 \text{ kg}$$

Thus, out of 42 kg S in the pyrites, 1.8 kg S is retained in the cinder in the form of SO_3.

Percentage of sulphur that remained

in the cinder on the basis of original charge $= \left(\frac{1.8}{42}\right) \times 100 = 4.29$ *Ans.* (a)

For finding out SO_3 content of roaster gas, oxygen balance is required. For these calculations, assume a new basis of 100 kmol of SO_3 – free roaster gases.

Amount of SO_2 in the roaster gases = 7.12 kmol

Amount of O_2 present in SO_2 = 7.12 kmol

Amount of O_2 in the gases (as such) = 10.6 kmol

Amount of N_2 in the roaster gases = 100 – (7.12 + 10.6) = 82.28 kmol

Amount of O_2 entering the

roaster along with $N_2 = \left(\frac{21}{79}\right) \times 82.28 = 21.88$ kmol

With the formation of SO_2, Fe gets converted to Fe_2O_3.

Therefore, O_2 in the cinder (in the form of Fe_2O_3) equivalent to SO_2 of the gases

$$= \left(\frac{3}{8}\right) \times 7.12 = 2.67 \text{ kmol}$$

Total O_2 accounted for = 7.12 + 10.60 + 2.67 = 20.39 kmol

Unaccounted O_2 = 21.88 – 20.39 = 1.49 kmol

According to Eq. (2), 8 kmol of SO_3 are formed for 15 kmol of O_2 consumed.

$$SO_3 \text{ formed} = \left(\frac{8}{15}\right) \times 1.49 = 0.795 \text{ kmol}$$

Sulphur in SO_2 = 7.12 kmol

Sulphur in SO_3 = 0.795 kmol

Total sulphur burnt = 7.12 + 0.795 = 7.915 kmol

Percentage of S roasted to $SO_3 = \left(\frac{0.795}{7.915}\right) \times 100 = 10.04$

However, it was found that 4.29% of the sulphur, charged to the roaster, was retained in the cinder.

Hence, Percentage of S going in

the roaster gas as SO_3 = 10.04 – 4.29 = 5.75%   *Ans.* (b)

SO_3 going into the roaster gases $= 0.795 \times \left(\frac{5.75}{10.04}\right) = 0.455$ kmol

The above data are calculated on the basis of the charge of 100 kmol SO_3-free roaster gases.

Now, again take the original basis of 100 kg pyrites. Out of 42 kg of S, the roasting of S to SO_2 is 37.78 kg (i.e., 89.96%) and the roasting of S to SO_3 is 4.22 kg (i.e., 10.04%).

$$SO_2 \text{ formed} = \left(\frac{37.78}{32}\right) = 1.181 \text{ kmol}$$

It is known that for 7.12 kmol of SO_2 in the roaster gas,

Air supplied = 82.28 + 21.88 = 104.16 kmol

For 1.181 kmol SO_2,

$$\text{Air supply} = \left(\frac{104.16}{7.12}\right) \times 1.181 = 17.28 \text{ kmol}$$

However, it is desired to roast 4 kg/s pyrites.

$$\text{Total air supplied} = \left(\frac{17.28 \times 4}{100}\right) = 0.6912 \text{ kmol/s}$$

$$\text{Specific volume of entering air} = 22.414 \times \left(\frac{100}{101.325}\right) \times \left(\frac{300}{273}\right)$$

$$= 24.309 \text{ m}^3/\text{kmol}$$

Volumetric flow rate of air = $24.309 \times 0.6912 = 16.802 \text{ m}^3/\text{s}$ \hfill *Ans.* (c)

Total roaster gases will be 100.455 kmol for 100 kmol of SO_3- free gases or for 104.16 kmol air supply.

Thus, for 0.6912 kmol air supply,

$$\text{Roaster gases} = \frac{(100.455 \times 0.6912)}{104.16} = 0.6666 \text{ kmol/s}$$

$$\text{Specific volume of roaster gases} = 22.414 \times \left(\frac{100}{101.325}\right) \times \left(\frac{798}{273}\right)$$

$$= 64.661 \text{ m}^3/\text{kmol}$$

Volumetric flow rate of roaster gases = $64.661 \times 0.6666 = 43.1 \text{ m}^3/\text{s}$ \hfill *Ans.* (d)

In the converter, SO_2 gets converted to SO_3 as per the reaction,

$$2SO_2 + O_2 = 2SO_3 \tag{3}$$

$$\text{Total } SO_2 \text{ entering the converter} = \frac{(7.12 \times 0.6666)}{100.455}$$

$$= 4.725 \times 10^{-2} \text{ kmol/s}$$

Since the conversion efficiency is 96%,

$$SO_2 \text{ converted to } SO_3 = 4.725 \times 10^{-2} \times 0.96 = 4.536 \times 10^{-2} \text{ kmol/s}$$

$$\text{Unconverted } SO_2 = (4.725 - 4.536)10^{-2}$$

$$= 1.89 \times 10^{-3} \text{ kmol/s}$$

$$\text{Amount of } O_2 \text{ consumed} = (4.536 \times 10^{-2})/2 = 2.268 \times 10^{-2} \text{ kmol/s}$$

Amount of O_2 in the gases   entering the converter

$$= \frac{(0.6666 \times 10.60)}{100.455} = 7.034 \times 10^{-2} \text{ kmol/s}$$

$$\text{Unreacted } O_2 = 7.034 \times 10^{-2} - 2.268 \times 10^{-2}$$

$$= 4.766 \times 10^{-2} \text{ kmol/s}$$

$$SO_3 \text{ formed} = 4.536 \times 10^{-2} \text{ kmol/s}$$

$$SO_3 \text{ entering the converter} = \left(\frac{0.455}{100.455}\right) \times 0.6666 = 3.019 \times 10^{-3} \text{ kmol/s}$$

$$\text{Total } SO_3 \text{ leaving the converter} = 4.536 \times 10^{-2} + 3.019 \times 10^{-3}$$

$$= 4.838 \times 10^{-2} \text{ kmol/s}$$

$$N_2 \text{ in the gases} = \left(\frac{82.28}{100.455}\right) \times 0.6666 = 0.546 \text{ kmol/s}$$

The analysis of the gases in given in Table 4.11.

Table 4.11 Composition of Converter Gases

Component	Inlet gas		Outlet gas	
	kmol/s	Volume %	kmol/s	Volume %
SO_2	4.725×10^{-2}	7.09	1.89×10^{-3}	0.29
O_2	7.034×10^{-2}	10.55	4.766×10^{-2}	7.41
SO_3	3.019×10^{-3}	0.45	4.838×10^{-2}	7.51
N_2	0.546	81.91	0.546	84.79
Total	0.6666	100.00	0.6439	100.00

Amount of SO_3 absorbed in the absorber = $4.838 \times 10^{-2} \times 0.98$

$$= 4.741 \times 10^{-2} \text{ kmol/s}$$

Absorption reaction is

$$SO_3 + H_2O = H_2SO_4 \tag{4}$$

Amount of H_2SO_4 produced = 4.741×10^{-2} kmol/s of 100% strength

Amount of 98% acid strength = $\dfrac{\left(4.741 \times 10^{-2} \times 98 \times 24 \times 3600\right)}{(0.98 \times 1000)}$

$$= 409.64 \text{ t/d} \qquad\qquad \textit{Ans. (f)}$$

Note: It may be noted that the bases for calculations were changed thrice in this example. This is required in many problems. However, all the different bases should not be confused with one another. For this reason the different bases should be clearly underlined while solving such problems.

Example 4.12 A mixture of pyrites and zinc sulphide ore is burnt in a burner. The mixture contains 75% pyrites and 25% zinc sulphide ore. The pyrites yield 92% FeS_2 and rest gangue. The zinc sulphide ore contains 68% ZnS and rest inerts. A sample of cinder yields 3.5% S. 70% of S in the cinder in the form of SO_3, absorbed in it, and the rest is unoxidised FeS_2. All percentages are by mass. Based on 100 kg of mixed charge, calculate: (a) the amount of cinder formed with its analyses, and (b) the percentage of the sulphur left in the cinder based on the total sulphur charged.

Solution Basis: 100 kg mixed charge
The charge consists of 75 kg pyrites and 25 kg zinc sulphide ore.
Pyrites: $\qquad\qquad\qquad FeS_2 = 75 \times 0.92 = 69$ kg

$$\text{Gangue} = 75 - 69 = 6 \text{ kg}$$

The roasting reactions are

$$4 FeS_2 + 11 O_2 = 2 Fe_2O_3 + 8 SO_2 \tag{1}$$

$$4 FeS_2 + 15 O_2 = 2 Fe_2O_3 + 8 SO_3 \tag{2}$$

Zince ore: $\qquad\qquad\qquad ZnS = 25 \times 0.68 = 17.0$ kg

$$\text{Inerts} = 25 - 17 = 8 \text{ kg}$$

The roasting reaction is

$$2 Zns + 3O_2 = 2 ZnO + 2 SO_2 \tag{3}$$

$$\text{Total inerts} = 8 + 6 = 14 \text{ kg}$$

Now assume a new basis of 100 kg cinder. It contains. 3.5% sulphur.

$$\text{Sulphur in the form of } SO_3 = 3.5 \times 0.7 = 2.45 \text{ kg}$$

$$\text{Sulphur in the form of } FeS_2 = 3.5 - 2.45 = 1.05 \text{ kg}$$

$$\text{Amount of } SO_3 \text{ in the cinder} = \left(\frac{2.45}{32}\right) \times 80 = 6.125 \text{ kg}$$

$$\text{Amount of } FeS_2 \text{ in the cinder} = \left(\frac{120}{64}\right) \times 1.05 = 1.969 \text{ kg}$$

$$\text{Sulphur compound-free cinder} = 100 - (6.125 + 1.969) = 91.906 \text{ kg}$$

This 91.906 kg comprises Fe_2O_3, ZnO and inerts. Now, for the original charge of 100 kg mixed feed,

$$ZnO = \left(\frac{81.4}{97.4}\right) \times 17 = 14.2 \text{ kg}$$

Let x be the weight of FeS_2 reacted.

$$\text{Unreacted } FeS_2 = (69 - x) \text{ kg}$$

$$\text{Amount of } Fe_2O_3 \text{ produced} = \frac{x \times 160}{120 \times 2} = 0.667\,x \text{ kg}$$

$$\text{Total S-free cinder} = 14.2 + 0.667\,x + 14$$

$$= 28.2 + 0.667x \text{ kg}$$

$$\text{Thus, } \frac{FeS_2 \text{ in cinder}}{\text{S - free cinder}} = \frac{(69 - x)}{(28.2 + 0.667x)}$$

But, this ratio is 1.969/91.906 as calculated before.

$$\frac{(69 - x)}{(28.2 + 0.667x)} = \frac{1.969}{91.906}$$

or

$$x = 67.43 \text{ kg}$$

$$\text{S-free cinder} = 14.2 + 0.667 \times 67.43 + 14 = 73.18 \text{ kg}$$

$$FeS_2 \text{ in the cinder} = 69 - 67.43 = 1.57 \text{ kg}$$

$$SO_3 \text{ in the cinder} = \left(\frac{6.125}{91.906}\right) 73.18 = 4.88 \text{ kg}$$

$$Fe_2O_3 \text{ produced} = 0.667\,x = 44.98 \text{ kg}$$

The composition of the cinder formed is given in Table 4.12.

Table 4.12 Composition of Cinder

Component	Cinder	
	kg	mass %
ZnO	14.20	17.83
Fe_2O_3	44.98	56.49
S as FeS_2	1.57	1.97
S as SO_3	4.88	6.13
Inerts	14.00	17.58
Total	79.63	100.00

Ans. (a)

$$\text{Sulphur charge in the burner} = \text{S in } FeS_2 + \text{S in Zns}$$

$$= \left(\frac{64}{120}\right) \times 69 + \left(\frac{32}{97.4}\right) \times 17 = 42.385 \text{ kg}$$

Amount of S in the cinder = $0.035 \times 79.63 = 2.787$ kg

Percentage of sulphur left in the cinder with respect to the total

sulphur charged to the burner = $\left(\dfrac{2.787}{42.385}\right) \times 100 = 6.58$ *Ans.* (b)

4.6 ELECTROCHEMICAL REACTIONS

Electrochemistry is an important branch of chemistry. The chlor-alkali industry, aluminium industry, copper industry, etc. are the typical examples of electro-chemical industries.

In an electrochemical cell, the amount of an electrolyte liberated depends on the current and time. Theoretically, the amount of current required to liberate 1 g eq of an electrolye at each pole is the *faraday* (F), which is equal to 96 485.309 coulombs/mol.

1 coulomb = 1 ampere.second

In actual practice, 1 faraday will liberate less than 1 g eq electrolyte. The ratio of the theoretical faraday consumption to the actual faraday consumption is defined as the current efficiency of the cell.

It may be noted that in electrochemical reactions, only the current is impor-tant for the liberation of the electrolyte. Hence, in most electrolytic cells, for maximum utilisation of the power, the vlotage is kept as low as possible while the current is kept to its maximum.

Example 4.13 In an electrochemical cell, the current is passed at the rate of 1130 amperes for 18 000 s through a solution containing copper sulphate. At the end of the process, 1.12 m^3 of oxygen (at NTP) is collected. Find (a) amount of copper liberated, and (b) the current efficiency of the cell.

Solution Basis : 1.12 m^3 of oxygen at NTP

At NTP, the specific volume of oxygen = 22.4 m^3/kmol

$$\text{Oxygen liberated} = 1.12 \text{ m}^3 = 1.12 \times \frac{1}{22.4} \text{ kmol}$$

$$\equiv 50 \text{ mol} \equiv 1600 \text{ g}$$

$$\text{Equivalent mass of oxygen} = \frac{16}{2} = 8$$

$$\text{Oxygen liberated} = \frac{1600}{8} = 200 \text{ g eq}$$

This electrochemical reactions taking place in the cell are:

$$CuSO_4 = Cu^{++} + SO_4^{--}$$

At the cathode: $\qquad Cu^{++} + 2e = SO_4$

At the anode: $\qquad SO_4^{--} - 2e = SO_4$

$$SO_4^{--} + 2 H_2O = H_2SO_4 + 2 OH^-$$

$$2 OH^- = H_2O + \frac{1}{2} O_2$$

Thus, $\qquad$ 1 mole of $O_2 \equiv 2$ moles of $CuSO_4$

$$\text{Equivalent mass of Cu} = \frac{63.5}{2} = 31.75$$

$$\text{Copper deposited} = \frac{(31.75 \times 1600)}{8} = 6350 \text{ g} \qquad \textit{Ans. (a)}$$

$$\text{Total energy passed through the solution in the cell} = \frac{(1130 \times 18\,000)}{96\,485} \text{ faradays}$$

$$\text{Theoretical liberation of Cu} = \left(\frac{1130 \times 18\,000 \times 31.75}{96\,485}\right)$$

$$= 6693.1 \text{ g}$$

$$\text{Current efficiency} = \left(\frac{\text{Cu liberated actually}}{\text{theoretical liberation of Cu}}\right) \times 100$$

$$= \left(\frac{6350}{6693.1}\right) \times 100 = 94.87\% \qquad \textit{Ans. (b)}$$

Example 4.14 Typical operating data on the Hooker-type diaphragm cell are as follows:

Power characteristics: 3.25 V, 15 000 A

$$\text{Brine feed} = 26.6\% \text{ NaCl by mass at}$$
$$338 \text{ to } 343 \text{ K (65 to 70°C)}$$

NaOH concentration in the cell liquor = 11.0% by mass

Salt/NaOH ratio in the cell liquor = 1.4:1.0 by mass

Temperature of the cell liquor = 360 K (87°C)

Production of NaOH = 514.1 kg/(d·cell)

Based on the above data, find: (a) the current efficiency of the cell, (b) the amounts of chlorine and hydrogen produced from the cell, and (c) the evaporation loss (of water) in the cell.

Solution Basis: 1 day operation of the cell

The reactions taking place in the cell are:

$$NaCl = Na^+ + Cl^-$$
$$H_2O = H^+ + OH^-$$
$$Na^+ + OH^- = NaOH^-$$
$$H^+ + e = \frac{1}{2} H_2$$
$$Cl^- - e = \frac{1}{2} Cl_2$$

$$\text{Total energy passed through the cell} = \frac{(15\,000 \times 3600 \times 24)}{96\,485}$$

$$= 13\,431.9 \text{ faraday/d}$$

$$\text{Theoretical (expected) NaOH formation} = \frac{(15\,000 \times 3600 \times 24 \times 40)}{(96\,485 \times 1000)}$$

$$= 537.3 \text{ kg/d}$$

$$\text{Current efficiency} = \left(\frac{\text{actual NaOH produced}}{\text{theoretical NaOH production}}\right) \times 100$$

$$= \left(\frac{514.1}{537.3}\right) \times 100 = 95.7\% \qquad \textit{Ans. (a)}$$

$$\text{Chlorine produced} = \left(\frac{35.5}{40}\right) \times 514.1 = 456.2 \text{ kg/d} \qquad \textit{Ans. (b-i)}$$

$$\text{Hydrogen produced} = \frac{514.1}{40} = 12.85 \text{ kg/d} \qquad Ans. \text{ (b-ii)}$$

Now, 40 g NaOH ≡ 58.5 g NaCl

$$\text{NaCl consumed in the reaction} = \left(\frac{58.5}{40}\right) \times 514.1 = 751.9 \text{ kg/d}$$

Cell liquor contains 11.0% NaOH.

$$\text{Total cell liquor} = \frac{514.1}{0.11} = 4673.6 \text{ kg/d}$$

NaCl that remained in the cell liquor = 514.1 × 1.4 = 719.7 kg/d

Total NaCl entering the system = 751.9 + 719.7 = 1471.6 kg/d

The original feed contains 26.6% NaCl.

$$\text{Brine feed rate} = \frac{1471.6}{0.266} = 5532.3 \text{ kg/d}$$

$$\text{Water consumed in the reaction} = \left(\frac{18}{40}\right) \times 514.1 = 231.3 \text{ kg/d}$$

Hence,

Loss of water due to evaporation = 5532.3 − (4673.6 + 231.3)

$$= 627.4 \text{ kg/d} \qquad Ans. \text{ (c)}$$

4.7 RECYCLING, PARALLEL AND BYPASSING OPERATIONS

The recycling operation with chemical reactions is common is industrial processes. This is mainly performed to utilise the valuable reactants to their maximum so that the loss of the reactants is minimised. However, various reasons for carrying out these operations are described in detail in Section 3.5. In most cases, the inerts enter with the fresh feed, which need to be limited to a desired level in the so-called *mixed or combined feed* of the fresh feed and recycle feed. For limiting the inerts, a portion of the recycle stream is purged.

For the overall material balance calculations, the recycling stream can be omitted as discussed in Chapter 3. After finding the flow rates of incoming and/ or outgoing streams, the recycling ratio can be easily calculated.

Parallel and bypassing operations are often encountered in industry. The materials balances of these operations are easier to evaluate than in the case of recycling operations.

Example 4.15 A fertiliser plant produces ammonia by reforming naphtha with steam. The synthesis gas, obtained from the methanator is passed through the converter after mixing with the recycle stream. Based on the operating parameters of the converter, the conversion per pass is limited to 25%. The composition of the fresh feed (synthesis make-up gas) is CH_4: 0.7%, Ar: 0.3%, H_2: 74.25% and N_2: 24.75% on mole basis. The converter outlet gases pass through the heat exchanger where it cools down. Later, the gases are passed through a chiller-cum-separator which separates 65% of the ammonia present in the converter outlet gas. Non-condensible gases and uncondensed ammonia are recycled back. In order to limit the concentration of inerts $(CH_4 + Ar)$ to 10 mole% in the mixed feed, a portion of the recycle stream is purged.

Based on a fresh feed rate of 100 kmol/s, calculate (a) the recycle feed rate and recycle ratio, (b) the purge gas rate, (c) the product ammonia rate, and (d) the compositions of various streams.

Solution

The process flow diagram is schematically represented in Fig. 4.2.

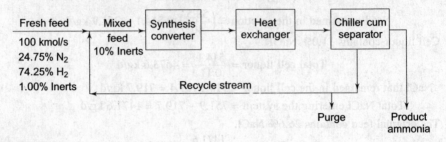

Fig. 4.2 Recycle Loop of Ammonia Synthesis

Basis: 100 kmol/s fresh feed

Let M, F and R respectively be the kmol/s of the mixed feed to the converter, fresh feed and recycle stream.

Material balance of feed: $F + R = M$

$$M = 100 + R \qquad (1)$$

Let a be the kmol/s of N_2 in the mixed feed.

$$H_2 \text{ in the mixed feed} = 3a \text{ kmol/s}$$

$$\text{Inerts (CH}_4 + \text{Ar) in the mixed feed} = 0.1 \text{ kmol/s}$$

$$\text{Ammonia in the mixed feed} = M - a - 3a - 0.1M = (0.9M - 4a) \text{ kmol/s}$$

$$\text{Chemical reaction: } N_2 + 3\,H_2 = 2\,NH_3$$

$$\text{Conversion per pass} = 25\%$$

$$N_2 \text{ reacted in the converter} = 0.25a \text{ kmol/s}$$

$$H_2 \text{ reacted in the converter} = 3 \times 0.25a = 0.75a \text{ kmol/s}$$

$$NH_3 \text{ produced in the converter} = 2 \times 0.25a = 0.50a \text{ kmol/s}$$

Total gas mixture leaving the converter $= M - 0.25a - 0.75a + 0.5a$

$$= (M - 0.5a) \text{ kmol/s}$$

Total NH_3 in the outlet gas $= 0.5a + 0.9M - 4a$

$$= (0.9M - 3.5a) \text{ kmol/s}$$

NH_3 separated in the separator $= (0.9M - 3.5a)\,0.65$

$$= (0.585M - 2.275a) \text{ kmol/s}$$

NH_3 uncondensed $= (0.9M - 3.5a)\,0.35$

$$= (0.315M - 1.225\,a) \text{ kmol/s}$$

The above values are listed in Table 4.13.

Table 4.13 Composition of Gas Mixture Leaving the Separator

Component	kmol/s
N_2	$0.75a$
H_2	$2.25a$
NH_3	$0.315M - 1.225a$
Inerts: (CH$_4$ + Ar)	$0.1M$
Total	$0.415M + 1.775a$

Let the purge be P kmol/s.

For the inerts level to be maintained in the fresh feed, the inerts exhausted out with the purge should equal the inerts in the fresh feed.

$$\text{Inerts in the purge} = \frac{0.1\,MP}{(0.415\,M + 1.775a)} \text{ kmol/s}$$

$$\text{Inerts in the fresh feed} = 100 \times 0.01 = 1.0 \text{ kmol/s}$$

Therefore, $0.1MP/(0.415M + 1.775a) = 1.0$ \hfill (2)

$$\text{Recycle stream} = (0.415M + 1.775a - P) \text{ kmol/s}$$

Substituting this value in Eq. (1),

$$100 + 0.415M - P + 1.775a = M \hfill (3)$$

Balance of nitrogen:

$$\text{Nitrogen lost in purge} = \frac{0.75aP}{(0.415M + 1.775a)} \text{ kmol/s}$$

$$\text{N}_2 \text{ in the recycle stream} = 0.75a - [0.75aP/(0.415M + 1.775a)] \text{ kmol/s}$$

$$\text{N}_2 \text{ in the fresh feed} = 24.75 \text{ kmol/s}$$

Hence, $0.75a - \left[\dfrac{0.75aP}{0.415M + 1.775a}\right] + 24.75 = a$ \hfill (4)

Equations (2), (3) and (4) need to be solved for evaluating a, M and P. Substituting the value of $0.415M + 1.775a = 0.1MP$ [from Eq. (2)] in Eq. (4),

$$0.75a - \left[\frac{0.75aP}{0.1MP}\right] + 24.75 = a$$

$$a = \frac{24.75\,M}{0.25\,M + 7.5} \hfill (5)$$

From Eq. (2), $\qquad\qquad\qquad P = (4.15\,M + 17.75a)/M$

Substituting the value of P in Eq. (3),

$$0.585M - 1.775a + (4.15M + 17.75a)/M = 100$$

or $\quad 0.585M^2 - 1.775aM + 4.15M + 17.75a = 100M$ \hfill (6)

Substituting the value of a from Eq. (5) into Eq. (6),

$$0.585M^2 - 1.775M\left[\frac{24.75\,M}{0.25\,M + 7.5}\right] - 95.85M + 17.75\left[\frac{24.75\,M}{0.25\,M + 7.5}\right] = 0 \hfill (7)$$

Simplifying Eq. (7)

$$0.146M^2 - 63.506M - 288.437 = 0$$

$$M = 439.468 \text{ kmol/s (only positive root)}$$

From Eq. (5), $\qquad\qquad\qquad a = \dfrac{24.75 \times 439.468}{0.25 \times 439.468 + 7.5}$

$$= 92.674 \text{ kmol/s}$$

From Eq. (2),

$$P = \frac{4.15 \times 439.468 + 17.75 \times 92.674}{439.467} = 7.893 \text{ kmol/s} \hfill \textit{Ans. (b)}$$

Recycle stream $R = 439.468 - 100.0 = 339.468$ kmol/s \hfill \textit{Ans. (a-1)}

$$\text{Recycle ratio} = \frac{339.468}{100} = 3.395 \text{ kmol/kmol fresh feed} \qquad \textit{Ans. (a-2)}$$

$$\text{Product NH}_3 \text{ rate} = 0.585M - 2.275\,a$$
$$= 0.585 \times 439.468 - 2.275 \times 92.674$$
$$= 46.256 \text{ kmol/s}$$

$$\text{Mass rate of NH}_3 \text{ product} = 46.256 \times 17.0305 = 787.77 \text{ kg/s} \qquad \textit{Ans. (c)}$$

The composition of various streams are given in Tables 4.14 and 4.15.

Table 4.14 Composition of Different Streams

Compo-	Fresh feed		Recycle stream		Mixed feed	
nent	kmol/s	mole%	kmol/s	mole%	kmol/s	mole%
N_2	24.75	24.75	67.924	20.01	92.674	21.09
H_2	74.25	74.25	203.772	60.03	278.022	63.26
$(CH_4 + Ar)$	1.00	1.00	42.947	12.65	43.947	10.00
NH_3	Nil	Nil	24.825	7.31	24.825	5.65
Total	100.00	100.00	339.468	100.00	439.468	100.00

Table 4.15 Composition of Different Streams

Component	Converter outlet stream		Gas stream after separator	
	kmol/s	mole%	kmol/s	mole/%
N_2	69.506	17.68	69.506	20.04
H_2	208.517	53.04	208.517	60.11
$(CH_4 + Ar)$	43.947	11.18	43.947	12.67
NH_3	71.162	18.10	24.906	7.18
Total	393.132	100.00	346.876	100.00

Note: The example illustrates the actual design calculations of a recycle loop. However, if it is assumed that the whole of ammonia formed in the converter is condensed and separated in the separator, the material balance calculations become simple. Solution of simultaneous equations can be made easy with Mathcad (refer Chapter 9).

Example 4.16 Methanol is produced by the reaction of carbon monoxide with hydrogen.

$$CO + 2 H_2 = CH_3OH \qquad (1)$$

The side reaction is

$$CO + 3 H_2 = CH_4 + H_2O \qquad (2)$$

At a pressure of 6.9 MPa and a temperature 574.6 K (301.5°C), the conversion per pass is 12.5% Of this amount, 87.5% is assumed to reach via Eq. (1) and 12.5% via Eq. (2). The stream leaving the reactor passes through a condenser and a separator. The carbon monoxide and hydrogen leaving this unit are recycled. The methane leaves as a gas and the liquid mixture of methanol and water passes to a distillation column for the concentration of methanol. Refer Fig. 4.3 for the process flow diagram.

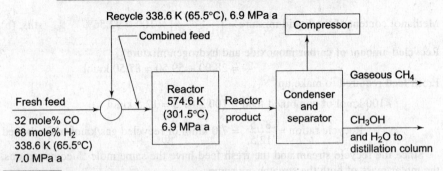

Fig. 4.3 Manufacture of Methanol

Compute: (a) the analysis, mole % and mass % of the hot gaseous stream leaving the reactor, (b) the methanol content, mass % of the liquid (methanol + water) stream, leaving the condenser and separator, (c) the recycle ratio, expressed as kg of carbon-monoxide and hydrogen recycled per kg of fresh gas, (d) the methane "off gas" expressed as a percentage by weight of the combined feed gas, and (e) the volumetric flow rate of the gaseous combined feed to the reactor, measured at 338.5 K (65.5°C) and 7 MPa a for a yield of 1 kg/s of methanol, assuming the ideal gas behaviour of the mixture.

Solution

Basis: 100 kmol combined feed

$$\text{Conversion per pass} = 12.5\%$$
$$\text{Total CO consumed} = 32 \times 0.125 = 4.0 \text{ kmol}$$
$$\text{CO consumed via Eq. (1)} = 4.0 \times 0.875 = 3.5 \text{ kmol}$$
$$\text{CO consumed via Eq. (2)} = 4.0 - 3.5 = 0.5 \text{ kmol}$$

It may be noted that H_2 is in excess and hence the conversion is based on CO which is the limiting component.

$$\text{CO unreacted} = 32 - 4 = 28 \text{ kmol}$$
$$H_2 \text{ consumed via Eq. (1)} = 2 \times 3.5 = 7.0 \text{ kmol}$$
$$H_2 \text{ consumed via Eq. (2)} = 3 \times 0.5 = 1.5 \text{ kmol}$$
$$\text{Total } H_2 \text{ consumed} = 7.0 + 1.5 = 8.5 \text{ kmol}$$
$$\text{Unreacted } H_2 = 68 - 8.5 = 59.5 \text{ kmol}$$
$$\text{Methanol formed} = 3.5 \text{ kmol}$$

Water and methane (each) produced = 0.5 kmol
The analysis of the hot gases is given in Table 4.16.

Table 4.16 Composition of Hot Gaseous Stream Leaving the Reactor

Component	n_i kmol	Mole%	Molar mass	Mass kg	Mass %
CO	28.0	30.43	28	784.0	75.97
H_2	59.5	64.68	2	119.0	11.53
CH_3OH	3.5	3.81	32	112.0	10.85
H_2O	0.5	0.54	18	9.0	0.87
CH_4	0.5	0.54	16	8.0	0.78
Total	92.0	100.00		1032.0	100.00

Ans. (a)

Methanol content of the liquid mixture $= \left[\dfrac{112}{112+9}\right] \times 100 = 92.56\%$ *Ans.* (b)

Recycled amount of carbor monoxide and hydrogen mixture
$$= 28.00 + 59.50 = 87.50 \text{ kmol}$$

Fresh feed required to make up

$$100 \text{ kmol of combined feed} = 100 - 87.5 = 12.5 \text{ kmol}$$

$$\text{Recycle ration} = \dfrac{87.5}{12.5} = 7.0 \text{ kmol of recycled gas/kmol of fresh feed}$$

Since the recycle stream and the fresh feed have the same mole % compositions, the molar mass of both the streams are same.

$$\text{Recycle ratio} = 7.0 \text{ kg recycled gas/kg fresh feed} \quad \textit{Ans. (c)}$$

$$\text{Methane produced} = 8 \text{ kg}$$

$$\text{Combined feed} = 32 \times 28 + 68 \times 2$$

$$= 1032 \text{ kg}$$

$$\text{Methane lost} = \left(\dfrac{8}{1032}\right) \times 100$$

$$= 0.78\% \quad \textit{Ans. (d)}$$

To produce 1 kg/s methanol,

$$\text{Molar flow rate of the combined feed} = \left(\dfrac{100}{112}\right) \times 1 = 0.8929 \text{ kmol/s}$$

$$\text{Based on ideal gas law}, V = \dfrac{RT}{p} = 8.314 \times \dfrac{338.5}{7000}$$

$$= 0.402 \text{ m}^3/\text{kmol}$$

Volumetric flow rate of the combined feed

$$= 0.402 \times 0.8929 = 0.359 \text{ m}^3/\text{s} \quad \textit{Ans. (e)}$$

Note: Considering high pressure (~ 7.0 MPa), use of ideal gas law may not be justified.

Example 4.17 In a partial demineralisation process (also called a blend process), the raw water is divided into two streams. One stream passes through the sodium ion exchanger while the other stream passes through the hydrogen ion exchanger. The process flow is shown in Fig. 4.4.

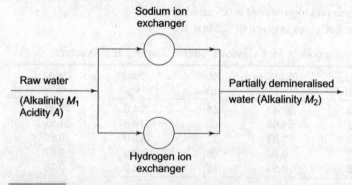

Fig. 4.4 Partial Demineralisation Process

In a particular partial demineraliser, the raw water analysis is observed to be as follows:

Total alkalinity (methyl-orange reading) = 550 mg/L as $CaCO_3$

Permanent hardness = Nil

Chlorides as Cl = 1312 mg/L

Sulphates as SO_4 = 43.2 kg/L

The mixed effluents of sodium ion and hydrogen ion exchangers were found to contain a total alkalinity of 50 mg/L as $CaCO_3$. Assume that both the ion exchangers are 100% efficient. Calculate the flow distribution of the water through the ion exchangers.

Solution

Since the water does not contain permanent hardness, the chlorides and sulphates are attached to sodium (assuming that the water does not contain potassium). When the raw water passes through the hydrogen ion exchanger, the chlorides and sulphates are converted to the corresponding mineral acids, i.e., HCl and H_2SO_4 respectively. The bicarbonates and carbonates produce weak carbonic acid (H_2CO_3). Thus, the decationated water shows free acidity. When the water passes through the softener (i.e., sodium ion exchanger), the Ca^{++} and Mg^{++} ions are replaced by Na^+ ion. This means that $Ca(HCO_3)_2$ and $Mg(HCO_3)_2$ get converted to $NaHCO_3$. The softened water will have the same total alkalinity when expressed in terms of equivalent $CaCO_3$ (although the actual alkalinity figure will vary).

The reactions taking place in the ion exchangers are summarised below.

Hydrogen ion exchanger:

$$NaCl + HRe = HCl + NaRe \tag{1}$$

$$Na_2SO_4 + 2\ HRe = H_2SO_4 + 2\ NaRe \tag{2}$$

$$Ca(HCO_3)_2 + 2\ HRe = 2\ H_2CO_3 + Ca(Re)_2 \tag{3}$$

$$Mg(HCO_3) + 2\ HRe = 2\ H_2CO_3 + Mg\ (Re)_2 \tag{4}$$

Sodium ion exchanger:

$$Ca(HCO_3)_2 + 2\ NaRe' = 2\ NaHCO_3 + Ca(Re')_2 \tag{5}$$

$$Mg\ (HCO_3)_2 + 2\ NaRe' = 2\ NaHCO_3 + Mg(Re')_2 \tag{6}$$

(Re and Re´ stand for resins)

Chlorides, expressed as equivalent $CaCO_3 = \left(\dfrac{50}{35.5}\right) \times 312 = 439.44$ mg/L

Sulphates, expressed as equivalent $CaCO_3 = \left(\dfrac{50}{48}\right) \times 43.2 = 45.0$ mg/L

Equivalent mineral acidity

(EMA) in raw water, $A = 439.44 + 45.0 = 484.44$ mg/L as $CaCO_3$

Let 100 L be the total raw water inlet to both the ion exchangers. Also let x L be the raw water inlet to the hydrogen ion exchanger.

Water input to sodium ion exchanger $= (100 - x)$ L

Free acidity in the demineralised water $= x\ (A + M_1)$ mg

where, M_1 is the total alkalinity of raw water.

Let M_2 be the total alkalinity of blend water.

Total alkalinity removed $= 100 \, (M_1 - M_2)$ mg

For the neutralisation to be balanced,

$$x \, (A + M_1) = 100 \, (M_1 - M_2)$$

$$\frac{x}{100} = \frac{(M_1 - M_2)}{(A + M_1)}$$

$$= \frac{(550 - 50)}{(484.44 + 550)}$$

$$x = 48.34$$

Thus,. 48.34 % of the total raw water passes through the hydrogen ion exchanger.

Note: This example illustrates the material balance calculations of the parallel flow operations. It may be noted that the final material balance equation could be written because all the values of acidity and alkalinity were expressed in terms of equivalent $CaCO_3$.

Consider another operation in which there is no sodium ion exchanger. A part of the raw water, however, passes through the hydrogen ion exchanger and the rest is bypassed to blend with decationated water. Will the flow distribution (i.e. 48.94%) change to attain 50 mg/L of the total alkalinity in the blend water? why?

Example 4.18 In Example 4.10, single reactor is considered for partial oxidation of methanol. In an innovative approach to boost the capacity of the existing plant, a second reactor is added in series[8] as shown in Fig. 4.5. Additional methanol is fed as bypass between the reactors and mixed with the gas mixture, leaving the first reactor in a static mixer.

Based on safety and catalyst life considerations methanol concentration is controlled at 6.25% (by volume) at the first reactor inlet while maintaining total wet molar gas mixture flow to the first reactor constant. Methanol concentration at the inlet of second reactor is maintained at 8.4% (by volume). Assume that conversion per pass in both the reactors in 99%, yield of formaldehyde is 90% and other secondary reactions are also unchanged. Also assume that the absorber can be revamped to take additional load of formaldehyde to produce bottom solution of 37% (by mass).

Make material balance of the new series reactors scheme. Calculate increase in the capacity achieved and % methanol bypassed to the second reactor.

Solution:

Basis: Gas mixture flow to Reactor I = 1488.1 kmol/h

$$CH_3OH \text{ in the gas mixture} = 1488.1 \times 0.0625$$

$$= 93.0 \text{ kmol/h}$$

$$\text{Ambient (wet) air flow} = 1488.1 - 93.0$$

$$= 1395.1 \text{ kmol/h}$$

$$\text{Dry air flow rate} = \frac{1395.1}{1.017\,72} = 1370.8 \text{ kmol/h}$$

$$\text{Moisture, entering with air} = 1395.1 - 1370.8$$

$$= 24.3 \text{ kmol/h}$$

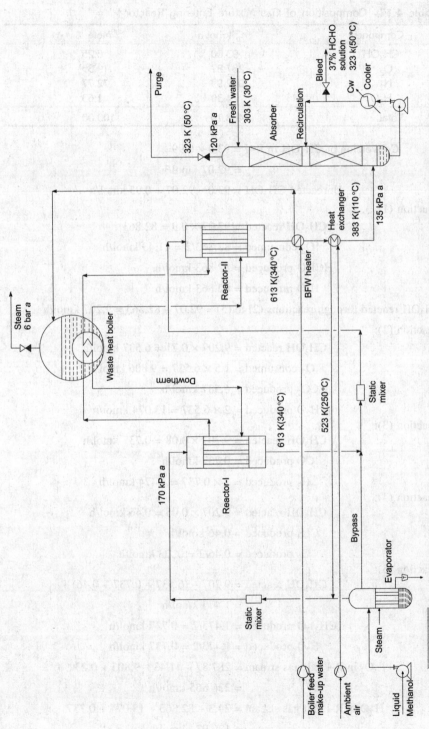

Fig. 4.5 Formaldehyde Production by Topsoe Series Reactor Process (Modified Formox Process)

Table 4.17 Composition of Gas Mixture Entering Reactor-I

Component	n_i, kmol/h	Mole %
CH_3OH	93.00	6.25
O_2	287.87	19.35
N_2	1082.93	72.77
H_2O	24.30	1.63
Total	1488.10	100.00

$$\text{Conversion of } CH_3OH \text{ in R–I} = 93.0 \times 0.99$$
$$= 92.07 \text{ kmol/h}$$
$$\text{Unreacted } CH_3OH = 93.0 - 92.07 = 0.93 \text{ kmol/h}$$

Reaction (1):

$$CH_3OH \text{ reacted} = 92.07 \times 0.9 = 82.863$$
$$O_2 \text{ consumed} = 82.863/2 = 41.43 \text{ kmol/h}$$
$$HCHO \text{ produced} = 82.863 \text{ kmol/h}$$
$$H_2O \text{ produced} = 82.863 \text{ kmol/h}$$

CH_3OH reacted through reactions (2) to (5) = 92.07 – 82.863 = 9.207 kmol/h

Reaction (2):

$$CH_3OH \text{ reacted} = 9.207 \times 0.71 = 6.537 \text{ kmol/h}$$
$$O_2 \text{ consumed} = 1.5 \times 6.537 = 9.806 \text{ kmol/h}$$
$$CO_2 \text{ produced} = 6.537 \text{ kmol/h}$$
$$H_2O \text{ produced} = 2 \times 6.537 = 13.074 \text{ kmol/h}$$

Reaction (3):

$$CH_3OH \text{ reacted} = 9.207 \times 0.08 = 0.737 \text{ kmol/h}$$
$$CO \text{ produced} = 0.737 \text{ kmol/h}$$
$$H_2 \text{ produced} = 2 \times 0.737 = 1.474 \text{ kmol/h}$$

Reaction (4):

$$CH_3OH \text{ reacted} = 9.207 \times 0.05 = 0.46 \text{ kmol/h}$$
$$CH_4 \text{ produced} = 0.46 \text{ kmol/h}$$
$$O_2 \text{ produced} = 0.46/2 = 0.23 \text{ kmol/h}$$

Reaction (5):

$$CH_3OH \text{ reacted} = 9.207 - (6.537 + 0.737 + 0.46)$$
$$= 1.473 \text{ kmol/h}$$
$$(CH_3)_2O \text{ produced} = 1.473/2 = 0.737 \text{ kmol/h}$$
$$H_2O \text{ produced} = 1.473/2 = 0.737 \text{ kmol/h}$$
$$O_2 \text{ in R-I exit gas stream} = 287.87 - 41.43 - 9.805 + 0.23$$
$$= 236.865 \text{ kmol/h}$$
$$H_2O \text{ in R-I exit gas stream} = 24.3 + 82.863 + 13.074 + 0.737$$
$$= 120.974 \text{ kmol/h}$$

Table 4.18 Composition of R-I Exit Gas Stream

Component	n_i, kmol/h	Mole%
CH_3OH	0.93	0.06
HCHO	92.07	5.96
CO_2	6.537	0.42
CO	0.737	0.05
H_2	1.474	0.10
CH_4	0.460	0.03
$(CH_3)_2O$	0.737	0.05
O_2	236.865	15.34
N_2	1082.930	70.15
H_2O	120.974	7.84
Total	1534.714	100.00

Let x kmol/h CH_3OH is added in between the reactors.

$$CH_3OH \text{ entering R-II} = 0.93 + x \text{ kmol/h}$$

$$\frac{0.93 + x}{1543.714 + x} = 0.084$$

or

$$x = 140.548 \text{ kmol/h}$$

$$CH_3OH \text{ entering R–II} = 140.548 + 0.93$$

$$= 141.478 \text{ kmol/h}$$

$$CH_3OH \text{ reacted in R–II} = 141.478 \times 0.99$$

$$= 140.063 \text{ kmol/h}$$

$$\text{Unreacted } CH_3OH = 141.478 - 140.063$$

$$= 1.415 \text{ kmol/h}$$

Reaction (1):

$$CH_3OH \text{ reacted} = 140.063 \times 0.9$$

$$= 126.057 \text{ kmol/h}$$

$$O_2 \text{ consumed} = 126.057/2 = 63.029 \text{ kmol/h}$$

$$HCHO \text{ produced} = 126.057 \text{ kmol/h}$$

$$H_2O \text{ produced} = 126.057 \text{ kmol/h}$$

CH_3OH reacted through reaction (2) to (5) = 140.063–126.057 = 14.006 kmol/h
Reaction (2):

$$CH_3OH \text{ reacted} = 14.006 \times 0.71 = 9.944 \text{ kmol/h}$$

$$O_2 \text{ consumed} = 9.944 \times 1.5 = 14.916 \text{ kmol/h}$$

$$CO_2 \text{ produced} = 9.944 \text{ kmol/h}$$

$$H_2O \text{ produced} = 2 \times 9.944 = 19.888 \text{ kmol/h}$$

Reaction (3):

$$CH_3OH \text{ reacted} = 14.006 \times 0.08 = 1.12 \text{ kmol/h}$$

$$CO \text{ produced} = 1.12 \text{ kmol/h}$$

$$H_2 \text{ produced} = 1.12 \times 2 = 2.24 \text{ kmol/h}$$

Reaction (4):

$$CH_3OH \text{ reacted} = 14.006 \times 0.05 = 0.7 \text{ kmol/h}$$
$$CH_4 \text{ produced} = 0.7 \text{ kmol/h}$$
$$O_2 \text{ produced} = 0.7/2 = 0.35 \text{ kmol/h}$$

Reaction (5):

$$CH_3OH \text{ reacted} = 14.006 - (9.944 + 1.12 + 0.7)$$
$$= 2.242 \text{ kmol/h}$$
$$(CH_3)_2O \text{ produced} = 2.242/2 = 1.121 \text{ kmol/h}$$
$$H_2O \text{ produced} = 2.242/2 = 1.121 \text{ kmol/h}$$
$$O_2 \text{ in R-II exit gas stream} = 236.865 - (63.029 + 14.916 - 0.35)$$
$$= 159.27 \text{ kmol/h}$$
$$H_2O \text{ in R-II exit gas stream} = 120.974 + 126.057 + 19.888 + 1.121$$
$$= 268.04 \text{ kmol/h}$$
$$HCHO \text{ in R-II exit gas stream} = 92.07 + 126.057$$
$$= 218.127 \text{ kmol/h}$$

Table 4.19 Composition of R-II Exit Gas Stream

Component	n_i, kmol/h	Mole %
CH_3OH	1.415	0.08
HCHO	218.127	12.43
CO_2	16.481	0.94
CO	1.857	0.11
H_2	3.714	0.20
CH_4	1.160	0.07
$(CH_3)_2O$	1.858	0.11
O_2	159.270	9.08
N_2	1082.930	61.71
H_2O	268.040	15.27
Total	1754.852	100.00

Material balance across absorber:

$$\text{Total HCHO produced} = 218.127 \times 30$$
$$= 6543.8 \text{ kg/h}$$
$$\text{Total } CH_3OH \text{ fed to both reactors} = 140.548 + 93$$
$$= 223.548 \text{ kmol/h}$$
$$CH_3OH \text{ bypassed} = \frac{140.548 \times 100}{223.548}$$
$$= 60.18\%$$
$$\text{Bottom solution flow rate} = \frac{6543.8}{0.37}$$
$$= 17\,686.0 \text{ kg/h}$$

$$\text{CH}_3\text{OH in bottom solution} = 1.415 \times 32$$
$$= 45.3 \text{ kg/h}$$
$$\text{H}_2\text{O entering the absorber} = 268.04 \times 18$$
$$= 4824.7 \text{ kg/h}$$
$$\text{Dry tail gas flow rate} = 1754.852 - (1.415 + 218.127 + 268.04)$$
$$= 1267.27 \text{ kmol/h}$$
$$\text{Moisture in tail gas} = 1267.27 \times 0.1146$$
$$= 145.229 \text{ kmol/h}$$
$$\equiv 2614.1 \text{ kg/h}$$
$$\text{Fresh water added} = 17\,686.0 - (6543.8 + 45.3 + 4824.7)$$
$$+ 2614.1$$
$$= 8886.3 \text{ kg/h}$$
$$\text{Increase in capacity} = \frac{(17\,686 - 9030.4)\,100}{9030.4}$$
$$= 95.85\% \qquad\qquad \textit{Ans.}$$

Table 4.20 Composition of Tail (Purge) Gas from Absorber

Component	n_i, kmol/h		Mole%	
	Dry	Wet	Dry	Wet
UC	25.07	25.07	1.98	1.77
O_2	159.27	159.270	12.57	11.28
N_2	1082.93	1082.930	85.45	76.67
H_2O	–	145.229	–	10.28
Total	1267.27	1412.499	100.00	100.00

4.8 METALLURGICAL APPLICATIONS

Complex reactions take place in the furnaces where the metal is extracted from the ore. It is difficult to treat individual reactions as seen in various examples cited above. Overall material balances are set for getting the desired information. Example 4.19 will demonstrate the application of stoichiometry in extractive ferrous metallurgy.

Example 4.19 A blast furnace makes pig iron containing 3.6% C, 1.4% Si and 95% Fe. The ore used contains 80% Fe_2O_3, 12% SiO_2 and 8% Al_2O_3. The coke analysis shows the presence of 10% SiO and 90%C. The flux used is pure $CaCO_3$. The exit gases contain 28% CO and 14% CO_2. The coke ratio is 1 kg/kg pig iron. Flux is 0.4 kg/kg pig iron. Calculate per tonne of pig iron: (a) the mass of the slag made, (b) the mass of the ore used, (c) the composition of slag, and (d) the volume of the air required at NTP.

Solution

Basis: 1 tonne (= 1000 kg) of pig iron

$$Coke = 1000 \text{ kg}$$

$$Flux = 400 \text{ kg}$$

$$\text{Fe in the pig iron} = 0.95 \times 1000 = 950 \text{ kg}$$

$$\text{Fe available per kg of ore} = \left(\frac{112}{160}\right) 0.8 = 0.56 \text{ kg}$$

$$\text{Ore required} = \frac{950}{0.56} = 1696.43 \text{ kg} \qquad \qquad \textit{Ans. (a)}$$

Silica balance: Si in the pig iron = $0.014 \times 1000 = 14$ kg as Si

$$SiO_2 \text{ present in the pig iron} = \left(\frac{60}{28}\right) \times 14 = 30 \text{ kg}$$

$$SiO_2 \text{ present in the ore} = 1696.43 \times 0.12 = 203.57 \text{ kg}$$

$$SiO_2 \text{ present in the coke} = 0.10 \times 1000 = 100 \text{ kg}$$

$$SiO_2 \text{ present in the slag} = 203.57 + 100 - 30 = 273.57 \text{ kg}$$

Al_2O_3 balance: Al_2O_3 present in the ore = $1696.43 \times 0.08 = 135.71$ kg

$$Al_2O_3 \text{ present in the slag} = 135.71 \text{ kg}$$

CaO balance:

CaO comes into the slag due to the decomposition of $CaCO_3$.

$$CaCO_3 \text{ fed to the furnace} = 400 \text{ kg}$$

$$\text{CaO present in the slag} = \left(\frac{56}{100}\right) \times 400 = 224 \text{ kg}$$

The composition of the slag is given in Table 4.21.

Table 4.21 Composition of Slag

Component	Mass, kg	Mass %
SiO_2	273.57	43.20
Al_2O_3	135.71	21.43
CaO	224.00	35.37
Total	633.28	100.00

Ans. (b) and (c)

Air requirement:

$$\text{Total carbon available} = \text{carbon present in the coke}$$

$$+ \text{ carbon present in the } CaCO_3$$

$$- \text{ carbon left over in pig iron}$$

$$= 0.90 \times 1000 + \left(\frac{12}{100}\right) \times 400 - 36$$

$$= 912 \text{ kg as C}$$

In the blast, the ratio of CO to CO_2 is 2:1. Therefore, two-thirds of 912 kg C will be burnt to CO and one-third to CO_2

Carbon converted to $CO_2 = \left(\dfrac{1}{3}\right) \times 912 = 304.0$ kg

Carbon converted to $CO = \left(\dfrac{2}{3}\right) \times 912 = 608.0$ kg

Oxygen required to form CO and $CO_2 = 608 \times \left(\dfrac{16}{12}\right) + 304 \times \left(\dfrac{32}{12}\right)$

$$= 810.68 + 810.67 = 1621.35 \text{ kg as } O_2$$

Thus, the total oxygen requirement is 1621.35 kg. However, a part of the oxygen is available from SiO_2, Fe_2O_3 and $CaCO_3$.

$$SiO_2 = Si + O_2$$
$$60 \quad 28 \quad 32$$

Oxygen derived from $SiO_2 = \left(\dfrac{32}{28}\right) \times 14 = 16$ kg

$$Fe_2O_3 = 2\,Fe + 3/2\,O_2$$
$$160 \quad 112 \quad 48$$

Oxygen derived from $Fe_2O_3 = \dfrac{1696.43 \times 0.8 \times 48}{160} = 407.15$ kg

$$CaCO_3 = CaO + CO_2$$
$$100 \quad 56 \quad 44$$

$$CO_2 = C + O_2$$
$$44 \quad 12 \quad 32$$

Oxygen derived form $CaCO_3 = \dfrac{400 \times 32}{100} = 128$ kg

Total oxygen available $= 16 + 407.15 + 128 = 551.15$ kg

Oxygen to be supplied from air $= 1621.35 - 551.15 = 1070.20$ kg

$$\equiv 33.44 \text{ kmol}$$

Air supplied $= \dfrac{33.44}{0.21} = 159.26$ kmol

At NTP, specific volume of air $= 22.414$ m^3/kmol

Volume of air supplied at NTP $= 159.26 \times 22.414 \times = 3569.6$ m^3 *Ans.* (d)

EXERCISES

4.1 In Exercise 3.22, decoking of a catalyst is described. Calculate mass % coke on the catalyst, assuming average composition of the coke to be $CH_{0.6}$ [*Ans.* 1.0%]

4.2 A pilot plant reactor was charged with 50 kg naphthalene and 200 kg (98% by mass) H_2SO_4. The reaction was carried out for 3 hours at 433 K (160°C). The reaction goes to near completion. The product distribution[9] was found to be 18.6% monosulphonate naphthalene and 81.4% disulphonate naphthalene. Calculate: (a) the quantities of monosulphonate (MSN) and disulphonate (DSN) products, and (b) the complete analysis of the product.

[*Ans.* (a) 19.51 kg MSN and 85.4 kg DSN
(b) 7.81% MSN, 34.16% DSN, 51.47% H_2SO_4 and 6.56% H_2O]

4.3 Dinitro-*o-sec*-butyl phenol (DNOSBP) is manufactured by the nitration of *sec*-butyl phenol (SBP) in presence of zinc chloride and hydrogen chloride.

After the reaction is complete, a sample from the reactor is analysed as follows:

Table 4.22 Analysis of Reactor Product

Component	Mass %
Nitric acid	15
sec-Butyl phenol	65
4,6 Dinitro-*o-sec*- butyl phenol (DNOSBP)	18
3,6 Dinitro-*p-sec*-butyl phenol (DNPSBP)	2

Calculate: (a) Conversion, and (b) Yield of *ortho* and *para* products.
[*Ans.* (a) Conversion = 41.2% (b) Yield of *o*-product = 90.04% and of *p*-product = 9.96%]

4.4. Ethyl alcohol is industrially produced by fermenation of molasses[10]. A sample of molasses contains 45% (mass) fermentable sugars (in the form of sucrose). The reactions taking place in the fermenter are as follows:

$$C_{12}H_{22}O_{11} \quad + \quad H_2O \quad = \quad C_6H_{12}O_6 \quad + \quad C_6H_{12}O_6$$

Sucrose   *d*-Glucose   *d*-Fructose

$$C_6H_{12}O_6 \quad = \quad 2\ C_2H_5OH \quad + \quad 2\ CO_2$$

Monosaccharide   Alcohol

Calculate the theoretical production of rectified spirit (having density of 0.785 kg/L) in liters per tonne of molasses.

[*Ans.* 308.41 L]

4.5 Selective dehydrogenation of alkanes to alkenes is a well established process. In this process, dehydrogenation of i-butane is carried out on a platinum impregnated catalyst at 50 kPa g and 773 K (500°C). The feed to the reactor is pure i-butane alongwith 0.75 kmol H_2 per kmol i-butane. Hydrogen stream contains 90% H_2 and 10% methane (by mole). Following reactions are known to take place.

$$i\text{-}C_4H_{10} \quad = \quad i\text{-}C_4H_8 \quad + \quad H_2 \qquad (1)$$
$$\text{i-Butane} \qquad \text{i-Butylene} \qquad \text{Hydrogen}$$

$$i\text{-}C_4H_{10} \quad = \quad C_3H_6 \quad + \quad CH_4 \qquad (2)$$
$$\text{i-Butane} \quad = \quad \text{Propylene} \qquad \text{Methane}$$

Literature reports 50% per pass conversion in a battery of three reactors with 88% yield of i-butylene. Calculate the composition of the product stream leaving the final reactor.

[*Ans.* (mole %) $i\text{-}C_4H_{10}$: 21..43%, $i\text{-}C_3H_8$: 18.86%,
C_3H_6: 2.57%, H_2: 51.01% and CH_4: 6.13%]

4.6 In the BASF oil quench process to manufacture acetylene, pure oxygen and pure methane are fed to the acetylene burner[11]. The cracked gas from the burner has the following composition:

H_2: 56.5% CH_4: 5.2%, C_2H_4: 0.3%, C_2H_2: 7.5%, C_3H_6: 0.5%,
CO: 25.8%, CO_2: 4.0% and O_2: 0.2% (mole% on dry basis).

Assume that formation of other compounds, such as aromatics, is negligible.

For 100 kmol cracked gas, calculate (a) methane requirement, (b) oxygen requirement, (c) production of water, (d) conversion of methane, and (e) yield of acetylene production.

[*Ans.* (a) 52.1 kmol CH_4, (b) 30.95 kmol O_2, (c) 27.7 kmol H_2O
(d) 90.02%, and (e) 31.98%]

4.7 The flue gas mixture is known to contain CO_2, O_2 and N_2 along with water vapour. In order to analyses the mixture, the gas is first passed through silica gel which absorbs the moisture. Later, the dry gas is passed through 1 L of caustic potash solution. Thus CO_2 is preferentially-absorbed in it. Finally, the mixture containing O_2 and N_2 is collected in 1 L flask at 101.325 kPa and 298.15 K (25°C). The increase in the mass of the silica gel due to moisture absorption was found to be 0.362 g. The caustic potash solution was analysed for carbonate formation. A volume of 10 mL of the solution was titrated against 0.012 N HCl solution. It was found that the phenolphthalein reading was 35.4 mL, while the total titration reading (with methyl orange indicator) was 38 mL. The increase in the mass of the flask was 1.16 kg. Bases on these observations, find: (a) the concentration of KOH and K_2CO_3 in the solution, (b) the Orsat (dry basis) analysis of the gas, and (c) the mass percentage composition of the wet gas.

[*Ans.* (a) 2191 mg/L KOH and 447 mg/L K_2CO_3 (b) 7.34% CO_2,
8.78% O_2 and 83.88% N_2 (by volume) (c) 10.65%
CO_2, 9.25% O_2, 77.39% N_2 and 2.71% H_2O (by mass)]

4.8 The analysis of limestone gives 60% $CaCO_3$, 33.5% $MgCO_3$ and rest inerts. It is treated with 12% aqueous sulphuric acid (by mass) to obtain pue CO_2. An excess of 15% of the acid over the stoichiometric amounts is used to ascertain that the reaction goes to completion. Based on the treatment of 500 kg limestone, calculate: (a) the amount of 100% (by mass) sulphuric acid required, (b) the amount of the residue, (c) the analysis of the residue left in the vessel, and (d) the moles of CO_2 produced.

[*Ans.* (a) 562 kg (b) 4964.2 kg (c) $CaSO_4$: 8.21%, $MgSO_4$: 4.82%,
H_2SO_4: 1.48%, H_2O: 84.84%,
Inerts 0.65% (by mass); (d) 5 kmol]

4.9 In the Deacon process for manufacturing chlorine, hydrochloric acid gas is oxidized with air. The reaction taking place is:

$$4\ HCl + O_2 = 2\ Cl_2 + 2\ H_2O$$

If the air is used in excess of 30% of that theoretically required, and if the oxidation is 80% complete, calculate the composition by volume of dry gases leaving the reaction chamber.

[*Ans.* HCl: 10.27%, O_2: 6.42%, Cl_2: 20.53%, and
N_2: 62.78% (by volume)]

4.10 The gaseous reaction A = 2 B + C takes place isothermally in a constant pressure reactor. Starting with a mixture of 75% A and 25% inerts (by volume), in a specified time the volume double. Calculate the conversion achieved.

[*Ans.* 66.67%]

4.11 The shift reaction is a very important reaction in the gas processing industry.

$$CO + H_2O = CO_2 + H_2$$

If a and b are the percent carbon monoxide in the dry inlet and outlet gas mixtures to and from the shift converter respectively, prove that moles of CO converted (x) per 100 moles of inlet gas mixture can be calculated by using the formula,

$$x = \frac{100(a-b)}{100+b}$$

4.12 The analysis of the gas entering the secondary converter in a contact sulphuric acid plant is 4% SO_2, 13% O_2 and 83% N_2 (on volume basis). The gas leaving the converter contains 0.45% SO_2 on SO_3-free basis (by volume). Calculate the percentage of SO_2 entering the converter getting converted to SO_3.

[*Ans.* 89.35%]

4.13 A mixture of pure carbon dioxide and hydrogen is passed over a nickel catalyst. The temperature of the catalyst bed is 588 K (315°C) and the reactor pressure is 2 MPa g. The analysis of the gases leaving the reactor showed CO_2: 57.1%, H_2: 41.1%, CH_4: 1.68% and CO: 0.12% (by volume) on a dry basis The reactions taking place in the reactor are:

$$CO_2 + 4\ H_2 = CH_4 + 2\ H_2O$$
$$\text{and} \quad CO_2 + H_2 = CO + H_2O$$

Find (a) the conversion of CO_2 per pass, (b) yield of CH_4 in terms of CO_2 reacted, and (c) the composition of the feed (volume basis)

[*Ans.* (a) 3.06% (b) 93.33%; (c) CO_2: 55.13%, H_2: 44.87% (volume basis)]

4.14 Acetaldehyde is oxidized over silica gel with the help of air. The mixture is passed over that catalyst at 387 K (114°C). The outgoing dry gases are found to contain 4.85% CO_2, 8.65% acetaldehyde, 14.9% acetic acid, 2.55% O_2 and 69.05% N_2 by volume (on dry basis). For carrying out dry analysis, water was first removed from the mixture. During the water removal, some acetic acid is also condensed.

Calculate: (a) the percentage conversion of acetaldehyde, (b) the percentage yield of acetic acid, (c) mass ratio of air to acetaldehyde in incoming feed, (d) the percentage removal of acetic acid during the removal of water, and (e) that actual analysis of the gases leaving the reactor.

[*Ans.* (a) 71.7% (b) 89% (c) 1.884:1 (d) 23.6% (e) CO_2: 4.43%, CH_3CHO: 7.90%, CH_3COOH: 17.82%, O_2: 2.33, N_2: 63.09% H_2O: 4.43% (vol. basis)]

4.15 It is desired to produce hydrogen from methane by partial oxidation in the presence of steam[12]. The reactor is charged with 100 kg of methane at 698 K (425°C), 100 kg of oxygen at 698 K (425°C) and 100 kg of steam at 1253 K (980°C). The product gases are assumed to leave the reactor at 1198 K (925°C) in chemical equilibrium. Based on kinetic considerations at 1198 K (925°C), the equilibrium constant value is 0.7,

i.e. $K_p = \dfrac{(y_{CO_2})(y_{H_2})}{(y_{CO})(y_{H_2O})} = 0.7$

where y stands for the mole fraction of the component. Calculate the kmol of various components present in the product gas.

[*Ans.* CO_2: 1.15, CO: 5.10, H_2: 13.65, and H_2O: 4.4, all in kmol]

4.16 Exercise 3.20 gives the analysis of water (Table 3.14). If the same water is treated with lime and soda ash, what will be the theoretical requirement of the chemicals?

[*Ans.* 159 mg/L of CaO]

4.17 The analysis of the water obtained from an underground source is given in Table 4.23.

Table 4.23 Analysis of Water

(a) Solids, mg/L	
Total solids	3071
Dissolved solids	2946
Suspended solids (by difference)	125

(Contd.)

Table 4.23 Contd.

(b) Alkalinity, expressed as $CaCO_3$ mg/L

Total alkalinity	250
Total carbonates	17.9
Total bicarbonates	232.1
Sodium bicarbonates (by difference)	Nil

(c) Hardness, expressed as $CaCO_3$, mg/L

Temporary hardness	232.6
Permanent hardness	623.4
Total hardness	856.0
Magnesium hardness	162.0

(d) Chlorides as Cl, mg/L — 1070
(e) Sulphates as SO_4, mg/L — 168.7

If this water is treated by the lime-soda method, calculate the theoretical dosages of chemicals required to be added to the water. Is it possible to give the actual concentrations of all components present in water?

[*Ans.* Requirement of lime = 130.3 mg/L; requirement of soda ash = 660.8 mg/L]

4.18 Raw water, described in Example 3.9 is to be softened in an ion exchange bed containing a strong cation exchange resin. It is proposed to soften raw water at the rate of 50 m³/h on a continuous basis. This is a batch process in which two ion exchange beds are utilised. One bed is in normal use for 8 hours (service cycle period) while another bed is under regeneration. Regeneration is carried out with the help of sodium chloride solution. In each of the beds, 4240 liters resin is loaded. From various considerations[13], the regeneration level is fixed at 60 kg NaCl/ m³ resin. Calculate the % excess NaCl used over the stoichiometric requirement in the softening process.

[*Ans.* 41.55% excess NaCl]

Note: The process flow sheet of the softening process is given in Fig. 3.2.

4.19 The composition of a sample of cotton seed oil is given in Table 4.24. This oil is saponified with caustic potash. For 100 kg oil, calculate: (a) the theoretical amount of KOH required, and (b) the amount of glycerine liberated after 100% saponification.

Table 4.24 Composition of Cotton Seed Oil[14]

Component	Chemical formula	Mass %
(i) Oleodipalmitin	C_3H_5 $(OOCH_{33}C_{17})$ $(OOCH_{31}C_{15})_2$	8
(ii) Oleopalmitostearin	C_3H_5—$(OOCH_{33}C_{17})$ $(OOCH_{35}C_{17})$ $(OOCH_{31}C_{15})$	5

(Contd.)

Table 4.24 Contd.

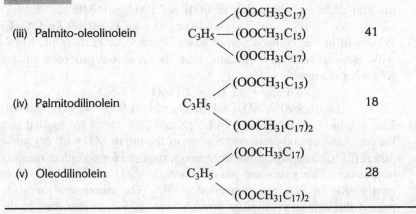

(iii)	Palmito-oleolinolein	C_3H_5 —— $(OOCH_{33}C_{17})$ / $(OOCH_{31}C_{15})$ \ $(OOCH_{31}C_{17})$	41
(iv)	Palmitodilinolein	C_3H_5 / $(OOCH_{31}C_{15})$ \ $(OOCH_{31}C_{17})_2$	18
(v)	Oleodilinolein	C_3H_5 / $(OOCH_{33}C_{17})$ \ $(OOCH_{31}C_{17})_2$	28

[*Ans.* (a) 19.525 kg (b) 10.693 kg]

4.20 Refined castor oil is analysed to have fatty acid composition (by mass) as under.

Palmitic acid: 1.4%, Stearic acid: 1.2%, Oleic acid: 4.5%,
Linoleic acid: 6.0% Linolenic acid: 0.5% and Ricinoleic acid: 86.4%
It is hydrogenated near to full saturation (having less than 3 Iodine value) and slip melting point of 358 K (85°C) for production of hydroxy stearic acid. Calculate: (a) Iodine value, and (b) theoretical hydrogenation requirement.   [*Ans.* (a) 85.9 (b) 7.586 $Nm^3/100$ kg oil]

Note: IUPAC Name of Ricinoleic acid is 12-hydroxy-9 octadecenoic acid and has a formula $CH_3(CH_2)_5$ CHOH CH_2 CH: $CH(CH_2)_7COOH$. Hydroxy stearic acid finds many industrial applications.

4.21 Used vegetable oil can be reacted with methanol to produce methyl esters which can be used as biodiesel in a diesel engine[15]. Used soybean oil is found to contain palmitic acid 46.04%, stearic acid 5.60%, oleic acid 21.94%, linoleic acid 23.22% and linolenic acid 3.20% (by mass). Methyl esters, produced by reaction at 343 K (70°C), can be used as biodiesel which meets requirements of high speed diesel (HSD) oil, conforming to IS: 1460. Its gross calorific value is found to be 39 920 kJ/kg at 298.15 K (25°C). Absence of sulphur and reduction of noxious compounds in exhaust gases from the engine makes it a 'green' fuel.

Calculate the stoichiometric requirements of methanol and production of methyl esters per kg soybean oil.

[*Ans.* (a) methanol requirement = 0.1136 kg per kg soybean oil
(b) methyl ester production = 1.005 kg per kg soybean oil]

4.22 Fatty acid methyl esters (FAME) can be hydrogenated to fatty alcohols (FOH) in a homogeneous phase by using propane at supercritical conditions[16]. FAME, derived in Exercise 4.21, are hydrogenerated over a fixed catalyst bed at 150 bar and 553 K (280°C). Reaction mixture contains 1% FAME, 20% H_2 and rest propane (by mole). Reactions go to 100% completion with near 100% selectivity to FOH in less than 800 ms. Calculate the production of FOH per 100 kg FAME.

[*Ans.* 90.1 kg FOH/100 kg FAME]

4.23 What will be the composition of gases obtained by burning pure FeS_2 with 60% excess air? Assume that the reaction proceeds in the following manner:

$$4 \, FeS_2 + 11 \, O_2 = 2 \, Fe_2O_3 + 8 \, SO_2$$

[*Ans.* 9.90%, SO_2, 8.17% O_2 and 81.93% N_2 (by volume)]

4.24 Zinc sulphide ore containing 74% ZnS and 26% inerts are roasted in a burner. Assume complete combustion of the ore to SO_2 with dry air at 300 K (27°C) and stoichiometric amount required for complete roasting of the ore. The gases are passed through V_2O_5 catalyst bed where nearly 98% of SO_2 gets converted to SO_3. The converter gases are passed through an absorption tower where all SO_3 is absorbed in the form of H_2SO_4 of 90% strength. It is desired to produce 1000 kg/h of 90% acid by spraying pure water at the top of the absorption tower. Calculate: (a) the analysis of the burner gases, (b) the analysis of the converter gases, (c) the quantity of the ore to be roasted per hour, and (d) the volumetric flow rate of air entering the converter in m^3/h.

[*Ans.* (a) 9.46% SO_2, 7.80% O_2, 82.74% N_2 (volume %)
(b) 0.20% SO_2, 9.72% SO_3, 3.32% O_2, 86.76% N_2 (by volume)
(c) 1232.7 kg/h (d) 2587 m^3/h]

4.25 A sample of iron pyrites contain 88% FeS_2 and rest gangue. It is roasted with air 150% in excess of the theoretical requirement for oxidiation of FeS_2 as per the reactions:

$$4 \, FeS_2 + 11 \, O_2 = 2 \, Fe_2O_3 + 8 \, SO_2$$
$$4 \, FeS_2 + 15 \, O_2 = 2 \, Fe_2O_3 + 8 \, SO_3$$

The residue of the burner contains 2.6% S. 40% of this sulphur is in the form of FeS_2 while the rest is in the form of SO_3 absorbed in the cinder. Also. assume that 92% of the sulphur burnt produces SO_2 and the rest 8% oxidizes to SO_3. Based on 100 kg pyrites charged, calculate: (a) the mass of the cinder produced, (b) the percentage of the sulphur lost in the cinder, (c) the analysis of the burner gas on SO_3-free basis, and (d) the volume of dry air required in m^3 at 300 K (27°C) and 100 kPa a (750 torr).

[*Ans.* (a) 74.4 kg (b) 4.11% (c) 5.59% SO_2, 13.03% O_2 and
81.38% N_2 (Volume %) (d) 589 m^3]

4.26 Magnesium ore (chiefly $MgCO_3$), containing 5% moisture is roasted with the help of flue gases in a furnace. The ratio of the dry flue gases to the ore is kept at 1.82 kg/kg. The analysis of the entering flue gases shows a composition of 12.8% CO_2, 6.1% O_2 and rest N_2 (volume % on dry basis). The exit gases from the furnace contain 24% CO_2 (by volume) on a dry basis. Based on the 100 kmol of dry gases entering the furnace, calculate: (a) the kmol of CO_2 added to flue gases, (b) the analysis of exit gases on a dry basis, and (c) the average molar mass of dry incoming and outgoing flue gases.

[*Ans.* (a) 14.74 kmol (b) CO_2: 24.0%, O_2: 5.33% and N_2: 70.67%
(c) 30.29 and 32.05, respectively]

4.27 Potassium iodide is electrolysed in an electrolytic cell. When a definite amount of current is passed through the cell liquor for 10 800 s, it was found that 127 g iodine was liberated at the anode. Calculate the theoretical current passed through the cell.

[*Ans.* 8.95 amperes]

4.28 In a silver electroplating plant, silver nitrate is used. When 1130 amperes were passed through $AgNO_3$ solution for 32 400 s, it was found that 2.0 m^3 oxygen (at NTP) was liberated at the anode. Calculate: (a) the amount of silver liberated in kg, and (b) the current efficiency of the cell.

[*Ans.* (a) 38.55 kg (b) 94.15%]

4.29 The addition of lime is being extensively used as a means of clarifying waste water. The limed waste water at *p*H of 11.8–12.0 is recarbonated by treatment with CO_2 to *p*H of 9.8–10.0 to remove ions:

$$Ca(OH)_2 + CO_2 = CaCO_3\downarrow + H_2O$$

However, this precipitation is rapid and $CaCO_3$ tends to deposit on some parts of the CO_2 absorber, lowering efficiency and causing maintenance problems.

A modified approach to the problem is to put a bypass of limed waste around the absorber to the clarifier[17] as shown in Fig. 4.6. Part of the feed stream goes through this bypass and the *p*H of the recarbonated stream is brought to 7.0 so that the carbonation forms bicarbonate instead of carbonate

$$Ca(OH)_2 + 2\ CO_2 = Ca(HCO_3)_2$$

Since $Ca(HCO_3)_2$ is soluble in water, it does not precipitate. The bicarbonate solution from the absorber subsequently meets the bypassed limed waste water. As a result, calcium is precipitated in the form of carbonate as per the reaction:

$$Ca(OH)_2 + Ca(HCO_3)_2 = 2\ CaCO_3\downarrow + 2H_2O$$

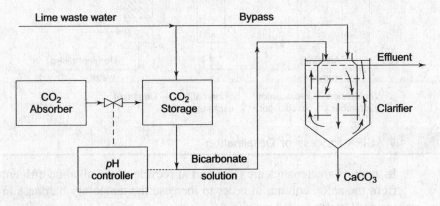

Fig. 4.6   Lime Clarification of Waste Water

This occurs in the clarifier, where $CaCO_3$ is conveniently removed. Assuming that the chemical reactions taking place in the absorber and the clarifier go to 100% completion, calculate the % of the incoming limed waste water flow bypassed to the clarifier

[*Ans.* 50%]

4.30 Refer Example 4.15.
(a) If conversion per pass is assumed to be 24% and ammonia separation is taken as 65%, calculate the purge rate.
(b) If conversion per pass is taken as 25% and ammonia separation is assumed to be 70%, calculate the purge rate.

[*Ans.* (a) 7.971 kmol/s, (b) 7.871 kmol/s]

Note: It may be noted that change in the conversion has pronounced effect on the purge rate over change in ammonia separation.

4.31 The use of weak ion exchange resins in the desalination processes offer advantages of very high regenation efficiency and lower rinse requirements. On the other hand, the ability of such resins to exchange ions is strongly influenced by the *p*H of the influents. Based on the buffer capacity of the CO_2/HCO_3 system, a process is developed for the desalination of saline water at the Bary Laboratory of the Water Research Institute, Italy, named as the SIRA process [18,19]. The process is shown in Fig. 4.7.

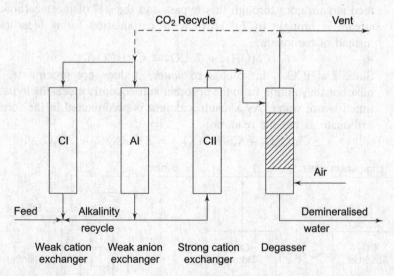

Fig. 4.7 SIRA Process of Desalination

Its main characteristics are (a) a partial recycle of the alkaline effluent from the anion column in order to increase the temporary hardness in the feed water as per reaction:

$$2\,RCOOH + Ca^{++} (or\ Mg^{++}) + 2\,HCO_3^- = (RCOO)_2Ca + H_2O + CO_2$$
$$or\ (RCOO)_2Mg$$

(b) a recycle of the CO_2 produced in the degasser (if necessary) to convert all the anions in the bicarbonate in the weak anion exchanger as per the reaction.

$$R'OH + NaCl + CO_2 = R'Cl + NaHCO_3$$

A third column, CII, containing strong cations can be used for obtaining complete demineralisation according to the reaction.

$$R''SO_3H + NaHCO_3 = R''SO_3Na + H_2O + CO_2$$

The effluent from CII flows to degasser where CO_2 is removed and recycled (if necessary). For producing potable water, column CII may not be necessary.

Let, A = feed water strong anions, meg/L
      M = feed water alkalinity, meq/L
      C = feed water cations, meq/L
      H = feed water hardness (total), meq/L
      X = alkalinity recyle flow rate from anion section/feed flow ratio
      Y = CO_2 recycle to anion section/CO_2 discharged in the product.

With the hypothesis that (a) leakage of strong ions (i.e., Ca and Mg from CI and Cl and SO_4 from AI) is nil, (b) cations are exchanged on the cationic column (CI) in quantum equal to the alkalinity contents of the feed water, and (c) (CO_2 is fed to the anionic column (AI) in a quantity equal to convert all the anions to bicarbonates, prove that

$$X = \frac{H-M}{C-H}$$

$$Y = \frac{A-H}{M}$$

and, $$(1+X)(1+Y) = \frac{A}{M}$$

Notes: 1. SIRA process offers the following advantages.

(a) Regeneration of CI can be carried out with low concentration of aqueous sulphuric acid solution, obtained by in-line dilution of the concentrated sulphuric acid solution, used for regeneration of CII in sodium from.

(b) Precipitation of hardness is avoided in the anionic column nearing exhaustion of cation column CI.

2. When A = H, i.e. strong anions and hardness are same, Y = 0 or CO_2 recycle is not necessary.

3. When M ≥ H, X = 0, thereby indicated that when feed water contains only temporary hardness, recycle of alkalinity is not necessary.

4.32 Refer Example 4.10. With a view to improve inherent safety of the plant, it is decided to recycle partially tail gas (shown as 'optional' in Fig. 4.1) from the absorber such that the concentration of oxygen in the feed gas to the reactor does not exceed 10% (by volume). Assume that conversion and yields are unchanged and total wet gas molar flow to the reactor also remains unchanged. Rework the material balance of the plant and calculate (a) ratio of recycle stream to purge stream,
(b) ratio of recycle stream to fresh air, and
(c) concentration of UC in purge stream on dry gas basis.

[*Ans.* (a) 2.042 kmol/kmol (b) 1.96 kmol/kmol
(c) UC = 3.37% (by volume)]

4.33 Cyclohexane can be produced by hydrogenation of benzene.[20]. The reaction can be written as

$$C_6H_6 + 3 H_2 = C_6H_{12}$$

Fresh benzene, make-up hydrogen stream, recycle hydrogen stream and recycle cyclohexane are mixed (ref. Fig. 3.5) and fed to a fixed bed catalytic reactor. Assume benzene as 100% pure while the make-up hydrogen stream contains 97.5% H_2 and 2.5% inerts (N_2 + CH_4). The heat of reaction is highly exothermic and to have effective control of the reaction temperature of 477.5 K (204.5°C) recycle of a definite amount of cyclohexane is maintained such that benzene concentration is limited at 18.5 mole% in the mixed feed. Also the mole ratio of hydrogen to benzene in the mixed feed is kept at 3.3. The heat of reaction is removed by boiling water outside the catalyst tubes.

Assume 100% conversion in the reactor. The reactor effluent is cooled and entire quantity of cyclohexane is condensed. Effluent form the cooler is sent to a separator where cyclohexane is separated from the mixture. A major portion of the gases from the separator will be recycled back to the reactor. A small portion of the offgasses is purged to bleed off the inerts from the recycle stream such that the total inerts are limited to the 10 mole% in the mixed feed.

For 100 kmol fresh benzene feed calculate the flows of purge, make-up hydrogen, recycle hydrogen and recycle cyclohexane streams.

[*Ans.* Purge stream = 12.139 kmol,
Make-up hydrogen stream = 312.139 kmol,
Recycle hydrogen stream = 71.915 kmol and
Recycle cyclohexane stream = 56.49 kmol]

4.34 Refer Exercise 4.33. As an energy conservation measure, it is decided to process the offgases from the separator by a cryogenic route in a cold-box. Product H_2 stream from the cold-box contains 90% of H_2 and 5% of inerts as compared to that contained in the offgases. Tail-gas stream containing 10% of hydrogen and 95% of inerts is purged out. For the revised conditions, calculate the flows of make-up hydrogen stream, recycle hydrogen stream, recycle cyclohexane stream and purge stream. Also calculate the inerts contents of the mixed feed.

[*Ans.* Purge stream = 10.769 kmol, Make-up H_2 stream = 303 kmol, Recycle H_2 stream = 27.404 kmol, Recycle cyclohexane stream = 102.236 kmol, Inerts content of mixed feed = 1.51 mole %]

Note: Cryogenic purification of cooler exit gas stream shows all-round improvement in process parameters.

4.35 In Halcon SD process to manufacture ethylene oxide, ethylene is directly oxidised by oxygen[21]. Ethylene concentration is maintained at 10% at the reactor inlet. Pure ethylene (100%) and oxygen with 97% purity are used as feedstocks. Both the gases are mixed with recycled gas and the mixed gas is then fed to a multi-tube reactor. The process is shown in shown in Fig. 4.8.

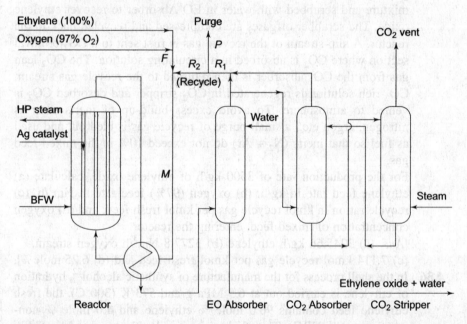

Fig. 4.8 Manufacture of Ethylene Oxide by Halcon SD Process

In the reactor, per pass conversion is 50% while the yield of ethylene glycol is 70% Carbon dioxide and water are the chief by-products while trace amounts of acetaldehyde and formaldehyde are also formed which may be neglected for stoichiometric calculations. Following reactions are known to take place

$$CH_2 = CH_2 + \frac{1}{2} O_2 = \underset{\underset{O}{\diagdown\diagup}}{CH_2 \!-\! CH_2} \qquad (1)$$

Ethylene   Ethylene Oxide

$$\underset{\text{Ethylene}}{CH_2 = CH_2} + 3\,O_2 = 2\,CO_2 + 2\,H_2O \qquad (2)$$

$$CH_2\!\!-\!\!CH_2 = CH_3CHO \qquad (3)$$
$$\diagdown_{\;\;O\;\;}\diagup$$

Ethylene Oxide   Acetaldehyde

$$CH_2 = CH_2 + O_2 = 2\,CH_2O \qquad (4)$$

Ethylene   Formaldehyde

The reactor is basically a heat exchanger in which the reaction is carried out at 2 MPa g and 523 K (250°C). Tubes are filled with silver catalyst while the reaction temperature is maintained by boiling water on the shell side, producing high pressure steam. The reactor effluent gas is cooled in a heat exchanger by exchanging heat with incoming gas mixture and scrubbed with water in EO Absorber to recover ethylene oxide. The scrubber offgases are compressed and recycled back to the reactor. A slip-stream of the recycle gas is first sent to a CO_2-removal section where CO_2 is absorbed in a circulating solution. The CO_2-lean gas from the CO_2 absorber is then returned to the recycle gas stream. CO_2-rich solution is regenerated in CO_2 stripper and desorbed CO_2 is vented to atmosphere. To avoid excess build-up of inerts such as nitrogen, argon etc., a small purge of recycle gas is bled out and used as fuel so that inerts (N_2 + Ar) do not exceed 10% in the mixed feed gas.

For the production rate of 3500 kg/h of ethylene oxide, calculate (a) ethylene feed rate in kg/h, (b) oxygen (97%) feed rate in Nm^3/h, (c) recycle ration in kmol recycle gas per kmol fresh feed, and (d) oxygen concentration of mixed feed, entering the reactor.

[*Ans.* (a) 3245.66 kg/h ethylene (b) 3277.8 Nm^3/h oxygen stream, (c) 7.114 kmol recycle gas per kmol fresh feed and (d) 6.25 mole%].

4.36 In the shell process for the manufacture of synthetic alcohol[22], hydration of ethylene is carried out at 6.5 MPa g and 573 K (300°C). the fresh ethylene feed contains 96.0 mole % ethylene and 4.0 mole % non-reactive gases (NRG). The ethylene is mixed with steam and heated in preheater. The preheated mixture is fed to a reactor which contains pellets of diatomaceous earth, impregnated with phosphoric acid. The steam input with fresh ethylene is so adjusted that the molar ratio of water to ethylene in the combined feed i.e. (fresh feed + recycle feed) is 0.65:1. At the operating conditions, the conversion per pass is only 5%, based on ethylene. The reaction taking place in the reactor is:

$$C_2H_{4(g)} + H_2O_{(g)} = C_2H_5OH_{(g)} \text{ (exothermic)}$$

Side reactions produce diethylether and acetaldehyde, which can be neglected for the purpose of calculations. The reactor effluents are first passed through the heat exchangers and then through a flash drum and a scrubber where practically all ethanol and water are removed from the gaseous mixture. The offgases from the scrubber are recycled back to the reactor. In order to limit the NRG concentration in the combined feed at 15 mole % based on ethylene plus NRG feed (excluding water), a small quantity of recycle stream is purged. The process flow diagram is shown in Fig. 4.9.

Compute, (a) the recycle ratio, (b) the purge rate per 100 kmol of fresh ethylene, (c) the percentage loss of ethylene based on unreacted ethylene from the reactor, (d) the composition of the gas mixtures ingoing to and outcoming from the reactor.

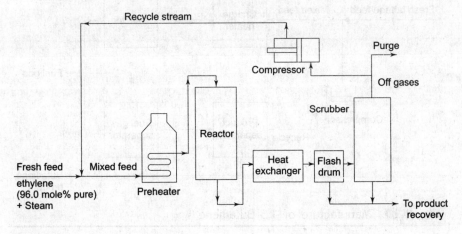

Fig. 4.9 Manufacture of Ethyl Alcohol by Hydration of Ethylene

[*Ans.* (a) Recycle ratio = 16.52 kmol per kmol fresh ethylene feed
(b) Purge = 25.526 kmol, (c) Loss = 1.52%,
(d) See Table 4.25]

Table 4.25 Composition of Reactor Exit Gases

Component	Gas mixture, ingoing to reactor		Gas mixture, outcoming from reactor	
	kmol	mole %	kmol	mole %
Ethylene	1489.41	54.83	1414.94	53.56
Water	968.12	35.64	893.65	33.82
NRG	258.92	9.53	258.92	9.80
Ethanol	–	–	74.47	2.82
Total	2716.45	100.00	2641.98	100.00

4.37 A plant produces 1,3-butadiene by dehydrogenation of *n*-butane using Houdry "one-step" process[22]. In this process, the heat of reaction is supplied by the burning of coke during the regeneration step of the process. The *n*-butane feed is preheated to about 868 K (595°C) and is passed through a brick-lined reactor containing a fixed bed of pelletised alumina-chromia catalyst. The absolute pressure in the reactor is maintained at around 20 kPa. The fresh n-butane feed is combined with the recycle feed and passed through the fuel gas separator system. The effluent gas mixture is then passed through a product separator where the butadiene is separated from the gases. The offgases from the product separator are recycled and mixed with the fresh feed. The simplified block diagram of the flow process is shown in Fig. 4.10. The composition of various gaseous streams are given in Table 4.26.

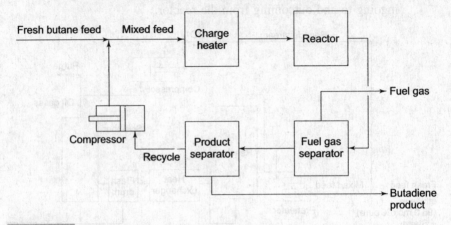

Fig. 4.10 Manufacture of 1,3-Butadiene

Calculate: (a) the recycle ratio, (b) the composition of recycle stream, and (c) the yield of butadiene based on n-butane consumption.

Table 4.26 Composition of Gaseous Streams

| Component | Composition, mole % | | | | |
	Fresh feed	Mixed feed (fresh + recycle)	Reactor effluent	Fuel gas	Butadiene product mixture
Hydrogen			22.05	73.57	
Methane			3.25	10.86	
Ethylene			1.16	3.83	
Ethane			1.08	3.56	
Propylene			1.32	4.39	
Propane			0.64	2.09	
iso-butane	1.5	3.84	2.50	–	
iso-butylene		6.94	4.93	0.24	
n-butylene		25.29	17.88	0.24	1.69
n-butane	98.5	63.59	30.91	0.45	–
1,3-butadiene	–	0.34	8.78	0.24	98.31
C5			0.16	0.56	
Coke			5.34	–	

[*Ans.* (a) Recycle ratio = 4.04 kmol per kmol fresh feed (b) *i*-butane: 4.42%, *i*-butylene: 8.66%, *n*-butylene; 31.55%, *n*-butane: 54.95% and 1,3-butadiene: 0.43% (mole %) (c) Yield of butadiene = 63.0%]

4.38 Flue gases from a steam generation plant, firing coal containing 1% (mass) sulphur, amounts to 265 000 m^3/h at 448 K (175°C) and 106.6 kPa a (800 torr). The gases are found to contain 1160 mg/m^3 SO_2 and 2.15 kg/s water vapour. It is necessary to remove sulphur dioxide from the flue gases by reacting it with aqueous soda-ash solution in an absorber[23].

$$Na_2CO_3 + SO_2 = Na_2SO_3 + CO_2$$

The scrubbing system is shown in Fig. 4.11. At first the flue gas is spray cooled in the quencher to 323 K (50°C) and directed downward into the circulating liquor. Gas bubbles through the liquor enters the adjacent absorber and travels upward through two sieve trays. A circulating pump pumps the solution to the absorber. A purge stream is maintained from the discharge of the pump to limit the solids (Na_2CO_3 + Na_2SO_3) concentration to 8% (mass) to avoid any precipitation in the absorber.

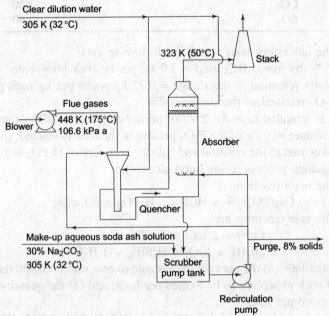

Fig. 4.11 Scrubbing of Sulphur Dioxide from Flue Gases

Soda ash is supplied in the form of aqueous 30% (mass) solution at 305 K (32°C) to the absorber pump. Dilution water is made-up at 305 K (32°C) in the quencher and the absorber as shown in the figure.

Gases leave the absorber at 323 K (50°C) and 101.325 kPa a (760 torr). Nearly 90% of SO_2 in the inlet gas is removed when 50% excess reactant is used in the system. Make the material balance of the system and calculate the flow rates of the make-up soda-ash solution, dilution water and purge solution.

[*Ans.* Make-up soda solution = 2545.7 kg/h, Dilution water = 17 270.3 kg/h, Purge = 10 626.9 kg/h]

4.39 Phosphoric acid is made by reacting the rock phosphate with hydrochloric acid. It is desired to use the rock phosphate, obtained from hilly areas near Udaipur, Rajasthan. The composition of the rock phosphate[24] is given in Table 4.27.

Table 4.27 Composition of Rock Phosphate of Rajasthan Region

Components	Analysis by mass %
P_2O_5	34.55
CaO	48.62
$Al_2O_3 + Fe_2O_3$	3.76
MgO	1.29
SiO_2	5.58
CaF_2	2.50
CO_2	1.30
SO_3	2.40

The laboratory tests reveal the following data[24].
25% (by mass) HCl used = 3.0 kg per kg rock phosphate
Water retention in the sludge = 0.22 kg water per kg rock phosphate
P_2O_5 retained in the sludge = 2%
It is intended to make 2 t/h of phosphoric acid of 80% strength.
Assume: (i) 95% of the P_2O_5 present in the rock is reacted, (ii) all CaF_2 takes part in the reaction and (iii) the recovery of H_3PO_4 is 97% by the leaching process (using butyl alcohol).
The main reaction:
$$Ca_3(PO_4)_2 + 6\ HCl = 2\ H_3PO_4 + 3\ CaCl_2$$
The side reactions are:
$$CaF_2 + 2\ HCl = 2\ HF + CaCl_2$$
$$6\ HF + SiO_2 = H_2SiF_6 + 2\ H_2O$$
Calculate: (a) the per cent excess acid excess acid used, (b) the quantity of rock phosphate to be treated per hour, and (c) the quantity of $CaCl_2$ formed per hour.

[*Ans.* (a) 40.71% (b) 3.64 t/h (c) 3.49 t/h]

4.40 In the manufacture of nitric acid, ammonia is oxidised to nitric oxide on a catalyst as per the following chemical reactions:

$$4\ NH_3 + 5\ O_2 = 4\ NO + 6\ H_2O \tag{1}$$

$$4\ NH_3 + 3\ O_2 = 2\ N_2 + 6\ H_2O \tag{2}$$

Nitric oxide is further oxidised to nitrogen dioxide which is absorbed in water to yield nitric acid

$$2\ NO + O_2 = 2\ NO_2 \tag{3}$$

$$2 \, NO_2 + \frac{1}{2} \, O_2 + H_2O = 2 \, HNO_3 \qquad (4)$$

Air is first preheated, mixed with superheated ammonia vapours and reacted over a catalyst gauze, composed of 90% Pt and 10% Rh (mass %), at a temperature of 1188 K (915°C) and 0.75 MPa g. The preheated air temperature is 533 K (260°C). The superheated ammonia enters the burner. Process flow is shown in Fig. 4.12.

Operating data of a plant[25] having a production capacity of 250 t/day of HNO_3 are given below.

Flow of primary air = 29 394 Nm^3/h (dry)

Flow of ammonia = 3266 Nm^3/h

Flow of secondary air = 8145 Nm^3/h (dry)

Vol.% NO in burner outlet gas = 9.27 (wet basis)

Vol.% NO in tail gas = 0.2 (dry basis)

Calculate, (a) the combustion efficiency, defined as the moles of ammonia consumed to produce NO to the moles of ammonia fed (can also be termed as the yield of NO), (b) the absorber efficiency, defined as NO consumed to NO fed to the absorber, and (c) the overall efficiency of the system, defined as the product of combustion efficiency and absorber efficiency.

[*Ans.* (a) 95.02% (b) 98.0% (c) 93.12%]

4.41 A blast furnace uses ore of the composition, Fe_2O_3: 90% and SiO_2: 10%. The coke fed the furnace has 90% C and 10% SiO_2. The flux is limestone containing 95% $CaCO_3$, 3% $MgCO_3$ and 2% SiO_2. The coke rate is 1 kg/kg of pig iron. The pig iron contains 4% C, 1% Si and rest Fe. The slag must contain 45% (CaO + MgO). Assume that no FeO is present in the slag. For 1000 kg of pig iron production, calculate the mass of limestone required.

All percentages are by mass.

[*Ans.* 354.1 kg limestone per tonne of pig iron]

REFERENCES

1. McCormach, H., *Ind. Engng. Chem.,* **29**(12): 1937, p. 1333.
2. Lowenheim, F. A. and M. K. Moran, *Faith, Keys and Clark's Industrial Chemicals,* 4th Ed., John Wiley & Sons, USA, 1975, p. 3.
3. Boffelli, S. O., *Ind. Engng. Chem.,* **53**(6): 1961, p. 428.
4. *Wealth of India,* Part I, Council of Scientific and Industrial Research, New Delhi, 1948, p. 89.
5. Levitt, B., *Oil, Fat and Soap,* Chemical Publication Co., USA, 1951, p. 58.
6. *Tappi,* **48**(1): 1965, p.167A.

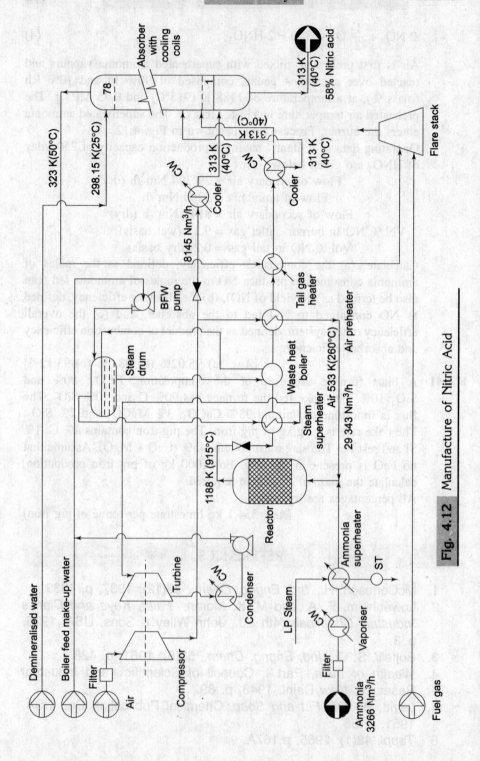

Fig. 4.12 Manufacture of Nitric Acid

7. Wolfgang Gerhartz, *Ullmann's Encyclopedia of Industrial Chemistry*, Vol. A11, 5th Ed., VCH Verlagsgesellschatt mbH, 1988, p. 625.
8. Private Communication with Haldor Topsoe, Denmark.
9. Simpson, W. A., and J. C. Olsen, *Ind. Engng. Chem.*, **29**(12): 1937, p. 1350.
10. Shreve, R. N. and J. A. Brink, Jr., *Chemical Process Industries*, 4th Ed., McGraw-Hill, USA, 1977, p. 530.
11. Wolfgang Gerhartz, *Ullman's Encyclopedia of Industrial Chemistry*, Vol. A1, 5th Ed., VCH Verlagsgesellschaft mbH, 1985, p. 110.
12. Edmister, W. C., *Hydrocarbon Processing*, **53**(8): 1973, p. 109.
13. Product Literature on "INDION 225" of Ion Exchange (India) Ltd., Mumbai.
14. Hilditch, T. P., *The Chemical Constitution of Natural Fats*, Chapman & Hall Ltd., U.K, 1949, p. 255.
15. Srivastava A. and R. Prasad, *Indian Chemical Engineer*, Section-B **44**(2), April–June 2002, p. 132.
16. Hark, S. van den and M. Harrord, *Ind. Engng. Chem. Research*, **40**, 2001, p. 5052.
17. Pinto, A. P., *Chem. Engng.*, **82**(2): Jan. 20, 1975, p. 125.
18. Boari, G., L. Liberti, C. Merli and R. Passino, *Proceedings of the Third International Symposium on Fresh Water from Sea*,2: 1970, p. 63.
19. Boari, G., L. Liberti and R. Passino, *Environmental Protection Engng.*, **1**(2): 1975.
20. Private Communication with Aspen Technology, Inc., USA.
21. Meyers, R. A., *Handbook of Chemicals Production Processes*, McGraw-Hill, USA, 1986, p. 15.
22. Stephenson, R. M., *Introduction to the Chemical Process Industries*, Van Nostrand Reinhold Co., USA, 1966.
23. *Power*, **121**(11): 1977, p. 51.
24. Chatterjee, M. K., *Chemical Age of India*, **24**(7): 1973, p. 428.
25. Jain, B. K. *Indian Chemical Engineer, Transactions*, **16**(3): 1974, p. 44.

Energy Balances

5.1 INTRODUCTION

Physical or chemical changes in matter are accompanied by enthalpy changes. Therefore, when a chemical reaction takes places, a change in enthalpy is invariably observed. In Chapters 3 and 4, the material balances with and without chemical reaction were considered. In this chapter, the energy balances related to these operations or reactions will be dealt with. Dilution of acid or alkali solutions, mixing of fluids, crystallization and other unit operations involve thermal changes. These physical processes will also be covered in this chapter.

5.2 ENERGY AND THERMOCHEMISTRY

When a definite amount of force is applied over a material object and if it is displaced in the direction of the force, mechanical work is said to be done on the object. This work can produce a property of the matter which is called *energy*. Thus, when a solid is forced upward, it results in an increase in potential energy. Similarly, due to friction between two solids, heat is generated, i.e. the loss of work done on the solid is converted into thermal energy. Thus, energy can be in different forms, e.g., potential energy, kinetic energy, thermal, electrical etc. Conversely, any form of energy can be converted into work, e.g., electricity can run mechanical machinery, potential energy can be utilized to run hydraulic turbines, thermal energy of a fuel can be beneficially utilized in a chemical process, chemical (internal) energy is utilised in softening or demineralisation of water, etc. Thus, basically the units of work and energy are same (refer Chapter 1).

When two substances are at different temperatures, it is known that heat flows from a hot substance to a relatively cold substance (*second law of thermodynamics*). Thus, heat is defined as a form of energy which is in transit between a hot source and a cold receiver and therefore has units of energy. The transmission of heat solely depends on the temperatures of the two substances. In other words, temperature can be termed as the level of thermal energy.

A substance possesses a definite quantity of energy due to the never-ending motion of its molecules. This quantity is by virtue of the presence, relative positions and movement of the molecules, and is defined as *internal energy*. The evaluation of internal energy involves the Einstein's theory and is beyond the scope of this book. To differentiate *external energy* from the internal energy, it can be said that the former is by virtue of the position and motion of the *whole* substance. Thus, external energy comprises of all mechanical energies. Since in chemical or physical changes, it is always the difference of the energies of two states which is important, the differential energy is commonly regarded as the useful quantity rather than absolute value. Enthalpy H of a particular substance is defined as

$$H = E + pV \tag{5.1}$$

where E is the internal energy, p pressure, and V volume.

Since p and V are the properties of the state of a system, H is again defined by the state only and is the external property.

In general, enthalpy is the energy possessed by a system due to its molecular arrangement while heat is the energy that flows due to a temperature gradient.

In this book, the terms "energy", "enthalpy" and "heat" are essentially used for thermal energy.

The science related with changes in energy, associated with a given chemical or physical process is called *thermochemistry*. The ultimate aim of thermochemistry is to determine thermodynamic properties, such as heat of formation, enthalpy, free energy, etc. Although calorimetric measurements from the major activity in thermochemistry, spectroscopic determination of the heats of dissociation of diatomic molecules, measurement of bond dissociation energies in polyatomic molecules by kinetic and electron impact studies, measurement of the equilibrium constant of a chemical reaction, statistical and other methods are also helpful in determining thermodynamic properties.

5.3 ENERGY BALANCES

The energy balance of a particular system can be achieved from the *first law of thermodynamics* which states that the total energy of an isolated system and its surrounding remains constant. The conversion of one form of energy into another is possible. When a system gains or loses energy, it must be exactly equal to the loss from or gain of energy by the surroundings. Thus, the first law of thermodynamics relates to the conservation of the energy. This concept can be understood clearly by considering the steady flow process of an incompressible fluid as shown in Fig. 5.1.

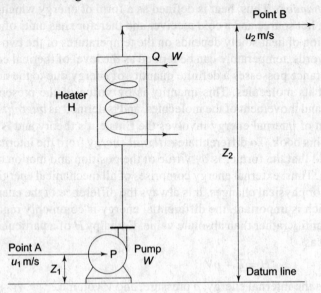

Fig. 5.1 Steady Flow Process of an Incompressible Fluid

In this process, the absolute pressure and velocity of the fluid at point A are p_1 and u_1 respectively. The fluid is pumped with the help of a pump P which does net work W on the fluid. The fluid receives heat Q in the heater H and comes out at point B with pressure p_2 and velocity u_2. Let E_1 and E_2 be the internal energies of the fluid at points A and B respectively.

$$\text{Total energy at point A} = E_1 + q_m \left[Z_1\left(\frac{g}{g_c}\right) + \frac{u_1^2}{2\alpha_1 g_c} + \frac{p_1}{\rho} \right]$$

where,

q_m = mass flow rate, kg/s

g = acceleration due to free fall (gravity)

= 9.806 65 m/s^2 at mean sea level

g_c = gravitational constant = 1 kg·m/(N·s^2)

u_1 = velocity, m/s

ρ = density of the fluid, kg/m^3

p_1 = pressure, N/m^2 (or Pa)

Z_1 = elevation from datum level, m

α_1 = kinetic energy correction factor

It is clear from the above equation that the total energy at point A is made of four different forms of the energy. The parameter E is the internal energy and depends entirely on the state and conditions of the fluid.

The quantity Z stands for potential energy, a form of mechanical energy, $u^2/(2\alpha g_c)$ is kinetic energy, another form of mechanical energy and p/ρ is pressure energy, yet another form of mechanical energy. These three forms of mechanical energy are expressed in pressure head terms (m of the fluid) and are converted to heat units with the help of J.

Energy added during the transport = mechanical work done by the pump

+ heat added by the heater

= $W + Q$

where W represents the mechanical work done by the pump (in J) and Q, the heat added by the heater (in J).

Instead of a pump, if a turbine is present in the system which is driven by the fluid, the mechanical work will be performed by the fluid on the turbine. As a result W will assume a negative sign.

Similarly, if a cooler is installed in the place of a heater, Q will assume a negative sign.

$$\text{Total energy at point } B = E_2 + q_m \left[Z_2 \left(\frac{g}{g_c} \right) + \frac{u_2^2}{2\alpha_2 g_c} + \frac{p_2}{\rho} \right]$$

According to the first law of thermodynamics,

Total energy in the fluid at A

+ energy gain during transport = total energy in the fluid at B

$$E_1 + q_m \left[Z_1 \left(\frac{g}{g_c} \right) + \frac{u_1^2}{2\alpha_1 g_c} + \frac{p_1}{\rho} \right] + Q$$

$$= E_2 + q_m \left[Z_2 \left(\frac{g}{g_c} \right) + \frac{u_2^2}{2\alpha_2 g_c} + \frac{p_2}{\rho} \right] \tag{5.2}$$

In Eq. (5.2), the friction losses are neglected.

Imagine a reactor R in the place of a heater H in Fig. 5.1. Let the flowing fluid be the mixture of reactants. In the reactor, reaction takes place and as a result, heat is absorbed from, or released to surroundings, depending on whether the reaction is endothermic or exothermic. This heat of reaction (refer Sec. 5.14) will take the place of Q with the proper sign in Eq. (5.2). It is clear that Eq. (5.2) accounts for the transformation of one form of energy into another form.

Often, in industrial chemical processes, changes in mechanical energies are absent or negligible. Under these circumstances, Eq. (5.2) reduces to thermal changes only and is called a heat balance. In other words, the change in internal energies amount to only a thermal change. Thus, a heat balance of a process is a simplified form of the energy balance, dealing with thermal changes only. This is normally a case with energy balances of the process industry.

Example 5.1 Water is pumped from the bottom of a well 50 m deep at the rate of 1 L/s into an atmospheric storage tank 10 m above the ground. To prevent freezing in the winters, a heater puts 52 kW into the water during its transfer from the well to the storage tank. Heat is lost from the whole system at the constant rate of 21 kW. A 1.5 BkW pump is used to pump the water. About 55% of the rated power goes into the work of pumping and the rest is dissipated as heat to the atmosphere. Assume the change in kinetic energy to be negligible. Calculate the changes in internal energies between the storage tank and the bottom of the well.

Solution   The flow system is shown in Fig. 5.2.

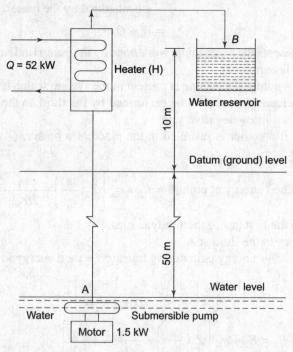

Fig. 5.2   Pumping of Water

Basis: Pumping 1 L/s of water

Heat added in the system = 52 kW

Heat lost to surroundings = 21 kW

Net heat gained by water, $\phi = 52 - 21 = 33$ kW

$$p_1 = p_2 = \text{atmospheric pressure} = 101\ 325\ \text{Pa}$$

$$Z_1 = -50\ \text{m}$$

$$Z_2 = 10\ \text{m}$$

$$g = 9.806\ 65\ \text{m/s}^2$$

$$g_c = 1\ \text{kg} \cdot \text{m/(N} \cdot \text{s}^2)$$

Density, $\rho = 1.0$ kg/L

Since the kinetic energy change is negligible, u_1 and u_2 can be neglected.

Net pump work done on the fluid (W) = $1.5 \times 0.55 = 0.825$ kW

It is required to find $(E_2 - E_1)$.

Writing the energy balance between A and B.

$$E_1 + q_m\left[\frac{p_1}{\rho} + Z_1\left(\frac{g}{g_c}\right)\right] + W + Q = E_2 + q_m\left[\frac{p_2}{\rho} + Z_2\left(\frac{g}{g_c}\right)\right]$$

Where q_m stands for the mass flow rate of water (1 kg/s).

Since $p_1 = p_2$

$$(E_2 - E_1) = W + Q + (Z_1 - Z_2)\left(\frac{g}{g_c}\right) q_m$$

$$= (0.825) + 33 + \left[(-50 - 10) \times \frac{9.806\ 65}{1000}\right]$$

$$= 0.825 + 33 - 0.588 = 33.237 \text{ kW}$$

The increase in internal energy will increase the temperature of water.   *Ans.*

Note: It may be noted that contribution of the potential energy and mechanical work done by the pump are very small and hence the change in internal energy due to these factors is quite small.

5.4 HEAT CAPACITY

In Chapter 1, the unit of heat (or enthalpy) is given as joule (J) in SI (Section 1.4.4). For any substance, the heat required to raise the temperature by 1 K of 1 kg of it, is defined as *heat capacity*. It is customary to define the heat capacity on a unit mass or on a unit mole basis the latter being known as *molar* (or *molal*) heat capacity. For pure water, heat capacity is 4.1855 kJ/(kg.K) at 288.15 K (15°C). *Specific heat* of a substance is the ratio of the heat capacity of a particular substance to that of water, usually at 277.15 K (4°C). For solids and liquids, heat capacity values on mass basis are normally used. However, molar values are not uncommon.

Consider the heat capacity of a gas. Its numerical value depends on the route followed for attaining a particular temperature. Normally, two routes are chosen, viz. the constant volume path and the constant pressure path.

Fundamentally $dQ = n \cdot C_m \cdot dT$ (5.3a)

where dQ is the change in heat, n the number of moles, C_m the molar heat capacity, and dT the change in temperature.

For $n = 1$ mole, $Q = C_m \cdot dT$ (5.3b)

For a constant volume process, $dQ = C_{mv} \cdot dT$ (5.4)

where C_{mv}, represents the molar heat capacity at constant volume.

Since the volume of the gas remains constant, no work is done on the gas. Hence,

$$dQ = dE$$ (5.5)

or $\qquad\qquad dE = C_{mv} \cdot dT$ (5.6)

This indicates that the change in internal energy equals the heat added at constant volume.

For a constant pressure process, $dQ = C_{mp} \cdot dT$ (5.7)

In this process, since the volume changes at constant pressure, Q is total heat content (or enthalpy) H of the gas.

$$dQ = dH$$

$$= dE + pdV$$

$$= C_{mp} \cdot dT \qquad (5.8)$$

For an ideal gas, it can be proved* that

$$C_{mp} - C_{mv} = R = \text{Gas constant} \qquad (5.9)$$

The ratio $\dfrac{C_{mp}}{C_{mv}}$ is denoted by γ and equals 1.4 for an ideal gas. The distinction of constant volume and constant pressure processes is not so important in the case of liquids and solids as the liquid or solid expands very little with increase in temperature. Therefore, heating or cooling at constant pressure nearly equals heating or cooling at constant volume for liquids and solids.

5.5 HEAT CAPACITY OF GASES AND SENSIBLE HEAT CHANGES IN GASES AT CONSTANT PRESSURE

As discussed in Sec. 5.4, the heat capacity at constant pressure is defined as

$$dQ = C_{mp} \cdot dT \qquad (5.10)$$

Integrating the above equation between the two temperatures,

$$Q = \int_{T_1}^{T_2} C_{mp} \cdot dT \qquad (5.11)$$

In order to evaluate Eq. (5.11), the value of C_{mp} should be known. For gases, C_{mp} at 101.325 kPa a** is expressed as a function of temperature (T) and is denoted by C_{mp}^0.

Although the calculations of enthalpy changes are accurate at 101.325 kPa a with published C_{mp}^0 data, they give fairly accurate enthalpy changes up to about 10 bar a for most of the gases. The effect of temperature on C_{mp}^0 can be expressed in graphical or tabular form or in an empirical equation form. Spencer[3] presented empirical equations as far back as 1948 based on the tabulated C_{mp}^0 data from API Research Project 44 (through April, 1947). Base

---

* For the proof of Eq. (5.9) a standard textbook on thermodynamics or physical chemistry should be referred such as those given in Ref. 1 and 2.

** That is, at standard atmospheric pressure in hypothetical idea state. Current literature reports the values at 1 bar a which may be taken as those for 1 atm.

data were since then constantly revised by API Research Project. A number of equations are developed on the basis of these data among which the most common form of the equation is the polynomial form.

$$C_{mp}^0 = a + bT + cT^2 \tag{5.12}$$

$$C_{mp}^0 = a + bT + cT^2 + dT^3 \tag{5.13}$$

$$C_{mp}^0 = A + BT + CT^2 + DT^{-2} \tag{5.14}$$

Thinh et al[4] utilized data compiled up to 1969 and presented constants of Eq. (5.13) for 408 hydrocarbons and related compounds. Yaws et al[5] presented constants of Eq. (5.13) for 700 organic compounds based on various references. Constants for Eq. (5.14) are given in Ref. 2. Physical properties package, called FLOWTRAN[6], developed by the Monsanto Company, USA, proposed a fourth order polynomial equation, generally valid in the range of 298.15 to 1500 K.

$$C_{mp}^0 = a + bT + cT^2 + dT^3 + eT^4 \tag{5.15}$$

Extensive data on constants have also been complied by Himmelblau[1]. Yuan and Mok[7,8] proposed the exponential equation:

$$C_{mp}^0 = a + be^{-c/T^n} \tag{5.16}$$

In Eqs. (5.12) to (5.16), constants do not necessarily have same values.

One specific claim of Eq. (5.16) is its versatility for use over a wide temperature range from 200 to 6000 K. Such a wide range is required to be split into three or more ranges for specifying the constants of Eq. (5.12) or Eq. (5.13). Yuan and Mok reported data for more than 30 hydrocarbons which were based on the data of the API Research Project 44 (1948). Thinh et al[9] used the data of the API Research Project 44 (1969) and obtained the constants of Eq. (5.16) for 221 hydrocarbons and two elements. This exponential model resulted in extremely low errors.

Many other equations have been developed for the estimation of C_{mp}^0. However, the data presented by Thinh et al[4] are accurate (up to 1500 K) as they are derived by minimising the sum of squares of percentage deviations. Also, Eq. (5.16) is not readily amenable for integration and hence requires the use of a programmable calculator or a computer.

The truncation of the polynomial equation for a given set of constants is normally not recommended. For example, Eq. (5.13) was truncated to a second order polynomial and the dT^3 term was omitted. The calculation of C_{mp}^0 with the reduced form of the equation and with the same constants were found to result in an error exceeding 2 – 3% above 500 K for the equation, valid in the range 298.15 K(25°C) to 1500 K.

Extensive data on constants for various equations are listed in Table 5.1.

In addition to the empirical equations, heat capacity data in the graphical form are given by Yaws[11] in MKS units.

Experimental data are not easily available for a number of substances for heat capacity of gases at high pressures. For this reason, a generalised approach is attempted by Weiss et al[12]. A graphical correlation in terms of the difference between the heat capacity under other operating conditions C_{mp} and the isobaric heat capacity in the ideal gas state C^0_{mo} (at zero absolute pressure) as a function of reduced temperature (T_r) and reduced pressure (p_r) is given in Fig. 5.3. For calculation of $\delta C_{mp} = C_{mp} - C^0_{mp}$ values, Benedict-Webb-Rubin Equation of State was used. δC_{mp} is also known as *residual heat capacity*.

It may clearly be noted that δC_{mp} is a point value. For calculating the enthalpy difference between given two temperature values at a given pressure, numerical integration will have to be adopted as a polynomial expression of δC_{mp} is not available in literature.

Another method for evaluation of δC_{mp} is given by Lee et al[13] which is based on a three parameters corresponding states principle. Values obtained by both the methods are generally in good agreement.

Ideal gas heat capacity C^0_{mp} referred to in Fig. 5.3 is for zero absolute pressure while the one reported in Table 5.1 is for a hypothetical ideal state at 101.325 kPa a. For the purpose of evaluation C_{mp} at high pressure, C^0_{mp} values from Table 5.1 may be used with caution.

δC_{mp} data from Fig. 5.3 are reliable for simple hydrocarbons and permanent light gases. For further discussion on the subject, the reader is advised to refer to Ref. 14.

Substituting C^0_{mp} in Eq. (5.13), for a polynomial equation of third order

$$Q = \int_{T_1}^{T_2} (a + bT + cT^2 + dT^3)\, dT$$

$$= a\,(T_2 - T_1) + \left(\frac{b}{2}\right)(T_2^2 - T_1^2) + \left(\frac{c}{3}\right)(T_2^3 - T_1^3)$$

$$+ \left(\frac{d}{4}\right)(T_2^4 - T_1^4) \tag{5.17}$$

This equation can be solved algebraically or with the help of Mathcad.

Example 5.2 Pure methane is heated from 303 K (30°C) to 523 K (250°C) at atmospheric pressure. Calculate the heat added per kmol methane, using data given in Table 5.1.

Solution Base: 1 kmol methane

$$T_1 = 303 \text{ K and } T_2 = 523 \text{ K}$$

(A) Reference 2: Using Eq. (5.17),

$$Q = 19.2494\,(523 - 303) + 52.1135 \times 10^{-3}\, \frac{[523^2 - 303^2]}{2}$$

$$+ 11.973 \times 10^{-6}\, \frac{[523^2 - 303^2]}{3} - 11.3173 \times 10^{-9}\, \frac{[523^2 - 303^2]}{4}$$

$$= 4234.9 + 4735.0 + 459.9 - 187.8 = 9242.0 \text{ kJ}$$

Table 5.1 Empirical Heat Capacity Equations for Gases

Form of equation:

$$C_{mp}^0 = a + bT + cT^2 + dT^3 + eT^4$$

where C_{mp}^0 = Ideal gas heat capacity at 101.325 kPa a (760 torr), kJ/(kmol·K)
and T = Absolute temperature, K

Compound	Formula	Molar mass	a	$b \times 10^3$	$c \times 10^6$	$d \times 10^9$	$e \times 10^{12}$	Range, K	Ref.
Inorganic Compounds									
Ammonia	NH₃	17.0305	27.55	25.6278	9.9004	-6.6864			6
			25.6503	33.4806	0.3518	-3.0832		298 – 1500	10
Argon	Ar	39.948	20.7723						6
Bromine	Br₂	159.808	33.6874	10.2992	-8.9025	2.6792			6
Carbon dioxide	CO₂	44.0095	19.0223	79.6291	-73.7067	37.4572	-8.133		
			30.664	-48.3885	382.5044	-492.6398		50 – 298	4
			21.3655	64.2841	-41.0506	9.7999		298 – 150	4
			37.174	23.2371	-7.3788	0.8213		1500 – 4000	4
			19.774	73.375	-56.02	17.155		298 – 1000	5
Carbon monoxide	CO	28.0101	29.0063	2.4924	-18.644	47.9892	-28.7266		
			29.1151	0.2456	-2.067	5.9026		50 – 298	4
			29.0277	-2.8165	11.6437	-4.7063		298 – 150	4
			27.4163	8.6192	-2.7046	0.3041		1500 – 4000	4
			30.842	-12.839	27.877	-12.709		298 – 1000	5
Chlorine	Cl₂	70.906	28.5463	23.8795	-21.3631	6.4726			6
Fluorine	F₂	37.9968	-24.9539	697.984	-3.2446	-528.857	270.246		6
Hydrogen	H₂	2.0159	17.6386	67.0055	-131.485	105.883	-29.1803		6
			19.6578	9.9027	289.2195	-741.5409		50 – 298	4
			28.6105	1.0194	-0.1476	0.769		298 – 1500	4
			25.4233	5.4355	-0.4974	-0.0054		1500 – 4000	4

(Contd.)

Table 5.1 Contd.

Compound	Formula	Molar mass	a	b × 10³	c × 10⁶	d × 10⁹	e × 10¹²	Range, K	Ref.
Hydrogen chloride	HCl	36.4609	30.3088	−7.609	13.2608	−4.3336			6
Hydrogen iodide	HI	127.9124	30.2697	−10.3319	25.946	−15.9529	3.1862		6
Hydrogen sulphide	H$_2$S	34.0809	34.5234	−17.6481	67.6664	−53.2454	14.0695		6
Oxygen	O$_2$	31.9988	29.8832	−11.3842	43.3779	−37.0082	10.1006		6
			29.1189	0.9952	−12.2586	40.1241		50 – 298	4
			26.0257	11.7551	−2.3426	−0.5623		298 – 1500	4
			18.4331	21.7174	−8.3048	1.1558		1500 – 4000	4
Ozone	O$_3$	47.9982	34.089	−23.1418	149.4231	43.8521		50 – 298	4
			20.5451	80.0947	−62.4369	16.9722		298 – 1500	4
Neon	Ne	20.1797	20.7723						6
Nitric oxide	NO	30.0061	29.7657	0.976	6.0987	−3.5881	0.5853		6
			29.4867	−2.0524	11.3379	−4.8195		298 – 1500	10
Nitrogen	N$_2$	28.0134	29.4119	−3.0068	5.4506	5.1319	−4.2531	298 – 1500	6
			29.5909	−5.141	13.1829	−4.968		298 – 1500	10
			31.1182	3.1969	−0.4052	0.0023		1500 – 4000	10
Nitrogen dioxide	NO$_2$	46.0055	25.1165	43.9956	−9.6172	−12.1653	5.4494	298 – 1500	6
			23.5804	53.5944	−31.4901	6.5394		298 – 1500	10
Nitrogen pentoxide	N$_2$O$_5$	108.0104	36.8193	259.7005	−215.4134	60.8531		298 – 1500	10
Nitrogen tetroxide	N$_2$O$_4$	92.0110	32.2558	189.6139	−138.303	35.908		298 – 1500	10
Nitrogen trioxide	N$_2$O$_3$	76.0116	37.4964	117.0169	−80.8775	20.137		298 – 1500	10
Nitrous oxide	N$_2$O	44.0128	20.5437	81.2993	−82.8968	49.8739	−11.2709	298 – 1500	6
			23.2082	63.6695	−42.3402	10.4061		298 – 1500	10
Sulphur (diatomic)	S$_2$	64.131	16.0581	4.7177	−2.9459	0.6668		298 – 1500	10
Sulphur dioxide	SO$_2$	64.0638	25.7725	57.8938	−38.0844	8.6063		800 – 1500	6
			24.7706	62.9481	−44.2582	11.122		298 – 1500	10
Sulphur trioxide	SO$_3$	80.0632	15.507	145.719	−113.253	32.4046		298 – 1500	6
			22.0376	121.624	−91.8673	24.3691		298 – 1500	10

(*Contd.*)

Table 5.1 Contd.

Compound	Formula	Molar mass	a	b × 10³	c × 10⁶	d × 10⁹	e × 10¹²	Range, K	Ref.
Water	H_2O	18.0153	34.0471	− 9.6501	32.9983	− 20.4467	4.3023	298 – 1500	6
			32.4921	0.0796	13.2107	− 4.5474		298 – 1000	10
			25.1584	21.2818	− 5.34	0.4825		1500 – 4000	10
Organic Compounds									
Acetaldehyde	CH_3CHO	44.0526	24.5377	76.013	136.254	− 199.942	75.9551	298 – 1500	6
			15.455	144.5	− 43.25	− 3.9835		298 – 1000	10
Acetic acid	CH_3COOH	60.0520	6.8995	257.068	− 191.771	75.7676	− 12.3175	298 – 1000	6
			4.828	254.68	175.26	49.509		298 – 1000	5
Acetylene (ethyne)	C_2H_2	26.0373	21.8212	92.058	− 65.2231	18.1959		298 – 1500	4
			22.5039	90.1238	− 63.7357	17.8644		298 – 1000	5
Aniline	$C_6H_5NH_2$	93.1265	15.812	128.15	− 127.85	50.589	235.694	298 – 1000	6
			− 2.2559	307.834	241.742	− 537.543			5
			− 40.502	637.93	− 513.08	163.31			
Benzene	C_6H_6	78.1118	18.5868	− 11.7439	1275.14	− 2079.84	1053.29	298 – 1500	6
			− 37.9852	490.4208	− 321.388	79.3646		298 – 1000	4
			− 43.781	523.29	376.27	106.61			5
Butadiene 1,2	C_4H_6	54.0904	17.2814	224.295	− 18.9688	− 102.998	44.4247	298 – 1500	6
			11.1997	272.361	− 146.8244	30.891		298 – 1000	4
			9.802	280.05	159.68	37.256			5
Butadiene 1,3	C_4H_6	54.0904	− 5.6322	312.606	− 2.8582	− 368.547	246.459	298 – 1500	6
			− 5.8354	353.1742	− 239.9229	62.5332		298 – 1000	4
			− 16.316	413.47	− 342.51	114.98			5
iso-Butane (methyl propane)	C_4H_{10}	58.1222	52.9035	− 107.178	1380.44	− 2066.67	1008.88	298 – 1500	6
			− 8.9133	419.5341	233.6331	51.0434		298 – 1500	4
			− 10.853	430.53	− 251.59	59.455		298 – 1000	5

(Contd.)

Table 5.1 Contd.

Compound	Formula	Molar mass	a	$b \times 10^3$	$c \times 10^6$	$d \times 10^9$	$e \times 10^{12}$	Range, K	Ref.
n-Butane	C_4H_{10}	58.1222	66.7088	−185.523	1528.44	−2187.92	1045.77	298–1500	6
			−2.4511	391.8275	−202.9882	40.7927		298–1000	4
Butene 1	C_4H_8	56.1063	−1.779	386.96	−193.25	34.833	124.165	298–1000	5
			9.2323	254.744	73.0443	−265.873		298–1500	4
cis-Butene 2	C_4H_8	56.1063	−2.3835	348.8153	−191.4879	41.2491		298–1000	5
			−4.02	357.67	−205.85	48.053		298–1500	4
			−7.8425	338.3705	−169.3661	32.239		298–1000	5
trans-Butene 2	C_4H_8	56.1063	−5.201	321.93	−139.37	15.605		298–1500	4
			9.2193	303.9495	−143.5319	25.4956		298–1000	5
			11.891	287.61	−114.33	9.5977		298–1500	4
n-Butyl alcohol (Butanol 1)	C_4H_9OH	74.1216	−2.07	429.749	−169.148	−73.744	61.4903	298–1500	6
			14.6837	360.4152	−133.0594	1.4778		298–1500	4
			7.913	396.63	−192.66	31.739		298–1000	5
Carbon disulphide	CS_2	76.141	33.0999	10.6167	275.934	−342.168	130.288	298–1000	6
			27.416	81.228	−76.63	26.724		298–1000	5
Carbon tetrachloride (Tetrachloromethane)	CCl_4	153.8227	8.9763	420.036	751.639	627.332	−199.811	273–1500	4
			50.1106	143.6852	−131.9483	39.3043		298–1000	5
			40.671	204.73	−226.88	88.383		298–1000	6
Chlorobenzene	C_6H_5Cl	112.5569	−2.7793	357.786	−23.148	−240.458	125.736	298–1000	6
			−31.032	549.48	430.53	131.7		298–1000	5
Chloroform (Trichloromethane)	$CHCl_3$	119.3776	31.8924	144.743	−111.583	30.721		273–1500	4
			30.2685	151.0778	−118.6769	33.1579		298–1000	5
Ethane	C_2H_6	30.069	23.975	189.18	−183.98	66.542		298–1500	4
			33.8339	−15.5175	376.892	−411.77	138.89	298–1000	6

(Contd.)

Table 5.1 Contd.

Compound	Formula	Molar mass	a	$b \times 10^3$	$c \times 10^6$	$d \times 10^9$	$e \times 10^{12}$	Range, K	Ref.
			5.4129	178.0872	-67.3749	8.7147		298 – 1500	4
			8.181	161.46	-40.071	-6.9421		298 – 1000	5
Ethyl alcohol (Ethanol)	C_2H_5OH	46.0684	17.6907	149.532	89.4815	-197.384	83.1747	273 – 1000	6
			10.4197	209.5142	-82.4825	3.9339		298 – 1000	4
			6.296	231.5	-118.56	22.218		298 – 1000	5
Ethyl benzene	$C_6H_5C_2H_5$	106.165	44.995	-45.8883	1832.28	-2919.74	1463.46	298 – 1500	6
			-36.7243	671.1231	-422.0211	101.1472		298 – 1500	4
			-43.087	706.76	-481.03	130.11		298 – 1000	5
Ethylene (Ethene)	C_2H_4	28.0532	16.8346	51.5193	216.352	-345.618	158.794	298 – 1500	6
			4.1261	155.0213	-81.5455	16.9755		298 – 1500	4
			3.798	156.5	-83.467	17.562		298 – 1000	5
Ethylene glycol	$C_2H_6O_2$	62.0678	35.8417	108.695	290.598	-452.216	186.584	298 – 1000	6
			29.226	287.87	-224.54	73.835		298 – 1000	5
Ethylene oxide (Epoxyethane)	C_2H_4O	44.0526	17.9573	34.3445	351.051	-478.345	190.011	298 – 1000	6
			-7.52	222.06	-125.6	25.918		298 – 1000	5
Ethyl amine	$C_2H_5NH_2$	45.0837	27.5175	62.6593	391.9	-527.782	206.496	298 – 1000	6
			3.68	274.96	158.26	38.088		298 – 1000	5
n-Hexane	C_6H_{14}	86.1754	42.7147	199.102	789.486	-1278.67	591.511	298 – 1000	6
			-4.4152	581.9233	-311.8584	64.9193		298 – 1500	4
			-4.738	582.41	-310.64	62.923		298 – 1000	5
Methane	CH_4	16.0425	38.387	-73.6639	290.981	-263.849	80.0679	298 – 1500	6
			19.2494	52.1135	11.973	-11.3173		298 – 1500	4
			25.36	16.868	71.312	-40.837		298 – 1000	5

(Contd.)

Table 5.1   Contd.

Compound	Formula	Molar mass	a	b × 10³	c × 10⁶	d × 10⁹	e × 10¹²	Range, K	Ref.
Methyl alcohol (Methanol)	CH_3OH	32.0419	34.4925	− 29.1887	286.844	− 312.501	109.833	273 – 1000	6
			24.8692	50.8755	58.6274	− 45.1266		298 – 100	4
			21.137	70.843	25.86	− 28.497			5
Methyl amine	CH_3NH_2	31.0571	12.5367	151.044	− 68.8093	12.345		298 – 1000	6
			16.086	121.42	− 22.822	− 9.0692	46.7507		5
Methyl chloride (Chloromethane)	CH_3Cl	50.4875	19.4308	59.6368	70.6089	− 117.502		298 – 1000	6
			13.5427	105.0548	− 47.4009	7.8612		273 – 1500	4
			13.728	102.3	− 40.602	3.442		298 – 1500	5
Methylene chloride (Dichloromethane)	CH_2Cl_2	84.9326	16.9092	140.4533	− 94.028	23.7905		273 – 1500	4
			11.87	172.27	− 149.25	52.283		298 – 1000	5
n-Pentane	C_5H_{12}	72.1488	83.1454	− 241.925	1946.53	− 2807.49	1352.76		6
			− 3.6266	487.4859	− 258.0312	53.0488		298 – 1500	4
			− 3.411	485.01	− 251.94	48.677		298 – 1000	5
Phenol	C_6H_5OH	94.1112	− 36.1498	566.519	− 411.357	93.903	18.0687	298 – 1000	6
			− 35.833	597.81	− 482.42	152.67			5
Propane	C_3H_8	44.0956	47.2659	− 131.469	1170	−1696.95	818.91	298 – 1000	6
			− 4.2227	306.264	− 158.6316	32.1455		298 – 1000	5
			− 5.338	310.24	− 164.64	34.691		298 – 1000	5
Propionic acid	C_2H_5COOH	74.0785	32.217	182.665	160.153	− 329.308	141.924	298 – 1000	6
Propylene (Propene)	C_3H_6	42.0797	24.3657	71.2795	338.448	− 515.275	230.475	298 – 1000	6
			3.7457	234.0107	− 115.1278	21.7353		298 – 1500	4
			5.084	225.64	− 99.926	13.311		298 – 1000	5
Propylene oxide	C_3H_6O	58.0791	− 7.868	322.82	− 194.98	46.455		298 – 1000	5

(Contd.)

Table 5.1 Contd.

Compound	Formula	Molar mass	a	b × 10³	c × 10⁶	d × 10⁹	e × 10¹²	Range, K	Ref.
Sytrene	C_8H_8	104.491	− 32.4471	631.898	− 398.206	46.5312	36.4421	298 – 1000	6
			− 36.914	665.26	− 485.05	140.88		298 – 1000	5
Toluene	$C_6H_5CH_3$	92.1384	31.82	− 16.1654	1444.65	− 2289.48	1135.73	298 – 1500	6
			− 35.1932	563.179	− 349.7963	82.5884		298 – 1000	4
			− 43.647	603.54	− 399.45	104.38		298 – 1000	5
m-Xylene (Dimethyl benzene 1,3)	C_8H_{10}	106.165	− 27.833	623.1759	− 366.4589	− 82.2828		298 – 1500	4
			− 29.154	629.32	374.51	84.789		298 – 1000	5
o-Xylene (Dimethyl benzene 1,2)	C_8H_{10}	106.165	− 15.1201	592.8425	− 341.4235	75.3348		298 – 1500	4
			− 15.859	595.72	344.22	75.312		298 – 1000	5
p-Xylene (Dimethyl benzene 1,4)	C_8H_{10}	106.165	− 26.733	609.0789	− 349.4772	76.4221		298 – 1500	4
			− 25.088	603.63	− 337.23	68.233		298 – 1000	5

(Reproduced with the permissions of (i) Monsanto Chemical Co., USA, (ii) Gulf Publishing Co., USA (iii) McGraw-Hill Inc., USA and (iv) Central Laboratory, Transport Ministry, Quebec, Canada.)

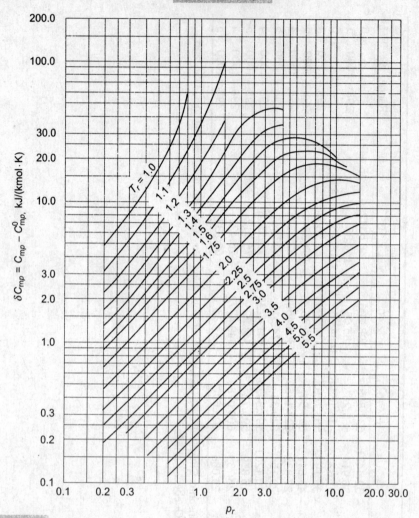

Fig. 5.3 Effects of Pressure on the Isobaric Heat Capacity of Gases

(Reproduced with the permission of the American Chemical Society, USA).
Mathcad Solution:

$$Q := \int_{303}^{523} (19.2494 + 52.1135 \cdot 10^{-3}\, T$$
$$+ 11.973 \cdot 10^{-6}\, T^2 - 11.3173 \cdot 19^{-9}\, T^3)\, dT$$

$$Q = 9.242 \cdot 10^3 \text{ kJ}$$

(B) Reference 3:

$$Q = 25.36\,(523 - 303) + 16.868 \times 10^{-3}\, \frac{\left[523^2 - 303^2\right]}{2}$$
$$+ 71.312 \times 10^{-6}\, \frac{\left[523^3 - 303^3\right]}{3} - 40.837 \times 10^{-9}\, \frac{\left[523^4 - 303^4\right]}{4}$$
$$= 5579.2 + 1532.6 + 2739.3 - 677.8 = 9173.3 \text{ kJ}$$

Mathcad Solution:

$$Q := \int_{303}^{523} (25.36 + 16.868 \cdot 10^{-3} \, T + 71.312 \cdot 10^{-6} \, T^2$$
$$- 40.837 \cdot 10^{-9} \, T^3) \, dT$$

$$Q = 9.173 \cdot 10^3 \text{ kJ}$$

(C) Reference 4.

$$Q = 38.387 \,(523 - 303) - 73.6639 \times 10^{-3} \, \frac{\left[523^2 - 303^2\right]}{2}$$
$$+ 290.981 \times 10^{-6} \, \frac{\left[523^3 - 303^3\right]}{3} - 263.849 \times 10^{-9}$$
$$\frac{\left[523^4 - 303^4\right]}{4} + 80.0679 \times 10^{-12} \, \frac{\left[523^5 - 303^5\right]}{5}$$

$$= 8445.1 - 6693.1 + 11\,177.3 + 4379.2 + 585.7 = 9135.8 \text{ kJ}$$

Mathcad solution:

$$Q := \int_{303}^{523} (38.387 - 73.6639 \cdot 10^{-3} \, T + 290.981 \cdot 10^{-6} \, T^2$$
$$- 263.849 \cdot 10^{-9} \, T^3 + 80.0679 \cdot 10^{-12} \, T^4) \, dT$$

$$Q = 9.136 \cdot 10^3 \text{ kJ}$$

Note: From the above calculations, it is evident that with different constants, the calculation differ to a certain extent and hence the use of reliable data is must.

Example 5.3 Calculate the heat added per kmol methane when it is heated from 303 K (30°C) to 523 K (250°C) at 25 bar a.

Solution 1 kmol methane at 25 bar a

For methane: $p_c = 46.04$ bar and $T_c = 190.5$ K (ref. Table 2.4)

$$p_r = 2.5/4.604 = 0.543$$

Residual enthalpy $\quad H - H^o = \int_{303}^{523} \delta C_{mp} \, dT$

Since only point values can be read from Fig. 5.3 for δC_{mp}, it is necessary to use a numerical method for integration.

The temperature range of 303 to 523 K can be divided into 4 intervals.

Temperature interval, $\Delta T = (523 - 303)/4$
$$= 55 \text{ K}$$

Table 5.2 Residual Heat Capacity Calculations

Temperature, K (°C)	Reduced temperature, T_r	Residual heat capacity δC_{mp}, kJ/(kmol·K) (read from Fig. 5.3)
303 (30)	1.59	2.6
358 (85)	1.879	1.5
413 (140)	2.168	1.0
468 (195)	2.457	0.7
523 (250)	2.745	0.52

According to Simpson's one-third rule,

$$H - H^0 = \frac{\Delta T}{3} \left(\delta C_{mp1} + 4\,[\delta C_{mp2} + \delta C_{mp4}] + 2[\delta C_{mp3}] + \delta C_{mp5}\right)$$

$$= \frac{55}{3} \left(2.6 + 4\,[1.5 + 0.7] + 2 \times 1.0 + 0.52\right) = 255 \text{ kJ/kmol}$$

Enthalpy required to be added for raising the temperature of methane from 303 to 523 K at 25 bar a,

$$H = 9173.3 + 255.2 = 9427.33 \text{ kJ/kmol} \qquad \qquad \textit{Ans.}$$

Note: Difference between the enthalpy values under ideal state conditions and at 2.5 MPa is 255.2 kJ/kmol which is about 2.7% of the correct enthalpy. Error becomes significant for high p_r and low T_r.

In the absence of reliable data on the heat capacity of many organic compounds (vapour/gas phase), various other data for estimation are available in literature[14]. Rihani and Doraiswamy[14] proposed an additive group method which is based on Eq. (5.12) and is applicable to many types of organic compounds. Another additive group method is given by Thinh, Duran and Ramalho[15] for a large number of hydrocarbons and is based on Eq. (5.18).

$$\Delta C^0_{mpc} = A + B_1\,e^{-C_1/T^{n_1}} - B_2\,e^{-C_2/T^{n_2}} \tag{5.18}$$

where, ΔC^0_{mpc} = contribution due to hydrocarbon group

and $A, B_1, B_2, C_1, C_2, n_1$ and n_2 are constants.

It is a modified form of Eq. (5.16), suggested by Yuan and Mok. This group contribution is the most accurate of all the methods. As the method is quite complicated, numerical techniques need to be employed. Detailed discussions on the group contribution methods is outside the scope of this book.

5.6 SENSIBLE HEAT CHANGES IN LIQUIDS

As mentioned earlier in Sec. 5.4, the heat capacities at constant pressure and constant volume of a liquid are nearly equal. In general, the heat capacity of a liquid increases with an increase in the temperature, although the variation of the heat capacity of a liquid with temperature is considered to be of less importance. This is because the temperature range in which the heating or cooling is performed is usually small.

For liquids, $dQ = m\,C_l\,dT$ \hfill (5.19)

where C_l is heat capacity of liquid [kJ/(kg · K)] and m is the mass of liquid (kg).

The heat capacity of a liquid can be expressed as a function of temperature.

Table 5.3 present data on molar liquid heat capacity from references 6, 11 and 16. Considering the third order polynomial equation (similar to Eq. (5.13)).

$$\int dQ = \int_{T_1}^{T_2} C_l\,dT \tag{5.20}$$

$$Q = a(T_2 - T_1) + \left(\frac{b}{2}\right)(T_2^2 - T_1^2) + \left(\frac{c}{3}\right)(T_2^3 - T_1^3)$$

$$+ \left(\frac{d}{4}\right)(T_2^4 - T_1^4) \tag{5.21}$$

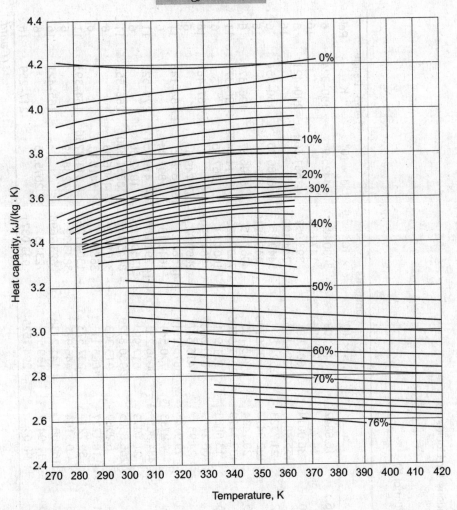

Fig. 5.4 Heat Capacity of Caustic Soda Solutions[17]

(Reproduced with the permission of Hooker Chemical Corporation, USA).

Luria and Benson[14] have proposed an accurate group contribution method for the estimation of the molar heat capacity of liquid hydrocarbons which is applicable below the normal boiling point.

Often, heat capacity data are available in the graphical or tabular form. For example, heat capacity plots for a number of aqueous solutions are available in literature. Figures 5.4 and 5.5 give the heat capacity of caustic soda solutions and sulphuric acid solutions respectively of different concentrations at different temperatures[17,18]. Figure 5.17 is another chart which gives heat capacity of mixed acids.

Table 5.3 (Empirical Heat Capacity Equations for Liquids

Form of equation:

$$C_l = a + bT + cT^2 + dT^3$$

where C_l = Liquid heat capacity, kJ/(kmol·K)

and T = Absolute temperature, K

Compound	Formula	Molar mass	a	$b \times 10^3$	$c \times 10^6$	$d \times 10^9$	Temp. Range K	Ref.
Acetaldehyde	C_2H_4O	44.0526	16.8842	810.208	−3080.85	4425.9	150–324	6
Acetic acid	$C_2H_4O_2$	60.0520	54.7	−22.0844	147.634		290–421	16
			−36.0814	604.681	−393.957	−561.602		6
Acetyl chloride	C_2H_3ClO	78.4922	155.48	−326.5951	744.199		160–354	16
			21.7323	1524.8	−5449.35	6980.35		6
Ammonia	NH_3	17.0305	102.94	−91.5796	446.3516		196–373	16
			20.1494	845.765	−4067.45	6606.87	196–373	6
Aniline	C_6H_7N	93.1265	−137.1179	2217.5586	−7907.6285	9811.4489		11
			−13.6683	931.971	−1604.01	1367.15		6
			206.27	−211.5065	564.2902		267–487	16
Argon	Ar	39.948	24.93	1416.64	−2869.02	−42 749.6	84–143	6
Benzene	C_6H_6	78.1118	−79.914	3875.2813	−42 566.2	162 688.2		11
			−7.2733	770.541	−1648.18	1897.94	279–523	6
Bromine	Br_2	159.808	−484.365	5056.235	−14 292.204	14 419.754		11
			21.1979	517.99	−1759.21	1952.66	266–553	6
Butadiene 1,2	C_4H_6	54.0904	−266.8805	2980.8129	8945.117	8851.3807		11
Butadiene 1,3	C_4H_6	54.0904	6.2582	913.303	3101.42	4386.33		6
			−16.1777	1085.11	3682.61	5410.41	164–393	6
1-Butanol (n-Butyl alcohol)	$C_4H_{10}O$	74.1216	85.721	237.573	−1304.7267	311.7756		11
			−0.5104	1446.97	3833.39	4288.49	165–421	6
Carbon dioxide	CO_2	44.0095	162.68	−141.2138	623.2696		217–259	16
			11.0417	1159.55	−7231.3	2075.75		6
			98.63	−294.1525	933.0371			16

(Contd.)

Table 5.3 Contd.

Compound	Formula	Molar mass	a	$b \times 10^3$	$c \times 10^6$	$d \times 10^9$	Temp. Range K	Ref.
Carbon disulphide	CS_2	76.141	17.4151	554.537	− 1723.46	15 501.9	161–349	6
			68.39	− 45.6772	243.2064			16
Carbon monoxide	CO	28.0101	14.9673	2143.97	− 32 470.3	15 804.2	68–112	6
			61.53	− 176.9687	2054.408			16
Carbon tetrachloride (Tetrachloromethane)	CCl_4	153.8227	12.2846	1094.75	− 3182.55	3425.24		6
			139.73	− 204.5003	586.787			16
Chlorine	Cl_2	70.906	15.412	723.104	− 3397.26	5262.36		6
			− 39.246	1401.2228	− 6047.226			11
Chlorobenzene	C_6H_5Cl	112.5569	− 11.5494	939.618	1898.5	8591.4	172–353	6
			150.41	− 142.546	464.2096	1791.89	228–435	16
Chloroform (Trichloromethane)	$CHCl_3$	119.3776	23.8419	755.531	− 2407.01	2842.62	210–364	6
			110.54	− 121.5667	441.0741			16
Ethanol (Ethyl alcohol)	C_2H_6O	46.0684	− 325.137	4137.87	− 14 030.7	17 035.4	159–381	6
			100.92	− 111.8386	498.54			16
Ethylene (Ethene)	C_2H_4	28.0532	− 39.959	730.3548	− 5887.003	14 834.966	104–233	11
Ethyl acetate	$C_4H_8O_2$	88.1051	4.2905	934.378	− 2640.0	3342.58		6
Ethylbenzene	C_8H_{10}	106.165	4.3143	900.174	− 1450.05	1433.6		6
Ethylene glycol	$C_2H_6O_2$	62.0678	31.0224	1100.34	− 2845.71	2889.21		6
			15.3	− 114.819	331.6842			16
Ethylene oxide	C_2H_4O	44.0526	7.4126	742.687	− 2713.2	3900.92	260–500	6
			79.81	− 27.5124	182.2322			16
Formaldehyde	CH_2O	30.0260	25.099	793.671	− 3826.91	6104.92	161–314	6
			77.73	− 56.6673	323.9887			16
Formic acid	CH_2O_2	46.0254	133.43	− 347.5111	785.7561		156–280	16
n-Hexane	C_6H_{14}	86.1754	31.421	976.058	− 2353.68	3092.73	282–404	6
Hydrogen peroxide	H_2O_2	34.0147	63.2314	170.7533	− 389.9272	372.4104	273–698	11
Hydrazine	N_2H_4	32.0452	− 621.733	6574.2164	− 20 138.569	20 970.409	275–473	11

(Contd.)

Table 5.3 Contd.

Compound	Formula	Molar mass	a	$b \times 10^3$	$c \times 10^6$	$d \times 10^9$	Temp. Range K	Ref.
Methanol (Methyl alcohol)	CH_4O	32.0419	− 258.25	3358.2	− 11 638.8	14 051.6	176–368	6
			74.86	− 102.315	406.6567	5515.01		16
Methyl chloride	CH_3Cl	50.4875	7.9961	798.5	− 3507.58		175–279	16
			72.77	− 44.0239	229.4864			16
Methylene chloride	CH_2Cl_2	84.9323	117.11	− 149.6366	616.2757	1218.97	178–343	6
			− 63.27	1243.34	− 1768.51			11
Naphthalene	$C_{10}H_8$	128.1735	− 757.746	6230.475	− 13 555.71	10 534.386	354–683	6
			33.6324	2904.98	− 32 658.3	120 828		11
Nitric oxide	NO	30.0061	− 2394.499	65 779.627	− 591 024.17	1786 075.2	109–138	11
			14.7141	2202.57	− 35 214.6	179 960		6
Nitrogen	N_2	28.0134	− 124.793	6975.028	− 90 158.135	393 765.98	63–113	11
			16.9925	1714.99	− 7839.62	12 001.7		6
Nitrogen dioxide	NO_2	46.0055	− 313.0	5657.775	− 11 888.25	13 246.19	262–413	11
			8.5894	1051.71	− 6392.8	13 326		6
Nitrous oxide	N_2O	44.0128	− 537.155	8152.228	36 393.88	55 521.39	182–303	11
			1105.01	− 33 363.6	35 021.1	1212 620		11
Oxygen	O_2	31.9988	− 61.4532	4332.673	− 52 932.565	211 100.59	55–143	6
			− 36.1614	1153.54	− 2122.91	1741.83		11
Phenol	C_6H_6O	94.1112	207.48	− 103.7491	274.0052		314–485	6
n-Pentane	C_5H_{12}	72.1488	65.4961	628.628	− 1898.8	3186.51		6
1-Propanol (n-Propyl alcohol)	C_3H_8O	60.0950	− 488.104	5786.32	− 18 872	22 003.5	147–400	16
			119.39	− 100.2081	501.3639			6
Propionic acid	$C_3H_6O_2$	74.0785	31.7072	930.795	− 2330.49	2457.4		6
			− 38.0191	1197.21	− 2195.65	1933.12		11
Styrene	C_8H_8	104.1491	− 137.5366	2383.124	− 6235.805	− 6253.25	243–598	11
Propylene (Propene)	C_3H_6	42.0797	82.9137	296.523	− 2963.469	7764.571	88–313	11

(Contd.)

Table 5.3 Contd.

Compound	Formula	Molar mass	a	$b \times 10^3$	$c \times 10^6$	$d \times 10^9$	Temp. Range K	Ref.
Sulphur dioxide	SO_2	64.0638	19.2884	845.429	– 3727.48	5653.65	200–423	6
Sulphur trioxide	SO_3	80.0632	– 153.877	2773.3755	– 10 803.826	14 175.33		11
Sulphur trioxide	SO_3	80.0632	16.2291	1374.62	– 5177.38	6886.34	290–473	6
Sulphur trioxide	SO_3	80.0632	– 1333.443	13 461.809	– 39 051.315	39 554.121		11
Toluene	C_7H_8	92.1384	1.8083	812.223	– 1512.67	1630.01	178–583	6
			– 56.3627	1768.423	– 5192.623	5497.39		11
Water	H_2O	18.0153	18.2964	472.118	– 1338.78	1314.24	273–623	6
			50.845	213.08	– 631.398	648.746		11
m-Xylene	C_8H_{10}	106.165	14.0673	870.264	– 1477.33	1511.93	225–573	11
			– 38.846	1699.3	– 4753.1	5086		6
o-Xylene	C_8H_{10}	106.165	14.8871	903.295	– 1550.98	1512.01	248–298	11
			– 199.626	3058.7	– 8254.7	7926.3		6
p-Xylene	C_8H_{10}	106.165	22.0553	811.839	– 1366.7	1442.16	287–598	11
			– 374.08	3976.9	– 9524	81 088.12		11

(Reproduced with the permissions of (i) Monsanto Chemical Co., USA and (ii) McGraw-Hill Inc., USA)

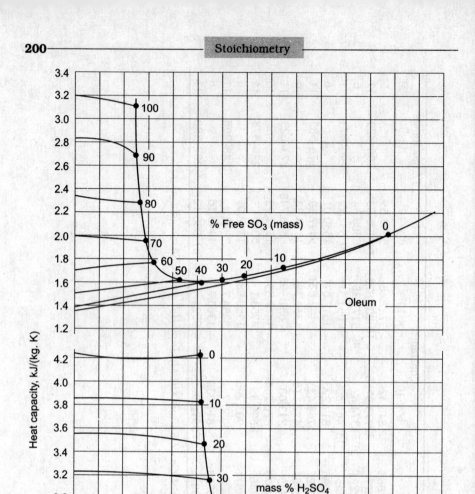

Fig. 5.5 Heat Capacity of Sulphuric Acid Solutions/Oleum[18]

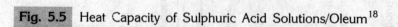

(Reproduced with the permission of Lurgi GmbH, Germany.)

Example 5.4 Toluene is heated from 290 K (17°C) to 350 K (77°C) at the rate of 0.25 kg/s. Calculate the heat required to be added to toluene using constants, given in Table 5.3.

Solution 0.25 kg/s toluene heated from 290 K to 350 K

$$\text{Molar flow rate, } q_m = \frac{0.25}{92} = 2.717 \times 10^{-3} \text{ kmol/s}$$

(A) Reference 6:

$$\phi = 2.717 \times 10^{-3} \left[1.8083 (350 - 290) + 812.223 \times 10^{-3} \frac{\left(350^2 - 290^2\right)}{2} \right.$$

$$\left. - 1512.67 \times 10^{-6} \frac{\left(350^3 - 290^3\right)}{3} + 1630.01 \times 10^{-9} \frac{\left(350^4 - 290^4\right)}{4} \right]$$

$$= 2.717 \times 10^{-3} [108.5 + 15\ 594.7 - 9321.1 + 3232.9]$$

$$= 2.717 \times 10^{-3} \times 9615 \text{ kJ/s} \equiv 26.124 \text{ kW} \qquad \qquad Ans.$$

(B) Reference 11:

$$\phi = 2.1717 \times 10^{-3} \left[-56.276 (350 - 290) + 1768.423 \times 10^{-3} \frac{\left(350^2 - 290^2\right)}{2} \right.$$

$$\left. - 5192.623 \times 10^{-6} \frac{\left(350^3 - 290^3\right)}{3} + 5497.39 \times 10^{-9} \frac{\left(350^4 - 290^4\right)}{4} \right]$$

$$= 2.717 \times 10^{-3} [-3376.6 + 33\ 901.4 - 31\ 947.5 + 10\ 886.5]$$

$$= 2.717 \times 10^{-9} \times 9463.8 \text{ kJ/s} \equiv 25.713 \text{ kW} \qquad \qquad Ans.$$

Both values differ by about 1.6%.
Mathcad can also be used to find ϕ.

Example 5.5 How much heat must be added in order to raise the temperature of a 20% (mass) caustic soda solution from 280 K (7°C) to 360 K (87°C).

Solution Basis: 1 kg 20% NaOH Solution
From Fig. 5.4, for 20% caustic soda solution,

$$C_{11} = 3.56 \text{ kJ/(kg} \cdot \text{K) at 280 K}$$

and $$C_{12} = 3.71 \text{ kJ/(kg} \cdot \text{K) at 360 K}$$

$$\text{Mean heat capacity, } C_{1m} = \frac{(3.56 + 3.71)}{2} = 3.635 \text{ kJ/(kg} \cdot \text{K)}$$

Heat required to raise the temperature

$$\text{of 1 kg 20\% NaOH solution} = 1 \times 3.635 (360 - 280)$$

$$= 290.8 \text{ kJ} \qquad \qquad Ans.$$

Example 5.6 Chlorinated diphenyl (Diphyl A-30*) is heated from 313 K (40°C) to 553 K (280°C) at the rate of 4000 kg/h in an indirectly fired heater. In this particular temperature range the heat capacity of the fluid is given by the equation

$$C_1 = 0.7511 + 1.465 \times 10^{-3} \, T \text{ kJ/(kg} \cdot \text{K)}$$

Where T is in K.

Also, the heat capacity data of Diphyl A-30 at 313 K (40°C) and 553 K (280°C) are 1.1807 and 1.5198 kJ/(kg·K) respectively[19].

---

* Registered Trade Mark of Bayer, Germany.

Calculate the heat to be supplied to the fluid in the heater using the heat capacity equation. Also, calculate the % error involved in using the mean heat capacity data for the heat change calculations.

Solution Basis: 1 kg Diphyl A-30
Sensible heat change,

$$Q = \int C_1 \, dT$$

$$= \int_{313}^{553} (0.7511 + 1.465 \times 10^{-3} \, T) \, dT$$

$$= 0.7511 (553 - 313) + 1.465 \times 10^{-3} \frac{(553^2 - 313^2)}{2}$$

$$= 180.26 + 152.24 = 332.50 \text{ kJ/kg}$$

For the mass flow rate of 4000 kg/h,

$$\phi = 4000 \times 332.50 = 133 \times 10^4 \text{ kJ/h} \equiv 369.44 \text{ kW} \qquad \textit{Ans. (a)}$$

$$C_{lm} = \frac{(1.1807 + 1.5198)}{2} = 1.3503 \text{ kJ/(kg·K)}$$

$$\phi = C_{lm} (T_2 - T_1)$$

$$= 1.3503 (553 - 313) = 324.06 \text{ kJ/kg}$$

$$\% \text{ error} = \left[\frac{324.06 - 332.50}{332.50} \right] \times 100 = -2.54 \qquad \textit{Ans. (b)}$$

The heat capacity of solids are lower than liquids and increase with the increase in temperature as is the case with liquids or gases. Extensive heat capacity data for solids (inorganic and organic) are given in Perry's Chemical Engineer's Handbook[20].

Number of methods are reported in literature for estimation of heat capacity of liquids, solutions and solids. A good summary of the methods can be found in Ref. 1 and 20. Only in the absence of non-availability of experimental data, these methods may be used with caution.

5.7 HEAT CAPACITY OF GASEOUS MIXTURES

In Sec. 5.5, the sensible heat change of a gas between two temperatures was considered. However, in practice, the mixtures of gases are often heated or cooled. The sensible heat change of a gaseous mixture can be calculated by calculating the mixture properties from the properties of pure gases present in the mixture. For ideal gas mixture the molar heat capacity of a gas mixture at a constant pressure is given by

$$C^0_{mp_{mix}} = \sum_1^n y_i C^0_{mpi} \qquad (5.22)$$

where y_i is the mole fraction of ith component and C^0_{mpi} is the molar heat capacity of the ith component. In this equation $C^0_{mp_{mix}}$ can be expressed as a function of temperature.

For real gas mixtures, Lee *et al*[13] have proposed an additive rule for estimation of critical properties which can be utilised for evaluation of residual heat capacity. This rule is different from Kay's additive rule for estimation of pseudo-critical properties (refer Example 2.21).

For a limited range of pressure and temperature, enthalpy of a real gas mixture can be represented by a model, incorporating $C^0_{mp_{mix}}$ and pressure parameter p. Carroll[21] have shown that simple equations can be accurate over a narrow range of pressure and temperature. Exercise 5.33 gives such an equation for sour gas mixture from a refinery. Such models should not be used beyond the specified range of conditions.

Example 5.7 Pyrites fines are roasted in a chamber plant for making sulphuric acid. The gases leaving the roaster are at 775 K (502°C) and have molar composition SO_2 7.09%, O_2 10.55%, SO_3 0.45% and N_2 81.91%. Calculate the heat content of 1 kmol gas mixture over 298.15 K (25°C), using the heat capacity data provided in Table 5.1.

Solution Basis: 1 kmol gas mixture

(a) In the first instance, take the value of $C^0_{mp} = f(T)$ given in Table 5.1.

$$\text{Heat change } Q = \int_{T_1}^{T_2} C^0_{mp_{mix}} \, dT$$

Sulphur dioxide:

$$y_{SO_2} \cdot C^0_{mp_{SO_2}} = 0.709\,(24.7706 + 62.9481 \times 10^{-3}\,T$$
$$- 44.2582 \times 10^{-6}\,T^2 + 11.122 \times 10^{-9}\,T^3)$$
$$= 1.7562 + 4.4630 \times 10^{-3}\,T - 3.1379$$
$$\times 10^{-6}\,T^2 + 0.7885 \times 10^{-9}\,T^3$$

Oxygen:

$$y_{O_2} \cdot C^0_{mp_{O_2}} = 0.1055\,(26.0257 + 11.7551 \times 10^{-3}\,T$$
$$- 2.3426 \times 10^{-6}\,T^2 - 0.5623 \times 10^{-9}\,T^3)$$
$$= 2.7457 + 1.2402 \times 10^{-3}\,T - 0.2471 \times 10^{-6}\,T^2$$
$$- 0.0593 \times 10^{-9}\,T^3$$

Sulphur trioxide:

$$y_{SO_3} \cdot C^0_{mp_{SO_3}} = 0.0045\,(22.0376 + 121.624 \times 10^{-3}\,T$$
$$- 91.8673 \times 10^{-6}\,T^2 + 24.3691 \times 10^{-9}\,T^3)$$
$$= 0.0992 + 0.5473 \times 10^{-3}\,T - 0.4134 \times 10^{-6}\,T^2$$
$$+ 0.1097 \times 10^{-9}\,T^3$$

Nitrogen:

$$y_{N_2} \cdot C^0_{mp_{N_2}} = 0.8191\,(29.5909 - 5.141 \times 10^{-3}\,T$$
$$+ 13.1829 \times 10^{-6}\,T^2 - 4.968 \times 10^9\,T^3)$$
$$= 24.2379 - 4.2110 \times 10^{-3}\,T + 10.7891 \times 10^{-6}\,T^2$$
$$- 4.0693 \times 10^{-9}\,T^3$$

Summing up

$$\Sigma y_i \cdot C^0_{mpi} = 28.833 + 2.0395 \times 10^{-3}\, T$$
$$+ 6.9997 \times 10^{-6}\, T^2 - 3.2304 \times 10^{-9}\, T^3$$
$$T_1 = 298.15 \text{ K and } T_2 = 775 \text{ K}$$

Using Eq. (5.17)

$$Q = 28.833\,(T_2 - T_1) + 2.0395 \times 10^{-3}\frac{\left(T_2^2 - T_1^2\right)}{2}$$
$$+ 6.9997 \times 10^{-6}\frac{\left(T_3^2 - T_1^3\right)}{3} - 3.2304 \times 10^{-9}\frac{\left(T_2^4 - T_1^4\right)}{4}$$
$$= 13\,749.0 + 536.4 + 1024.2 - 285.0$$
$$= 15\,024.6 \text{ kJ/kmol} \qquad\qquad Ans.$$

5.8 HEAT CAPACITY OF LIQUID MIXTURES

For immiscible liquid mixture, pure component values are additive and a weighted average is used for calculations. For miscible systems, additivity is not generally true although for similar substances and for systems with small heats of mixing, additivity gives fairly good results. As indicated in Sec. 5.6 earlier, a number of plots are available for aqueous solutions in literature. The heat capacity of mixtures of liquid metals or fused salts can be predicted within about 10% accuracy by the additivity rule.

For petroleum oils, American Petroleum Institute have compiled extensive data[22]. For a defined liquid hydrocarbon mixture, additivity rule is recommended by API. Thus, for immiscible liquid mixtures and also for liquid hydrocarbon mixture,

$$C_1 = \Sigma\, x_i\, C_{1i} \qquad\qquad (5.23)$$

where
x_i = mass fraction of ith component and

C_{1i} = heat capacity of ith component.

For petroleum fractions, API gravity is the parameter used to find the heat capacity at atmospheric pressure[1].

Example 5.8 A mixture of aniline and water, containing 11.8 (mass %) aniline, is subcooled in the overhead condenser of the distillation column from 373 K to 313 K (100 to 40°C) with the help of cooling water at the rate 8000 kg/h. Find the heat removal rate of the sub-cooling zone of the condenser.

Solution Basis: 8000 kg/h mixture is to be cooled.

Aniline and water are practically immiscible in each other and hence the additivity rule can be used for calculations.

Aniline in the mixture = $0.118 \times 8000 = 944$ kg/h ≡ 10.151 kmol/h

Water in the mixture = $8000 - 944 = 7056$ kg/h ≡ 392 kmol/h

Use the data provided in Table 5.3 (Ref. 16 for aniline and Ref. 11 for water).

$$T_1 = 373 \text{ K and } T_2 = 313 \text{ K}$$

Heat extraction rate,

$$\phi = 10.151 \left[206.27 \, (T_1 - T_2) - 211.5065 \times 10^{-3} \frac{(T_1^2 - T_2^2)}{2} \right.$$

$$\left. + 564.2902 \times 10^{-6} \frac{(T_1^3 - T_2^3)}{3} \right] + 392 \left[50.845 \, (T_1 - T_2) \right.$$

$$+ 213.08 \times 10^{-3} \frac{(T_1^2 - T_2^2)}{2} - 631.398 \times 10^{-6} \frac{(T_1^3 - T_2^3)}{3}$$

$$\left. + 648.746 \times 10^{-9} \frac{(T_1^4 - T_2^4)}{4} \right]$$

$$= 10.151 \, (12\,376.2 - 4352.8 + 3993.4)$$

$$+ 392 \, (3050.7 + 4385.2 - 4468.4 + 1581.4)$$

$$= 10.151 \times 12\,016.8 + 392 \times 4548.9$$

$$= 121\,982.5 + 1783\,168.8 = 1905\,151.3 \text{ kJ/h} \equiv 529.21 \text{ kW}$$

Heat capacity of aniline and water at 298.15 K are 2.0515 and 4.1868 kJ/(kg·K) respectively[20]. If it is assumed to be constant over the temperature range of 313 K to 373 K,

$$\phi = (944 \times 2.0515 + 7056 \times 4.1868) \, (373 - 313)$$

$$= (1936.6 + 29\,542.1) \, (60) = 1888\,722 \text{ kJ/h} \equiv 524.65 \text{ kW}$$

$$\text{Error} = (529.21 - 524.65) \, \frac{100}{529.21} = 0.86\%$$

This error is quite low. It indicates that in most cases of liquids, the variation of heat capacity with respect to the temperature is quite small.

5.9 LATENT HEATS

When matter changes from one phase to another, the latent heat is either absorbed or rejected. For example, ice melts at 273.15 K (0°C) by supplying heat to produce water. Similarly, water at 101.325 kPa (760 torr) and 373.15 K (100°C) produces vapour if heat is continuously supplied to it. The former is called the latent heat of fusion, while the latter is called the latent heat of vaporization. In some cases, such as iodine crystals, camphor, dry ice, etc. vapour is produced from the solids, the process being called sublimation. The heat supplied for such a phase change process is called the latent heat of sublimation.

The heat supplied to melt the solid to liquid or removed to convert the liquid into solid per kilogram is called the *latent heat of fusion*, represented by symbol λ_f.

The heat supplied to convert liquid to vapour at a constant pressure (at the corresponding boiling point) is called the *latent heat of vaporization*, represented by symbol λ_v.

In the case of liquids/vapours, the boiling/saturation point changes with changes in pressure, and hence the latent heat of vaporization also varies with pressure. From the foregoing discussion it is clear that the units of latent heat are kJ/kg. As in the case of heat capacity, molar latent heats are expressed in kJ/mol.

The variation of the latent heat of vaporization with pressure/temperature is of considerable interest to the process industry. For this, a reliable equation for the correlation of pressure and the corresponding saturation temperature must be available.

An equation proposed by Antoine is as follows:

$$\log_{10} p_v = A - \frac{B}{(T + C)} \quad \text{or} \tag{5.24}$$

$$\ln p_v = A - \frac{B}{(T + C)} \tag{5.25}$$

where p_v is the vapour pressure in kPa, T is the temperature in K and A, B and C are constants. In these equations, constants do not necessarily have same values.

A graph having $\log p_v$ (or $\ln p_v$) on y-axis and $1/T$ on x-axis is called the *Cox chart*. In another words, it is a representation of Antoine equation in the graphical form.

It is observed that barring some of the compounds (such as organic sulphur compounds), the Antoine equation is proved to give the vapour pressure in the range of 1 to 200 kPa (10 to 1500 torr) of a variety of compounds well within the experimental uncertainty. Table 5.4 gives values of A, B and C for Eq. (5.24) and Eq. (5.25) for various compounds[6,23,24]. The representation of vapour pressure over a wider range of pressure, however, requires the use of a more complex equation of four or more parameters such as the one given by Yaws[25].

Example 5.9 Calculate vapour pressure of (a) *n*-hexane at 305 K (32°C) and (b) water at 395 K (122°C) using Antoine constants given in Table 5.4.
Solution
(a) Vapour pressure of *n*-hexane: T = 305 K

Reference 24: $$\log_{10} p_v = 5.9951 - \left[\frac{1168.70}{(305 - 48.95)}\right] = 1.4308$$

or $$p_v = 26.96 \text{ kPa}$$

Reference 6: $$\ln p_v = 14.0568 - \left[\frac{2825.42}{(305 - 42.7089)}\right] = 3.2847$$

or $$p_v = 26.70 \text{ kPa}$$

Reference 24 gives $$p_v = 200 \text{ torr} = 26.66 \text{ kPa at } 304.75 \text{ K } (31.6°C)$$

(b) Vapour pressure of water: T = 395 K

Reference 24:
$$\log_{10} p_v = 7.0436 - \left[\frac{1636.90}{(395 - 48.25)} \right] = 2.3229$$

or
$$p_v = 210.33 \text{ kPa}$$

Reference 6:
$$\ln p_v = 16.5362 - \left[\frac{3985.44}{(395 - 38.9974)} \right] = 5.3412$$

or
$$p_v = 208.76 \text{ kPa}$$
Steam Tables (Appendix-A-III.2) gives $p_v = 211.45$ kPa at 395 K.

The latent heat of vaporization can be calculated from the Antoine constants B and C and the second virial coefficient[2,24]. Reader is advised to refer the book by Zwolinski and Wilhoit for the correlation. Another method is given in Ref. 14 which also uses Antoine constants for calculation of latent heat of vaporization.

For reliable estimation of latent heat of vaporization, the following equation, proposed by Watson is recommended

$$\frac{\lambda_v}{\lambda_{v_1}} = \left[\frac{T_c - T}{T_c - T_1} \right]^n \tag{5.26}$$

where
λ_v = latent heat of vaporization at T K,

λ_{v_1} = latent heat of vaporization at T_1, K.

T_c = critical temperature, K and

n = characteristic constant of equation = 0.38

The Watson equation is simple and reliable. Values of T_c, λ_{v_1} and T_1 are given in Table 5.5. It may be noted that T_1 is usually selected as the normal boiling point T_B in Table 5.5 in most cases as experimental data for many compounds for λ_v at T_B are available. In absence or non-availability of value of λ_v at T_B, Riedel equation[2] is useful

$$\frac{\lambda_v}{RT_B} = \frac{1.092(\ln p_c - 5.6182)}{0.930 - T_{Br}} \tag{5.27}$$

where
λ_v = latent heat of vaporization, kJ/kmol

p_c = critical pressure, kPa

T_{Br} = reduced pressure at $T_B = T_B/T_c$

R = 8.314 51 kJ/(kmol·K)

Riedel equation is quite accurate and error rarely exceeds 5%.

Example 5.10 For *o*-xylene, Calculate (a) latent heat of vaporization at T_B using Riedel equation and (b) latent heat of vaporization at 298.15 (25°C) using Watson equation.

Table 5.4 Antoine Constants

Forms of equation:
Form 1: Eq. (5.24)
Form 2: Eq. (5.25)

where p_v = Vapour pressure, kPa
and T = Absolute saturation temperature, K

Compound	Chemical formula	Molar mass	A	B	C	Temp. range K	Form of equation	Ref.
Acetaldehyde (Ethanal)	C_2H_4O	44.0526	7.1304	1600.00	− 18.6500	273 – 307	1	23
			15.1206	2845.25	− 22.0670		2	6
Acetic acid (Ethanoic acid)	$C_2H_4O_2$	60.0520	6.5127	1533.30	− 50.8500	303 – 400	1	23
			15.8667	4097.86	− 27.4937		2	6
Acetic anhydride	$C_4H_6O_3$	102.0886	6.2744	1444.70	− 73.3500	336 – 413	1	23
Acetone (2-propanone)	C_3H_6O	58.0791	6.2834	1231.20	− 41.3500	311 – 329	1	23
			14.7171	2975.95	− 34.5228		2	6
Acetylene (Ethyne)	C_2H_2	26.0373	6.2248	711.00	− 19.7500	143 – 177	1	24
			5.7043	936.80	− 43.3500	192 – 206	1	23
			14.8321	1836.66	− 8.4521		2	6
Aniline (Phenylamine)	C_6H_7N	93.1265	6.4450	1731.50	− 67.0500	375 – 458	1	23
Ammonia	NH_3	17.0305	15.0205	4103.52	− 62.7983		2	6
Argon	Ar	39.948	15.4940	2363.24	− 22.6207		2	6
Benzene	C_6H_6	78.1118	13.9153	832.78	2.3608		2	6
			6.0306	1211.00	− 52.3500	281 – 377	1	24
Butadiene (1,2)	C_4H_6	54.0904	14.1603	2948.78	− 44.5633		2	6
			6.5231	1219.90	− 13.3500	204 – 239	1	24
			6.1187	1041.10	− 30.8500	239 – 303	1	24
Butadiene (1,3)	C_4H_6	54.0904	14.4754	2580.48	− 22.2012		2	6
			6.1605	998.10	− 27.9500	193 – 212	1	24
			5.9749	930.40	− 34.2500	212 – 288	1	24

(Contd.)

Table 5.4 Contd.

Compound	Chemical formula	Molar mass	Antoine constants			Temp. range K	Form of equation	Ref.
			A	B	C			
Butadiene (1,3)	C_4H_6	54.0904	14.0719	2280.96	-27.5956		2	6
n-Butane	C_4H_{10}	58.1222	5.9339	935.90	-34.4500	195 - 292	1	24
			13.9836	2292.44	-27.8623		2	6
i-Butane (Methylpropane)	C_4H_{10}	58.1222	6.0354	946.40	-26.4500	187 - 280	1	24
			13.8137	2150.23	-27.6228		2	6
n-Butyl alcohol (1-butanol)	$C_4H_{10}O$	74.1216	6.4886	1305.20	-99.7500	362 - 399	1	23
			14.6961	2902.96	-102.9116		2	6
iso-butyl alcohol (2-butanol)	$C_4H_{10}O$	74.1216	6.3262	1157.00	-104.8500	345 - 380	1	23
			15.4994	3246.51	-82.6994		2	6
Carbon dioxide	CO_2	44.0095	8.7947	1295.50	-3.9500	154 - 196	1	23
			15.3768	1956.25	-2.1117		2	6
Carbon disulphide	CS_2	76.141	6.0677	1169.10	-31.5500	276 - 353	1	23
			15.2388	3549.90	15.1796		2	6
Carbon monoxide	CO	28.0101	13.8722	769.93	1.6369		2	6
Carbon tetrachloride (Tetrachloromethane)	CCl_4	153.8227	6.0467	1235.20	-44.2500	293 - 251	1	23
			14.6247	3394.46	-10.2163		2	6
Chlorine	Cl_2	70.906	14.1372	2055.15	-23.3117		2	6
Chlorobenzene	C_6H_5Cl	112.5569	6.1030	1431.10	-55.5500	335 - 405	1	23
			14.3050	3457.17	-48.5524		2	6
Chloroform (Trichloromethane)	$CHCl_3$	119.3776	14.5014	2938.55	-36.9972		2	6
Cyclohexane	C_6H_{12}	84.1595	5.9662	1201.50	-50.5500	280 - 378	1	24
			13.7865	2794.58	-49.1081		2	6
Cyclohexanol	$C_6H_{12}O$	100.1589	5.3802	912.90	-164.0500	367 - 434	1	23
Chloromethane (Methyl chloride)	CH_3Cl	50.4875	6.2184	948.60	-23.8500	198 - 278	1	23
			14.3114	2170.02	-25.2701		2	6
Dichlorobenzene (1,2)	$C_6H_4Cl_2$	147.0020	6.2687	1704.49	-53.734		1	23

(Contd.)

Table 5.4 Contd.

Compound	Chemical formula	Molar mass	Antoine constants			Temp. range K	Form of equation	Ref.
			A	B	C			
Dichlorobenzene (1,3)	$C_6H_4Cl_2$	147.0020	6.165	1607.05	-59.772		1	23
Dichlorobenzene (1,4)	$C_6H_4Cl_2$	147.0020	6.1457	1590.88	-62.924		1	23
Dichloromethane (Methylene chloride)	CH_2Cl_2	84.9326	8.8506	2979.50	-122.3500	303 – 313	1	23
Diethanolamine	$C_4H_{11}NO_2$	105.1356	7.2637	2327.90	-98.7500	467 – 514	1	23
Diethylamine	$C_4H_{11}N$	73.1368	4.9265	583.30	-129.0500	304 – 334	1	23
Diethylether	$C_4H_{10}O$	74.1216	6.0452	1064.10	-44.3500	212 – 293	1	23
			14.1675	2563.73	-39.3707		2	6
Dimethylamine	C_2H_7N	45.0837	6.2070	960.20	-51.4500	202 – 280	1	23
Dimethylether	C_2H_6O	46.0684	6.1009	889.30	-31.1500	195 – 248	1	23
			14.3448	2176.84	-24.6733		2	6
Ethane	C_2H_6	30.069	5.9594	663.70	-16.6500	130 – 198	1	24
			13.8797	1582.18	-13.7622		2	6
Ethyl alcohol (Ethanol)	C_2H_6O	46.0684	7.2371	1592.90	-46.9500	292 – 367	1	23
			16.1952	3423.53	-55.7152		2	6
Ethyl acetate	$C_4H_8O_2$	88.1051	14.5813	3022.25	-47.8833		2	6
Ethyl benzene	C_8H_{10}	106.165	6.0821	1424.3	-59.95		1	23
Monoethanolamine	C_2H_7NO	61.0831	6.5817	1577.70	-99.7500	338 – 444	1	23
Ethylchloride (Chloroethane)	C_2H_5Cl	64.5141	6.1114	1030.00	-34.5500	217 – 285	1	23
			14.2656	2458.21	-30.6994		2	6
Ethyl mercaptan (Ethanethiol)	C_2H_6S	62.1340	6.0770	1084.50	-411.7500	224 – 329	1	24
			14.2423	2616.51	-36.3192		2	6
Ethylene (Ethene)	C_2H_4	28.0532	5.8725	585.00	-18.1500	120 – 182	1	23
			13.8182	1427.22	-14.3080		2	6
Ethylene glycol	$C_2H_6O_2$	62.0678	7.2157	2088.90	-69.7500	323 – 473	1	23
			16.1847	4493.79	-82.1026		2	6
Ethylene oxide	C_2H_4O	44.0526	6.2533	1054.50	-35.3500	225 – 285	1	23

(Contd.)

Table 5.4 Contd.

Compound	Chemical formula	Molar mass	Antoine constants			Temp. range K	Form of equation	Ref.
			A	B	C			
(Epoxy ethane)	C_2H_4O	44.0526	14.5116	2478.12	− 33.1582		2	6
Formaldehyde	CH_2O	30.0260	6.3207	970.60	− 29.0500	164 – 295	1	23
			14.3483	2161.33	− 31.9756		2	6
Formic acid	CH_2O_2	40.0254	6.7067	1699.20	− 12.4500	310 – 374	1	23
Furfural	$C_5H_4O_2$	96.0841	16.7802	5365.88	5.6186		2	6
Glycerol	$C_3H_8O_3$	92.0938	5.2899	1036.10	− 245.0500	456 – 534	1	23
n-Hexane	C_6H_{14}	86.1754	5.9951	1168.70	− 48.9500	248 – 365	1	23
			14.0568	2825.42	− 42.7089		2	6
Hydrazine	N_2H_4	32.0452	6.9378	1684.00	− 45.1500	288 – 343	1	23
Hydrogen	H_2	2.0159	12.7844	232.32	8.0800		2	6
Hydrogen chloride	HCl	36.4609	14.7081	1802.24	− 9.6678		2	6
Hydrogen cyanide	HCN	27.0253	6.6531	1329.50	− 12.7500	257 – 319	1	23
			15.4856	3151.53	− 8.8383		2	6
Hydrogen sulphide	H_2S	34.0819	14.5513	1964.37	− 15.2417		2	6
Methane	CH_4	16.0425	5.8205	405.40	− 5.3500	92 – 120	1	24
			13.5840	968.13	− 3.7200		2	6
Methyl alcohol (Methanol)	CH_4O	32.0422	7.2059	1582.30	− 33.4500	288 – 357	1	23
			16.4948	3593.39	− 35.2249		2	6
Methyl amine	CH_5N	31.0571	6.4618	1011.50	− 39.8500	190 – 267	1	23
Methyl bromide (Bromomethane)	CH_3Br	94.9385	6.2157	1046.10	− 28.2500	203 – 277	1	23
Methyl ethyl ketone	C_4H_8O	72.1057	6.1885	1261.30	− 51.1500	315 – 362	1	23
			14.2173	2831.82	− 57.3831		2	6
Naphthalene	$C_{10}H_8$	128.1705	6.1356	1733.70	− 71.2500	359 – 523	1	24
			13.7520	3701.48	− 85.8319		2	6
α-Naphthol	$C_{10}H_8O$	144.1699	6.6405	2227.40	− 74.9500	414 – 555	1	23

(Contd.)

Table 5.4 Contd.

Compound	Chemical formula	Molar mass	Antoine constants			Temp. range K	Form of equation	Ref.
			A	B	C			
β-Naphthol	$C_{10}H_8O$	144.1699	5.5328	2162.30	−82.8500	417 − 561	1	23
Nitric oxide	NO	30.0061	6.9196	1319.11	−14.1427		2	6
Nitrobenzene	$C_6H_5NO_2$	123.1094	6.2405	1746.60	−71.3500	407 − 484	1	23
Nitrogen	N_2	28.0134	13.4477	648.22	−2.8540		2	6
Nitrogen dioxide	NO_2	46.0055	21.9837	6615.35	86.8780		2	6
Nitrous oxide	N_2O	44.0128	14.2447	1547.56	−23.9090		2	6
Oxygen	O_2	31.9988	5.8124	318.70	−6.4500	55 − 100	1	23
			13.6835	780.26	−4.1758		2	6
n-Pentane	C_5H_{12}	72.1488	6.0012	1075.80	−39.9500	223 − 331	1	24
			13.9778	2554.60	−36.2529		2	6
Propane	C_3H_8	44.0956	5.9289	803.80	−26.1500	165 − 247	1	24
			15.7097	1872.82	−25.1011		2	6
Propionic acid	$C_3H_6O_2$	74.0785	15.4276	3761.14	−66.0009		2	6
n-Propyl alcohol (1-propanol)	C_3H_8O	60.0950	6.8691	1437.70	−74.6500	333 − 377	1	23
			15.2175	3008.31	−86.4909		2	6
iso-Propyl alcohol (2-propanol)	C_3H_8O	60.0950	6.8651	1359.50	−75.6500	325 − 362	1	23
			15.6491	3109.34	−73.5459		2	6
Propylene (Propene)	C_3H_6	42.0797	5.9445	785.00	−26.1500	161 − 242	1	24
			13.8782	1875.25	−22.9101		2	6
Phenol	C_6H_6O	94.1112	6.2579	1516.80	−98.1500	380 − 455	1	23
			15.2767	4027.98	−76.7014		2	6
Pyridine	C_5H_5O	79.0999	6.1661	1373.80	−58.1500	340 − 426	1	23
Sytrene	C_8H_8	104.491	6.1911	1507.40	−58.1500	303 − 418	1	23
Sulphur dioxide	SO_2	64.0638	14.9404	2385.00	−32.2139		2	6
Sulphur trioxide	SO_3	80.0632	13.8467	1777.66	−125.1972		2	6

(Contd.)

Table 5.4 Contd.

Compound	Chemical formula	Molar mass	Antoine constants			Temp. range K	Form of equation	Ref.
			A	B	C			
Toluene (Methyl benzene)	C_7H_8	92.1384	6.0795	1344.80	-53.6500	280-410	1	24
			14.2515	3242.38	-47.1806		2	6
Water	H_2O	18.0153	7.3092	1791.30	-35.0500	273-302	1	24
			7.2643	1767.30	-36.8500	303-312	1	24
			7.2136	1739.40	-39.0500	313-322	1	24
			7.1713	1715.40	-41.0500	323-332	1	24
			7.1365	1695.20	-42.7500	333-342	1	24
			7.1095	1678.90	-44.1500	343-352	1	24
			7.0883	1665.90	-45.3500	353-362	1	24
			7.0733	1656.40	-46.2500	363-372	1	24
			7.0436	1636.90	-48.2500	373-423	1	24
			16.5362	3985.44	-38.9974		2	6
m-Xylene (Dimethyl benzene)	C_8H_{10}	106.165	6.1340	1462.30	-58.0500	301-439	1	24
			14.1146	3360.81	-58.3463		2	6
o-Xylene (Dimethyl benzene)	C_8H_{10}	106.165	6.1238	1474.70	-59.4500	305-445	1	24
			14.1257	3412.02	-58.6824		2	6
p-Xylene (Dimethyl benzene)	C_8H_{10}	106.165	6.1154	1453.40	-57.8500	300-439	1	24
			14.0891	3351.69	-57.6000		2	6

(Reproduced with the permissions of (i) Monsanto Chemical Co., USA (ii) Thermodynamics Research Centre, USA and (iii) Elsevier Scientific Publishing Co., The Netherlands.)

Solution

(a) For *o*-xylene, $p_c = 3730$ kPa and $T_c = 630.3$ K

$$T_B = 417.5 \text{ K}$$

$$T_{Br} = \frac{417.5}{630.3} = 0.662$$

$$\lambda_v = 8.314\,51 \times 417.5 \left[\frac{1.092(\ln 3730 - 5.6182)}{(0.930 - 0.662)} \right]$$

$$= 36\,860 \text{ kJ/kmol}$$

Ref. 24 gives $\lambda_v = 36\,819$ kJ/kmol.

(b) $\qquad T_1 = 298.15$ K

$$\lambda_{v_1} = 36\,819 \left[\frac{630.3 - 298.15}{630.3 - 417.5} \right]^{0.38} = 43\,606 \text{ kJ/kmol}$$

Ref. 25 and Ref. 24 give $\lambda_{v_1} = 43\,580$ kJ/kmol and 43 430 kJ/kmol at 298.15 K (25°C) respectively.

Nomographs are available in literature[20] for the estimation of the latent heat of vaporization or fusion.

Some of the compounds are extensively used in industry for heating and cooling. Steam, thermic fluids, refrigerants etc. are commonly used in the process industry. It is rather inconvenient to handle equations for vapour pressure, saturation temperature and latent heat of vaporization calculations for such compounds. Tables are found to be more convenient in practice.

Steam tables in Appendix III give the latent heat of water at different temperatures/pressures. In the steam tables, h denotes the sensible heat of water over 273.16 K (0.01°C). The latent heat of vaporization is λ_v and the total heat of steam is given by H. For saturated steam,

$$H = h + \lambda_v \qquad (5.28)$$

For wet steam having dryness fraction x [i.e. $(1 - x)$ kg moisture present in 1 kg moist (wet) steam],

$$H = h + x\lambda_v \qquad (5.29)$$

In the case of superheated steam, total heat,

$$H = h + \lambda_v + C_{pm} (T - T_s) \qquad (5.30)$$

where C_{pm} is the mean heat capacity of steam in kJ/(kg·K), T the temperature of superheated steam in K, and T_s the saturation temperature of steam corresponding to pressure in K.

Relationship of saturation vapour pressure (p_v) of a pure liquid at temperature T is not directly proportional as can be seen from Eq. (5.24) or Eq. (5.25). Therefore, estimation of saturation vapour pressure at intermediate temperature T can be accurately calculated by

$$\ln \frac{p_s}{p_{s_1}} = \frac{T_2(T - T_1)}{T(T_2 - T_1)} \ln \frac{p_{s_2}}{p_{s_1}} \qquad (5.31)$$

where $\qquad p_s =$ saturation vapour pressure at T

$\qquad\qquad p_{s_1} =$ saturation vapour pressure at T_1

Table 5.5 Correlation Constants for Latent Heat of Vaporization [Eq. (5.26)]

Compound	Formula	Molar mass	T_c, K	T_1, K	λ_{v_1} kJ/kmol	Range, K	Ref.
Acetaldehyde	C_2H_4O	44.0526	461.0	293.8 (T_B)	25 732	50–461	25
Acetic acid	$C_2H_4O_2$	60.0520	592.71	391.3 (T_B)	23 681	290–594	25
Acetone	C_3H_6O	58.0791	508.1	329.4 (T_B)	29 121	178–508	25
Acetylene (Ethyne)	C_2H_2	26.0373	308.33	192.4 (T_B)	16 674	192–309	25
Ammonia	NH_3	17.0305	405.5	239.7 (T_B)	23 346	195–405	11
Aniline	C_6H_7N	93.1265	699.0	457.2	418 40	267–699	25
Argon	Ar	39.948	150.69	87.3	6 520	84–150	11
Benzene	C_6H_6	78.1118	562.16	353.3 (T_B)	30 761	278–562	25
Bromine	Br_2	159.808	588.0	331.9	29 980	266–588	11
1-2-Butadiene	C_4H_6	54.0904	443.7	284.0 (T_B)	24 267	137–444	25
1,3-Butadiene	C_4H_6	54.0904	425.0	268.7 (T_B)	22 468	164–425	25
n-Butane	C_4H_{10}	58.1222	425.18	273.0 (T_B)	22 393	135–425	25
i-Butane (2-methyl propane)	C_4H_{10}	58.1222	408.15	261.5 (T_B)	21 297	114–408	25
n-butyl alcohol (1-butanol)	$C_4H_{10}O$	74.1216	563.05	390.6 (T_B)	43 095	165–563	25
Carbon dioxide	CO_2	44.0095	304.12	216.6 (T_B)	15 326	217–304	25
Carbon disulphide	CS_2	76.141	552.0	319.0 (T_B)	26 736	161–552	25
Carbon monoxide	CO	28.0101	132.85	81.6 (T_B)	6 042	68–133	25
Chlorine	Cl_2	70.9056	416.90	239.1	20 662	172–417	11
Chlorobenzene	C_6H_5Cl	112.5569	632.40	405.1 (T_B)	36 547	228–632	25
Chlorodifluoromethane (R-22)	$CHClF_2$	86.4684	369.3	232.4 (T_B)	20 192	113–369	25

(Contd.)

Table 5.5 Contd.

Compound	Formula	Molar mass	T_c, K	T_1, K	kJ/kmol	Range, K	Ref.
Chloroform (Trichloromethane)	$CHCl_3$	119.3776	536.50	334.3 (T_B)	29 706	210–536	25
Chlorotrifluoromethane (R-13)	$CClF_3$	104.4589	302.0	191.7 (T_B)	15 506	92–254	25
Cyclohexane	C_6H_{12}	84.1616	553.5	353.9 (T_B)	29 957	280–302	25
Dichlorodifluoromethane (R-12)	CCl_2F_2	120.9132	384.95	243.3 (T_B)	19 966	115–385	25
Dichlorofluoromethane (R-21)	CCl_2FH	102.9227	451.58	282.1 (T_B)	24 937	138–452	25
Diethyl ether	$C_4H_{10}O$	74.1228	466.74	307.7 (T_B)	26 694	157–467	25
Ethane	C_2H_6	30.0696	305.42	184.6 (T_B)	14 707	190–305	25
Ethanol (Ethyl alcohol)	C_2H_6O	46.069	53.92	351.5 (T_B)	38 744	159–514	25
Ethyl acetate	$C_4H_8O_2$	88.1063	523.2	349.8 (T_B)	32 217	190–523	25
Ethylbenzene	C_8H_{10}	106.1674	617.20	409.3 (T_B)	35 564	178–617	25
Ethylene (Ethene)	C_2H_4	28.0538	282.34	169.4 (T_B)	13 544	104–282	25
Ethylene glycol	$C_2H_6O_2$	62.0684	607.0	470.5 (T_B)	52 509	260–469	25
Ethylene oxide (Epoxy ethane)	C_2H_4O	44.0526	469.0	283.8 (T_B)	225 606	161–607	25
n-Hexane	C_6H_{14}	86.1754	507.5	341.9 (T_B)	28 853	178–508	25
Hydrogen bromide	HBr	80.9119	363.20	217.7	17 613	186–363	11
Hydrogen chloride	HCl	36.4609	324.70	188.1	16 149	159–325	11
Hydrogen iodide	HI	127.9124	424.00	237.7	17 079	222–424	11
Methane	CH_4	16.0425	190.56	111.6 (T_B)	8 180	91–191	25

(Contd.)

Table 5.5 Contd.

Compound	Formula	Molar mass	T_c, K	T_1, K	λ_{v_1} kJ/kmol	Range, K	Ref.
Methanol (Methyl alcohol)	CH_3OH	32.0419	512.64	337.8 (T_B)	32 254	176–513	25
Methyl chloride (R-40) (Chloro methane)	CH_3Cl	50.4875	416.25	249.2 (T_B)	21 442	175–416	25
Methylene chloride (R-30) (Dichloro methane)	CH_2Cl_2	84.9326	510.00	313.2 (T_B)	27 991	178–510	25
Methyl ethyl ketone (2-butanone)	C_4H_8O	72.1057	536.78	352.6 (T_B)	31 213	186–537	25
Naphthalene	$C_{10}H_8$	128.1705	748.4	491.1 (T_B)	43 263	354–748	25
Nitric oxide	NO	30.0061	180.00	121.4	13 818	109–180	11
Nitrogen	N_2	28.0134	126.09	77.4	5 348	63–126	11
Nitrogen dioxide	NO_2	46.0055	431.00	294.4	19 069	262–431	11
Nitrous oxide	N_2O	44.0128	309.60	183.7	16 566	182–310	11
Oxygen	O_2	31.9988	154.58	90.2	6 891	55–155	11
n-Pentane	C_5H_{12}	72.1488	469.70	309.2 (T_B)	25 773	143–470	25
Phenol	C_6H_6O	94.1112	694.20	454.9 (T_B)	45 606	314–694	25
Propane (R-290)	C_3H_8	44.0956	369.82	231.1 (T_B)	18 774	86–370	25
1-Propanol (n-propyl alcohol)	C_3H_8O	60.095	536.78	370.4 (T_B)	41 756	147–537	25
Propylene (Propene)	C_3H_6	42.0797	364.85	225.7 (T_B)	18 410	88–365	25
Styrene	C_8H_8	104.1491	647.00	418.2 (T_B)	36 819	243–647	25
Sulphur dioxide	SO_2	64.0638	430.80	263.2	24 945	200–431	11
Sulphur trioxide	SO_3	80.0632	491.00	318.0	42 903	290–491	11
Toluene	C_7H_8	92.1384	591.79	383.7 (T_B)	33 179	178–592	25

(Contd.)

Table 5.5 Contd.

Compound	Formula	Molar mass	T_c, K	T_1, K	λ_{v_1} kJ/kmol	Range, K	Ref.
Trichlorofluoromethane (R-11)	CCl_3F	137.3681	471.2	297.1 (T_B)	24 769	162–471	25
Water	H_2O	18.0153	647.11	373.15 (T_B)	40 677	273–647	11
m-Xylene	C_8H_{10}	106.165	617.05	412.2 (T_B)	36 359	225–617	25
o-Xylene	C_8H_{10}	106.165	630.30	417.5 (T_B)	36 819	248–630	25
p-Xylene	C_8H_{10}	106.165	616.20	411.4 (T_B)	35 982	286–616	25

(*Reproduced with the permissions of (i) Gulf Publishing Co., USA and (ii) McGraw-Hill Inc., USA.*)

and p_{s_2} = saturature vapour pressure at T_2

Eq. (5.31) could be quite useful in interpolation of steam tables.

For interpolation of enthalpy values, linear relationship with temperature gives satisfactory results.

Example 5.11 Refer Appendix III and calculate saturation pressure of steam at 565.15 K (292°C).

Solution From Appendix III.2,

$$p_{s_1} = 75 \text{ bar a and } T_1 = 563.65 \text{ K } (290.5°C)$$

and $p_{s_2} = 80 \text{ bar a and } T_2 = 568.12 \text{ K } (294.97°C)$

for $T = 565.15 \text{ K } (292°C)$,

$$\ln \frac{p_s}{75} = \frac{568.12(565.15 - 563.65)}{565.65(568.12 - 563.65)} \ln \frac{80}{75}$$

or $p_s = 76.65 \text{ bar a}$

JSME Steam Tables report $p_s = 76.65$ bar a at $T = 565.15$ K (292°C).

Linear interpolation will yield $p_s = 76.68$ bar a.

Heating and cooling are commonly encountered in the process industry. Steam is the most widely used heating medium. Apart from steam, organic heat transfer fluids are also used. Figure 5.6 gives the temperature range for various heat transfer fluids and electrical heating systems. Diphenyl-diphenyl oxide eutectic* is another versatile vapour phase heating medium. Properties of this eutectic mixture are given in Table 5.6.

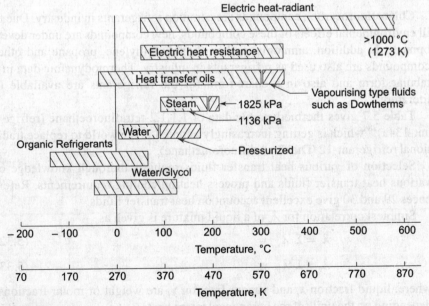

Fig. 5.6 Temperature Range for Selected Heat Transfer Media[27]

---

* Dowtherm A of The Dow Chemical Company, USA.

Table 5.6 Characteristic Data of Eutectic Mixture of Diphenyl (26.5% v/v) and Diphenyl Oxide (73.5% v/v)[26]

Temperature		Saturation pressure, p_s	Density (kg/m³)		Enthalpy, kJ/kg		
°C	K	kPa a	Liquid	Vapour	Sensible h	Latent λ_v	Total H
100	373	0.5	995	0.027	147.3	364.8	512.1
120	393	1.31	978	0.067	184.1	356.1	540.2
140	413	3.09	961	0.151	221.7	347.3	569.0
160	433	6.61	943	0.306	260.7	338.9	599.6
180	453	13.1	925	0.579	300.4	330.1	630.5
200	473	24.9	907	1.025	341.4	321.7	663.1
220	493	41.7	888	1.717	383.3	313.4	696.7
240	513	68.6	869	2.742	426.8	304.2	731.0
257.1	**530.25**	**101.325**	**852**	**3.957**	**464.8**	**296.2**	**761.0**
260	533	107.9	849	4.194	471.1	295.0	766.1
280	553	163.1	828	6.210	516.7	284.9	801.6
300	573	237.9	807	8.911	563.6	274.0	837.6
320	593	336.5	784	12.48	611.7	262.3	874.0
340	613	463.3	761	17.12	660.7	250.2	910.9
360	633	623.0	736	23.10	711.3	236.8	948.1
380	653	820.9	709	30.87	762.7	222.6	985.3
400	673	1063.0	680	40.98	815.5	206.3	1021.8

(Courtesy: The Dow Chemical Company, USA)

Chlorofluorocarbon compounds are common refrigerants in industry. Due to ill environmental effects of these compounds, new compounds are under development. In addition, ammonia, carbon dioxide, ethylene, propane and other compounds are also used as refrigerants in industry. Thermodynamic data in a tabular form and also in a chart form for the refrigerants are available in literature[27].

Table 5.7 gives thermodynamic data of 1,1,1,2-tetrafluoroethane (refrigerant-134a)[28] which is getting increasingly adopted in the world to replace traditional refrigerant-12 (Dichloro-difluoromethane).

Selection of various heat transfer fluids requires thorough knowledge of various heat transfer fluids and process heating/cooling requirements. References 29 and 30 give excellent account on heat transfer fluids.

Simplest correlation for λ_v of a liquid mixture is given as

$$\lambda_v = \Sigma \, \lambda_{v_i} \, x_i \qquad (5.32)$$

$$\lambda_v = \Sigma \, \lambda_{v_i} \, y_i \qquad (5.33)$$

where, liquid fraction x_i and vapour fraction y_i are weight or molar fractions, depending on the units of the component latent heats.

For organic mixtures, above equations represent the data within 15%. For other mixtures and extreme temperature-pressure conditions the error can be quite high.

Table 5.7 Thermodynamic Properties of Refrigerant[28] R-134a
Chemical name: 1,1,2-Tetrafluoroethane (CH_2FCF_3)

Temperature		Saturation pressure, p_s bar	Liquid density kg/m³ ρ_l	Specific volume of vapour V_v, m³/kg	Enthalpy kJ/kg		Entropy kJ/(kg·K)	
°C	K				h	H	S_l	S_v
−40	233.15	0.512 2	1414.8	0.360 95	148.57	374.16	0.7973	1.7649
−30	243.15	0.843 6	1385.9	0.225 96	161.10	380.45	0.8498	1.7519
−26.07[b]	**247.08**	**1.013 25**	**1374.3**	**0.190 16**	**166.07**	**382.90**	**0.8701**	**1.7476**
−24	249.15	1.112 7	1368.2	0.174 10	168.70	384.19	0.8806	1.7455
−22	251.15	1.216 0	1362.2	0.160 10	171.26	385.43	0.8908	1.7436
−20	253.15	1.326 8	1356.2	0.147 44	173.82	386.66	0.9009	1.7417
−18	255.15	1.445 4	1350.2	0.135 97	176.39	387.89	0.9110	1.7399
−16	257.15	1.572 1	1344.1	0.125 56	178.97	389.11	0.9211	1.7383
−14	259.15	1.707 4	1338.0	0.116 10	181.56	390.33	0.9311	1.7367
−12	261.15	1.851 6	1331.8	0.107 49	184.16	391.55	0.9410	1.7351
−10	263.15	2.005 2	1325.6	0.099 63	186.78	392.75	0.9509	1.7337
−8	265.15	2.168 4	1319.3	0.092 46	189.40	393.95	0.9608	1.7323
−6	267.15	2.341 8	1313.0	0.085 91	192.03	395.15	0.9707	1.7310
−4	269.15	2.525 7	1306.6	0.079 91	194.68	396.33	0.9805	1.7297
−2	271.15	2.720 6	1300.2	0.074 40	197.33	397.51	0.9903	1.7285
0	273.15	2.926 9	1293.7	0.069 35	200.00	398.68	1.0000	1.7274
2	275.15	3.145 0	1287.1	0.064 70	202.68	399.84	1.0097	1.7263
4	277.15	3.375 5	1280.5	0.060 42	205.37	401.00	1.0194	1.7252
6	279.15	3.618 6	1273.8	0.056 48	208.08	402.14	1.0291	1.7242
8	281.15	3.874 9	1267.0	0.052 84	210.80	403.27	1.0387	1.7233
10	283.15	4.144 9	1260.2	0.049 48	213.53	404.40	1.0483	1.7224
12	285.15	4.428 9	1253.3	0.046 36	216.27	405.51	1.0579	1.7215

(Contd.)

Table 5.7 Contd.

Temperature		Saturation pressure, p_s bar	Liquid density kg/m³ ρ_l	Specific volume of vapour V_v, m³/kg	Enthalpy kJ/kg		Entropy kJ/(kg · K)	
°C	K				h	H	S_l	S_v
14	287.15	4.727 6	1246.3	0.043 48	219.03	406.61	1.0674	1.7207
16	289.15	5.041 3	1239.3	0.040 81	221.80	407.701	1.0770	1.7199
18	291.15	5.370 6	1232.1	0.038 33	224.59	408.78	1.0865	1.7191
20	293.15	5.715 9	1224.9	0.036 03	227.40	409.84	1.0960	1.7183
24	297.15	6.456 6	1210.1	0.031 89	233.05	411.93	1.1149	1.7169
28	301.15	7.267 6	1194.9	0.028 29	238.77	413.95	1.1338	1.7155
32	305.15	8.153 0	1179.3	0.025 16	244.55	415.90	1.1527	1.7142
36	309.15	9.117 2	1163.2	0.022 41	250.41	417.78	1.1715	1.7129
40	313.15	10.165	1146.5	0.019 99	256.35	419.58	1.1903	1.7115
44	317.15	11.300	1129.2	0.017 86	262.38	421.28	1.2091	1.7101
48	321.15	12.527	1111.3	0.015 98	268.49	422.88	1.2279	1.7086
52	325.15	13.852	1092.6	0.014 30	274.71	424.35	1.2468	1.7070
56	329.15	15.280	1073.0	0.012 80	281.04	425.68	1.2657	1.7051
60	333.15	16.815	1052.4	0.011 46	287.49	426.86	1.2847	1.7031
64	337.15	18.464	1030.7	0.010 26	294.08	427.84	1.3039	1.7007
68	341.15	20.234	1007.7	0.009 17	300.84	428.61	1.3234	1.6979
72	345.15	22.130	983.1	0.008 18	307.79	429.10	1.3430	1.6945
76	349.15	24.159	956.5	0.007 28	314.96	429.27	1.3631	1.6905

[b] normal boiling point (T_B)

Reference state: h = 200 kJ/kg and S_l = 1.0000 kJ/(kg · K) at 273.15 K(0 °C)

(Reproduced with permission of the American Society of Heating, Refrigerating and Air-Conditioning Engineers, Inc., Atlanta, USA.)

For latent heat of fusion, attempts to obtain general correlations have been unsuccessful. Table 5.8 gives the latent heat of fusion of common compounds.

Table 5.8 Latent Heat of Fusion

Compound	Formula	Melting Point		Latent heat of fusion λ_f kJ/kg
		K	°C	
Acetic acid	CH_3COOH	289.85	16.7	195.5
Acetone	C_3H_6O	178.45	– 94.7	99.6
Benzene	C_6H_6	278.65	5.5	126.0
Carbon tetrachloride	CCl_4	250.35	– 22.8	16.1
Chloroform	$CHCl_3$	209.65	– 63.5	77.0
Cyclohexane	C_6H_{12}	279.65	6.5	31.8
Diethylether	$C_2H_5OC_2H_5$	156.85	– 116.3	98.6
Ethanol	C_2H_5OH	159.05	– 114.1	108.9
Ethyl acetate	$CH_3COOC_2H_5$	189.55	– 83.6	118.9
n-Heptane	C_7H_{16}	182.55	– 90.6	140.2
n-Hexane	C_6H_{14}	177.85	– 95.3	151.9
Methanol	CH_3OH	175.45	– 97.7	100.5
1-Propanol	C_3H_7OH	146.95	– 126.2	86.5
2-Propanol	C_3H_7OH	184.65	– 88.5	90.1
Toluene	C_7H_8	178.15	– 95.0	71.9
Water	H_2O	273.15	0.0	333.7
m-Xylene	C_8H_{10}	225.25	– 47.9	444.2
o-Xylene	C_8H_{10}	248.05	– 25.1	444.2
p-Xylene	C_8H_{10}	286.45	13.3	444.2

Extensive data on latent heat of fusion are given in Perry's Chemical Engineers' Handbook[20].

The latent heat of sublimation is the sum of the latent heats of vaporization and fusion where both the latent heats are at the same temperature.

5.10 ENTHALPY CHANGES FOR PURE SUBSTANCES AND THEIR MIXTURES IN IDEAL STATES

In chemical plants different types of mixtures are encountered. Mostly these are liquid and gaseous mixtures. In this section a general methodology for calculating enthalpies of different types of mixtures is described.

5.10.1 Generalized Procedure

The following steps may be followed when enthalpy of a stream (an ideal fluid or an ideal mixture) is required:

(a) The composition of the stream is fixed from the material balance of the process. Also the pressure and temperature of the stream are known or can be fixed depending on the process requirements.

(b) Enthalpy of substances are calculated relative to a particular temperature. This temperature, T_0 which can be selected based on convenience and is called the *reference temperature*. This may not be the same for all the streams of the plant. Generally, 298.15 K(25°C) is taken as the reference temperature for calculating the enthalpy but the processes involving stream and using enthalpies given in Steam Tables (Appendix-A III), 273.16 K (0.01°C) is taken as the reference temperature. In petroleum industry, 288.7 K (15.56°C or 60°F) is used as the reference temperature for many calculations.

(c) Based on the data available in para (a), the fluid can be classified into following categories:

  (i) Pure substances and
  (ii) Mixtures

   Enthalpies of the process fluids in ideal state can then be calculated as described below.

5.10.2 Pure Substances

If the stream contains a pure substance, the enthalpy depends on the temperature and the state of the substance. As the degree of freedom is only one for a pure substance, only one variable is required to know the state of the substance. Thus, if the pressure or temperature of the substance is known, its state can be found. For the given pressure, the saturation temperature, T_s, of the substance can be found from published data or from correlations like the Antoine equation [(Eq. (5.24) or Eq. (5.25)].

If the temperature, $T < T_s$, then the state of the substance is liquid and if $T > T_s$, the state is superheated vapour (i.e. gas). For example, at atmospheric pressure, water will be liquid at ambient temperature.

After finding the state of the substance the enthalpy of an ideal substance (in kJ/kg) can be calculated from the following equation:

(i) For liquids, $H_L = m \displaystyle\int_{T_0}^{T} C_1 \, dT$ (5.34)

and

(ii) For vapour, $H_V = \displaystyle\int_{T_0}^{T_s} C_1 \, dT + \lambda_v + \int_{T_s}^{T} C_p^0 \, dT$ (5.35)

where λ_v = Latent heat of vaporization at T_s.

If molar heat capacity data are used, conversion with the help of molar mass will be required.

The integral in the above equations can be solved by using methods described in Sec. 5.5 and 5.6 while the latent heat of vaporization at different temperatures can be evaluated by using methods described in Sec. 5.9. For certain common compounds (e.g. steam, refrigerants, heat transfer fluids etc.), enthalpy values are read from the tables (as described in Sec. 5.9) and substituted in Eq. (5.34) or Eq. (5.35).

5.10.3   Ideal Mixtures

The mixtures, encountered in the chemical plants, can be divided into three types, with respective criteria for ideality, as follows:

(i) Ideal Gas Mixture
Gas mixture following ideal-gas law is defined as the *Ideal Gas Mixture*. At low pressure (say up to 10 bar) a gas mixture may be considered as an ideal gas mixture. For an ideal gas mixture, the mixture enthalpy depends only on the enthalpy of the individual ideal gas which comprises the gas mixture. The enthalpy of the ideal gas mixture can be calculated as described in Sec. 5.7. In other words

$$H^{ig}_{mix} = \Sigma\, y_i H^{ig}_i \tag{5.36}$$

where H^{ig}_i is the enthalpy of the ith component in ideal state at the prevalent pressure and temperature and y_i is the mole fraction of the ith component in the gas mixture.

(ii) Ideal Liquid Solution
Ideal liquid solution follows Raoult's law (Sec. 2.6). Its heat of mixing (Sec. 5.16) is zero. The enthalpy of the ideal liquid solution is given by

$$H_{sol} = \Sigma\, x_i H_i \tag{5.37}$$

where H_i is the enthalpy of the ith component (in pure state) at the mixture temperature (and pressure) and x_i is the mole fraction of the ith component. Usually the effect of pressure on liquid enthalpy is quite small.

(iii) Ideal Vapour-Liquid Mixture
When the vapour phase is an ideal gas and the liquid phase is an ideal solution, the equilibrium vapour-liquid mixture can be described by simple and useful Raoult's law (Sec. 2.6). In other words, an equilibrium vapour-liquid mixture which follows Raoult's law is defined as ideal vapour-liquid mixture. When a system consists of saturated liquid and saturated vapour phases co-existing in equilibrium, the enthalpy of the mixture is the sum of the enthalpies of the individual phases.

As the degrees of freedom for a mixture are more than one (depending on the number of components in the mixture), more than one variable are required to be specified for defining the state of mixture. It can be established by using the composition, pressure and temperature data. From the known composition and pressure, the bubble point (T_{BB}) and dew point (T_{DP}) temperatures can be found by using the methods shown in Sec. 5.10.4. The state of the mixture can then be judged from Table 5.9.

When the temperature is between bubble point and dew point, the mixture is an equilibrium vapour-liquid mixture. For calculating the enthalpy of such ideal mixtures the fraction of total mixture in saturated vapour condition (V), is required to be known. Also the compositions of the saturated vapour and liquid phases are required. These can be found by the equilibrium $p - T$ (also known as flash) calculations, described in Sec. 5.11.

$$H^{Vi}_{mix} = (1 - V) H_{sol} + V \cdot H^{ig}_{mix} \qquad (5.38)$$

for mixtures, which are non-ideal, calculations are complex and the reader is advised to refer any standard textbook on thermodynamics (Refs. 2 and 14).

Table 5.9 State of Vapour-liquid Mixtures

Condition	State of mixture
$T < T_{BB}$	Subcooled liquid mixture
$T = T_{BB}$	Saturated liquid mixture
$T_{BB} < T < T_{DP}$	Equilibrium vapour-liquid mixture
$T = T_{DP}$	Saturated vapour mixture
$T > T_{DP}$	Superheated vapour mixture

5.10.4 Bubble Points and Dew Points of Ideal Mixtures

When a liquid mixture is heated from a subcooled state a constant pressure, the vaporization occurs over a range of temperatures unlike vaporization of a pure substance which occurs at a constant temperature at a given pressure. For any mixture the two limiting temperatures of the above range are known as *bubble point* and *dew point*.

Figure 5.7 shows T vs. x, y of n-pentane for the n-pentane/n-hexane system at 101.325 kPa (760 torr) considering the mixture to be an ideal one.

When the mixture is heated from point L, the mixture temperature follows path LM. At M, the liquid mixture is saturated and a slight increase in temperature will form a bubble of vapour. Hence the point M is called the bubble point.

As the heating process continues beyond M, the temperature rises, the amount of vapour increases and the amount of liquid decreases. During this process, the vapour and liquid phase compositions change along the paths MN and MN', respectively. Finally as the point N is approached, the liquid phase is reduced to minute drops (called dew) and at point N, the liquid phase is completely vaporized to a saturated vapour phase. Hence the point N is called the *dew point*.

Further heating above point N, increases the temperature of the vapour phase and the vapour gets superheated (path NO).

When a vapour-liquid mixture is present, amounts of both phases can be calculated by a tie-line method. A horizontal line at point Q on Fig. 5.7 is the tie-line. By geometric principles,

$$\frac{\text{Amount of liquid mixture}}{\text{Amount of vapour mixture}} = \frac{a}{b} \qquad (5.39)$$

For an ideal mixture, the bubble and dew points can be calculated using the Raoult's law. For a given pressure and composition, the bubble point and dew point and the composition at respective points are calculated by the iterative calculations shown below:

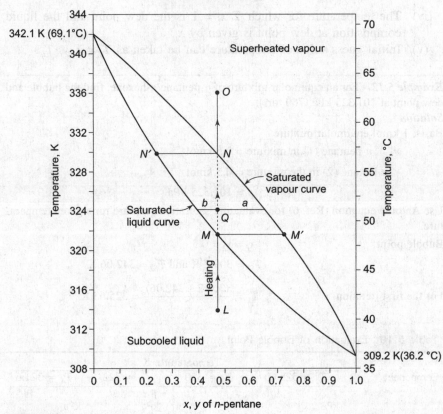

Fig. 5.7 Vapour-liquid Equilibrium Diagram (or $T/t - x, y$ Diagram) for
n-Pentane/n-Hexane

(a) Bubble Point
(i)   For a liquid mixture of known composition, assume a temperature and
      find the vapour pressure of all the components present in the mixture
      (p_{is}) at this temperature.
(ii) Calculate $y_i = x_i \cdot p_{is}/p$
      where p is the total pressure.
(iii) Σy_i should be 1. If $\Sigma y_i \neq 1$, then a new temperature should be assumed
      and the above calculations be repeated.
(iv) The temperature for which $\Sigma y_i = 1$ is the bubble point. Also the vapour
      composition at bubble point is given by y_i.
(v)   Initial guess value of temperature can be taken as $T_i = \Sigma (x_i \cdot T_{is})$. Where
      T_{is} is the saturation temperature of ith component at a total pressure p.

(b) Dew Point
(i)   For a vapour mixture of known composition, assume a temperature and
      find the vapour pressures of all components (p_{is}) at this temperature.
(ii) Calculate $x_i = y_i \cdot p/p_{is}$.
(iii) Σx_i should be 1. If $\Sigma x_i \neq 1$, then a new temperature should be assumed
      and the above calculations be repeated.

(iv) The temperature for which $\Sigma\, x_i = 1$ is the dew point and the liquid composition at dew point is given by x_i.

(v) Initial guess value of temperature can be taken as $T_i = \Sigma\, y_i \cdot T_{is}$.

Example 5.12 For an equimolar mixture of n-pentane/n-hexane, find the bubble and dew point at 101.325 kPa (760 torr).

Solution

Basis: 1 kmol equimolar mixture

$$n\text{-pentane (1) in mixture} = 0.5 \text{ kmol}$$

$$n\text{-hexane (2) in the mixture} = 0.5 \text{ kmol}$$

$$p = 101.325 \text{ kPa}$$

Use Antoine equation (Ref. 6) for evaluating saturation pressure for a given temperature.

Bubble point:
$$x_i = x_2 = 0.5$$
$$T_{S1} = 309.2 \text{ K and } T_{S2} = 342.06 \text{ K}$$

For the first iteration,
$$T_1 = \frac{(309.2 + 342.06)}{2} = 325.63 \text{ K}$$

Table 5.10 Evaluation of Bubble Point

Component		\multicolumn{8}{c}{Temperature, K}							
		$T_1 = 325.63$		$T_2 = 320$		$T_3 = 322$		$T_4 = 321.6$	
	x_i	P_{si} kPa	y_i	P_{si} kPa	y_i	P_{si} kPa	y_i	P_{si} kPa	y_i
n-pentane(1)	0.5	172.41	0.851	144.71	0.714	154.12	0.761	152.20	0.751
n-hexane (2)	0.5	58.57	0.289	47.82	0.236	51.44	0.254	50.70	0.250
$\Sigma\, y_i$			1.140		0.950		1.015		1.001

Bubble point, $\qquad\qquad\qquad T_{BB} = 321.6 \text{ K } (48.6°\text{C})$ ⠀⠀⠀⠀*Ans.* (a)

Dew point: $\qquad\qquad\qquad y_1 = y_2 = 0.5 \qquad y_i \cdot p = 50.6625$

for first iteration, $\qquad\qquad T_1 = 325.63 \text{ K}$

Table 5.11 Evaluation of Dew Point

Component	y_i	\multicolumn{6}{c}{Temperature, K}					
		$T_1 = 325.63$		$T_2 = 328$		$T_3 = 330$	
		P_{si} kPa	x_i	P_{si} kPa	x_i	P_{si} kPa	x_i
n-pentane (1)	0.5	172.41	0.294	185.228	0.274	196.606	0.258
n-hexane (2)	0.5	58.57	0.865	63.635	0.796	68.177	0.743
$\Sigma\, x_i$	1.0		1.159		1.070		1.001

Dew point, $\qquad\qquad\qquad\qquad T_{DP} = 330 \text{ K } (57°\text{C})$ ⠀⠀⠀⠀*Ans.* (b)

Note: For accurate determination of the bubble/dew point for a binary mixture, temperature (T) vs. $\Sigma\, y_i$ or $\Sigma\, x_i$ may be plotted respectively for different iterations. At a unity value of $\Sigma\, y_i$ or $\Sigma\, x_i$, bubble point or dew point is read. Figure 5.8 is the plot for n-pentane and n-hexane mixture.

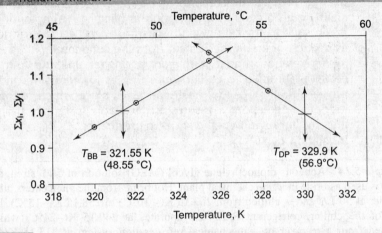

Fig. 5.8 Graphical Determination of Bubble Point and Dew Point

Example 5.13 A hot air drying machine (called a stenter) in a textile industry uses 8 bar a steam at the rate of 1000 kg/h. The condensate at its saturation temperature is discharged to the atmosphere through a steam trap. Assume that there is no loss of heat to the surroundings. Calculate the quantity of flash steam produced at the atmospheric pressure due to the let down of the pressure.

Solution Basis: 1000 kg/h condensate at the saturation temperature corresponding to 8 bar a.

The thermodynamic properties of steam at 101.3 kPa and 8 bar a can be had from the steam table (Appendix III.2).

The condensate has enthalpy equal to 720.94 kJ/kg before the trap. After discharge, at atmospheric pressure, it cannot have enthalpy more than 419.06 kJ/kg. Thus, the additional heat of condensate is converted into the latent heat of vaporization and thereby flashing takes place.

Let x be the quantity in kg of the flash steam produced.

$$\text{Condensate at 101.3 kPa a} = (1000 - x)\ \text{kg}$$

$$\text{Total heat of condensate before flashing} = 1000 \times 720.94 = 720\,940\ \text{kJ/h}$$

$$\text{Total heat of condensate after flashing} = (1000 - x)\,419.06$$

$$\text{Total heat of flash steam} = x \times 2676.0\ \text{kJ/h}$$

$$2676.0x + (1000 - x)\,419.06 = 720\,940$$

$$2256.94\,x = 720\,940 - 419\,060 = 301\,880$$

$$x = 133.76\ \text{kg/h} \qquad\qquad Ans.$$

Note: 1. Flashing of the condensate has assumed importance as a result of the energy crisis. In most of the industries, it is now an accepted practice to utilise the flash steam. Boiler blow down is flashed to produce low-pressure steam. Atmospheric pressure steam, produced from flashing of low-pressure condensate, can be compressed in a thermocompressor (see Exercise 5.14) to a sufficiently high pressure for utilisation in heaters. A simple, nomograph such as the one given by Sisson[31] can be used for quick estimation of the flashed steam from the condensate.

2. In refrigeration, liquid refrigerant at higher pressure from receiver is throttled to chiller, operating at low pressure. In this process, flashing of the refrigerant takes place which results in loss of refrigeration. Measures are available to reduce flashing thereby improving coefficient of performance (COP) of the refrigeration cycle.

Example 5.14 Aqueous monoethylene glycol (MEG) solution of 50% strength (by mass) is used as brine in a fine chemical plant. Hot brine from the plant enters tubes of a chiller at 50 L/s and is chilled from 263.15 K(– 10°C) to 258.15 K(–15°C). In the shell of the chiller, refrigerant R-134a evaporates at 249.15 K(–24°C) which is supplied from a receiver of a mechanical refrigeration system at 313.15 K(40°C) through an expansion valve. Density and specific heat of aqueous MEG solution are 1.08 kg/L and 3.08 kJ/(kmol·K) respectively in the desired temperature range. Calculate the flow of saturated vapours of R-134a from the evaporator.

Solution

Brine flow, $\qquad\qquad\qquad q_{vl} = 50$ L/s

$$q_m = 50 \times 1.08 = 54 \text{ kg/s}$$

Heat transfer in the chiller, $\qquad \phi = 54 \times 3.08 (263.15 - 258.15)$

$$= 831.6 \text{ kJ/s or kW}$$

From Table 5.7, latent heat of vaporization at 249.15 K,

$$\lambda_v = 384.19 - 168.70$$
$$= 25.49 \text{ kJ/kg}$$

Evaporation rate of R-134a in chiller,

$$q_{m2} = 831.6/215.49$$
$$= 3.859 \text{ kg/s}$$

Enthalpy of liquid R-134a at 313.15 K = 256.35 kJ/kg

Let x kg/s be flash vapours formed due to isoenthalpic expansion of liquid at 313.15 K to 249.15 K.

$$256.35 (3.859 + x) = 168.7 \times 3.859 + x \times 384.19$$

or $\qquad\qquad\qquad x = 2.649$ kg/s

Total flow of R-134a vapours from the chiller

$$= 3.859 + 2.646$$
$$= 6.505 \text{ kg/s} \qquad\qquad Ans.$$

Note: Flashing of 2.646 kg/s R-134a represents nearly 40% of total vapour flow.

Example 5.15 Compression of chlorine is carried out to liquefy it in the chloralkali industry[32]. The suction temperature of chlorine gas to the compressor plays an important role in determining the size and power requirement of the compressor. In order to keep the ingoing gas temperature low, the dry cellhouse gas (refer Example 6.16) available at 103 kPa a and 313 K (40°C) is passed through a wash column in which gas bubbles through liquid chlorine. Saturated gas at 101 kPa a leaves the wash column and is compressed in the first stage of the compressor. Compressed gas at 225 kPa g is discharged from the first stage and is cooled in an intercooler to 313 K (40°C) with the help of cooling water. Gas at 215 kPa g enters the second stage of the compressor and is further compressed to 560 kPa g. An aftercooler is provided to cool the gas to 313 K (40°C) with the help of cooling water. A chiller provided on the downstream of the aftercooler liquefies the gas at 530 kPa g. A portion of liquid chlorine is recycled to the wash column. Cooling water is supplied at 305 K (32 °C) and a temperature rise of 8 K is permitted in the cooler. Figure 5.9 schematically represents the compression system. For a liquefaction plant having 0.116 kg/s ($\approx$ 10 t/d) capacity, calculate: (a) the recycle ratio in terms of the amount of liquid chlorine recycled to the wash column to the fresh chlorine gas, entering the wash column, (b) cooling water requirements of the intercooler and aftercooler and (c) the refrigeration load of the chiller.

Solution

Basis: Liquefaction capacity = 0.116 kg/s

The final saturated product is withdrawn at 510 kPa g. Similarly, mixed feed is fed to the first stage as saturated vapours. Therefore saturation temperatures are required to be calculated for both these pressures. Using Eqs (5.24) and (5.26), saturation temperatures and latent heats of vaporization can be calculated.

$$p_1 = 101 \text{ kPa a}$$

Using Antoine equation,

$$T_{s_1} = 239.15 \text{ K } (-34°C)$$

Using Watson equation,

$$\lambda_{v_1} = 20\,662 \text{ kJ/kmol} = 291.4 \text{ kJ/kg}$$
$$p_2 = 530 \text{ kPa g} = 631.3 \text{ kPa a}$$

From Ref. 11,

$$T_{s_2} = 290.75 \text{ K } (17.6°C)$$

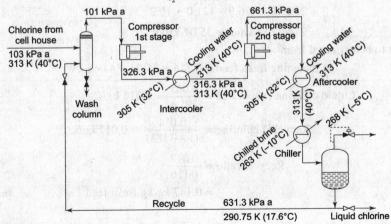

Fig. 5.9 Liquefaction of Chlorine

Using Watson equation,

$$\lambda_{v_2} = 18\ 136 \text{ kJ/kmol} = 255.8 \text{ kJ/kg}$$

Since the lowest temperature in the system is 239.15 K, it can be taken as the base temperature. The sensible heat of saturated chlorine vapours at 101 kPa a and 239.15 K ($-34°C$) = 0 kJ/kg. The sensible heat of liquid chlorine at 290.75 K (17.6°C) can be calculated using Eq. (5.21) and Table 5.3.

$$T_1 = 239.15 \text{ K} \qquad T_2 = 290.75 \text{ K}$$

$$H_1 = \int_{T_1}^{T_2} C_{ml}\, dT$$

$$= -39.246\, (T_2 - T_1) + 1401.223\, \frac{\left(T_2^2 - T_1^2\right)10^{-3}}{2}$$

$$- 6047.226\, \frac{\left(T_2^3 - T_1^3\right)10^{-6}}{3} + 8591.4\, \frac{\left(T_2^4 - T_1^4\right)10^{-9}}{9}$$

$$= -2025.1 + 19\ 448.8 - 21\ 973.8 + 8323.5$$

$$= 3773.4 \text{ kJ/kmol}$$

Let x be the quantity of liquid chlorine which will be flashed per kg of liquid chlorine at 631.3 kPa a.

$$3773.4 = x \times 20\ 662$$

$$x = 0.183 \text{ or } 18.3\% \text{ flashing}$$

Now the sensible heat to be extracted of the fresh chlorine feed

$$H_2 = \int_{T_3}^{T_1} C_{mp}^0\, dT \qquad\qquad \text{(Ref. Table 5.1)}$$

$$T_3 = 313 \text{ K}$$

$$H_2 = 28.5463\, (T_3 - T_1) + 23.8795 \times 10^{-3}\, \frac{\left(T_3^2 - T_1^2\right)}{2}$$

$$- 21.3631 \times 10^{-6}\, \frac{\left(T_3^3 - T_1^3\right)}{3} + 6.4726 \times 10^{-9}\, \frac{\left(T_3^4 - T_1^4\right)}{4}$$

$$= 2108.1 + 486.9 - 121.0 + 10.2$$

$$= 2484.2 \text{ kJ/kmol} \equiv 35.04 \text{ kJ/kg}$$

Heat to be extracted from

$$\text{the incoming fresh feed} = 0.116 \times 35.04 = 4.065 \text{ kW}$$

$$\text{Liquid chlorine evaporated} = \frac{4.065}{291.4} = 0.014 \text{ kg/s}$$

$$\text{Recycled chlorine} = \frac{0.014}{(1 - 0.183)} = 0.017 \text{ kg/s}$$

$$\text{Recycle ratio} = \frac{0.017}{0.116}$$

$$= 0.147 \text{ kg/kg fresh feed} \qquad\qquad Ans.\ (a)$$

Mixed feed, entering 1st stage = 0.116 + 0.017 = 0.133 kg/s

First stage compression:

For adiabatic compression,

$$\frac{T_4}{T_1} = \left(\frac{p_2}{p_1}\right)^{(\gamma-1)/\gamma} \tag{5.40}$$

where γ = ratio of heat capacity at constant pressure to that at constant volume

= 1.355 for chlorine   (Ref. 20)

$p_2 = 326.3$ kPa a

$p_1 = 101$ kPa a

$$T_4 = 239.15 \left(\frac{326.3}{101}\right)^{\frac{(1.355-1)}{1.355}} = 239.15 \, (3.2037)^{0.262}$$

$$= 325.15 \text{ K} \equiv 52°\text{C}$$

$T_5 = 313$ K after intercooler

Enthalpy, removed in the intercooler,

$$H_3 = \frac{0.133}{70.9054} \int_{T_5}^{T_4} (28.5463 + 23.8795 \times 10^{-3}\, T$$

$$- 21.3631 \times 10^{-6}\, T^2 + 6.4726 \times 10^{-9}\, dT$$

$$= 1.876 \times 10^{-3} \, (346.8 + 92.6 - 26.4 + 2.6) = 0.8 \text{ kW}$$

$$\text{Cooling water flow rate} = \frac{0.8}{8 \times 4.1868} = 0.023 \text{ kg/s} \qquad \textit{Ans. (b-i)}$$

2nd stage compression:

$$\frac{T_6}{T_5} = \left(\frac{p_4}{p_3}\right)^{0.262}$$

$p_3 = 316.3$ kPa a after intercooler

$p_4 = 560$ kPa g = 661.3 kPa a

$$T_6 = 313 \left(\frac{661.3}{316.3}\right)^{0.262}$$

$$T_6 = 379.7 \text{ K} \equiv 106.6°\text{C}$$

This gas is cooled top 313 K (40°C) in the aftercooler.

$$H_4 = 1.876 \times 10^{-3} \int_{T_5}^{T_6} C_{mp}^0 \, dT$$

$$= 1.876 \times 10^{-3} \, [28.5463 \, (T_6 - T_5) + 23.8795 \times 10^{-3} \, \frac{\left(T_6^2 - T_5^2\right)}{2}$$

$$- 21.3631 \times 10^{-6} \, \frac{\left(T_6^3 - T_5^3\right)}{3} + 6.4726 \times 10^{-9} \, \frac{\left(T_6^4 - T_5^4\right)}{4}]$$

$$= 1.876 \times 10^{-3} \, (1904.0 + 551.7 - 171.5 + 18.1) = 4.32 \text{ kW}$$

$$\text{Cooling water flow rate} = \frac{4.32}{8 \times 4.1868} = 0.129 \text{ kg/s} \qquad \textit{Ans. (b-ii)}$$

Total cooling water requirement = 0.129 + 0.023 = 0.152 kg/s

The gas at 313 K is to be further cooled to and liquefied at 290.75 K with the help of chilled water.

Heat removal rate (i.e. refrigeration requirement),

$$h_5 = 1.876 \times 10^{-3} \int_{T_2}^{T_5} C_{mp}^0 \, dT + 0.133 \, \lambda_{v2}$$

$$= 1.876 \times 10^{-3} \left[28.5463 \, (T_5 - T_2) + 23.8795 \times 10^{-3} \frac{(T_5^2 - T_2^2)}{2} \right.$$

$$\left. -21.3631 \times 10^{-6} \frac{(T_5^3 - T_2^3)}{3} + 6.4726 \times 10^{-9} \frac{(T_5^4 - T_2^4)}{4} \right]$$

$$+ 0.133 \times 255.8$$

$$= 11.876 \times 10^{-3} [635.2 + 160.4 - 43.3 + 4.0] + 34.02$$

$$= 35.44 \text{ kW} \qquad \textit{Ans. (c)}$$

Note: In this example, the use of various equations outlined in previous sections was demonstrated. It can be seen that empirical equations lead to tedious calculations. Tabular thermodynamic properties (such as Tables 5.6 and 5.7) based on an definite reference temperature are therefore preferred over empirical equations.

Example 5.16 Tin in melted in an open pan using a jacket. The jacket is fed with the vapours of an eutectic mixture of diphenyl-diphenyl oxide at 171 kPa a. Tin is fed to the pan at 303 K (30°C). Calculate the quantity of eutectic mixture of the diphenyl-diphenyl oxide condensed per 100 kg of tin melted at its melting temperature. Assume no subcooling of vapours.

Data for Tin[20]:

$$\text{Molar mass, } M = 118.7$$

$$\text{Melting point} = 505 \text{ K}$$

$$\text{Latent heat of fusion, } \lambda_f = 7201 \text{ kJ/kmol}$$

$$\text{Heat capacity of solid tin, } C_{ms} = 21.14 + 0.02T \text{ kJ/(kmol·K)}$$

where T is in K.

Data on diphenyl-diphenyl oxide are given in Table 5.6.

Solution Basis: 100 kg tin

For melting tin, the temperature of tin must be raised from 303 K to the melting point (505 K). At the melting point, the heat of fusion must be supplied to melt it.

Sensible heat for raising the temperature,

$$Q_1 = n \int_{T_1}^{T_2} C_{ms} \, dT$$

$$n = \frac{100}{118.70} = 0.8425 \text{ kmol}$$

$$T_1 = 303 \text{ K}, \quad T_2 = 505 \text{ K}$$

$$Q_1 = 0.8425 \int_{T_1}^{T_2} (21.14 + 0.02T) \, dT$$

$$= 4972.9 \text{ kJ}$$

Latent heat supply

$$Q_2 = n \times \lambda_f$$

$$= 0.8425 \times 7201 = 6066.8 \text{ kJ}$$

Total heat supply

$$Q = Q_1 + Q_2$$

$$= 4972.9 + 6066.8$$

$$= 11 \, 039.7 \text{ kJ}$$

This amount of heat is supplied by condensation of the diphenyl-diphenyl oxide vapours at 171 kPa. At this pressure, latent heat, $\lambda_v = 278$ kJ/kg. Since no subcooling is allowed, only latent heat transfer takes place.

$$\text{Amount of vapour condensed} = \frac{11 \, 039.7}{278} \approx 39.7 \text{ kg} \qquad \textit{Ans.}$$

Example 5.17 In a chemical plant, the demand of steam keeps fluctuating. To permit steady operation of the boiler, a steam accumulator of volume 45 m³ is used. Water and steam are present at equilibrium in the accumulator at 6 bar g. When the accumulator is in operation, 85% of the tank volume is filled with water, the remaining being steam. The accumulator is well-insulated. During two plant holidays, the accumulator stores the steam and water but does not have the incoming and outgoing steam flows. Under these circumstances, the accumulator loses the heat at the rate of

$$Q = 0.045 \, (T_s - T_a) \text{ kW}$$

where, T_s is the temperature of steam inside the accumulator and T_a is the ambient temperature in K.

If the average ambient temperature is 300 K (27 °C), calculate the time in hours by which the pressure of steam and will be 5 bar g inside the accumulator.

Solution This illustration is a case of an unsteady-state process, because the rate of heat loss depends on the temperature of the steam inside the accumulator. As soon as some heat is lost, the vapour-liquid equilibrium in the accumulator changes and the pressure is reduced. Correspondingly, the saturation temperature of steam also varies. This in turn reduces the heat loss. Such a problem can be solved by numerical integration. For illustration, four different temperatures/pressures are taken. The properties of steam at these four pressures (see Appendix III.2) are given in Table 5.12.

Table 5.12 Properties of Steam

| Pressure | Saturation temperature | Density, kg/m³ | | Enthalpy, kJ/kg | | |
| | | Liquid | Steam | Sensible | Latent | Total |
kPa a	K	ρ_L	ρ_G	h	λ_v	H
701.3	438.2	902.30	3.674	697.38	2064.7	2762.1
666.7	436.0	904.31	3.502	688.53	2071.4	2759.9
634.0	434.0	906.28	3.339	679.82	2078.0	2757.8
601.3	432.1	908.30	3.176	670.78	2084.7	2755.5

I.   At 6 bar g (i.e. 701.3 kPa a), the volume occupied by the water is 85%.

Volume of water in the accumulator $= 0.85 \times 45 = 38.25 \text{ m}^3$

Volume occupied by steam in the accumulator $= 0.15 \times 45 = 6.75 \text{ m}^3$

Total weight of both the fluids in the accumulator $= 38.25 \times 902.30 + 6.75$
$$\times\ 3.674$$

$$= 34\ 512.975 \text{ kg water} + 24.8 \text{ kg steam}$$
$$= 34\ 537.775 \text{ kg}$$

Total thermal energy accumulated in the accumulator,
$$H_1 = 34\ 512.975 \times 697.38 + 24.800 \times 2762.1$$
$$= 24\ 137\ 159 \text{ kJ over } 273.16 \text{ K}$$

II.   Now, when the temperature of steam water mixture drops to 436 K, the proportions of steam and water in the accumulator will change. Let x be amount of steam present in the accumulator at 436 K. Since total mass is constant,

Water in the accumulator $= (34\ 537.775 - x_1) \text{ kg}$

However, the total volume occupied by both the fluids remains unchanged, i.e., 45 m³.

$$\frac{x_1}{3.502} + \frac{(34\ 537.775 - x_1)}{904.31} = 45 \quad \text{or} \quad x_1 = 23.93 \text{ kg steam}$$

Quantity of water $= 34\ 537.775 - 23.93$
$$= 34\ 513.85 \text{ kg}$$

Total enthalpy at $H_2 = 34\ 513.85 \times 688.53 + 23.93 \times 2759.9$
$$= 23\ 829\ 866 \text{ kJ}$$

Loss in enthalpy between 438.2 K and 436 K, $H_1 - H_2 = 307\ 293 \text{ kJ}$

III.   Temperature of fluids in the accumulator = 434 K

$$\frac{x_2}{3.339} + \frac{(34\ 537.775 - x_2)}{906.28} = 45 \quad \text{or} \quad x_2 = 23.09 \text{ kg steam}$$

Quantity of water $= 34\ 514.685 \text{ kg}$

Total enthalpy at $H_3 = 34\ 514.685 \times 679.82 + 23.09 \times 2757.8$
$$= 23\ 527\ 451 \text{ kJ}$$

Loss in enthalpy between 436 K and 434 K, $H_2 - H_3 = 302\ 415 \text{ kJ}$

IV.   Temperature of fluids in the accumulator = 432.1 K

$$\frac{x_3}{3.176} + \frac{(34\ 537.775 - x_3)}{908.30} = 45 \quad \text{or} \quad x_3 = 22.23 \text{ kg steam}$$

Quantity of water = 34 515.545 kg

Total enthalpy at H_4 = 34 515.545 × 670.78

+ 22.23 × 2755.5

= 23 213 592 kJ

Change in enthalpy $H_3 - H_4$ = 313 859 kJ

Temperature fall calculations:

I.   Average steam temperature in the range 438.2 K and 436 K,

$$T_{s1} = \frac{(438.2 + 436)}{2} = 437.1 \text{ K}$$

$$T_a = 300 \text{ K}$$

$$Q_1 = 0.045 (437.1 - 300) = 6.1695 \text{ kW}$$

$$\equiv 22\ 210.2 \text{ kJ/h}$$

$$\text{Time } \theta_1 = \frac{307\,293}{22\,210.2}$$

$$= 13.836 \text{ h}$$

II. $$T_{s2} = \frac{(436 + 434)}{2} = 435 \text{ K}$$

$$Q_2 = 0.045 (435 - 300)$$

$$= 6.075 \text{ kW} \equiv 21\ 870 \text{ kJ/h}$$

$$\text{Time } \theta_2 = \frac{302\,415}{21\,870} = 13.828 \text{ h}$$

III. $$T_{s3} = \frac{(434 + 432.1)}{2} = 433.05 \text{ K}$$

$$Q_3 = 0.045 (433.05 - 300)$$

$$= 5.987\ 254 \text{ kW} \equiv 21\ 554.1 \text{ kJ/h}$$

$$\text{Time } \theta_3 = \frac{313\,859}{21\,554.1}$$

$$= 14.561 \text{ h}$$

Total time $\theta = \Sigma\ \theta_i$

$$= 13.836 + 13.828 + 14.561 = 42.225 \text{ h } Ans.$$

Without numerical integration, the problem can be solved as follows:

Total enthalpy change between 438.2 K and 432.1 K, $H_1 - H_4$ = 923 567 kJ

Average temperature of fluids in the accumulator = $\dfrac{(438.2 + 432.1)}{2} = 435.15$ K

$$Q = 0.045 (435.15 - 300) = 6.081\ 75 \text{ kW} \equiv 21\ 894.3 \text{ kJ/h}$$

$$\text{Time } \theta = \frac{923\ 567}{21\ 894.3} = 42.183 \text{ h} \qquad\qquad Ans.$$

Example 5.18 High pressure carbon dioxide, available in the urea plant of a fertilizer factory, is used to manufacture dry ice. Pure carbon dioxide is available at 20 MPa a and 430 K (130°C). It is cooled in a cooler with the help of cooling water to 313 K (40°C). Cooled gas is throttled to 3.9 MPa a as a result of which a part of the carbon dioxide is liquefied. The mixture of gas and liquid is taken to a carbon dioxide liquefier which utilises ammonia refrigerant at 268 K (– 5°C). Liquefied carbon dioxide exchanges heat with revert gas and the latter is vented at 273 K (0°C). Subcooled liquid is throttled to atmospheric pressure in the snow tower to produce dry ice. Sublimed carbon dioxide gas is reverted through the exchanger and vented to the atmosphere. Figure 5.10 depicts the process schematically. Calculate (a) yield of dry ice, based on carbon dioxide fed to the water cooler, (b) per cent liquefaction, achieved by throtting cooled gas (at 313 K) to 3.9 MPa a, assuming pressure drop in the water cooler to be negligible and (c) temperature of gas being vented to the atmosphere.

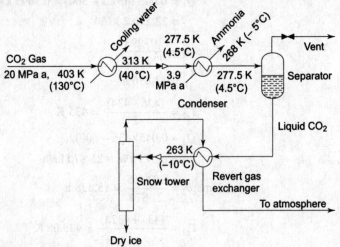

Fig. 5.10   Manufacture of Dry Ice

Solution   Basis: 100 kg/h feed gas at 20 MPa a and 430 K (130°C).

Since the pressure is quite high, the data given in Table 5.1 can lead to grossly erroneous results. Therefore real heat capacity data are required. At 20 MPa a, the heat capacity data are as follows:

Table 5.13   Real Heat Capacity Data for CO_2[33]

Pressure, MPa a	Heat capacity, kJ/(kg·K)		
	Temperature K (°C)		
	403 (1300)	313 (40)	277.6 (4.5)
20	2.060	2.244	1.938
3.9	1.072	1.252	–

Average heat capacity at 20 MPa a in the range 313 to 403 K = $\dfrac{(2.060 + 2.244)}{2}$

$$= 2.152 \text{ kJ/(kg·K)}$$

Heat removed in water cooler, $\phi_1 = 100 \times 2.152\,(403 - 313)$

$$= 19\,368 \text{ kJ/h} \equiv 5.38 \text{ kW}$$

If data contained in Table 5.1 (Ref. 2) are used;

$$T_1 = 313 \text{ K}$$

$$T_2 = 403 \text{ K}$$

$$Q_1 = 21.3655\,(T_2 - T_1) + 64.2841 \times 10^{-3}\,\frac{(T_2^2 - T_1^3)}{2}$$

$$- 41.0506 \times 10^{-6}\,\frac{(T_2^3 - T_1^3)}{3} + 9.7999 \times 10^{-9}\,\frac{(T_2^4 - T_1^4)}{4}$$

$$= 1922.9 + 2071.2 - 476.0 + 41.1 = 3559.2 \text{ kJ/kmol}$$

$$\phi_1 = \frac{(3559.2 \times 100)}{44}$$

$$= 8089.1 \text{ kJ/h} \equiv 2.25 \text{ kW}$$

It can be seen that a gross error will be introduced in the design of the cooler if data of Table 5.1 are used.

When the gas is throttled from 20 MPa a and 313 K (40°C) to 3.9 MPa a, cooling/liquefaction will take place due to the Joule-Thompson effect. At first, saturation temperature and latent heat of vaporization of carbon dioxide, corresponding to 3.9 MPa a are required to be found. Using data of Table 5.4 and 5.5:

$$T_s = 277.6 \text{ K (4.5°C)} \hspace{2cm} \text{(Ref. 20)}$$

Using Watson equation $\lambda_v = 221.3 \text{ kJ/kg}$

Let x be the amount of liquefied gas (in kg/h).

$$\text{Uncondensed gas} = (100 - x) \text{ kg/h}$$

Assume the base temperature as 277.6 K (4.6°C).
Average heat capacity of gas at 20 MPa a

$$\text{between 313 K and 277.6 K} = \frac{(2.244 \times 1.938)}{2} = 2.901 \text{ kJ/(kg·K)}$$

Sensible heat of gas at 313 K over 277.6 K = 100 (313 - 277.6) 2.091

$$= 7402.1 \text{ kJ/h} \equiv 2.056 \text{ kW}$$

Sensible heat of saturated liquid CO_2 at 277.6 K = 0

Total enthalpy of saturated vapour CO_2 at 277.6 K = 221.3 kJ/kg

$$221.3\,(100 - x) = 7402.1$$

$$x = 66.55 \text{ kg}$$

$$\text{Liquefaction due to throttling} = 66.6\% \hspace{1cm} \textit{Ans.} \text{ (b)}$$

The balance liquefaction is achieved in CO_2 liquefier. Liquid CO_2 at 277.6 K (4.6°C) leaves the liquefier and enters the revert gas exchanger. It leaves the exchanger at 263 K (- 10°C). Use data contained in Table 5.3 (Ref. 11).

$$\phi_2 = \left[3555.4 \,(T_3 - T_2) + 46\,902.2 \times 10^{-3} \,\frac{\left(T_3^2 - T_2^2\right)}{2} \right.$$
$$\left. -\, 201\,812 \times 10^{-6} \,\frac{\left(T_3^3 - T_2^3\right)}{3} + 289\,832 \times 10^{-9} \,\frac{\left(T_3^4 - T_2^4\right)}{4} \right] \frac{100}{44}$$

$$T_3 = 277.6 \text{ K}$$
$$T_2 = 263 \text{ K}$$
$$\phi_2 = 1487 \times 2.2727 = 3379.5 \text{ kJ/h} \equiv 0.94 \text{ kW}$$

Liquid CO_2 is throttled to atmospheric pressure at 194.75 K (– 78.4°C). Let y be the amount of dry ice formed (in kg/h) for 100 kg/h saturated liquid to be expanded to atmospheric pressure.

$$\text{Sublimed vapours} = (100 - y) \text{ kg}$$

Heat of sublimation[20] at 194.75 K = 573.8 kJ/kg

Heat of fusion[20] at 215.65 K = 180.8 kJ/kg

Assuming that heat of fusion at 194.75 K is the same as that at 215.65 K,

Latent heat of vaporization at 194.75 K = 573.8 – 180.8

$$= 393 \text{ kJ/kg}$$

Based on Table 5.3, the heat capacity of liquid CO_2 in the range 263 K to 194.75 K is 2.093 kJ/(kg·K).

Take the base temperature as 263 K (– 10°C).

Enthalpy of liquid CO_2 at 263 K = 0 kJ/kg

Enthalpy of dry ice at 194.75 K = $y \times 2.093$ (194.75 – 263) – $y \times 180.8$

$$= -\,323.6 \, y \text{ kJ/h}$$

Enthalpy of CO_2 vapours at 194.75 K = (100 – y) 2.093 [194.75 – 263]

$$+ (100 - y) \, 393 = 250.2 \,(100 - y) \text{ kJ/h}$$

Enthalpy of inlet liquid = enthalpy of gas + enthalpy of solid CO_2

$$0 = -\,323.6 \, y + 250.2 \,(100 - y)$$

$$y = 43.6 \text{ kg/100 kg of inlet liquid } CO_2$$

$$\text{Yield} = 43.6\% \hspace{3cm} \textit{Ans. (a)}$$

Heat picked up by reverted gas = 3379.5 kJ/h = 0.94 kW

Reverted gas = 53.4 kg/h

Temperature of gas entering

the exchanger T_4 = 194.75 K

If T_5 is the temperature of the gas leaving the exchanger,

$$3379.5 = \left(\frac{56.0}{44}\right) \left[30.6643 \,(T_5 - T_4) - 48.3885 \times 10^{-3} \,\frac{\left(T_5^2 - T_4^2\right)}{2} \right.$$
$$\left. +\, 382.5044 \times 10^{-6} \,\frac{\left(T_5^3 - T_4^3\right)}{3} - 492.6398 \times 10^{-9} \,\frac{\left(T_5^4 - T_4^4\right)}{4} \right]$$

The equation can be solved by trial-and-error method (or by Mathcad).

$$T_5 = 273.6 \text{ K} \quad \text{i.e. } 0.6°C \hspace{3cm} \textit{Ans. (c)}$$

The above example can be easily solved by the pressure-enthalpy (p-H) diagram of CO_2. Refer Fig. 5.11[34]. A point representing 3.9 MPa a and 263 K (– 10°C) is located on it. The constant enthalpy path (i.e. vertical line) is followed till the horizontal line representing 101.3 kPa a is crossed. This clearly gives 0.56 mass fraction of gaseous CO_2. In other words, dry ice formation is 0.44 kg/kg of liquid CO_2. This agrees well with the calculated yield of 0.436 kg/kg. Diagrams are thus very useful in finding final conditions under various operating conditions, such as adiabatic letdown, constant enthalpy letdown, etc.

Example 5.19 A sulphur burner in a sulphite pump mill burns 200 kg of pure sulphur per hour[35]. The gases leave the burner at 1144 K (871°C) and are cooled before being sent to an absorption tower. As a primary cooler, a waste heat boiler is employed for producing saturated steam at 15 bar a. The temperature of the feed water to the boiler is 15 K lower than that of saturated steam at 15 bar a and the temperature of the gas mixture leaving the boiler is 463 K(190°C). Assume 10% excess air, complete combustion, no heat loss to the surroundings and no SO_3 formation. Calculate the amount of steam produced.

Solution Basis: 200 kg/h sulphur firing

$$\text{Molar feed rate of sulphur} = \frac{200}{32} = 6.25 \text{ kmol/h}$$

The reaction is:

$$S + O_2 = SO_2$$

$$\text{Theoretical oxygen required} = 6.25 \text{ kmol/h}$$

$$\text{Actual oxygen supplied} = 6.25 \times 1.1 = 6.875 \text{ kmol/h}$$

$$\text{Air supply to the burner} = \frac{6.875}{0.21} = 32.738 \text{ kmol/h}$$

$$N_2 \text{ entering the burner with air} = 32.738 - 6.875 = 25.863 \text{ kmol/h}$$

$$SO_2 \text{ formed} = 6.25 \text{ kmol/h}$$

The burner effluent gases will contain 6.25 kmol/h SO_2, 0.625 kmol/h O_2 and 25.863 kmol/h N_2.

$$T_1 = 1144 \text{ K} \quad \text{and} \quad T_2 = 463 \text{ K}$$

Assume base temperature to be 298 K.

$$\Sigma\, C^0_{mpi} = [6.25 \times 24.7706 + 0.625 \times 26.0257 + 25.863 \times 29.5909]$$

$$+ [6.25 \times 62.9481 + 0.625 \times 11.7551 - 25.853 \times 5.141]10^{-3}\, T$$

$$+ [- 44.2585 \times 6.25 - 0.625 \times 2.3426 + 25.863 \times 13.1829]10^{-6}\, T^2$$

$$+ [6.25 \times 11.122 - 0.625 \times 0.5623 - 25.863 \times 4.968]10^{-9}\, T^3$$

$$= 930.3919 + 267.8108 \times 10^{-3}\, T + 62.8714 \times 10^{-6}\, T^2 - 59.3263 \times 10^{-9}\, T^3$$

Enthalpy removed in the WHB, $\phi = \displaystyle\int_{T_2}^{T_1} (\Sigma n_i . C^0_{mpi})\, dT$

$$= 788\ 799.2 \text{ kJ/h} \equiv 219.11 \text{ kW}$$

Enthalpy to be supplied for

steam generation = sensible heat for raising temperature of 15 K

+ latent heat of vaporization at 15 bar

$$H = 15 \times 4.1868 + 1945.2 = 2008 \text{ kJ/kg}$$

Amount of steam generated, $q_m = \phi/H$

$$= \frac{788\,799.2}{2008}$$

$$= 392.8 \text{ kg/h} \qquad\qquad Ans.$$

Example 5.20 Calculate (a) enthalpy of equimolar liquid mixture of n-pentane and n-hexane and (b) enthalpy of equimolar vapour mixture of the same components at 101.325 kPa.

Solution Bubble point and dew point of the equimolar liquid and vapour mixture are calculated (in Example 5.12) to be 321.6 K (48.6°C) and 330.0 K (57°C) respectively.

Enthalpy of liquid mixture at T_{BB}:

Assume a reference temperature (T_0) as 298.15 K (25°C). Table 5.3 give constants of the polynomial equation for liquid heat capacities.

Enthalpy of n-pentane at T_{BB}, $H_1 = 65.4961 \, (321.6 - 298.15)$

$$+ 628.628 \times 10^{-3} \frac{\left(321.6^2 - 298.15^2\right)}{2}$$

$$- 1898.8 \times 10^{-6} \frac{\left(321.6^3 - 298.15^3\right)}{3}$$

$$+ 3186.51 \times 10^{-9} \frac{\left(321.6^4 - 298.15^4\right)}{4}$$

$$= 4078.1 \text{ kJ/kmol}$$

Enthalpy of n-hexane at T_{BB}, $H_2 = 31.421 \, (321.6 - 298.15)$

$$+ 976.058 \times 10^{-3} \frac{\left(321.6^2 - 298.15^2\right)}{2}$$

$$- 2353.68 \times 10^{-6} \frac{\left(321.6^3 - 298.15^3\right)}{3}$$

$$+ 3092.73 \times 10^{-9} \frac{\left(321.6^4 - 298.15^4\right)}{4}$$

$$= 4717.4 \text{ kJ/kmol}$$

$$H_{sol} = 0.5 \, H_1 + 0.5 \, H_2$$

$$= 0.5 \times 4078.1 + 0.5 \times 4717.4$$

$$= 4397.8 \text{ kJ/kmol} \qquad\qquad Ans.\ (a)$$

Enthalpy of vapour mixture at T_{DP}

Pure component enthalpy in vapour state comprises sensible enthalpy of liquid from T_0 to T_{DP} and latent heat of vaporization at T_{DP}. For evaluation of the latent heat, Watson equation (Eq. 5.26) can be used.

Latent heat of vaporisation of n-pentane,

$$\lambda_{v_1} \text{ at } T_{DP} = 25\,773 \left(\frac{469.7 - 330}{469.7 - 309.2}\right)^{0.38}$$

$$= 24\,448.9 \text{ kJ/kmol}$$

Latent heat of vaporisation of *n*-hexane,

$$\lambda_{v_2} \text{ at } T_{DP} = 28\,853 \left(\frac{507.5 - 330}{507.5 - 341.9} \right)^{0.38}$$

$$= 29\,624.0 \text{ kJ/kmol}$$

Enthalpy of *n*-pentane vapour at T_{DP}

$$H_1^{ig} = \int_{T_0}^{T_{DP}} C_{l1}\, dT + \lambda_{v_1}$$

$$= 65.4961\,(330 - 298.15)$$

$$+ 628.628 \times 10^{-3} \left(\frac{330^2 - 298.15^2}{2} \right)$$

$$- 1898.8 \times 10^{-6} \left(\frac{330^3 - 298.15^3}{3} \right)$$

$$+ 3186.51 \times 10^{-9} \frac{\left(330^4 - 298.15^4 \right)}{4} + 24\,448.9$$

$$= 5581.3 + 24\,448.9 = 30\,030.2 \text{ kJ/kmol}$$

Enthalpy of *n*-hexane vapour at T_{DP}

$$H_2^{ig} = \int_{T_0}^{T_{DP}} C_{l2}\, dT + \lambda_{v_2}$$

$$= 31.421\,(330 - 298.15)$$

$$+ 976.058 \times 10^{-3} \frac{\left(330^2 - 298.15^2 \right)}{2}$$

$$- 2353.68 \times 10^{-6} \frac{\left(330^3 - 298.15^3 \right)}{3}$$

$$+ 3092.73 \times 10^{-9} \frac{\left(330^4 - 298.15^4 \right)}{4} + 29\,624.0$$

$$= 6452.4 + 29\,624.0 = 36\,076.4 \text{ kJ/kmol}$$

$$H_{mix}^{ig} = 0.5 \times H_1^{ig} + 0.5 \times H_2^{ig}$$

$$= 0.5 \times 30\,032.2 + 0.5 \times 36\,076.4$$

$$= 33\,053.3 \text{ kJ/kmol} \hspace{2cm} \textit{Ans. (b)}$$

5.11 EQUILIBRIUM FLASH CALCULATION OF A MULTICOMPONENT SYSTEM

A single component system as well as a binary system were discussed in Sec. 5.10. Calculations of a multicomponent system are quite complex. The amount of each of the several components in the liquid and vapour states in equilibrium are required to be calculated. The cryogenic separation of gases involve such calculations. The separation of hydrogen, helium, argon, etc. are classical examples of the cryogenic process. The liquefaction of natural gas, partial condensation of vapours, depressurisation of a liquid below its vapour pressure, etc. are other operations in which equilibrium flash calculations are involved. Normally these calculations are done by trial and error. Basic formulae are derived from the material balance and vapour-liquid equilibrium relationships and follow the guidelines given in Sec. 5.10. An important source of vapour-liquid equilibrium data for the hydrocarbons is the Engineering Data Book[36] published by the Gas Processors Suppliers Association. References 2 and 37 may also be referred for the vapour-liquid equilibrium calculations.

For 1 kmol of the total fluid (vapour + liquid),

Let

N_i = kmol of the ith component in the total fluid

V = kmol of vapours

L = kmol of liquid

x_i = mole fraction of the ith component in the liquid

y_i = mole fraction of the ith component in the vapour

L_i = kmol of the ith component in the liquid

V_i = kmol of the ith component in the vapour

K_i = equilibrium constant

$$= y_i/x_i \quad \text{by definition} \tag{5.41}$$

$$N_i = L_i + V_i \tag{5.42}$$

$$= Lx_i + Vy_i$$

$$= Lx_i + VK_ix_i$$

$$= x_i (L + VK_i) \tag{5.43}$$

$$x_i = L_i/L \tag{5.44}$$

$$N_i = \frac{L_i}{L} (L + VK_i) \tag{5.45}$$

$$L_i = \frac{LN_i}{(VK_i + L)} \tag{5.46}$$

$$= \frac{N_i}{\left(\dfrac{V}{L} K_i + 1\right)} \tag{5.47}$$

$$L_i = \frac{N_i}{\left(\dfrac{1-L}{L} K_i + 1\right)} \tag{5.48}$$

Trial-and-error methods differ slightly in format and presentation. A commonly-employed approach is to assume L. Since N_i is known from feed data, L_i can be calculated for each of the components. ΣL_i is compared with the assumed value of L. Iterations are repeated till the assumed L and calculated $L(= \Sigma L_i)$ are in agreement. For ideal fluids, according to Dalton's law,

$$\bar{p}_i = y_i\, p \qquad (5.49)$$

and according to Raoult's law

$$\bar{p}_i = x_i\, p_i \qquad (5.50)$$

where
$\bar{p}_i$ = partial pressure of the ith component

p = total pressure

p_i = vapour pressure of the ith component

Thus, for an ideal fluid,

$$K_i = \frac{y_i}{x_i} = \frac{p_i}{p} = \frac{\text{Vapour pressure of the } i\text{th component}}{\text{total pressure}} \qquad (5.51)$$

Example 5.21 A mixture[38] containing 45.1% propane, 18.3% *iso*-butane and 36.6% *n*-butane (on mole basis) is flashed at 366 K (93°C) and 24 bar a. At these conditions, the respective K values are 1.42, 0.86 and 0.72. Calculate the liquid fractions after flashing.

Solution Basis: 1 kmol of the mixture

Table 5.14 Flashing of Propane-Butane Mixture

Comp-onent	N_i kmol	K_i	Values of L_i for trial values of L				Mole % in liquid fraction
			$L = 0.8$ kmol	0.6 kmol	0.5 kmol	0.4 kmol	
C_3H_8	0.451	1.42	0.3328	0.2317	0.1864	0.1441	36
iso-C_4H_{10}	0.183	0.86	0.1506	0.1163	0.0984	0.0799	20
n-C_4H_{10}	0.366	0.72	0.3102	0.2476	0.2128	0.1760	44
Total	1.000		0.7936	0.5956	0.4796	0.4000	100

Sample calculations for C_3H_8: For $L = 0.8$

$$\left(\frac{1-L}{L}\right) K_i + 1 = \left(\frac{1-0.8}{0.8}\right) 1.42 + 1 = 1.355$$

$$L_i = \frac{0.451}{1.355} = 0.3328$$

Liquid fraction will contain 36% C_3H_8, 20% *iso*-C_4H_{10} and 44% *n*-C_4H_{10} (on mole basis).

Ans.

Example 5.22 A basic flow sheet of the conventional process for cryogenic gas separation from the oil refinery off gas is given in Fig. 5.12. Feed gas contains a number of acid gases, including carbon dioxide and hydrogen sulphide. These impurities are removed by chemical wash process. After the removal of a bulk of the impurities, trace constituents and water are completely eliminated and dried by adsorption. The final cleaned-up feed gas containing 60% H_2, 20% CH_4 and 20%

C_2H_6 (on mole basis) enters the cold box where it is cooled and condensed in two plate-and-fin type brazed aluminium exchangers. The major portion of the hydrocarbons is liquefied at 147.5 K (– 125.5°C) in the first heat exchanger and collected in the first separator. The condensate from the first separator is then throttled to 4.5 bar a and evaporated and reverted through the first exchanger.

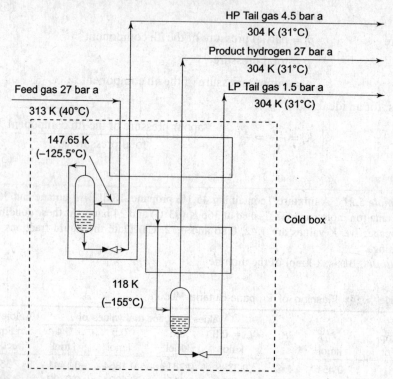

Fig. 5.12 Hydrogen Recovery from Refinery Off Gases

The gas leaving the first separator is further cooled in the second separator to 118 K (– 155°C). This low temperature makes it necessary that the condensate is throttled to low pressure, say 1.5 bar a. This mixture is evaporated and reverted through both the heat exchangers while the incoming feed gas is cooled and partially liquefied. Feed gas enters at 27 bar a and at 313 K (40°C) at the rate of 12 000 Nm³/h and product hydrogen (at ~ 27 bar a) and tail gas streams (at 4.5 bar a and 1.5 bar a) leave the cold box at 304 K (31.°C). Calculate the recovery and purity of hydrogen stream.

Use the following data:

Solution Basis: Feed gas = 12 000 Nm³/h = 535.4 kmol/h

First gas separator: incoming feed gas is cooled to 147.65 K (– 125.5°C) in the first heat exchanger by exchanging heat with reverted gases and sent to the first gas separator.

$$T = 147.65 \text{ K}$$

Calculate K_i using data given in Table 5.15.

Table 5.15 Equilibrium Constants[39] (K) at 27 bar a

Equation: $\log_{10} K = A/T + B$, where T = temperature in K

Component	A	B	Temperature range, K
Methane	− 378.9	2.1686	110-200
	− 302.2	1.5134	100-110
	− 214.5	0.638	90-100
Ethane	− 756.0	2.83	157-200
	− 752.0	2.75	90-157
Hydrogen	120.5	0.611	90-200
Nitrogen	− 257.0	2.379	110-200
	− 242.5	2.241	90-110

Table 5.16 Flashing in First Gas Separator

Gas	K_i	N_i kmol	$L_1 =$ 0.5	$L_2 =$ 0.3636	$L_3 =$ 0.3285	$L_4 =$ 0.3190	$L_5 =$ 0.3163	V_i kmol	Mole fraction in vapour
H_2	26.8	0.6	0.0216	0.0125	0.0108	0.0103	0.0102	0.5898	0.8617
CH_4	0.4	0.2	0.1429	0.1176	0.1100	0.1079	0.1073	0.0927	0.1355
C_2H_4	0.0045	0.2	0.1991	0.1984	0.1982	0.1981	0.1981	0.0019	0.0028
Total		1.0	0.3636	0.3285	0.3190	0.3163	0.3156	0.6844	1.0000

Values of L_i for trial values of L

Table 5.17 HP Tail Gas Stream

HP Tail gas stream (liquid from first gas separator)

Gas	kmol/h	Nm^3/h	Vol. %
H_2	5.46	122.4	3.23
CH_4	57.45	1287.7	34.00
C_2H_4	106.06	1377.2	62.77
Total	168.97	3787.3	100.00

Second gas separator: Vapours (366.43 kmol/h) under pressure from the first gas separator are taken to the second gas exchanger, cooled to 118 K (− 155°C) and sent to the second gas separator.

$$T = 118 \text{ K}$$

Calculate K_i using data given in Table 5.15.

Table 5.18 Flashing In Second Gas Separator

Gas	K_i	N_i kmol	$L_1 =$ 0.1	$L_2 =$ 0.0798	$L_3 =$ 0.0709	$L_4 =$ 0.06	V_i kmol
H_2	42.9	0.8617	0.0022	0.0017	0.0015	0.0013	0.8606
CH_4	0.09	0.1355	0.0748	0.0664	0.0621	0.0561	0.0792
C_2H_4	2.38×10^{-4}	0.0028	0.0028	0.0028	0.0028	0.0028	0
Total		1.0000	0.0798	0.0709	0.0664	0.0602	0.9398

Values of L_i for trial values of L

Table 5.19 Product Hydrogen and LP Tail Gas Streams

Gas	Product hydrogen stream			LP tail gas stream		
	kmol/h	Nm^3/h	mole %	kmol/h	Nm^3/h	mole %
H$_2$	315.35	7068.3	91.58	0.48	10.8	2.17
CH$_4$	29.01	650.2	8.42	20.56	460.8	93.16
C$_2$H$_6$	0	0	0	1.03	23.1	4.67
Total	344.36	7718.5	100.00	22.07	494.7	100.00

Ans.

Example 5.23 Chlorination of benzene is carried out in a single stage co-current continuous reactor. The reaction pressure and temperature are kept at 150 kPa a and 328 K (55°C). The reactions taking place in the reactor are:

Benzene   Chlorine   MCB   Hydrochloric acid

MCB   Chlorine   1,4-DCB   Hydrochloric acid

The reactor is supplied with chlorine at the rate of 0.4 kmol Cl$_2$ per kmol benzene. Conversion of benzene in the reactor is 37% while yield of monochlorobenzene (MCB) is 91.89%. Liquid product coming out of the reactor is in equilibrium with the gas mixture leaving the reactor. Establish the material balance.

Solution Basis: 100 kmol/h of benzene feed rate

$$Cl_2 \text{ feed rate} = 0.4 \times 100 = 40 \text{ kmol/h}$$

From the reactions, it is clear that 1 kmol of chlorine produces 1 kmol of HCl,

$$\text{HCl production rate} = 40 \text{ kmol/h}$$

$$\text{Benzene consumed} = 37 \text{ kmol/h}$$

$$\text{MCB production rate} = 100 \times 0.37 \times 0.9189 = 34 \text{ kmol/h}$$

$$\text{1,4-DCB production rate} = 37 - 34 = 3 \text{ kmol/h}$$

$$\text{Unreacted benzene} = 100 - 37 = 63 \text{ kmol/h}$$

Overall material balance:

If L is the liquid product rate (kmol/h) and V is the vapour flow rate (kmol/h),

$$N_t = L + V = 40 + 34 + 3 + 63 = 140 \text{ kmol/h}$$

Vapours, leaving the reactor, will have hydrogen chloride gas (1), benzene (2), MCB (3) and 1,4-DCB (4). Let y be the mole fraction of each component in gaseous mixture and x be the mole fraction of each component in the liquid product. Assume ideal behaviour of gas and liquid mixtures.

$$y_i = \frac{p_i}{p_t}\, x_i = K_i x_i$$

$$x_i = \frac{N_i}{L + VK}$$

$$= \frac{N_i}{L + (N_t - L)\cdot K_i}$$

$$= \frac{N_i}{L(1 - K_i) + N_t K_i}$$

$$\Sigma\, x_i = 1$$

Since the vapour pressure of hydrogen chloride is very high at 328 K, K_i for HCl will be so high that x_i may be taken as nil. Use Antoine constant from Table 5.4 for calculation of vapour pressures of other components. At 140 kPa and 328 K (55°C), $K_2 = 0.2892$, $p_2 = 43.386$ kPa, $K_3 = 0.0472$, $p_3 = 7.084$ kPa, $K_4 = 0.0093$, and $p_3 = 1.394$ kPa.

Assume a value of L. Calculate x_2 to x_4. Sum of mole fractions in liquid state should be equal to one. If not unity, iterate L.

$$\frac{63}{(1-0.2892)L + 140 \times 0.2892} + \frac{34}{(1-0.0472)L + 140 \times 0.0472}$$

$$+ \frac{3}{(1-0.0093)L + 140 \times 0.0093} = 1$$

$$\frac{63}{0.7108L + 40.488} + \frac{34}{0.9528L + 6.608} + \frac{3}{0.9907L + 1.302} = 1$$

By trail-and-error or by Mathcad,

$$L = 90.53 \text{ kmol/h}$$

$$V = 140 - 90.5 = 49.47 \text{ kmol/h}$$

Table 5.20 Composition of Liquid and Vapour Mixtures

Component	Product mixture N_i kmol/h	Vapour, V kmol/h	mol %	Liquid, L kmol/h	mol %
Benzene	63.0	8.600	17.38	54.400	60.09
MCB	34.0	0.855	1.73	33.145	36.61
1,4-DCB	3.0	0.015	0.03	2.985	3.30
HCl	40.0	40.000	80.86	–	–
Total	140.0	49.470	100.00	90.530	100.00

Ans.

5.12 ENTHALPY CHANGES ACCOMPANYING CHEMICAL REACTIONS

In Secs .5.1 to 5.11 the enthalpy changes of physical processes were considered. However, when chemical reactions take place, either heat is absorbed or evolved.

Three types of reactions are of interest, viz. combustion, formation and the reaction of one or more substances to form other compounds. In Chapter 7 the combustion of fuels will be described in detail. In this Chapter, the discussion will be restricted to the heat of formation and heat of reaction.

5.12.1 Standard Heat of Formation and Standard Heat of Combustion

Heat of formation is defind as the isothermal enthalpy change in a synthesis reaction from the elements in their standard states. This enthalpy change can be exothermic (i.e. evolution of enthalpy) or can be endothermic (i.e. absorption of enthalpy). Take a look at the synthesis reaction:

$$N_2 + 3\,H_2 \rightarrow 2\,NH_3$$

In this reaction, elements react to form ammonia and therefore it is a representation of a formation reaction.

Consider another reaction in which phosphorous pentoxide is dissolved in water to produce phosphoric acid.

$$P_4O_{10} + 6\,H_2O \rightarrow 4\,H_3PO_4$$

This is not the formation reaction for the purpose of calculation of enthalpy of formation.

In reality only a few formation reactions can be actually carried out (e.g. ammonia synthesis) and therefore the enthalpy of formation is usually determined indirectly. Combustion reaction easily lends itself to experimental investigation and the methods are well known for evaluation of heat of combustion.

Data on heat of combustion can be conveniently utilised for the calculation of heat of formation. Due to this reason, often heat of formation and heat of combustion data are tabulated side-by-side.

For tabulating the data, *standard states* need to be defined. Following standard states represent a normal choice.

Phase	Reference standard state
Solid	Pure crystalline at 298.15 K (25°C)
Liquid	Pure at 298.15 K (25°C) and 1 bar a
Gas	Pure at 298.15 K (25°C) and 1 bar a

In Appendix IV, standard heat of formation (ΔH_f°) and standard heat of combustion (ΔH_c°) are tabulated. Units employed are kJ/mol which can be easily converted to other units like kJ/kg, kJ/L etc. Most data are extracted from the thermodynamic tables, published by the Thermodynamics Research Centre, USA and the NBS Tables of Chemical Thermodynamics Properties, published by the National Institute of Standards and Technology, USA. These are considered very reliable data. Although the tabulated data correspond to 298.15 K (25°C), data are reported in literature corresponding to 0 K (– 273.15°C), 273.15 K (0°C) and 291.15 (18°C).

Data on ΔH_f^0 are useful in evaluating the heat of reaction as will be discussed in Sec. 5.14. More discussion on ΔH_c^0 is given in Chapter 7 (Ref. Sec. 7.3).

Example 5.24 Calculate the heat of formation of ethylene gas at 298.15 K (25°C) using the heat of combustion data.

Solution The values of heats of combustion of carbon, hydrogen and ethylene are listed in Appendix IV.

The combustion reaction are

$$2\,C_{(g)} + 2\,O_{2(g)} = 2\,CO_{2(g)} \tag{A}$$

$$2\,H_{2(g)} + O_{2(g)} = 2\,H_2O_{(g)} \tag{B}$$

$$C_2H_{4(g)} + 3\,O_{2(g)} = 2\,CO_{2(g)} + 2\,H_2O_{(g)} \tag{C}$$

Add Eqs. (A) and (B), and from the sum, subtract Eq. (C).

$$2\,C_{(g)} + 2\,O_{2(g)} + 2\,H_{2(g)} + O_{2(g)} - C_2H_{4(g)} - 3\,O_{2(g)}$$
$$= 2\,CO_{2(g)} + 2\,H_2O_{(g)} - 2\,CO_{2(g)} - 2\,H_2O_{(g)}$$

Simplifying, $2\,C_{(g)} + 2\,H_{2(g)} = C_2H_{4(g)}$ (D)

Thus, it is clear that the algebraic sum of relevant heats of combustion (with proper signs) gives the heat of formation of ethylene.

Heat of formation of ethylene gas $(\Delta H_f^0$ = Heat of combustion of carbon (solid)

> or heat of formation of $CO_{2(g)}$ + Heat of combustion of hydrogen (gas) or heat of formation of $H_2O_{(g)}$ – heat of combustion of ethylene (gas)

$$= -2 \times 393.51 - 2 \times 241.82 + 1323.1$$

$$= 52.44 \text{ kJ/mol}$$

From Appendix IV.2, the standard heat of formation of ethylene gas is 52.5 kJ/mol which is in close agreement with the calculated figure.   *Ans.*

Example 5.25 Find standard heat of formation data of gaseous diethyl ether from Appendix AIV.2 and calculate latent heat of vaporization using data from Table 5.4 at 298.15 K (25°C). With these data, calculate the standard heat of formation of liquid diethyl ether.

Solution λ_{v_1} at 307.7 K (34.55°C) = 26 694 kJ/kmol Ref. Table 5.5. T_c = 466.74 K

Latent heat of vaporization

$$\text{at 298.15 K (25°C), } \lambda_{v_2} = 26\,694 \left(\frac{466.74 - 298.15}{466.74 - 307.7} \right)^{0.38}$$

$$= 27\,292 \text{ kJ/kmol} \equiv 27.292 \text{ kJ/mol}$$

Standard heat of formation of gaseous diethyl ether,

$$\Delta H_{f(g)}^\circ = -252.0 \text{ kJ/mol}$$

Therefore, standard heat of formation of liquid diethyl ether,

$$\Delta H_{f(l)}^\circ = -252.0 - 27.292 = -279.292 \text{ kJ/kmol}$$

$$\text{Reported } \Delta H_{f(l)}^\circ = -279.2 \text{ kJ/mol} \qquad\qquad\qquad \textit{Ans.}$$

Example 5.26 A sample of motor spirit (83 octane) has an API gravity of 64. The net heat of combustion of motor spirit (liquid) is determined to be 44 050 kJ/kg at 288.7 K. Calculate the heat of formation of the motor spirit at 298.15 K (25°C).

Solution Basis 1 kg motor spirit

The carbon to hydrogen weight ratio of petroleum fraction is given by the following formula[22]

$$\frac{C}{H} = \frac{74 + 15\,G}{26 - 15\,G} \tag{5.52}$$

where   G = specific gravity of petroleum fraction at 288.7 K (15.6°C or 60°F)

$$= \frac{141.5}{(131.5 + 64)} = 0.724 \qquad\qquad \text{[Ref. Eq. (2.15)]}$$

$$\frac{C}{H} = \frac{74 + 15 \times 0.724}{26 - 15 \times 0.724} = 5.605$$

$$\text{Carbon content of motor spirit} = \frac{5.605}{6.605}$$

$$= 0.8486 \text{ kg} \equiv 0.070\,72 \text{ kmol}$$

$$\text{Hydrogen content of motor spirit} = 1 - 0.8486$$

$$= 0.1514 \text{ kg} \equiv 0.0757 \text{ kmol}$$

$$\text{Oxygen required for complete combustion} = 0.070\,72 + \left(\frac{0.0757}{2}\right)$$

$$= 0.108\,57 \text{ kmol}$$

Motor spirit (l)	+	$O_2(g)$	=	$CO_2(g)$	+	$H_2O(g)$
1 kg		0.10 857 kmol		0.070 72 kmol		0.0757 kmol
ΔH_{f1}^0		$\Delta H_{f2}^0 = 0$		ΔH_{f3}^0		ΔH_{f4}^0

Assume net heat of combustion at 288.7 K to be same as the heat of reaction at 298.15 K.

$$\Delta H_R^0 = \Delta H_c^0$$

$$= -44\,050$$

$$= -0.070\,72 \times 393.51 \times 1000 - 241.82 \times 0.0757 \times 1000 - \Delta H_{f1}^0$$

$$\Delta H_{f1}^0 = +44\,050 - 27\,829 - 18\,306 = -2085 \text{ kJ/kg} \qquad\qquad Ans.$$

A number of group contribution methods are available for the estimation of the standard heat of formation and the standard heat of combustion of a compound. These methods are summarised in literature[14]. Among these, the method proposed by Thinh and coworkers[40] is quite accurate for hydrocarbons.

5.12.2   Effect of Temperature on Heat of Formation

As is the case with heat capacity, heat of formation varies with temperature. A generalised equation for calculation of heat of formation at any temperature T in K is

$$\Delta H_f = \Delta H_f^\circ + \int_{298.15}^{T} \Delta C_{mp}^0 \, dT \tag{5.53}$$

where ΔC_{mp}^0 represents the algebraic sum of the heat capacities of the compound and the constituent elements in their standard states using appropriate stoichiometric co-efficients (ref. Sec. 4.4). It may be noted that ΔC_{mp}^0 is not residual heat capacity (δC_{mp}) as defined in Sec. 5.5. While using appropriate ΔC_{mp}^0 data for elements, care should be exercised in referring to the standard states of these elements. For example, standard state of carbon, sulphur and iodine is solid while that of bromine is liquid and that of hydrogen and chlorine is gas.

As the method, represented by Eq. (5.53) is tedious, attempts are made to represent the relation of the heat of formation with the temperature, in a polynomial form.

Yaws et al[41] have presented data for 700 organic compounds in the second order polynomial form.

$$\Delta H_f = a' + b'T + c'T^2 \tag{5.54}$$

Values of a', b' and c' permit direct calculations of the heat of formation at a given temperature. In most cases, the average deviation of correlation and data are claimed to be less than 0.2 kJ/mol.

5.13 ABSOLUTE ENTHALPY

As such enthalpy has no absolute value. Only change in enthalpy can be calculated. In order to account for variations of ΔH_f° with temperature, a new function ($H^\circ - H_0^\circ + \Delta H_{f0}^\circ$) is developed. In this function, ΔH_{f0}° stands for heat of formation of the compound from its elements at 101.325 kPa and 0 K ($-273.15°C$), H° for enthalpy of the compound at T K, and ΔH_0° for enthalpy of the compound at 0 K ($-273.15°C$). As this new function is the enthalpy of the compound over 0 K (the lowest thermodynamic temperature), it is termed as *absolute enthalpy* in this book.

United Catalyst Inc., USA have reported the value of ($H^\circ - H_0^\circ + \Delta H_{f0}^\circ$) for various compounds[42] at different temperatures. These data are given in Table 5.21. This new function is extremely useful and allows speedy calculations of enthalpy change during any physical and/or chemical process. This is particularly so in cases where chemical reactions cannot be accurately written. For example, in steam-hydrocarbon reforming reactions the exact extent of individual reactions taking place in the reformer is not easy to be spelled out. However, the product gas stream analysis is solely determined by the chemical equilibrium. Under such circumstances, the initial and final compositions and conditions (such as pressure and temperature) are well known. With the data on ($H^\circ - H_0^\circ + \Delta H_{f0}^\circ$), the enthalpy changes of such reactions can be easily evaluated. The value of ($H^\circ - H_0^\circ + \Delta H_{f0}^\circ$) can be converted into mean heat capacity data. For such conversions, a reference temperature is required to be fixed, e.g., 298.15 K (25°C). The difference in the values of ($H^\circ - H_0^\circ + \Delta H_{f0}^\circ$) between the desired temperature and base temperature gives the enthalpy change between the two temperatures. When this enthalpy difference is divided by the temperature difference, the mean heat capacity is evaluated. Mean heat capacity data for combustion gases are given in Table 7.14. Example 5.27 will indicate the method.

Enthalpy values of various compounds are extensively tabulated in literature at different pressures and temperatures. These data permit calculations of enthalpy changes of processes involving changes in pressure.

$(H° - H_0°)$ is called enthalpy above 0 K $(- 273.15°C)$ which can be calculated using ΔC_{mp}^0 data valid up to 0 K $(- 273.15°C)$, considering ideal gas. However, for evaluation of this function at different pressure and temperature, a generalised correlation based on three-parameter corresponding states principle is presented by Lee and Kesler[13]. For use of this procedure, the reader is advised to refer the original article or Ref. 2.

Table 5.21 Absolute Enthalpy of Gases in Ideal State Conditions[42]

Temperature		Absolute enthalpy $(H° - H_0° + \Delta H_{f0}°)$ kJ/kmol			
K	°C	Nitrogen N_2	Oxygen O_2	Hydrogen H_2	Carbon monoxide CO
273.15	0.00	7 905	7 878	7 683	– 105 978
298.15	25.00	8 613	8 597	8 407	– 105 271
400.00	126.85	11 541	11 603	11 363	– 102 340
500.00	226.85	14 479	14 666	14 272	– 99 387
600.00	326.85	17 478	17 830	17 194	– 96 361
700.00	426.85	20 537	21 086	20 131	– 93 267
800.00	526.85	23 656	24 423	23 088	– 90 107
900.00	626.85	26 833	27 833	26 070	– 86 885
1000.00	726.85	30 066	31 305	29 079	– 83 603
1100.00	826.85	33 355	34 830	32 119	– 80 265
1200.00	926.85	36 699	38 399	35 196	– 76 874
1300.00	1026.85	40 096	42 003	38 313	– 73 433
1400.00	1126.85	43 545	45 630	41 473	– 69 946
1500.00	1226.85	47 045	49 273	44 681	– 66 415

Temperature		Absolute enthalpy $(H° - H_0° + \Delta H_{f0}°)$ kJ/kmol			
K	°C	Carbon dioxide CO_2	Water H_2O	Sulphur dioxide SO_2	Sulphur trioxide SO_3
273.15	0.00	– 385 097	– 230 070	– 348 938	– 444 062
298.15	25.00	– 384 158	– 229 252	– 347 992	– 442 759
400.00	126.85	– 380 118	– 225 843	– 343 911	– 437 046
500.00	226.85	– 375 835	– 222 379	– 339 575	– 430 849
600.00	326.85	– 371 268	– 218 799	– 334 953	– 424 131
700.00	426.85	– 366 448	– 215 101	– 330 082	– 416 950
800.00	526.85	– 361 405	– 211 284	– 325 000	– 409 365
900.00	626.85	– 356 167	– 207 346	– 319 746	– 401 437
1000.00	726.85	– 350 766	– 203 286	– 314 357	– 393 224
1100.00	826.85	– 345 231	– 199 103	– 308 873	– 384 785
1200.00	926.85	– 339 593	– 194 796	– 303 331	– 376 180
1300.00	1026.85	– 333 880	– 190 363	– 297 769	– 367 469
1400.00	1126.85	– 328 122	– 185 802	– 292 225	– 358 710
1500.00	1226.85	– 322 351	– 181 113	– 286 738	– 349 962

(Contd.)

Table 5.21 Contd.

Temperature		Absolute enthalpy $(H° - H_0° + \Delta H_{f0}°)$, kJ/kmol			
K	°C	Ammonia	Nitrous oxide	Nitric oxide	Nitrogen dioxide
		NH_3	N_2O	NO	NO_2
273.15	0.00	− 29 616	93 524	98 322	45 856
298.15	25.00	− 28 751	94 505	99 044	46 779
400.00	126.85	− 24 997	98 699	102 042	50 751
500.00	226.85	− 20 962	103 117	105 067	54 954
600.00	326.85	− 16 599	107 817	108 170	59 426
700.00	426.85	− 11.925	112 784	111 345	64 136
800.00	526.85	− 6 958	118 003	114 589	69 054
900.00	626.85	− 1 713	123 459	117 897	74 149
1000.00	726.85	3 792	129 138	121 265	79 389
1100.00	826.85	9 539	135 025	124 688	84 744
1200.00	926.85	15 512	141 105	128 163	90 183
1300.00	1026.85	21 693	147 363	131 686	95 675
1400.00	1126.85	28 066	153 784	135 251	101 190
1500.00	1226.85	34 613	160 354	138 854	106 695

Temperature		Absolute enthalpy $(H° + H°0 + \Delta H°_{f0})$ kJ/kmol			
K	°C	Hydrogen sulphide	Carbon disulphide	Methane	Ethane
		H_2S	CS_2	CH_4	C_2H_6
273.15	0.00	− 72.670	− 5 844	− 57 770	− 58 620
298.15	25.00	− 71 852	− 4 644	− 56 960	− 57 348
400.00	126.85	− 68 387	378	− 53 206	− 51 315
500.00	226.85	− 64 785	5 509	− 48 845	− 44 137
600.00	326.85	− 60 993	10 818	− 43 863	− 35 813
700.00	426.85	− 57 021	16 286	− 38 305	− 26 441
800.00	526.85	− 52 877	21 893	− 32 219	− 16 115
900.00	626.85	− 48 571	27 620	− 25 650	− 4 934
1000.00	726.85	− 44 111	33 449	− 18 646	7 006
1100.00	826.85	− 39 507	39 358	− 11 252	19 608
1200.00	926.85	− 34 768	45 330	− 3 516	32 775
1300.00	1026.85	− 29 902	51 345	4 517	46 412
1400.00	1126.85	− 24 920	57 383	12 800	60 421
1500.00	1226.85	− 19 829	63 425	21 286	74 705

(Contd.)

Example 5.27 The values of $(H° - H_0° + \Delta H_{f0}°)$ are listed in Table 5.21 for styrene at 298.15 K (25°C) and 600 K (327°C). Calculate the mean heat capacity between the two temperatures.

Solution Basis: 1 kmol styrene

Enthalpy change between 298.15 K and 600 K = 241 749 − 189 398

$$= 52\ 351 \text{ kJ/mol}$$

$$C°_{mpm} = \frac{52\ 351}{(600 - 298.15)}$$

$$= 173.4 \text{ kJ/(kmol} \cdot \text{K)} \qquad Ans.$$

Table 5.21 Contd.

Temperature		Absolute enthalpy, $(H° - H°_0 + \Delta H°_{f0})$ kJ/kmol			
K	°C	Propane C_3H_8	n-Butane $n\text{-}C_4H_{10}$	i-Butane $i\text{-}C_4H_{10}$	n-Pentane $n\text{-}C_5H_{12}$
273.15	0.00	− 68 896	− 80 996	− 87 877	− 93 812
298.15	25.00	− 67 080	− 78 546	− 85 450	− 90 834
400.00	126.85	− 58 434	− 67 003	− 73 961	− 76 755
500.00	226.85	− 48 114	− 53 376	− 60 326	− 60 069
600.00	326.85	− 36 133	− 37 666	− 44 563	− 40 790
700.00	426.85	− 22 644	− 20 062	− 26 871	− 19 161
800.00	526.85	− 7 800	− 756	− 7 452	4 577
900.00	626.85	8 247	20 065	− 13 494	30 183
1000.00	726.85	25 345	42 210	35 764	57 415
1100.00	826.85	43 339	65 489	59 160	86 030
1200.00	926.85	62 078	89 713	83 479	115 789
1300.00	1026.85	81 409	114 693	108 520	146 448
1400.00	1126.85	101 179	140 237	134 083	177 766
1500.00	1226.85	121 235	166 158	159 966	209 502

Temperature		Absolute enthalpy $(H° - H°_0 + \Delta H°_{f0})$ kJ/kmol			
K	°C	Ethylene C_2H_4	Propylene C_3H_6	Butadiene 1,2 C_4H_6	Butadiene 1,3 C_4H_6
273.15	0.00	70 158	47 246	189 852	139 270
298.15	25.00	71 239	48 818	191 780	141 345
400.00	126.85	76 268	56 205	200 816	150 892
500.00	226.85	82 119	64 906	211 401	161 862
600.00	326.85	88 800	74 922	223 499	174 267
700.00	426.85	96 235	86 134	236 930	187 962
800.00	526.85	104 348	98 424	251 513	202 802
900.00	626.85	113 066	111 673	267 067	218 641
1000.00	726.85	122 311	125 763	203 410	235 333
1100.00	826.85	132 010	140 575	283 410	252 734
1200.00	926.85	142 085	155 990	300 362	270 698
1300.00	1026.85	152 463	171 891		289 079
1400.00	1126.85	163 068	188 157		307 732
1500.00	1226.85	173 824	204 672		326 511

(Contd.)

Example 5.28 The cryogenic separation of hydrogen from a refinery gas mixture is described in Example 5.22. Enthalpies of various streams are given in Table 5.22.

Table 5.22 Enthalpies of Gases[43]

Gas conditions	Enthalpy, kJ/kg*		
	Hydrogen	Methane	Ethane
27 bar a and 313 K	4428	− 3537	− 1934
27 bar a and 304 K	4302	− 3559	− 1956
4.5 bar a and 304 K	4291	− 3537	− 1900
1.5 bar a and 304 K	4226	− 3534	− 1894

*Above 0 K.

Calculate the heat infiltration which can be permitted in the cold box.

Table 5.21 Contd.

Temperature		Absolute enthalpy $(H° - H_0° + \Delta H°_{f0})$ kJ/kmol			
K	°C	Acetylene C_2H_2	Methanol CH_3OH	Ethanol C_2H_5OH	n-Propanol C_3H_7OH
273.15	0.00	236 213	– 180 149	– 205 628	– 216 632
298.15	25.00	237 351	– 179 072	– 203 811	– 214 323
400.00	126.85	242 241	– 174 130	– 195 536	– 203 604
500.00	226.85	247 422	– 168 462	– 186 129	– 191 160
600.00	326.85	252 947	– 162 049	– 175 553	– 176 986
700.00	426.85	258 786	– 154 954	– 163 915	– 161 254
800.00	526.85	264 910	– 147 240	– 151 315	– 144 133
900.00	626.85	271 288	– 138 971	– 137 859	– 125 795
1000.00	726.85	277 890	– 130 210	– 123 649	– 106 411
1100.00	826.85	284 685		– 108 789	– 86 150
1200.00	926.85	291 645		– 93 383	– 65 185
1300.00	1026.85	298 738		– 77 534	– 43 686
1400.00	1126.85	305 934		– 61 346	– 21 823
1500.00	1226.85	313 203		– 44 922	

Temperature		Absolute enthalpy $(H° - H_0° + \Delta H°_{f0})$ kJ/kmol			
K	°C	i-Propanol C_3H_7OH	Formalde- hyde $HCHO$	Acetalde- hyde CH_3CHO	Acetone CH_3COCH_3
273.15	0.00	– 235 063	– 103 023	– 144 129	– 186 057
298.15	25.00	– 232 733	– 102 193	– 142 835	– 184 142
400.00	126.85	– 221 954	– 98 477	– 136 775	– 175 268
500.00	226.85	– 209.484	– 94 336	– 129 683	– 164 984
600.00	326.85	– 195 310	– 89 742	– 121 580	– 153 279
700.00	426.85	– 179 595	– 84 732	– 112 581	– 140 285
800.00	526.85	– 162 502	– 79 343	– 102 805	– 126 136
900.00	626.85	– 144 195	– 73 611	– 92 369	– 110 965
1000.00	726.85	– 124 837	– 67 572	– 81 391	– 94 905
1100.00	826.85	– 104 591	– 61 264		– 78 091
1200.00	926.85	– 83 620	– 54 721		– 60 655
1300.00	1026.85	– 62 088	– 47 981		– 42 731
1400.00	1126.85	– 40 158	– 41 081		– 24 452
1500.00	1226.85	– 17 993	– 34 056		– 5 951

(Contd.)

Solution

Basis: 12 000 Nm^3/h (= 535.4 kmol/h) feed gas

Enthalpy of feed, $\phi_1 = 535.4 \dfrac{(0.6 \times 4428 \times 2 - 0.2 \times 3537 \times 16 - 0.2 \times 1934 \times 30)}{3600}$

$$= - 2618.81 \text{ kW}$$

Enthalpy of product hydrogen stream, $\phi_2 = \dfrac{(315.35 \times 4302 \times 2 - 29.01 \times 3559 \times 16)}{3600}$

$$= 294.81 \text{ kW}$$

Table 5.21 Contd.

Temperature		Absolute enthalpy ($H° - H°_0 + \Delta H°_{f0}$), kJ/kmol			
K	°C	Benzene	Toluene	Ethyl benzene	Styrene
		C_6H_6	C_7H_8	C_8H_{10}	C_8H_8
273.15	0.00	112 278	88 263	76 827	186 280
298.15	25.00	114 397	90 912	80 119	189 398
400.00	126.85	124 642	103 665	95 830	204 143
500.00	226.85	137 046	119.052	114 612	221 605
600.00	326.85	151 546	137 007	136 405	241 749
700.00	426.85	167 919	157 265	160 899	264 299
800.00	526.85	185 938	179 558	187 781	288 982
900.00	626.85	205 380	203 618	216 741	315 524
1000.00	726.85	226 019	229 179	247 466	343 649
1100.00	826.85	247 630	225 972	279 645	373 084
1200.00	926.85	269 990	283 731	312 967	403 554
1300.00	1026.85	292 872	312 189	347 120	434 786
1400.00	1126.85	316 052	341 077	381 793	466 504
1500.00	1226.85	339 306	370 129	416 674	498 434

(Reproduced with the permission of United Catalysts Inc., USA)

Enthalpy of HP tail gas,

$$\phi_3 = \frac{(5.46 \times 4291 \times 2 - 57.45 \times 3537 \times 16 - 106.06 \times 1900 \times 30)}{3600}$$

$$= -2569.38 \text{ kW}$$

Enthalpy of LP tail gas, $\phi_4 = \dfrac{(0.48 \times 4226 \times 2 - 20.56 \times 3534 \times 16 - 1.03 \times 1894 \times 30)}{3600}$

$$= -338.06 \text{ kW}$$

Let heat infiltration to cold box = ϕ_5

$$\phi_1 + \phi_5 = \phi_2 + \phi_3 + \phi_4$$

$$-2618.82 + \phi_5 = 294.81 - 2569.38 - 338.06$$

$$\phi_5 = 6.19 \text{ kW} \qquad\qquad Ans.$$

Note: The heat infiltration rate of 6.19 kW is reasonable for this size of cold box. However, because of seasonal variation in the ambient temperature, the heat infiltration rate can vary and hence a hydrogen injection facility into the LP tail gas stream is normally provided.

5.14 STANDARD HEAT OF REACTION

An understanding of the heat of formation enables one to evaluate the standard heat of a chemical reaction at 298.15 K (25°C). Consider the reaction between A and B to produce C and D.

$$n_a \, A + n_b \, B = n_c \, C + n_d \, D \tag{5.55}$$

where n_a, n_b, n_c, and n_d are number of moles of A, B, C and D respectively. For this reaction, the standard heat of reaction, ΔH_R° is defined as

$$\Delta H_R^\circ = \text{Enthalpy of products} - \text{enthalpy of reactants}$$

$$= \Sigma(n_i \cdot \Delta H_{fi}^\circ)_{\text{Products}} - \Sigma(n_i \cdot \Delta H_{fi}^\circ)_{\text{Reactants}} \tag{5.56}$$

$$= n_c \, \Delta H_{fc}^\circ + n_d \, \Delta H_{fD}^\circ - n_a \, \Delta H_{fA}^\circ - n_b \, \Delta H_{fB}^\circ$$

where ΔH_{fi}° is the standard heat of formation of the ith component. If the values of ΔH_{fi}° are used at some other temperature (but all values at one particular temperature only), ΔH_R will be available at the corresponding temperature. In general,

$$\Delta H_R = \Sigma(n_i \cdot \Delta H_{fi})_{\text{Products}} - \Sigma(n_i \cdot \Delta H_{fi})_{\text{Reactants}} \tag{5.57}$$

When ΔH_R is positive, the reaction is said to be endothermic, i.e., it absorbed heat during the course of reaction and, if (ΔH_R) is negative, the reaction is termed as exothermic, i.e. heat will be evolved during the course of the reaction.

Example 5.29 In the production of sulphuric acid from anhydrite, the gypsum is roasted with clay to obtain sulphur dioxide and cement clinker. The reaction proceeds as follows.

$$3 \, CaSO_{4(s)} + SiO_{2(s)} = 3 \, CaO \cdot SiO_2(g) + 3 \, SO_{2(g)} + 3/2 \, O_{2(g)}$$

Calculate the heat of reaction at 298.15 K (25°C).

Solution Basis: 1 mol $SiO_{2(s)}$ reacted

Table 5.23 Thermodynamic Data

Component	Phase	ΔH_f° at 298.15 K (25°C) kJ/mol
$CaSO_4$	Solid	– 1432.7
SiO_2	Solid (amorphous)	– 903.5
$3 \, CaO.SiO_2$	Solid (clinker)	– 2879.0
SO_2	Gas	– 296.81
O_2	Gas	0.0

Standard heat of reaction

at 298.15 K, $\Delta H^\circ{}_R = \Sigma(n_i \cdot \Delta H_{fi})_{\text{Products}} - \Sigma(n_i \cdot \Delta H_{fi})_{\text{Reactants}}$

$$= \left[- 2879.0 + 3 \, (- 296.81) + \left(\frac{3}{2} \right) \times 0 \right]$$

$$- [3 \, (- 1432.7) + 1 \, (- 903.5)]$$

$$= (- 2879.0 - 890.43) - (4298.1 - 903.5)$$

$$= 1432.17 \text{ kJ/mol } SiO_2 \equiv 477.39 \text{ kJ/mol } CaSO_4 \quad Ans.$$

Since ΔH_R° is positive, the reaction is highly endothermic.

Example 5.30 Calculate the standard heat of reaction at 298.15 K (25°C) when gaseous ammonia is dissolved in water to form 2% by mass of its solution for the regeneration of weak anion exchanger of a water treatment plant.

Solution Basis: 100 kg of 2% ammonia solution

In the solution, 2 kg ammonia (as NH_3) and 98 kg water are present. However, the ammonia is usually present as NH_4OH.

$$NH_{3(g)} + H_2O_{(l)} = NH_4OH_{(l)}$$

Using data given in Appendix IV.1,

$$\Delta H_R^\circ = -361.20 - (-45.94 - 285.83)$$

$$= -361.20 + 331.77 = -29.43 \text{ kJ/mol } NH_3 \text{ dissolved}$$

Since ΔH_R° is negative, the dissolution is exothermic.

$$\text{Ammonia present in the solution} = \frac{2}{17.0305} \text{ kmol}$$

$$\text{Heat of dissolution} = \frac{29.43 \times 2 \times 1000}{17.0305}$$

$$= \frac{3456.1 \text{ kJ}}{100 \text{ kg solution}} \text{ at 298.15 K} \qquad \textit{Ans.}$$

5.14.1 Effect of Temperature on Heat of Reaction

In Examples 5.29 and 5.30, the heat of reaction is calculated at 298.15 K (25°C) using the data on the standard heat of formation. However, in actual practice, reactants and products are at temperature other than 298.15 K (25°C). When the heat balance is to be made with reactants and products at 1 bar a pressure but at temperatures other than 298.15 K (25°C), the following procedure is recommended (Fig. 5.13).

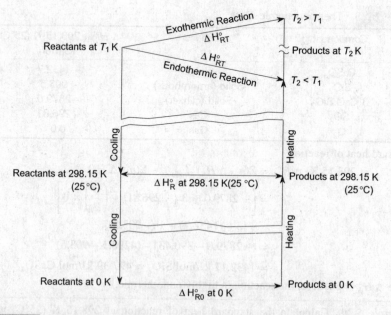

Fig. 5.13 Effect of Temperature on Heat of Reaction at 1 bar Absolute Pressure

Consider again the reaction,

$$n_a\,A + n_b\,B = n_c\,C + n_d\,D \qquad (5.55)$$

There can be two possibilities. In one case, both the reactants and products are at T K, while in another case both are at different temperatures, say the reactants enter the reactor at T_1 K while products leave it at T_2 K. In either case, the method of calculation is essentially the same.

Step 1: Assume that reactants are cooled to 298.15 K (25°C). Calculate the enthalpy of (ΔH_1) of reactants at T_1 K over 298.15 K (25°C).

Step 2: Calculate the standard heat of reaction (ΔH_R^o) using data given in Appendix IV. If more than one reaction is taking place, the standard heat of reaction for each of them should be calculated and summed up algebraically.

Step 3: Assume that products are heated from 298.15 K (25°C) to temperature T_2 K. Calculate the enthalpy (ΔH_2) of products at T_2 K over 298.15 K (25°C).

The *algebraic* sum of enthalpies of all the three steps yield the heat balance, as enthalpies are point (state) functions.

Case (a): $T_1 = T_2 = T$

For this case, the heat balance yields the heat of reaction at T K. It is possible to develop an empirical relation for the heat of reaction at T K using the empirical equation for heat capacity as described below.

$$\Delta H_1 = \int_{T_0}^{T_1} (\Sigma n_i \cdot C_{mpi}^0)_{\text{Reactants}}\, dT \qquad (5.58)$$

$$\Delta H_2 = \int_{T_0}^{T_2} (\Sigma n_i \cdot C_{mpi}^0)_{\text{Products}}\, dT \qquad (5.59)$$

Now at constant pressure (at 1 bar),

$$\Delta H_{RT}^o = \Delta H_R^o - \Delta H_1 + \Delta H_2 \qquad (5.60)$$

where ΔH_R^o is the heat of reaction at reference temperature.

$$\Delta H_2 - \Delta H_1 = \int_{T_0}^{T_2} (\Sigma n_i \cdot C_{mpi}^0)_{\text{Products}}\, dT - \int_{T_0}^{T_1} (\Sigma n_i \cdot C_{mpi}^0)_{\text{Reactants}}\, dT \quad (5.61)$$

When $T_1 = T_2 = 298.15$ K and $T_0 = 0$ K, (refer Fig. 5.13)

$$\Delta H_{R0}^o = \text{Standard heat of reaction at 0 K}$$

$$= \Delta H_R^o + (\Delta H_2 - \Delta H_1)$$

$$= \Delta H_R^o + \int_{298.15}^{0} (\Delta a + \Delta b\,T + \Delta c\,T^2 + \Delta d\,T^3)\, dT \qquad (5.62)$$

where Δ represents the algebraic summation of constants of heat capacity equation (Table 5.1) for the products and the reactants.

When $T_0 = 0$ K and $T_1 = T_2 = T$,

$$\Delta H_{RT}^o = \Delta H_{R0}^o + \int_{0}^{T} (\Delta a + \Delta b\,T + \Delta c\,T^2 + \Delta d\,T^3)\, dT$$

or
$$\Delta H_{RT}^\circ = \Delta H_{R0}^\circ + \Delta a\, T + \left(\frac{\Delta b}{2}\right) T^2 + \left(\frac{\Delta c}{3}\right) T^3 + \left(\frac{\Delta d}{4}\right) T^4 \quad (5.63)$$

Equations (5.58) to (5.62) are entirely general and can be used for any chemical reaction. For finding ΔH_R°, the heat of reaction at 298.15 K (25°C) is calculated by using data of the standard heat of formation [Appendix (IV)] and substituting in Eq. (5.56). Care must be taken to use correct data, taking into account phase changes, if any.

Example 5.31   Obtain an expression relating the heat of reaction and the temperature of the reaction

$$SO_{2(g)} + \frac{1}{2}\, O_2(g) = SO_{3(g)}$$

Using the same expression, calculate the heat of reaction at 775 K (502°C).
Solution   Basis: 1 kmol SO_2 reacted

$$\Delta a = 22.036 - 24.771 - 0.5\,(26.026) = -15.748$$
$$\Delta b \times 10^3 = 121.624 - 62.948 - 0.5\,(11.755) = 52.799$$
$$\Delta c \times 10^6 = -91.867 - (-44.258) - 0.5\,(-2.343) = -45.438$$
$$\Delta d \times 10^9 = 24.369 - 11.122 - 0.5\,(-0.562) = 13.528$$
$$\Delta H_R^\circ = -395\,720 - (-296\,810) = -98\,910 \text{ kJ/kmol}$$

$$\Delta H_{R0}^\circ = \Delta H_R^\circ + \int\limits_{298.15}^{0} (-15.748 + 52.799 \times 10^{-3}\, T - 46.438 \times 10^{-6}\, T^2$$
$$+ 13.528 \times 10^{-9}\, T^3)\, dT$$

$$= -98\,910 + 15.748 \times 298.15 - 52.799 \times 10^{-3}\, \frac{(298.15)^2}{2}$$
$$+ 46.438 \times 10^{-6}\frac{(298.15)^3}{3} - 13.528 \times 10^{-9}\, \frac{(298.15)^4}{4}$$
$$= -98\,910 + 4695 - 2347 + 410 - 27$$
$$= 96\,178 \text{ kJ/kmol} \qquad\qquad \textit{Ans.} \text{ (a)}$$

$$\Delta H_{RT}^\circ = 96\,178 - 15.748\, T + 26.4 \times 10^{-3}\, T^2 - 15.48 \times 10^{-6}\, T^3 + 3.382 \times 10^{-9}\, T^4$$

Substituting $T = 775$ K
$$\Delta H_R^\circ = -96\,178 - 12\,205 + 15\,857 - 7206 + 1220$$
$$= -98\,512 \text{ kJ/kmol} \qquad\qquad \textit{Ans.} \text{ (b)}$$

Case (b): $T_1 \ne T_2$.

For this case, the heat balance calculations are best illustrated by the following example.

Example 5.32   In Table 5.24 the compositions of the incoming and outgoing gas mixtures to and form a converter are given. Assume that the sulphur burner gases enter the converter at 800 K (527°C) and the outgoing gases leave it at 875 K (602°C). Intercoolers are installed in the catalyst beds of the converter.

Table 5.24 Composition of Converter Gases

Components	Inlet gas kmol/h	Outlet gas kmol/h
SO_2	8.851	0.351
O_2	13.200	8.950
SO_3	0.984	9.484
N_2	102.400	102.400
Total	125.435	121.185

Calculate the heat transfer taking place in the intercoolers, using (a) heat capacity data and (b) the data of $(H° - H_0° + \Delta H_{f0}°)$ from Table 5.21.
Solution Basis: 125.435 kmol/h inlet gas mixture (n_1)

Table 5.25 Heat Capacity Equation Constants for Incoming Gas Mixture

Component	n_i kmol/h	$a_i \cdot n_i$	$b_i \cdot n_i \times 10^3$	$c_i \cdot n_i \times 10^6$	$d_i \cdot n_i \times 10^9$
SO_2	8.851	219.245	557.154	− 391.729	98.441
O_2	13.200	343.539	155.167	− 30.922	− 7.422
SO_3	0.948	21.685	119.678	− 90.397	23.997
N_2	102.400	3030.108	− 526.438	1349.929	− 508.723
Total	125.435	3614.577	305.561	836.881	− 393.707

Enthalpy of ingoing gas mixture at 800 K over 298.15 K,

$$\phi_1 = 3614.577 (800 - 298.15)$$
$$+ 305.561 \times 10^{-3} \frac{(800^2 - 298.15^2)}{2}$$
$$+ 836.881 \times 10^{-6} \frac{(800^3 - 298.15^3)}{3}$$
$$- 393.707 \times 10^{-9} \frac{(800^4 - 298.15^4)}{4}$$
$$= 1814\ 518 + 84\ 212 + 135\ 445 - 39\ 541$$
$$= $$
$$1994\ 634 \text{ kJ/h} \equiv 554.07 \text{ kW}$$

Table 5.26 Heat Capacity Equation Constants for Outgoing Gas Mixture

Component	n_i kmol/h	$a_i \cdot n_i$	$b_i \cdot n_i \times 10^3$	$c_i \cdot n_i \times 10^6$	$d_i \cdot n_i \times 10^9$
SO_2	0.351	8.694	22.095	− 15.535	3.904
O_2	8.950	232.930	105.208	− 20.966	− 5.033
SO_3	9.484	209.005	1153.482	− 871.269	231.117
N_2	102.400	3030.108	− 526.438	1349.929	− 508.723
Total	121.185	3480.737	754.347	442.159	− 278.735

Enthalpy of outgoing gas mixture at 875 K over 298.15 K,

$$\phi_2 = 3480.737\,(875 - 298)$$

$$+ 754.347 \times 10^{-3}\,\frac{\left(875^2 - 298.15^2\right)}{2}$$

$$+ 442.159 \times 10^{-6}\,\frac{\left(875^3 - 298.15^3\right)}{3}$$

$$- 278.735 \times 10^{-9}\,\frac{\left(875^4 - 298.15^4\right)}{4}$$

$$= 2008\,385 + 255\,278 + 94\,837 - 40\,298$$

$$= 2318\,203 \text{ kJ/h} \equiv 643.95 \text{ kW}$$

$$\Delta H_R^\circ = -98\,910 \text{ kJ/kmol } SO_2 \text{ reacted \quad (Ref. Example 5.31)}$$

Total heat of reaction at 298.15 K,

$$\phi_3 = n_{SO_2 \text{ (reacted)}} \cdot \Delta H_R^\circ$$

$$= (8.8511 - 0.351)\,\frac{(-98\,910)}{3600} = -233.54 \text{ kW}$$

$$\text{Net enthalpy change} = \phi_2 + \phi_3 - \phi_1$$

$$= 643.95 - 233.54 - 554.07$$

$$= -143.66 \text{ kW (exothermic)}$$

Thus, during the reaction, enthalpy equivalent to -143.66 kW is to be removed from the system in order to maintain the temperature of the outgoing gas mixture at 875 K (602°C). *Ans. (a)*

Table 5.27 Absolute Enthalpy Data

Component	Ingoing gas mixture mixture at 800 K		Outgoing gas mixture at 875 K	
	n_i kmol/h	$n_i \cdot (H^\circ - H_0^\circ + \Delta H_{f0}^\circ)$ kW	n_i kmol/h	$n_i \cdot (H - H_0^\circ + \Delta H_{f0}^\circ)$ kW
SO_2	8.851	− 799.05	0.351	− 31.30
O_2	13.200	89.55	8.950	67.08
SO_3	0.984	− 111.89	9.484	− 1067.78
N_2	102.400	672.88	102.400	740.66
Total	125.435	− 148.51	121.185	− 286.35

Enthalpy change $= -286.34 - (-148.51) = -137.83$ kW \qquad *Ans. (b)*

Error between two answers is 7.75%.

Example 5.33 Refer Example 4.4. Assume that the moisture in ingoing ambient air is 0.015 kg/kg dry air. The mixture of ethanol-air is fed to the reactor at 335 K (62°C). Make enthalpy balance across the reactor.

Solution Basis: 100 kmol outgoing gas mixture from scrubber

Moisture entering with ambient air $= 3127.7 \times 0.015 = 46.92$ kg

$$\equiv 2.61 \text{ kmol}$$

Total water in the reactor effluent $= 40.2 + 2.61 = 42.81$ kmol

$$= \Sigma n_i \cdot (H^\circ - H_0^\circ + \Delta H_{f0}^\circ)_{\text{Products}} -$$

$$\Sigma n_i \cdot (H^\circ - H_0^\circ + \Delta H_{f0}^\circ)_{\text{Reactants}}$$

Table 5.28 Enthalpy of Reactants at 335 K (62°C)

Component	n_i kmol	$(H_0 - H_0^\circ + \Delta H_{f0}^\circ)$, kJ/kmol	$n_i \cdot (H^\circ - H_0^\circ + \Delta H_{f0}^\circ)$ kJ
C_2H_5OH	135.99	– 200 817	– 27 309 104
N_2	85.2	9 672	824 054
O_2	22.65	9 685	218 881
H_2O	2.61	– 224 977	– 587 190
Total	246.45		– 26 853 359

Table 5.29 Enthalpy of Products at 720 K (447°C)

Component	n_i kmol	$(H_0 - H_0^\circ + \Delta H_{f0}^\circ)$, kJ/kmol	$n_i \cdot (H^\circ - H_0^\circ + \Delta H_{f0}^\circ)$ kJ
C_2H_5OH	89.09	– 161 395	– 14 378 681
N_2	85.2	21 161	1 802 900
O_2	2.1	21 753	45 682
CO_2	0.7	– 365 439	– 255 808
CO	2.3	– 92 635	– 213 061
H_2	7.1	20 722	147 129
CH_4	2.6	– 37 088	– 96 428
CH_3CHO	44.1	– 110 626	– 4 878 598
H_2O	42.81	– 214 338	– 9 175 793
Total	276.00		– 27 002 658

From Tables 5.28 and 5.29,

Net heat of reaction, ΔH_R = – 27 002 658 – (– 26 853 359) = – 149 299 kJ

$$\equiv 605.9 \text{ kJ/kmol total reactants (exothermic)}$$

$$= 3183.3 \text{ kJ/kmol } C_2H_5OH \text{ reacted (exothermic)}$$

The net heat of reaction (exothermic) is quite small and it can be attributed to heat losses from the system. Hence the reaction can be termed as near isenthalpic or adiabatic. *Ans.*

Example 5.34 Refer Example 4.10. Make heat balance of the system and calculate saturated steam generation at 6 bar a assuming that the boiler is fed with water at 303 K (30°C). Also assume constant molar heat capacity (at constant pressure) as 65.8 and 48.2 kJ/(kmol · K) for gaseous dimethyl ether and formaldehyde, respectively. If the Dowtherm circuit operates at atmospheric pressure, calculate its circulation rate.

Solution Calculate standard heat of reaction using standard heat of formation (Appendix-IV) for all five reactions.

$$\Delta H_{R1}^\circ = -241.82 - 108.6 - (-200.94)$$

$$= -149.48 \text{ kJ/mol } CH_3OH$$

$$\Delta H_{R2}^\circ = -393.51 - 241.82 - (-200.94)$$

$$= -434.39 \text{ kJ/mol } CH_3OH$$

$$\Delta H_{R3}^\circ = -110.53 - (-200.94)$$

$$= +90.41 \text{ kJ/mol } CH_3OH$$

$$\Delta H^\circ_{R4} = -74.52 - (-200.94)$$
$$= +126.42 \text{ kJ/mol } CH_3OH$$
$$\Delta H^\circ_{R5} = -184.0 - 241.82 - (-2 \times 200.94)$$
$$= -23.94 \text{ kJ/2 mol } CH_3OH$$
$$\equiv -11.97 \text{ kJ/mol } CH_3OH$$

Total heat of reaction at 298.15 K,

$$\Delta H^\circ_R = 11.375 \, (-149\,480) + 8.786 \, (-434\,390)$$
$$+ 0.99 \, (+99\,410) + 0.610 \, (+126\,420) + 1.98 \, (-11\,970)$$
$$= -20\,320\,839 \text{ kJ/h}$$
$$\equiv 5644.68 \text{ kW}$$

For evaluation of enthalpy of ingoing gas mixture to the reactor, heat capacity data are tabulated below.

Table 5.30 Heat Capacity Data of Reactor Inlet Gas Mixture

Component	n_i, kmol/h	Heat capacity (C^0_{mpi}) equation constants			
		$n_i \cdot a_i$	$n_i \cdot b_i \times 10^3$	$n_i \cdot c_i \times 10^6$	$n_i \cdot d_i \times 10^9$
CH_3OH	125.00	3108.7	6359.4	7328.4	−5640.8
O_2	281.27	7320.2	3306.4	−658.9	−158.2
N_2	1058.10	31310.1	−5439.7	13948.8	−5256.6
H_2O	23.73	771.0	1.9	313.5	−107.9
Total	1488.10	42510.0	4228.0	20931.8	−1163.6

From the above Table 5.30, heat capacity of input air,
$$C^0_{mpa} = 39\,401.3 - 2131.4 \times 10^{-3} T + 13\,603.4 \times 10^{-6} T^2$$
$$- 5522.7 \times 10^{-9} T^3$$
and, heat capacity of input methanol,
$$C^0_{mpme} = 3108.7 + 6359.4 \times 10^{-3} T + 7328.4 \times 10^{-6} T^2$$
$$- 5640.8 \times 10^{-9} T^3$$
In similar fashion, heat capacity data of reaction exit gas stream are given in Table 5.31.

Table 5.31 Heat Capacity Data of Reactor Exit Gas Stream

Component	n_i, kmol/h	Heat capacity (C^0_{mpi}) equation constants			
		$n_i \cdot a_i$	$n_i \cdot b_i \times 10^3$	$n_i \cdot c_i \times 10^6$	$n_i \cdot d_i \times 10^9$
CH_3OH	1.25	31.1	63.6	73.3	−56.4
HCHO	111.375	5368.3	—	—	—
CO_2	8.786	187.7	564.8	−360.7	86.1
CO	0.99	28.7	−2.8	11.5	−4.7
H_2	1.98	56.6	2.0	−0.3	1.5
CH_4	0.619	11.9	32.3	7.4	−7.0
$(CH_3)_2O$	0.99	65.1	—	—	—
O_2	212.712	5536.0	2500.5	−498.3	119.6
N_2	1058.100	31310.1	−5439.7	13948.8	−5256.6
H_2O	153.667	4993.0	12.2	2030.0	−698.8
Total	1550.469	47588.5	−2267.1	15211.7	−5816.3

Reactor exit gas stream is cooled from 613.15 K (340°C) to 383.15 K (110°C), preheating ingoing air.

$$\text{Heat duty of heat exchanger, } \phi_4 = \int_{383.15}^{613.15} C_{mpi}^0 \, dT$$

$$= 11\ 395\ 056 \text{ kJ/h}$$

$$\equiv 3165.29 \text{ kW}$$

Air enters the heat exchanger at 308.15 K (35°C) and leaves it at T_1 K.

$$\int_{308.15}^{T_1} C_{mpa}^0 \, dT = 11\ 395\ 056$$

Solving by Mathcad, $T_1 = 588$ K or 315°C

Evaporator heat duty:

Liquid methanol enters evaporator at 308.15 K (35°C) and at 170 kPa a.

Using Antoine equation (Eq. 5.24),

$$\log 170 = 7.2059 - \frac{1582.30}{T - 33.45}$$

or $\qquad\qquad T = 351.47$ K or 78.32°C

Using Watson equation (Eq. 5.26) and data of Table 5.5,

$$\frac{\lambda_v}{35\ 254} = \left(\frac{512.64 - 351.47}{512.64 - 337.8} \right)^{0.38}$$

$$\lambda_v = 32\ 710 \text{ kJ/kmol at 351.47 K}$$

Thus, liquid methanol will have to be first heated from 308.15 K to 351.47 K and then supplied λ_v for evaporation. Heat capacity data of liquid methanol can be taken from Table 5.3.

Heat duty of evaporator,

$$\phi_1 = 125 \int_{308.15}^{351.47} C_{ml} \, dT + 125 \times 32\ 710$$

$$= 462\ 513 + 4088\ 750$$

$$= 4551\ 263 \text{ kJ/h} \equiv 1264.24 \text{ kW}$$

Assume use of saturated steam at 4.5 bar a.

λ_v of steam = 2119.7 kJ/kg $\qquad$ (Refer Appendix III.2)

$$\text{Steam consumption in evaporator} = \frac{4551\ 263}{2119.7}$$

$$= 2147.1 \text{ kg/h}$$

Methanol vapours at 351.47 K and hot air at 588 K mix in a static mixer. Let the temperature of mixed stream be T_2.

$$\int_{351.47}^{T_2} C_{pmme}^0 \, dT = \int_{T_2}^{588} C_{pma}^0 \, dT$$

Solving by Mathcad $T_2 = 554.1$ K or $281.1°$C

Assume reference temperature, $T_0 = 298.15$ K

Enthalpy of reactor input gas stream,

$$\phi_2 = \int_{298.15}^{554.1} C^0_{mpr} \, dT$$

$$\phi_2 = 12\ 080\ 393 \text{ kJ/h}$$

$$\equiv 3355.66 \text{ kW}$$

Enthalpy of reactor exit gas stream,

$$\phi_3 = \int_{298.15}^{613.15} C^0_{mpi} \, dT$$

$$= 15\ 505\ 407 \text{ kJ/h}$$

$$\equiv 4307.06 \text{ kW}$$

$$\text{Heat transfer in reactor} = 12\ 080\ 393 + 20\ 320\ 839 - 15\ 505\ 407$$

$$= 16\ 895\ 825 \text{ kJ/h}$$

$$\equiv 4693.28 \text{ kW}$$

From Table 5.6, λ_v of Dowtherm-A at 101.325 kPa a = 296.2 kJ/kg

$$\text{Dowtherm circulation rate} = \frac{16\ 895\ 825}{296.2}$$

$$= 57\ 042 \text{ kg/h}$$

This heat is picked up by Dowtherm-A and used in generation of saturated steam at 6 bar a.

Enthalpy required for steam generation = 2755.3 − 126   (Appendix-III.2)

$$= 2629.3 \text{ kJ/kg}$$

$$\text{Steam generated, } \dot{m}_s = \frac{16\ 895\ 825}{2629.3}$$

$$= 6426.0 \text{ kg/h} \qquad \textit{Ans.}$$

5.14.2 Effect of Pressure on Heat of Reaction

In Sec. 5.14.1, the effect of temperature on the heat of reaction at 1 bar pressure is described. Usually, the effect of pressure on the heat of reaction is insignificant at relatively low pressures. However, a number of reactions take place at very high pressures, such as ammonia synthesis, methanol synthesis, etc. For such reactions, correction needs to be applied. Enthalpies given by Canjar[43] are useful for such calculations. The following example will illustrate the correction procedure.

Example 5.35 Synthesis gas enters the converter at 728 K (455°C) containing 5 mole % ammonia. The molar ratio of nitrogen to hydrogen is 1:3. The operating pressure is 415 bar a. The conversion per pass is 18.3%. The product stream leaves the converter at 823 K (550°C). Calculate the heat to be removed from the converter[44].

Solution Basis: 100 kmol inlet gas mixture

Reaction; $N_2 + 3 H_2 = 2 NH_3$

NH_3 entering the mixture = 5 kmol

$N_2 : H_2 = 1 : 3$ (mole ratio

Total moles of $(N_2 + H_2) = 100 - 5 = 95$ kmol

N_2 in the inlet gas mixture $= \dfrac{95}{4} = 23.75$ kmol

H_2 in the inlet gas mixture $= \dfrac{(95 \times 3)}{4} = 71.25$ kmol

Per pass conversion = 18.3%

N_2 reacted = 23.75 × 0.183 = 4.35 kmol

H_2 reacted = 4.35 × 3 = 13.05 kmol

NH_3 produced = 4.35 × 2 = 8.7 kmol

Table 5.32 Enthalpy Balance **without** Pressure Correction

Component	n_i kmol	Temperature, K(°C)	Absolute enthalpy, $(H_0 - H_0^\circ + \Delta H_{f0}^\circ)_i$ kJ/kmol	Total enthalpy, $n_i \cdot (H_0 - H_0^\circ + \Delta H_{f0}^\circ)$ kJ
Inlet to reactor:				
H_2	71.25	728 (455)	+ 20 959	+ 1493 329
N_2	23.75	728 (455)	+ 32 410	+ 508 495
NH_3	5.00	728 (455)	− 10 535	− 52 675
Total	100.00	—	—	+ 1949 149
Outlet from reactor:				
H_2	71.25 − 13.05 = 58.2	823 (550)	+ 23 774	+ 1383 647
N_2	23.75 − 4.35 = 19.4	823 (550)	+ 24 387	+ 473 108
NH_3	5 + 8.7 = 13.7	823 (550)	− 5 752	− 78 802
Total	91.3	—	—	+ 1777 953

Net heat of reaction = 1777 953 − 11949 149

= − 171 196 kJ (exothermic)

Table 5.33 Enthalpy Balance **with** Pressure Correction

Component	kmol	Temperature K(°C)	Enthalpy correction due to high pressure[44], δH_i kJ/kmol	Absolute enthalpy with correction, $(H_0 - H_0^\circ + \Delta H_{f0}^\circ + \delta H_i)_i$ kJ/kmol	Total enthalpy, $n_i \cdot (H_0 - H_0^\circ + \Delta H_{f0}^\circ + \delta H_i)_i$ kJ
Inlet to reactor:					
H_2	71.25	728 (455)	+ 700	+ 21 659	+ 1543 204
N_2	23.75	728 (455)	+ 700	+ 22 110	+ 525 113
NH_3	5.00	728 (455)	− 3720	− 14 255	− 71 275
Total	100.00	—	—	—	+ 1997 042

Contd.

Table 5.33 Contd.

Component	n_i kmol	Temperature K(°C)	Enthalpy correction due to high pressure[44], δH_i kJ/kmol	Absolute enthalpy with correction, $(H_0 - H_0^\circ + \Delta H_{f0}^\circ + \delta H_i)_i$ kJ/kmol	Total enthalpy, $n_i \cdot (H_0 - H_0^\circ + \Delta H_{f0}^\circ + \delta H_i)_i$ kJ
Outlet from reactor:					
H_2	58.2	823 (550)	+ 700	+ 24 474	+ 1424 387
N_2	19.40	823 (550)	+ 700	+ 25 807	+ 486 688
NH_3	13.7	823 (550)	− 2580	− 8 332	− 114 148
Total	91.3		—	—	+ 1796 927

$$\text{Net heat of reaction} = 1796\ 927 - 1997\ 042$$
$$= -200\ 115 \text{ kJ (exothermic)}$$
$$\% \text{ Error} = \left(\frac{200\ 115 - 171\ 196}{200\ 115}\right) 100$$
$$= 14.45 \qquad \qquad Ans.$$

Enthalpy correction due to pressure or *residual enthalpy* can be calculated by knowing p_r and T_r by Lee-Kesler[13] method. If H is the enthalpy of a compound at a given p and T, residual enthalpy,

$$\delta H = H^0 - H \qquad \qquad (5.64)$$

Residual enthalpy of the real gas can also be calculated by numerical integration of residual heat capacity values as described in Sec. 5.5.

5.15 ADIABATIC REACTIONS

When a system does not give heat to the surroundings nor does it receive from the surroundings, it is called an *adiabatic* process or operation. More correctly speaking, the system is called *isenthalp*, as reversible adiabatic processes also obey constant entropy criterion. In this book, adiabatic process will be considered as the one in which the heat is contained within a system without loss or addition of heat to or from the outside source.

When adiabatic reactions take place, two observations can be made.

(a) If the reaction is exothermic, the temperature of the product stream rises. In this case, the total heat content of the product stream equals the heat content of reactants plus the heat of reaction.

All oxidation reactions are exothermic. Similarly, the dilution of sulphuric acid or caustic soda solution is exothermic.

(b) If the reaction is endothermic, the temperature of the product stream decreases. In this case, the total enthalpy of the product stream equals the total enthalpy of reactants minus the heat of reaction.

Industrially important steam-hydrocarbon reforming reaction, thermal reduction of hydrogen sulphide to sulphur, dehydrogenation of ethylbenzene, etc. are endothermic. The dissolution of common salt in water is also endothermic.

The temperature of products under adiabatic conditions of reaction is called the *adiabatic reaction temperature.*

In actual industrial practice, except for a few reactions, the reaction temperatures are controlled either by the addition or removal of heat as the case may be. This is because of conflicting demands from kinetic and thermodynamic considerations. When such a temperature control is provided, the reaction becomes non-adiabatic. Oxidation reactions are practically irreversible and hence they can be carried out without the control of temperature. When the fuel is burnt (i.e. combustion reaction), the adiabatic reaction temperature is called the *adiabatic flame temperature* because it represents the flame temperature. Even in well-insulated furnaces and boilers, the heat is lost due to radiation from the surface. Hence, the *actual flame temperature* is less than the adiabatic flame temperature.

Chapter 7 gives calculations of flame temperatures.

Example 5.36 In a commercial process, chlorine is manufactured by burning hydrogen chloride gas using air. The reaction taking place in the burner is:

$$4\ HCl_{(g)} + O_{2(g)} = 2\ H_2O_{(g)} + 2\ Cl_{2(g)}$$

For good conversion, air is used in 35% excess of that theoretically (stoichiometrically) required. Assume that the oxidation is 80% complete and the dry air and hydrogen chloride gas enter the burner at 298.15 K (25°C). Calculate (a) the composition of dry gases leaving the burner and (b) the adiabatic reaction temperature of the product gas steam.

Solution Basis: 4 kmol hydrogen chloride gas

Theoretical O_2 requirement = 1 kmol

Actual O_2 supply = $1 \times 1.35 = 1.35$ kmol

Nitrogen supply through air = $\left(\dfrac{79}{21}\right) \times 1.35 = 5.08$ kmol

Total air supply = $1.35 + 5.08 = 6.43$ kmol

Conversion in the burner is 80%.

HCl burnt = $0.8 \times 4 = 3.2$ kmol

Table 5.34 Composition of Product Gas Stream

Component	Product gas stream, kmol Wet (n_i)	Dry	Composition on dry basis (mole %)
HCl	4 – 3.2 = 0.8	0.8	9.96
O_2	1.35 – 0.8 = 0.55	0.55	6.85
Cl_2	0.8 × 2 = 1.6	1.60	19.93
H_2O	0.8 × 2 = 1.6	—	—
N_2	5.08	5.08	63.26
Total	9.63	8.03	100.00

Ans. (a)

Now assume base temperature to be 298.15 K (25°C).

Enthalpy of the reactants

at 298.15 K (25°C), $\Delta H_1 = 0$ kJ

Standard heat of reaction

at 298.15 K (25°C), $\Delta H_R^0 = -241.82 \times 2 - 4.0 \,(-92.31)$

$= -114.4$ kJ/mol O_2 consumed

This represents the exothermic nature of the reaction.

Total heat liberated $= 114.4 \times 1000 \times 0.8 = 91\,520$ kJ

Total enthalpy of product stream $\Delta H_2 = 0 + 91\,520 = 91\,520$ kJ

Table 5.35 Heat Capacity Equation Constants for Product Gas Stream

Component	n_i kmol	Heat capacity equation constants			
		$a_i \cdot n_i$	$b_i \cdot n_i \times 10^3$	$c_i \cdot n_i \times 10^6$	$d_i \cdot n_i \times 10^9$
HCl	0.8	24.247	-6.087	10.609	-3.467
O_2	0.55	14.314	6.465	-1.288	-0.309
Cl_2	1.6	45.674	38.207	-34.181	10.356
H_2O	1.6	51.987	0.127	21.137	-7.276
N_2	5.08	150.322	-26.116	66.969	-25.237
Total	9.63	286.544	12.596	63.246	-25.933

Enthalpy of product stream

over 298.15 K (25°C), $\displaystyle \Delta H_2 = \int_{298.15}^{T} (\,286.544 + 12.596 \times 10^{-3}\,T$

$+\, 63.246 \times 10^{-6}\,T^2 - 25.933 \times 10^{-9}\,T^3)\,dT$

$= 91\,520$

Solving by Mathcad

T = Adiabatic reaction temperature

$= 599.5$ K or 326.5°C   *Ans.* (b)

Note: The product gas stream contains HCl and H_2O which condense when cooled. Acid gas dew point can be calculated by a method, given by Ganapathy[45]. At atmospheric pressure (101.325 kPa), this dew point is calculated to be 346.5 K (73.5°C). For more discussion on the acid dew point, refer Sec. 7.7.

Example 5.37 Dehydrogenation of ethylbenzene (EB) is commercially employed to manufacture styrene. The reaction is carried out in the gas phase with steam over a catalyst[46], consisting primarily of iron oxide with potassium as a promoter. The reaction is endothermic and is carried out adiabatically at near atmospheric pressure.

Main reaction: $C_6H_5CH_2CH_3 = C_6H_5CH{:}CH_2 + H_2$ (A)

Competing reactions; $C_6H_5CH_2CH_3 = C_6H_6 + C_2H_4$ (B)

$$C_6H_5CH_2CH_3 = 8\,C + 5\,H_2 \tag{C}$$

$$C_6H_5CHCH_2 + 2\,H_2 = C_6H_5CH_3 + CH_4 \tag{D}$$

Fresh EB is mixed with recycled EB, vaporized and superheated to 811 K (538°C). To prevent coke formation [reaction (C)], one mole of EB is mixed with 15 moles of superheated steam at 978 K (705°C). Large dilution of steam also supplies necessary heat of reaction.

Overall conversion is 35%. Net yield of styrene is 90%. Yields of benzene and toluene are 3% and 6% respectively. Assume that 11% of EB converted forms coke by reaction (C). Calculate the adiabatic reaction temperature at the outlet of the reactor.

Solution   Basis: 1 kmol EB vapours entering the reactor at 811 K

Steam mixed with EB = 15 kmol

Table 5.36 Heat Capacity Equation Constants for Reactants

Component	n_i kmol	$n_i \cdot a_i$	$n_i \cdot b_i \times 10^3$	$n_i \cdot c_i \times 10^6$	$n_i \cdot d_i \times 10^9$
EB	1.0	– 36.72	671.12	– 422.02	101.15
H$_2$O	15.0	487.38	1.19	198.16	– 68.21
Total	16.0	450.66	672.31	– 223.86	32.94

Let T_1 K be the temperature of reactant gas stream.

$$\int_{811.15}^{T_1} (-36.72 + 671.12 \times 10^{-3}\,T - 422.02 \times 10^{-6}\,T^2 + 101.15 \times 10^{-9}\,T^3)\,dT$$

$$= \int_{T_1}^{978.15} (487.38 + 1.19 \times 10^{-3}\,T + 198.16 \times 10^{-6}\,T^2 - 68.21 \times 10^{-9}\,T^3)\,dT$$

Solving by Mathcad, $T_1 = 929.72$ K or 656.57°C

Reference temperature, $T_0 = 298.15$ K

Enthalpy of reactants at 929.72 K over 298.15 K,

$$H_1 = \int_{298.15}^{929.72} C_{mp1}^0\,dT$$

$$= 493\,405 \text{ kJ}$$

EB reacted = 0.35 kmol

Styrene in product stream = 0.35 × 0.9 = 0.315 kmol

Benzene produced by reaction (B) = 0.35 × 0.03

$$= 0.0105 \text{ kmol}$$

Ethylene produced by reaction (B) = 0.0105 kmol

Carbon formation by reaction (C) = 0.35 × 0.01

$$= 0.0035 \text{ kmol}$$

Carbon will deposit on the catalyst and will not appear in the product gas mixture stream.

Toluene produced by reaction (D) = 0.35 × 0.06

$$= 0.021 \text{ kmol}$$

$$= CH_4 \text{ produced}$$

$$= \text{styrene reacted by reaction (D)}$$

$$= \text{EB reacted by reaction (A)}$$

Total hydrogen produced = 0.315 + 0.021 + 0.0035 × 5 – 0.021 × 2

$$= 0.315 \text{ kmol}$$

Heat of reactions at 298.15 K:

Reaction (A): $\Delta H^\circ_{R1} = 148.30 - 29.92$

$$= 118.38 \text{ kJ/mol EB}$$

Reaction (B): $\Delta H^\circ_{R2} = 82.93 + 52.50 - 29.92$

$$= 105.51 \text{ kJ/mol EB}$$

Reaction (C): $\Delta H^\circ_{R3} = -29.92 \text{ kJ/mol EB}$

Reaction (D): $\Delta H^\circ_{R4} = 50.17 - 74.52 - 148.30$

$$= -172.65 \text{ kJ/mol styrene}$$

Total heat of reaction,

$$\Delta H^0_R = 1000 [118.38 (0.315 + 0.021) + 105.51 \times$$
$$0.0105 - 29.92 \times 0.0035 - 172.65$$
$$\times 0.021]$$

$$= 37\ 153 \text{ kJ} \quad \text{(endothermic)}$$

Table 5.37 Heat Capacity Equation Constants for Products

Component	n_i kmol	$n_i \cdot a_i$	$n_i \cdot b_i \times 10^3$	$n_i \cdot c_i \times 10^6$	$n_i \cdot d_i \times 10^9$
EB	0.6500	– 23.87	436.23	– 274.31	65.75
Styrene	0.3150	– 11.63	209.56	– 152.79	44.38
C_6H_6	0.0105	– 0.40	5.15	– 3.37	0.83
C_7H_8	0.0210	– 0.74	11.83	– 7.35	1.73
H_2	0.3115	8.91	0.32	– 0.05	0.24
CH_4	0.0210	0.40	1.09	0.25	– 0.24
C_2H_4	0.0105	0.04	1.63	– 0.86	0.18
H_2O	15.0000	487.38	1.19	198.16	– 68.21
Total	16.3395	460.09	667.00	240.32	44.66

Let T_2 be the temperature of product gas stream, leaving the reactor.

$$\text{Enthalpy of products} = \int_{298.15}^{T_2} C^0_{mp2} \, dT$$

$$= 493\ 405 - 37\ 153$$

$$= 456\ 252 \text{ kJ}$$

Solving by Mathcad,

$$T_2 = 886.49 \text{ K or } 613.34°C \qquad\qquad Ans.$$

5.16 THERMOCHEMISTRY OF MIXING PROCESSES

It is a common experience that when a solute (either solid, liquid or gas) is dissolved in a solvent to make its solution, enthalpy change takes place When a solid or gas is dissolved in the solvent (liquid), the heat evolved or absorbed is called the *heat of solution*, more correctly, the *heat of dissolution*. When two liquids are mixed, the heat effect is termed as the *heat of mixing*. Both are also known as *excess enthalpy*. These heat changes are measured at constant temperature usually at 291.15 K (18°C) or 298.15 K (25°C) and at atmospheric pressure or at 1 bar. It is expressed in different forms, e.g., kJ/kmol solution, kJ/kg solution, kJ/kmol solute, kJ/kg solute, etc. The heat of solution of an ideal solution is zero.

Basically, the heat of solution is defined as the heat change associated with the system when one mole of solute is dissolved in a definite number of moles of solvent, keeping the temperature constant and the pressure at 101.3 kPa a (760 torr). The number of moles of solvent vary from 100 to 1800 and even more. When the number of moles is very high, the heat of solution at infinite dilution is obtained. Since the measurement of the heat of solution is made in a calorimeter, practical difficulty is observed in measuring the temperature changes when a large number of moles of the solvent are present. Therefore, from the practical point of view, the number of moles is usually restricted to about 200.

The heat effect can be exothermic (realized by the evolution of heat) or endothermic (realized by the absorption of heat). The common nomenclature used in most literature is a little confusing and hence needs clarification.

When solids dissolve in a solvent, the exothermic heat of solution is given a *positive* sign and vice versa. This is the convention followed in Perry's Chemical Engineers' Handbook (Ref. 20).

In the case of liquids, it is the other way round, i.e. the exothermic heat of dissolution is given a *negative* sign and vice versa.

The above convention will be followed in this book.

Let H_1 and H_2 be the enthalpies of two pure components mixed together. Let H^E represent the total heat of solution while the total enthalpy of the final solution is assumed to be H_m.

$$H^E = n_1 H_1 + n_2 H_2 - H_m (n_1 + n_2) \qquad\qquad (5.65)$$

where n_1 and n_2 are the number of moles of the two components mixed together. Consistent units need be employed in the above equation.

Different systems will now be considered in the light of the above equation.

5.17 DISSOLUTION OF SOLIDS

Dissolution of solids in water is a very common process in the industry, the well known examples being the dissolution of caustic soda, common salt, etc. Data are reported in literature of the heat of solution of solids in water at 291.15 K (18°C)[20].

Crystallization is the reverse process of dissolution. For all practical purposes, the heat of solution with a reverse sign is taken as heat of crystallization. Most data on the heat of crystallization indicate exothermic operation.

Example 5.38 The heat absorbed when $Na_2CO_3.10H_2O$ is dissolved isothermally at 291.15 K (18°C) in a large quantity of water is 67.91 kJ per mol solute[20]. Calculate the heat of crystallization of 1 kg $Na_2CO_3.10H_2O$.

Solution As indicated earlier, the heat of crystallization is just the opposite of the heat of solution.

Heat of solution of $Na_2CO_3.10H_2O$ at 291.15 K

$$= -67.91 \text{ kJ/mol solute (endothermic)}$$

Molar mass of $Na_2CO_3.10H_2O = 286.141$

$$\text{Heat of crystallization} = \frac{67\,910}{286.141}$$

$$= 237.33 \text{ kJ/kg solute (exothermic)} \qquad Ans.$$

Example 5.39 Calculate the heat of crystallization of $Na_2SO_4.10H_2O$ using the data of heat of formation. Standard heat of formation of $Na_2SO_{4(c)}$ and $Na_2SO_4.10H_2O(c)$ are -1387.08 and -4327.26 kJ/mol respectively.

Solution From Appendix IV, ΔH_f^0 of $H_2O_{(1)} = -285.82$ kJ/mol

The crystallization reaction can be written as

$$Na_2SO_{4(c)} + 10\ H_2O_{(1)} = Na_2SO_4.10\ H_2O_{(c)}$$

Using the thermodynamic laws of the heat of reaction,

$$\text{Heat of crystallization} = -4327.26 - (-1387.08 - 10 \times 285.82)$$

$$= -81.98 \text{ kJ/mol (exothermic)}$$

The above heat of crystallization is also called the heat of hydration. *Ans.*

Note: The heat of solution of $Na_2SO_4.10H_2O$ is reported[20] to be -78.461 kJ/mol (endothermic). Therefore the heat of crystallization is $+78.461$ kJ/mol (exothermic). This value is lower than the value obtained in Example 5.39. Such a discrepancy is due to the neglect of the heat of dilution in the calculation of the heat of crystallization.

It is known that the boiling point of a solution is higher than the boiling point of the solvent at a definite pressure. Also, the enthalpy of a solution at different temperatures is different from that of enthalpy of a pure solvent. This is because of the effect of the heat of dissolution of the solute into the solvent and of the different heat capacity of the solution as compared to the solvent. A chart giving the relation between the enthalpy of the solution and the concentration of the solution is called an enthalpy-concentration diagram. Figure 5.14 is the enthalpy-concentration diagram of $NaOH$-H_2O system. On the diagram, various isotherms are plotted. Such diagrams are useful in the evaluation of (a) the heat required to be added to or removed from the solution when heating or cooling of the solution is carried out and (b) the temperature of the resultant mixture when two different solutions having different concentrations and temperatures are mixed together by tie-line method.

The following example will help clarify the applications.

Example 5.40 find the temperature of 25% NaOH solution, prepared by diluting 46% NaOH lye at 298.15 K (25°C) with water at 308 K (35°C). All percentages are by mass.

Solution On the chart (Fig. 5.14), place A representing 46% NaOH lye at 298.15 K (25°C). Place point B representing pure water (0% NaOH) at 308 K (35°C). Join the points A and B. The tie-line AB intersects the vertical axis at 25% concentration to an isotherm of 329.5 K (56.5°C)   *Ans.*

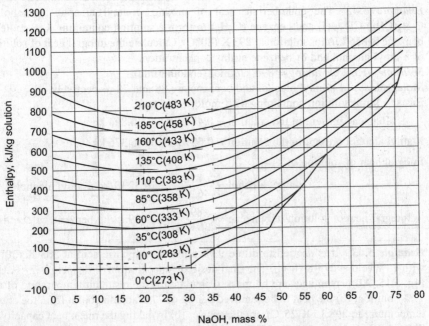

Fig. 5.14 Enthalpy-concentration Diagram for $NaOH$-H_2O System[47]

(Reproduced with permission of John Wiley & Sons, Inc., USA.)

Example 5.41 How much heat is to be added in order to raise the temperature of a 20% NaOH solution from 280 K (8°C) to 360 K (87°C)? Compare the value with that calculated in Example 5.5.

Solution Refer Fig. 5.14.

Heat content of 20% NaOH solution at 280 K, H_1 = 34 kJ/kg solution

Heat content of 20% NaOH solution at 360 K, H_2 = 314 kJ/kg solution

Heat to be added to the solution = $H_2 - H_1$ = 314 – 34

= 280 kJ/kg solution

Ans. (a)

The value of 280 kJ/kg compared with 290.8 kJ/kg, calculated in Example 5.5, gives 3.4% lower value.

5.18 LIQUID-LIQUID MIXTURE

The heat of dissolution of one liquid into another is calculated in a manner similar to that of solid-liquid system. Enthalpy-concentration diagrams can also be plotted for a liquid-liquid system. Such a diagram representing H_2SO_4-H_2O system is given in Fig. 5.15. Similar diagrams for mixed acids, ammonia-water system and benzene-toluene system are given in Figs 5.18, 5.19 and 6.1, respectively.

Example 5.42 The endothermic heat of mixing *n*-amyl alcohol [pentanol-1, $C_2H_5(CH_2)_2CH_2OH$] and benzene (C_6H_6) to form a solution containing 47.3 mole % benzene is 816 kJ/mol solution at 293 K (20°C). Calculate the integral heat of solution of *n*-amyl alcohol and of benzene at this concentration.

Solution Heat of mixing = 896 kJ/kmol (endothermic)

Molar masses of *n*-amyl alcohol and benzene are 88 and 78 respectively.

Basis: 1 kmol solution containing 47.3 mole % benzene.

Benzene present in the solution = 0.473 × 78 = 36.894 kg

n-amyl alcohol present in the solution = 0.527 × 88 = 46.376 kg

Integral heat of solution of

$$n\text{-amyl alcohol} = \frac{896}{46.376} = 19.32 \text{ kJ/kg } n\text{-amyl alcohol}$$

$$\text{Integral heat of solution of benzene} = \frac{896}{36.894} = 24.29 \text{ kJ/kg benzene} \qquad Ans.$$

Example 5.43 It is desired to dilute 93% aqueous sulphuric acid at 303 K (30°C) with 15% acid at 273 K (0°C). The final desired concentration of the acid is 77%. Use Fig. 5.15. All percentages are by mass. Calculate (a) the resultant temperature of the 77% solution, (b) the heat to be removed per kg of 77% acid to cool it from the above temperature to 298.15 K(25°C), (c) the answer (b) by taking the mean heat capacity of 77% H_2SO_4 between 293 K (20°C) and its boiling point, (d) by material balance the quantity of 15% acid to be mixed up with 100 kg 93% acid for getting 77% acid product, (e) the answer (d) by using Fig. 5.15 and applying co-ordinate geometry principles.

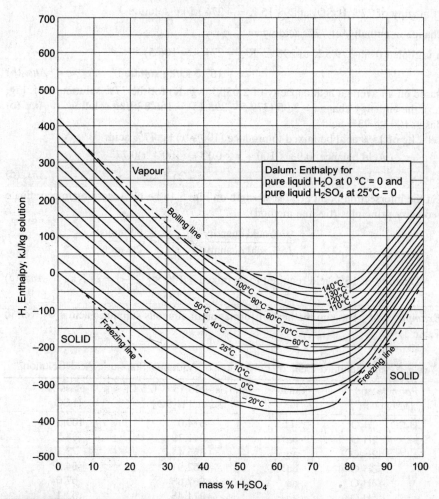

Fig. 5.15 Hx diagram for H_2SO_4/H_2O (Redrawn from data of Techni-cal Note 270-3, National Bureau of Standards[48], USA, 1968 and Ref. 49 and 50.)

Solution Refer to Fig. 5.15.

Place point *A* to represent 93% H_2SO_4 at 303 K (25°C) and point *B* to represent 15% H_2SO_4 at 273 K (0°C). Join *A* and *B*. The tie-line *AB* intersects the vertical line representing 77% H_2SO_4 at 379.5 K (106.5°C).

Thus, the resultant temperature of 77% solution will be 379.5 K, if no heat is lost to the surrounding during the mixing.

Enthalpy of 77% H_2SO_4 at 379.5 K = – 106.5 kJ/kg solution

From Fig. 5.5,

Heat capacity of 77% acid at 379.5 K = 2.06 kJ/(kg · K)

Heat capacity of 77% acid at 298.15 K =1.94 kJ/(kg· K)

Enthalpy of 77% H_2SO_4 at 298.15 K = $- 274$ kJ/kg solution

Change in enthalpy of 77% acid when

it is cooled from 379.5 K to 298.15 K = $- 274 - (- 106.5)$

$$= - 167.5 \text{ kJ/kg solution} \qquad Ans. \ (b)$$

Based on an average heat capacity of 2.05 kJ/(kg· K) for the 77% solution (Ref. Fig. 5.5), the enthalpy change = 2.05 (379.5 – 298.15) = 166.8 kJ/kg solution   *Ans.* (c)

Basis: 100 kg 93% acid

Let x kg of 15% acid be mixed to produce $(100 + x)$ kg 77% acid.

Acid balance: $0.93 \times 100 + x \times 0.15 = (100 + x)0.77$

$$x = 25.8 \text{ kg} \qquad Ans. \ (d)$$

Let the intersection point at 77% strength on Fig. 5.15 be C. According to coordinate geometry principles (tie-line method),

$$\frac{93\% \text{ acid quantity}}{15\% \text{ acid quantity}} = \frac{CB}{CA} = \frac{9.9 \text{ units}}{2.5 \text{ units}}$$

Quantity of 15% acid required to be mixed = $100 \times \left(\dfrac{2.5}{9.9} \right) = 25.3$ kg   *Ans.* (e)

Example 5.44 Data on the heat of formation of aqueous sulphuric acid are given in Table 5.38.

Table 5.38 Standard Heat of Formation of Aqueous Sulphuric Acid Solution[48]

Formula and Description	State	ΔH_f^0 at 298.15 K (25°C) kJ/mol H_2SO_4	Mass % H_2SO_4
H_2SO_4, $0H_2O$	l	– 814.0	100.0
$1H_2O$	aq	– 841.79	84.5
$2H_2O$	aq	– 855.44	73.1
$3H_2O$	aq	– 862.91	64.5
$4H_2O$	aq	– 867.88	57.6
$5H_2O$	aq	– 871.48	52.1
$6H_2O$	aq	– 874.22	47.6
$7H_2O$	aq	– 876.37	43.8
$8H_2O$	aq	– 878.08	40.5
$9H_2O$	aq	– 879.43	37.7
$10H_2O$	aq	– 880.53	35.3
$12H_2O$	aq	– 882.13	31.2
$15H_2O$	aq	– 883.62	26.6
$20H_2O$	aq	– 884.92	21.4
$25H_2O$	aq	– 885.59	17.9
$30H_2O$	aq	– 885.98	15.4
$40H_2O$	aq	– 886.46	12.0
$50H_2O$	aq	– 886.77	9.82
$75H_2O$	aq	– 887.29	6.77
$100H_2O$	aq	– 887.64	5.16
$150H_2O$	aq	– 888.19	3.50
$200H_2O$	aq	– 888.63	2.65

(*Source: National Institute of Standards and Technology, USA*)

Solve Example 5.43 with the above data assuming that both acids are available at 298.15 K (25°C).

Solution Basis: 100 kg 93% acid and 25.8 kg 15% acid

Since, the interpolation of heat of formation for intermediate concentration is required, data given in Table 5.38 are plotted in Fig. 5.16.

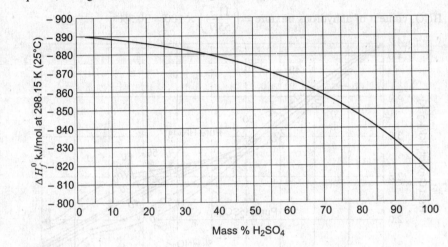

Fig. 5.16 Heat of Formation of Sulphuric Acid Solution

For 93% H_2SO_4, $\Delta H_f^0 = -830$ kJ/mol H_2SO_4

For liquid 100% H_2SO_4, $\Delta H_f^0 = -814.0$ kJ/mol H_2SO_4

Heat of solution, $H_1 = -830 - (-814.0) = -16$ kJ/mol H_2SO_4

For 15% H_2SO_4, $\Delta H_f^0 = -886.2$ kJ/mol H_2SO_4

Heat of solution, $H_2 = -886.2 - (-814.0) = -72.2$ kJ/mol H_2SO_4

For 77% H_2SO_4, $\Delta H_f^0 = -851.0$ kJ/mol H_2SO_4

Heat of solution, $H_3 = -851.0 - (-814.0) = -37$ kJ/mol H_2SO_4

Using Eq. (5.65), heat evolved $= \dfrac{1000}{98.0785} [-93 \times 16 - 25.8$
$$\times 0.18 \times 72.2 + 125.8 \times 0.77 \times 37]$$
$$= 10.1959 [-1488.0 - 335.3 + 3584.0]$$
$$= 17\,592 \text{ kJ}/125.8 \text{ kg solution}$$
$$= 142.7 \text{ kJ/kg solution at } 298.15 \text{ K} \qquad \textit{Ans.}$$

Another important unit process in organic industry is nitration. This reaction is usually carried out with the help of mixed acids. Figures 5.17 and 5.18 are useful in evaluating the enthalpy changes taking place during the mixing and also during the nitration reaction. The following examples clarify the use of these figures.

Example 5.45 In Example 3.8, a mixed acid is produced by blending the three acids. If all the acids are available at 308.15 K (35°C), calculate the heat to be removed to maintain the temperature of the final mixed acid at 308.15 K (35°C).

Solution Basis: 1000 kg mixed acid

For calculating the heat removal, the enthalpies of each of the acids to be mixed are calculated as follows

(a) Spent acid at 308.15 K (35°C):

Total acid content of spent acid = 11.3 + 44.4 = 55.7%

$$\text{HNO}_3 \text{ content of anhydrous mixture} = \left(\frac{11.3}{55.7}\right) \times 100 = 20.3\%$$

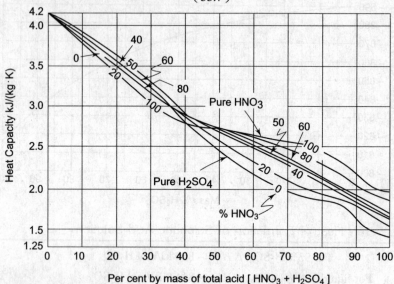

Fig. 5.17 Heat Capacity of Aqueous Mixed Acids[51]

Locate 55.7% on the x-axis and then draw a vertical line which intersects the curve representing the 20.3% HNO_3 content. Read the enthalpy of the mixture equal to -296.7 kJ/kg at 273.15 K (0°C) from Fig. 5.18.

Similarly, the heat capacity (C_{11}) of the mixture is found to be 2.45 kJ/(kg·K) from Fig. 5.17.

Enthalpy of spent acid $H_1 = -296.7 + 2.45 (308.15 - 273.15) = -210.95$ kJ/kg

(b) Aqueous 90% HNO_3 at 308.15 K (35°C):

Total acid content = 90%

HNO_3 content of anhydrous acid = 100%

Enthalpy at 273.15 K (0°C) = -87.8 kJ/kg

$$C_{12} = 2.2 \text{ kJ/(kg·K)}$$

Enthalpy of 90% HNO_3 $H_2 = -87.8 + 2.2 (308.15 - 273.15) = -10.8$ kJ/kg

(c) Aqueous 98% H_2SO_4 at 308.15 K (35°C):

Total acid content = 98%

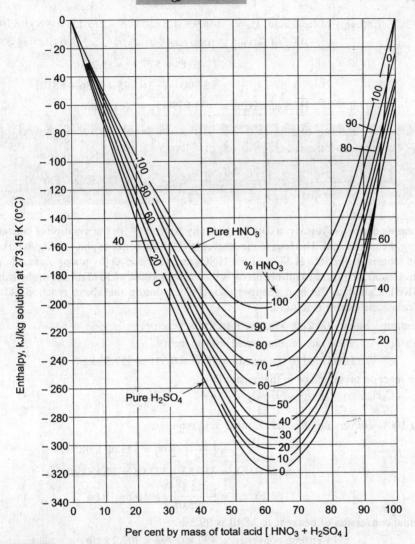

Fig. 5.18 Enthalpy-concentration Diagram for Mixed Acids[51]

(*Both figures are reproduced with permission of Pergamon Press Ltd., UK*)

HNO_3 content of anhydrous acid = 0%

Enthalpy at 273.15 K (0°C) = – 35.5 kJ/kg

$$C_{13} = 1.45 \text{ kJ/(kg} \cdot \text{K)}$$

Enthalpy of 98% $H_2 SO_4$ H_3 = – 35.5 + 1.45 (308.15 – 278.15) = 15.25 kJ/kg

This value agrees well with the value read from Fig. 5.15.

(d) Final mixed acid at 308.15 K (35°C) :

Total acid content = 92%

$$HNO_3 \text{ content of anhydrous acid} = \left(\frac{32}{92}\right) \times 1100$$

$$= 34.8\%$$

Enthalpy at 273.15 K (0°C) = – 148.9 kJ/kg

$$C_{14} = 1.8 \text{ kJ/(kg} \cdot \text{K)}$$

Enthalpy of final acid, $H_4 = -148.9 + 1.8 (308.15 - 273.15) = -85.9$ kJ/kg

Heat of mixing $= 1000 (-85.9) - [76.3 (-210.95) + 345.9$

$(-10.8) + 577.7 (+15.25)]$

$= 85\,900 - [-16\,095 - 3736 + 8810]$

Heat of mixing $= -74\,879$ kJ   (exothermic)   *Ans.*

Note: In case the exothermic heat is not removed from the system, the fortified mixed acid will attain a temperature

$$= \left[\frac{74\,879}{(1000 \times 1.8)} + 308.15 \right] = 349.75 \, K (76.6°C)$$

Example 5.46 A typical run data are given by Albright[52] for the nitration of benzene using the mixed acid. The feed to the reactor is 400 kg/h benzene and 1135 kg/h mixed acid (consisting of 56% H_2SO_4, 31.5% HNO_3 and 12.5% H_2O (by mass). Assume that conversion of benzene to nitrobenzene is 99.3% with 100% yield of mononitrobenzene (MNB). Calculate the heat changes taking place during the above reaction. Also, calculate the excess acid used.

Solution   Basis: 400 kg/h benzene feed to the reactor

Feed rate of mixed acid = 1135 kg/h

HNO_3 fed to the reactor $= 1135 \times 0.315 = 357.53$ kg/h

The reaction taking place in the reactor is

C_6H_6	+	HNO_3	=	$C_6H_5NO_2$	+	H_2O
78		63		123		18

For 100% conversion of benzene, nitric acid required

$$= \left(\frac{63}{78} \right) \times 400 = 323.08 \text{ kg/h}$$

Excess $HNO_3 = 357.53 - 323.08 = 34.45$ kg/h

$$\% \text{ Excess} = \left(\frac{34.45}{323.08} \right) \times 100 = 10.66 \qquad \textit{Ans. (a)}$$

Actual conversion of benzene to MNB is 99.3%

Benzene converted $= 400 \times 0.993 = 397.2$ kg/h

$$HNO_3 \text{ consumed} = \left(\frac{63}{78} \right) \times 397.2 = 320.82 \text{ kg/h}$$

$$\text{Water formed} = \left(\frac{18}{78} \right) \times 397.2 = 91.66 \text{ kg/h}$$

The composition of spent acid at the end of the reaction is given in Table 5.39.

Table 5.39 Composition of Spent Acid

Component	kg/h	mass %
HNO_3	357.53 − 320.82 = 36.71	4.05
H_2O	141.87 + 91.66 = 233.53	25.78
H_2SO_4	633.60	70.17
Total	905.84	100.00

Feed mixed acid:

$$\text{Total acid content} = 56 + 31.5 = 87.5\%$$

$$HNO_3 \text{ content of anhydrous acid} = \left(\frac{31.5 \times 100}{86.5}\right) = 36\%$$

$$H_1 \text{ at } 273.15 \text{ K } (0°C) = -186.5 \text{ kJ/kg}$$

$$C_{11} = 1.88 \text{ kJ/(kg} \cdot \text{K)}$$

$$H'_1 \text{ at } 298.15 \text{ K } (25°C) = -186.5 + 1.88 (298.15 - 273.15) = -139.5 \text{ kJ/kg}$$

Spent acid:

$$\text{Total acid content} = 70.17 + 4.05 = 74.22\%$$

$$HNO_3 \text{ content of anhydrous acid} = \frac{(4.05 \times 100)}{74.22} = 5.5\%$$

$$H_2 \text{ at } 273.15 \text{ K } (0°C) = -288.9 \text{ kJ/kg}$$

$$C_{12} = 1.96 \text{ kJ/(kg} \cdot \text{K)}$$

$$H'_2 \text{ at } 298.15 \text{ K } (25°C) = -288.9 + 1.95 (298.15 - 273.15) = -239.9 \text{ kJ/kg}$$

Pure HNO_3:

$$H_3 \text{ at } 273.15 \text{ K } (0°C) = 0 \text{ kJ/kg}$$

$$C_{13} = 1.98 \text{ kJ/(kg} \cdot \text{K)}$$

$$H'_3 \text{ at } 298.15 \text{ K } (25°C) = 1.98 (298.15 - 273.15) = 49.5 \text{ kJ/kg}$$

Standard heat of reaction:

The heat of formation of mono-nitrobenzene is + 12.50 kJ/mol at 298.15 (25°C). For other compounds, refer Appendix IV.

$$\Delta H_R^0 = -285.83 + 12.50 - (-174.10 + 49.08)$$

$$= -148.31 \text{ kJ/mol}$$

$$\text{Benzene reacted} = \frac{397.2}{78.1118} = 5.085 \text{ kmol/h}$$

$$\text{Total heat changes} = 905.84 \, H'_2 + 320.82 \, H'_3 - 1135 \, H'_1$$
$$+ 5.085 \, \Delta H_R^0$$

$$= 905.84 \, (-239.9) + 320.82 \, (49.5)$$

$$- 1135 \, (-139.5) + 5.085 \, (-148.31) \, 1000$$

$$= -217 \, 311 + 15 \, 881 + 158 \, 333 - 754 \, 156$$

$$= -797 \, 253 \text{ kJ/h}$$

$$\equiv -221.46 \text{ kW (exothermic)} \qquad \textit{Ans. (b)}$$

5.19 GAS-LIQUID SYSTEM

Absorption and desorption of gases in liquids are commonly encountered in the process industry. Enthalpy changes are invariably associated with these unit operations.

Enthalpy concentration diagram for ammonia-water is given in Fig. 5.19. This diagram is useful in determining the equilibrium vapour composition of aqueous ammonia solution. Also, it can be used to determine the final tempera-ture of aqueous solution prepared by mixing liquid or gaseous ammonia in water or by diluting strong aqueous solution. It is quite useful in establishing material and energy balances of an ammonia absorption refrigeration system (refer Example 8.4) which is becoming increasingly popular for utilization of low level heat such as low pressure steam, flue gases from a furnance, etc.

In addition, data on the heat of formation for the ammonia-water system are presented in Table 5,40 which can be also be used for mixing calculations.

Table 5.40 Standard Heat of Formation of Aqueous Ammonia Solution[48]

Formula and Description	State	ΔH_f^0 at 298.15 K (25°C) kJ/mol NH_3	Mass % NH_3
$NH_3, 0H_2O$	g	– 45.94	100.0
$1H_2O$	aq	– 75.36	48.6
$2H_2O$	aq	– 77.66	32.1
$5H_2O$	aq	– 79.27	15.9
$10H_2O$	aq	– 79.81	8.63
$20H_2O$	aq	– 80.02	4.51
$50H_2O$	aq	– 80.15	1.85
$100H_2O$	aq	– 80.19	0.94
$\infty\ H_2O$	aq	– 79.69	0.0

Note: Number of the first column indicates number of moles of water, mixed with one mole of ammonia.

(*Source: National Institute of Standards and Technology, USA*)

Example 5.47 Ammonia vapours (100%) from a nitrogenous fertilizer solution plant at the rate of 140 kg/h are taken to a vent scrubber. Vapours enter the scrubber at 101.3 kPa a (760 torr) and 323 K (50°C). Water is sprayed at the top of the scrubber at 303 K (30°C). Assume (a) complete absorption of ammonia and (b) 15% NH_3 (mass) strength of the solution. Calculate the temperature of resultant solution (i) with the help of Fig. 5.19 and (ii) with the help of data given in Table 5.40 and assuming average heat capacity of 15% ammonia solution to be 4.145 kJ/(kg· K).

Solution Enthalpy of ammonia gas at 101.3 kPa a(760 torr) and 323 K (50°C)

$$= 1548 \text{ kJ/kg with } T_0 = 195.45 \text{ K}(-77.7°C) \qquad \text{(Ref. 54)}$$

Place point A to represent ammonia gas having enthalpy of 1548 kJ/kg. Point B represents liquid water at 303 K (30°C). Tie-line AB intersects 15% aqueous ammonia solution axis at 373 K (100°C). *Ans.* (i)

For 15% NH_3,

$$\Delta H_f^0 = -79.3 \text{ kJ/mol } NH_3 \qquad \text{(Ref. Table 5.40)}$$

for gaseous NH_3,

$$\Delta H_f^0 = -45.94 \text{ kJ/mol } NH_3$$

$$\text{Heat of solution} = -79.3 - (-45.94) = -33.36 \text{ kJ/mol } NH_3$$

$$\text{Total heat generated} = \frac{33\,360 \times 140}{17.0305} = 274\,236 \text{ kJ/h}$$

$$\equiv 76.18 \text{ kW}$$

$$\text{Aqueous solution rate} = \frac{140}{0.15} = 933.33 \text{ kg/h}$$

$$\text{Rise in temperature} = \frac{274\,236}{(4.145 \times 933.33)} = 70.9 \text{ K}$$

$$\text{Temperature of aqueous solution} = 70.9 + 303 = 373.9 \text{ K} \qquad \textit{Ans.} \text{ (ii)}$$

Example 5.48 Solve Example 5.30 with the help of data given in Table 5.40.
Solution For 2% NH_3 (mass),

$$\Delta H_f^0 = -80.14 \text{ kJ/mol } NH_3$$

For gaseous NH_3

$$\Delta H_f^0 = -45.94 \text{ kJ/mol } NH_3$$

$$\text{Heat of solution} = -80.14 - (-45.94) = -34.2 \text{ kJ/mol } NH_3$$

$$\text{Heat generated for making 2\% solution} = 34\,200 \times \frac{2}{17.0306}$$

$$= 4016.3 \text{ kJ/00 kg solution} \qquad Ans.$$

$$\text{Error introduced in Example 5.30} = \left(\frac{4016.3 - 3456}{4016.3}\right) 100 = 14\%$$

Note: It may be seen that an error of the order of 14% is introduced by using the heat of reaction instead of data on the actual heat of formation. This is because the latter data are determined experimentally and also take into consideration heat of mixing.

Example 5.49 Refer Example 4.10 and Example 5.34. It is reported in literature[55] that the exothermic heat of solution of formaldehyde gas in water is substantially independent of concentration and has a value of 62.75 kJ/mol HCHO at 298.15 K (25°C) up to a concentration of about 40% (by mass) of HCHO. Considering a small concentration of methanol in absorber feed gas, its heat of solution may be neglected.

Assume heat capacity of 37% HCHO solution to be 3.45 kJ/(kg·K). Make heat balance of the absorber and calculate the heat duty of the cooler.
Solution Enthalpy of gas mixture, entering the absorber

$$\phi_5 = \phi_3 - \phi_4$$

$$= 15\,505\,407 - 11\,395\,056$$

$$= 4110\,351 \text{ kJ/h}$$

$$\equiv 1141.77 \text{ kW}$$

Heat evolved by absorption, $\phi_6 = 111.375 \times 62.75 \times 1000$

$$= 6988\,781 \text{ kJ/h}$$

$$\cong 1941.33 \text{ kW}$$

Table 5.41 Heat Capacity Data of Absorber Exit Gas Stream

Component	n_i kmol/h	Heat capacity ($C°_{mpab}$) equation constants			
		$n_i \cdot a_i$	$n_i \cdot b_i \times 10^3$	$n_i \cdot c_i \times 10^6$	$n_i \cdot d_i \times 10^9$
CO_2	8.786	187.7	564.8	−360.7	86.1
CO	0.990	28.7	−2.8	11.5	−4.7
H_2	1.980	56.6	2.0	−0.3	1.5
CH_4	0.619	11.9	32.3	7.4	−7.0
$(CH_3)_2O$	0.990	65.1			
O_2	212.712	5 536.0	2500.5	−498.3	119.6
N_2	1058.167	31 310.1	−5439.7	13 948.8	−5256.6
H_2O	147.167	4 781.8	11.7	1 994.2	−669.2
Total	1431.344	41 978.0	−2331.2	15 052.6	−5730.3

Enthalpy of absorber exit gas stream,

$$\phi_7 = \int_{298.15}^{323.15} C°_{mpab}\, dT$$

$$= 1063\ 375\ \text{kJ/h}$$

$$\equiv 295.38\ \text{kW}$$

Enthalpy of fresh water, $\phi_8 = 5532.15 \times 4.1868\ (303.15 - 298.15)$

$$= 115\ 810\ \text{kJ/h}$$

$$= 32.17\ \text{kW}$$

Enthalpy of formaldehyde solution, ϕ_9

$$= 9030.4 \times 3.45\ (323.15 - 298.15)$$

$$= 778\ 872\ \text{kJ/h}$$

$$= 216.35\ \text{kW}$$

Heat removal in the cooler

$$= \phi_5 + \phi_6 + \phi_8 - \phi_7 - \phi_9$$

$$= 1141.77 + 1941.33 + 32.17 - 295.38 - 216.35$$

$$= 2603.54\ \text{kW} \hspace{2cm} \textit{Ans.}$$

5.20 HEAT OF SOLUTION BY PARTIAL MOLAL QUANTITIES

Any extensive property G can be obtained by a knowledge of partial molal quantities. Let a mixture of m compounds have partial molal quantities $\overline{G}_1, \overline{G}_2, \ldots$ At any given temperature and pressure, these quantities are defined as

$$\overline{G} = \left(\frac{\partial G}{\partial n_1}\right)_{T,p,n_2,n_3 \ldots n_m} \hspace{2cm} (5.66)$$

$$\ldots\ldots\ldots\ldots\ldots\ldots\ldots\ldots\ldots\ldots$$

$$\overline{G}m = \left(\frac{\partial G}{\partial n_m}\right)_{T,p,n_2,n_3 \ldots n_{m-1}} \hspace{2cm} (5.67)$$

Combining all of them,

$$dG = \left\{\frac{\partial G}{\partial n_1}\right\} dn_1 + \left\{\frac{\partial G}{\partial n_2}\right\} dn_2 + \ldots + \left\{\frac{\partial G}{\partial n_m}\right\} dn_m$$

$$= \overline{G}_1\, dn_1 + \overline{G}_2\, dn_2 + \ldots + \overline{G}_m\, dn_m \hspace{1.5cm} (5.68)$$

For a binary system,

$$dG = \overline{G}_1\, dn_1 + \overline{G}_2\, dn_2 \hspace{2cm} (5.69)$$

Since $\overline{G}_1$ and $\overline{G}_2$ are always constant for a given concentration and for a given temperature of a given solution and are independent of the quantity of past history of the solution, the partial molal quantities are intensive properties of the solution. A table of partial molal quantities can be used to calculate the corresponding extensive property of the solution.

Enthalpy of the mixture of the solution is the extensive property which can be obtained from partial molal enthalpy (intensive property) of component.

In Table 5.42, the partial molal heats of solution at 291.15 K (18°C) of the SO_3–H_2O system are given. $\bar{H}_1$ and $\bar{H}_2$ are the respective partial molal heats of solution of H_2O and SO_3.

$$\text{Enthalpy of mixture, } H_m = n_1 \bar{H}_1 + n_2 \bar{H}_2 \qquad (5.70)$$

Table 5.42 Partial Molal Heats of Dilution of Sulphur Trioxide (Liquid) in Water (Liquid)[56]

Mole fraction of SO₃	Mass percent			Enthalpy, kJ/mol		
	SO_3	H_2SO_4	Free SO₃ (based on H_2SO_4)	ΔH/mol solution	$\bar{H}_1$/mol water in solution	$\bar{H}_2$/mol SO₃ in solution
(1)	(2)	(3)	(4)	(5)	(6)	(7)
0.00[a]	0.0	0.0	–			– 181.079
0.02	8.33	10.2	–	– 3.266	– 0.042	– 161.192
0.04	15.60	19.1	–	– 6.322	– 0.084	– 157.005
0.05	19.00	23.2	–	– 7.913	– 0.335	– 156.168
0.07	25.1	30.8	–	– 10.969	– 0.879	– 154.074
0.10	33.6	40.5	–	– 15.282	– 2.093	– 134.438
0.15	44.0	53.8	–	– 21.562	– 3.559	– 125.981
0.20	52.6	64.4	–	– 27.758	– 5.066	– 117.691
0.25	59.7	73.1	–	– 32.657	– 10.844	– 98.683
0.30	65.6	80.6	–	– 36.802	– 16.663	– 83.317
0.35	70.5	86.4	–	– 39.649	– 21.604	– 73.269
0.40	74.8	91.6	–	– 41.868	– 26.502	– 64.812
0.45	78.4	96.1	–	– 43.585	– 32.657	– 56.940
0.50[c]	81.6	100.0	–	– 44.338	– 44.338	– 44.338
0.52	82.5	–	6.4	– 43.752	– 66.654	– 22.609
0.55	84.5	–	15.4	– 42.287	– 71.887	–18.213
0.60	87.0	–	29.0	– 39.230	– 81.643	– 10.886
0.65	89.2	–	41.2	– 35.672	– 81.643	– 10.886
0.70	91.2	–	52.1	– 32.155	– 84.908	– 9.295
0.75	93.0	–	62.0	– 27.675	– 97.762	– 4.229
0.80	94.7	–	71.0	– 22.944	– 98.641	– 3.977
0.85	96.2	–	79.2	– 17.794	– 100.274	– 3.349
0.90	97.6	–	86.7	– 12.686	– 113.923	– 1.633
0.95	98.8	–	93.6	– 6.699	– 129.791	– 0.042
1.00[b]	100.0	–	100.0	–	– 154.912	–

[a]Heat of solution of 1 mol SO_3 in an infinite amount of water.
[b]Heat of solution of 1 mol water in an infinite amount of SO_3.
[c]Heat of formation of pure H_2SO_4 liquid.
Basis: At reference temperature of 291.15 K (18°C),

for H_2O (1), $\bar{H}_1$ =0.0 kJ/mol for SO_3 (1), $\bar{H}_2$ = 0.0 kJ/mol

(Reproduced with the permission of the American Chemical Society, USA)

Example 5.50 A solution containing 96.1% H_2SO_4 is diluted with pure water to form 23.2% H_2SO_4 solution. Using partial molal quantities given in Table 5.42, calculate heat of dilution at 291.15 K (18°C).

Also calculate the temperature of 23.2% solution after dilution. All percentage by mass.

Solution Basis: 100 kg 96.1% H_2SO

From Table 5.42, it is clear that 100 kg 96.1% H_2SO_4 solution contains 78.4 kg SO_3 and 21.6 kg water.

$$SO_3 \text{ in the solution} = \frac{78.4}{80.063} = 0.98 \text{ kmol}$$

$$H_2O \text{ in the solution} = \frac{21.6}{18.015} = 1.2 \text{ kmol}$$

The resultant solution has 23.2% H_2SO_4, i.e., 100 kg 23.2% H_2SO_4 contains 19 kg SO_3 and 81 kg water.

$$\text{Mass of the resultant solution after dilution} = \frac{78.4}{0.19} = 412.63 \text{ kg}$$

$$\text{Water added for dilution} = 412.63 - 100 = 312.53 \text{ kg}$$

$$\text{In the resultant solution, water} = \frac{(412.63 - 78.4)}{18.015} = 18.57 \text{ kmol}$$

The dilution process can be written as:

0.98 kmol SO_3 in 1.2 kmol H_2O

$$+ \ 17.37 \text{ kmol } H_2O = 0.98 \text{ kmol } SO_3 \text{ in } 18.57 \text{ kmol } H_2O$$

In terms of enthalpies,

Total enthalpy of original

solution + enthalpy of water

$$+ \text{ enthalpy of mixing } H^E = \text{total enthalpy of final solution}$$

The enthalpies of aqueous acids can be calculated using the partial molal enthalpies given in Table 5.42.

Total enthalpy of original

$$\text{solution (96.1\% acid) at 291.15 K} = 0.98 \times (-56\ 940) + 1.2\ (-32\ 657)$$

$$= -55\ 801 - 39\ 188 = -94\ 989 \text{ kJ}$$

Total enthalpy of resultant

$$\text{solution (23.2\% acid) at 291.15 K} = 0.98 \times (-156\ 168) + 18.57\ (-335)$$

$$= -153\ 045 - 6221 = -159\ 266 \text{ kJ}$$

$$\text{Enthalpy of water at 291.15 K} = 0 \text{ kJ (basis of the table)}$$

$$H^E = -159\ 266 - (-94\ 989)$$

$$= -64\ 277 \text{ kJ/100 kg original acid}$$

$$\equiv -642.77 \text{ kJ/kg original acid}$$

From Fig. 5.5,

$$\text{Average specific heat} = 3.43 \text{ kJ/kg} \cdot \text{K})$$

$$\text{Rise in temperature} = \frac{64\,277}{(412.63 \times 3.43)} = 45.4 \text{ K}$$

Final temperature of the resultant solution = 45.4 + 291.15 = 336.55 K (63.4°C)

Check: Using Fig. 5.15 it can be found that the resultant temperature of final solution is 336 K (63°C).

Alternative Route:

(Moles of original aqueous acid) × (heat of solution of original aqueous acid) + (moles of water) × (enthalpy of water) + enthalpy of mixing

$$H^E = \text{(moles of final acid)} \times \text{(heat solution of final acid)}$$
$$H^E = (18.57 + 0.98)\,(-7913)$$
$$\qquad - (1.2 + 0.98)\,(-43\,585)$$
$$\qquad = -1154\,699 + 95\,105$$
$$\qquad = -59\,684 \text{ kJ/100 kg original acid} \qquad\qquad \textit{Ans.}$$

Example 5.51 Refer Example 5.50. Instead of water at 291.15 K (18°C), if ice at 273.15 K (0°C) is added, what will be the heat of dilution?

Solution Basis: 100 kg original acid

Latent heat of fusion of ice at 273.15 K = 333.7 kJ/kg   (Refer Table 5.8)

Enthalpy of ice with reference to 291.15 K = 333.7 − 18.015 × 4.1868

$$= -408.8 \text{ kJ/kg}$$
$$H^E = -64\,277 + 408.8 \times 312.63$$
$$= \frac{63\,534}{100\,\text{kg}} \text{ original solution}$$

This means that 635.34 kJ/kg of original acid need be supplied to maintain the temperature 291.15 K of the original acid.   *Ans.*

Example 5.52 Refer Example 5.51. What is the quantity of ice required to be added in 96.2% acid for dilution so that the heat of dilution is zero?

Solution Basis: 100 kg original acid

Let x kg be the ice required. The ice should absorb all the exothermic heat of dilution.

$$410.4\,x = 64\,277$$

Therefore, $x = 156.62$ kg

This means that if 156.62 kg ice and (312.63 − 56.62) = 156.01 kg water at 291.15 K are added, the temperature of the resultant solution will rise over 291.15 K.

Partial molal excess enthalpy can be derived from *excess enthalpy* of the solution. By definition, excess enthalpy is the difference between the actual enthalpy and the enthalpy for an ideal solution at the same temperature and pressure. In other words, excess enthalpy of an ideal solution is zero.

The thermodynamic treatment of the excess properties and partial molal properties are outside the scope of the book. However, this subject is dealt in sufficient details in Refs. 2 and 20. Thermodynamics Research Centre, USA publishes International Data Series[57] for a number of binary systems of non-electrolyte organic substances.

Excess enthalpy data can be easily transformed into partial molal excess enthalpy. Normally excess enthalpy is plotted against mole % concentration of the component for a given temperature. At a desired concentration, a tangent is drawn on the graph and the intercepts on the y-axis give partial molal excess enthalpies.

5.21 DATA SOURCES

There are a number of institutions in the world which have compiled thermodynamic data for organic and inorganic compounds. Among these, Thermodynamics Research Centre (TRC), USA is one of the oldest and highly respected data centres in the world. The TRC Thermodynamic Tables (formerly the API Research Project 44 and the Manufacturing Chemists Association Research Project) are the most favourably cited source of evaluated thermophysical and thermodynamic information (Ref. 58). Founded by Dr. F. D. Rossini, in 1942 the Centre is constantly engaged in updating the information.

Design Institute for Physical Property Data (DIPPD), sponsored by the American Institute for Chemical Engineers (AIChE), USA is also actively engaged in compiling the physical, thermodynamic and transport properties of various compounds. Further supplements are periodically published covering data on additional chemicals.

National Institute of Standards and Technology (NIST), USA is yet another source which have brought out Technical Note-270 series on Selected Values of Chemical Thermodynamic Properties of organic and inorganic compounds (Ref. 59).

Monsanto Co., USA compiled a physical properties package, called FLOWTRAN[6]. Compilation by Yaws and his colleagues are also popular in the chemical process industry (Ref. 60).

In addition to above, there are large number of other data source such as DECHEMA databooks, Ullmann's Encyclopedia of Industrial Chemistry, Perry's Chemical Engineers' Handbook[20], etc. A series of tables are published by the Commission on Thermodynamics and Thermochemistry of the Physical Chemistry Division of the International Union of Pure and Applied Chemistry (IUPAC)[61], compiling internationally agreed values of the thermodynamic properties of liquids and gases. Reader may refer the relevant references for obtaining the requisite data for process engineering calculations.

EXERCISES

5.1 A thermic fluid (derived from a petroleum stock) is used as a heating medium in a particular process. A pump sucks the thermic fluid at atmospheric pressure and 473 K (200°C). The circulation rate is 10 000 L/h. The fluid discharged from the pump, passes through a heater (coil type) where it receives the heat from the product gases of combustion.

The heat transfer rate is 232.6 kW. The motor of the pump consumes 1.1 kW. The overall mechanical efficiency of the pump and motor is 50%. The pressure of the fluid at the outlet of the heater is 100 kPa g. Assume (i) negligible kinetic energy changes, (ii) negligible potential energy changes, (iii) negligible friction losses and (iv) no heat loss to the surrounding. If the mean specific gravity and mean heat capacity of the fluid are 0.75 and 2.68 kJ/(kg·K) respectively at the operating conditions, calculate the outlet temperature of the fluid.

[*Ans.* 541.7 K (241.7°C)]

5.2 Temperature of pure oxygen is raised from 350 to 1500 K. Calculate the amount of heat to be supplied for raising the temperature of 1 kmol oxygen using the following C_{mp}^0 data given in Table 5.1[4,6] and the absolute enthalpies given in Table 5.21.

[*Ans.* (i) 39 122.6 kJ; Ref. 4 (ii) 39 066 kJ; Ref. 6
(iii) 39 146 kJ; Table 5.21]

5.3 Heat capacity data for gaseous SO_2 are reported in Table 5.1[6,10] and also by the following equation[62].

$$C_{mp}^0 = 43.458 + 10.634 \times 10^{-3}\, T - 5.945 \times \frac{10^5}{T^2}$$

Calculate the heat required to raise the temperature of 1 kmol pure sulphur dioxide from 300 to 1000 K (27 to 727°C), using the above three equations. Also calculate the same by using absolute enthalpies given in Table 5.21.

[*Ans.* (a) 34 164.6 kJ/kmol (Ref. 6)
(b) 34 385.8 kJ/kmol (Ref. 10)
(c) 33 871.9 kJ/kmol (Ref. 62)
(d) 33 564 kJ/kmol (Table 5.21)]

5.4 In a fertilizer plant, naphtha (C: H = 6:1) is used as the feedstock. The gas mixture coming out of the absorber has the following composition by volume on dry basis: CH_4: 0.25%, CO: 0.38% CO_2: 0.10%, H_2: 74.62%, N_2: 24.35% and Ar: 0.3%.

The gas mixture contains 0.0126 kmol water vapour per kmol of the dry gas mixture. The mixture comes out at 343 K (70°C) and is passed through a methanator preheater where it is heated to 618 K (345°C). Calculate the heat duty of the preheater per 100 kmol of the dry gas mixture. If the above gas mixture is saturated with water vapour when it comes out of the absorber, find the total pressure of the gas mixture at the inlet of the preheater.

[*Ans.* (a) 818 230 kJ, based on data of Table 5.1
(b) 817 114 kJ, based on data of Table 5.21
(c) 25.05 bar a]

5.5 A heat exchanger for cooling a hot hydrocarbon liquid uses 10 000 kg/h of cooling water, which enters the exchanger at 294 K (21°C). The hot oil at the rate of 5000 kg/h enters at 423 K (150°C) and leaves at

338 K (65°C) and has an average heat capacity of 2.51 kJ/(kg·K). Calculate the outlet temperature of water.

[*Ans.* 319.5 K (46.5°C)]

5.6 A mixture of isomeric diphenyl-diphenyloxides (Diphyl DT*) is used as a thermic fluid in a liquid phase heating system[19]. The thermic fluid enters an indirect fired heater at 453 K (180°C) and leaves it at 553 K (260°C). The heat capacity of the fluid is given by

$$C_1 = 1.436 + 0.002\ 18\ T\ \text{kJ/(kg·K)}$$

where T is in K.

(i) Calculate the supply of heat in the heater per kg of the liquid heated.

(ii) If the heat capacity of Diphyl DT at 453 K (180°C) and 533 K (260°C) are 2.03 and 2.206 kJ/(kg·K) respectively, how much error will be involved in the computation of heat load using the mean heat capacity value?

[*Ans.* (i) 200.4 kJ/kg (ii) − 15.5%]

5.7 Liquid benzene, C_6H_6 at 303 K (30°C) is mixed and dissolved continuously in liquid toluene, C_7H_8 at 373 K (100°C) in molar proportion 3:2 in an insulated mixing tank. If the heat of mixing is assumed to be zero, what is the temperature of the mixed solution?

Table 5.43 Heat Capacity Data[20] for Benzene and Toluene

Temperature K (°C)	Heat capacity (C_l), kJ/(kg · K)	
	Benzene	Toluene
283 (10)	1.591	1.524
338 (65)	2.018	—
358 (86)	—	2.236

Assume the variation of the heat capacity is linear with temperature, i.e.

$$C_1 = a + bT\ \text{kJ(kg·K)}$$

where a and b are constants

[*Ans.* 336.6 K (63.6°C)]

(b) Solve the problem by using data given in Table 5.3.

[*Ans.* 334.3 K (61.3°C)]

5.8 Using Antoine equation, calculate vapour pressure of

(a) acetic acid at 316 K (43°C) (Ref. 23) and

(b) sulphur trioxide at 293.5 K (20.5°C) (Ref. 6)

[*Ans.* (a) 5.37 kPa; (b) 26.694 kPa]

5.9 Using Watson equation, calculate latent heat of vaporization of

(a) acetone at 313 K (40°C) and

(b) carbon disulphide at 413 K (140°C)

[*Ans.* (a) 30 109 kJ/kmol; (b) 21 971 kJ/kmol]

* Registered trade mark of Bayer, Germany.

5.10 Using Antoine equation, calculate the normal boiling point (T_B) of chlorobenzene. Also calculate its latent heat of vaporization at T_B using Riedel equation.

[*Ans.* (a) 404.85 K (131.85°C) (b) 35 490 kJ/kmol]

5.11 Naphthalene is evaporated in a jacketed closed vessel. Pure naphthalene is fed to the vessel at 303 K (30°C) and is vaporised at atmospheric pressure by condensing the eutectic mixture of diphenyl-diphenyl oxide vapours in the jacket at 171 kPa a. Assume no subcooling of the vapours. Calculate the quantity of eutectic mixture of diphenyl oxide condensed per 100 kg naphthalene evaporated.

Data on Naphthalene[20]:

Formula: $C_{10}H_8$

$$\text{Molar mass} = 128.1735$$

$$\text{Melting point} = 353.2 \text{ K } (80.2°C)$$

$$\text{Boiling point} = 491 \text{ K } (218°C)$$

$$\text{Latent heat of fusion, } \lambda_f = 150.7 \text{ kJ/kg}$$

$$\text{Latent heat of vaporization, } \lambda_v = 316.1 \text{ kJ/kg}$$

Heat capacity of solid naphthalene,

$$C_s = -0.092 + 0.0046 \, T \text{ kJ/(kg} \cdot \text{K)}$$

where T is the temperature in K

Table 5.44	Heat Capacity of Liquid Naphthalene	
Temperature, K(°C)		C_l kJ/(kg $\cdot$ K)
353 (80)		1.738
473 (200)		2.135

Assume linear relationship of C_l with T and use the same for evaluating the heat load. Use data given in Table 5.6.

[*Ans.* 277.1 kg eutectic mixture]

5.12 Superheated steam at a pressure of 4.4 bar a and 543 K (216°C) is available from one source at the rate of 10 000 kg/h. Another source supplies saturated 4.4 bar a steam at the rate of 7500 kg/h. Both the streams are mixed. Assuming no heat loss, calculate the conditions of steam after mixing.

[*Ans.* 4.4 bar a, 489 K (216°C), Superheated]

5.13 Superheated steam is available at 5 bar a and 523 K (250°C), Calculate the quantity of water needed to be sprayed at 303 K (30°C) for saturating 100 kg superheated steam.

[*Ans.* 8.15 kg]

5.14 A cylinder drying range (in a textile mill) uses saturated steam at 310 kPa a. The low pressure steam is obtained by pressure reduction from steam source at 780 kPa a and desuperheating with condensate saturated at atmospheric pressure. The let down system is shown in Fig. 5.20.

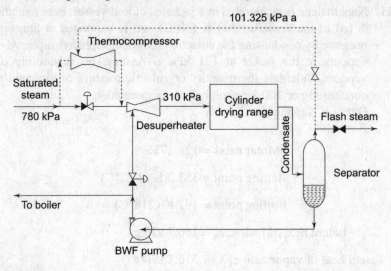

101.325 kPa a

Thermocompressor

Saturated steam
780 kPa

310 kPa

Cylinder drying range

Desuperheater

Flash steam

Condensate

Separator

To boiler

BWF pump

Fig. 5.20 Efficient Use of Steam in a Cylinder Drying Range

As a part of an energy saving drive, it is proposed to compress the flash steam at atmospheric pressure through a steam jet thermocompressor (an ejector) with the help of motive 780 kPa a saturated steam. This proposed modification is indicated in dotted lines in Fig. 5.20. Calculate the percentage reduction in steam consumption of 780 kPa a with the use of the thermocompressor.

[*Ans.* 6.35%]

5.15 In a fertilizer plant, partial oxidation of naphtha yields the gas mixture having the composition on a dry basis:
H_2: 55.7%, CO: 34.5%, CO_2: 2.8%; CH_4: 0.5% and N_2: 6.5% (by volume)
Steam to dry gas mixture is 1.85 on molar basis.
The temperature of the gas mixture is 1473 K (1200°C). The hot gases are passed through a waste heat boiler (WHB) in which they are cooled to 573 K (300°C) by heat exchange with water. Saturated steam is produced at 40 bar g. Based on 100 kmol of gas mixture, calculate the amount of steam generated. Assume that water is fed at 20 K lower than its saturation temperature (why?) and there is no heat loss to surroundings.

[*Ans.* 5452 kg]

5.16 Liquid ammonia is stored at 705 kPa a in a tank. It is discharged to an atmospheric storage. Calculate the percentage flash vapours produced letting down the pressure.

Table 5.45 Properties of Ammonia[54]

Pressure, kPa a	Saturation temperature K (°C)	Enthalpy, kJ/kg		
		Sensible h	Total H	Latent λ_v
705	287.15 (14)	265.56	1475.1	1209.6
101.3	239.82 (–33.3)	49.1	1418.7	1369.6

[Reference state: h = 200 kJ/kg at 273.15 K(0°C)]

[*Ans.* 15.47%]

5.17 In Fig. 5.21 a two-stage compressor is demonstrated to liquefy ammonia vapours. This is a common system for atmospheric ammonia storage facility. These vapours are sucked at 108.4 kPa a (saturated) at the rate of 100 kg/h. Compressed vapours from the first stage are taken to a flash cooler where liquid ammonia obtained from the aftercooler of the second stage is sprayed. The product rate from the flash cooler is 100 kg/h liquid ammonia at 276 K (3°C). The cooled vapours are sucked in the second stage. The vapours discharged by the second stage are cooled in the aftercooler in which the cooling water enters at 305 K (32°C). Calculate (a) the quantity of liquid ammonia obtained from the after cooler and (b) the flow rate of cooling water in the aftercooler in kg/s assuming a rise of 8 K.

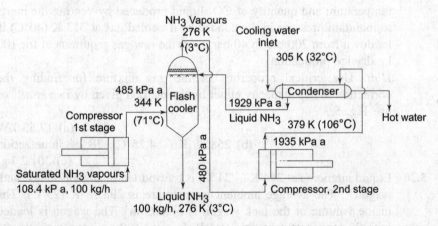

Fig. 5.21 Liquefaction of Ammonia

Use data of Table 5.46.

[*Ans.* (a) 137.13 kg/h, (b) 1.402 kg/s]

5.18 Pure liquid carbon dioxide is available at 273.15 K (0°C). It is required at 1.0 MPa g and 313 K (40°C) for purging purpose. Using the p–H diagram for CO_2 (Fig. 5.11), (a) calculate the percent vapour formed by pressure reduction from saturation pressure to 10 bar g and (b)

Table 5.46 Properties of Ammonia[54]

Conditions of ammonia vapours	Pressure kPa a	Saturation temperature K(°C)	Enthalpy, kJ/kg		
			Sensible h	Total H	Latent λ_v
Saturated	108.37	241 (– 32)	54.97	1420.65	1365.68
Superheated	485.0	344 (71)		1632.68	
Saturated	480.0	276 (3)	213.92	1464.93	1251.00
Superheated	1935.0	379 (106)		1663.91	
Saturated	1930.3	321 (48)	431.07	1491.07	1060.00

calculate the enthalpy required to be provided in a vaporiser to achieve final gas at 313 K (40°C).

[*Ans.* (a) 27.7% (b) 311 kJ/kg CO_2]

5.19 In Example 5.18, pure CO_2 was assumed to be available at 200 bar a for dry ice production. Assume now that the composition of dry gas is as follows:

CO_2: 94.7%, H_2: 1.5%, N_2: 3.0% and O_2: 0.8% (by volume)

Also consider that CO_2 condenser (shown in Fig. 5.10), employing ammonia as refrigerant, is not used. Calculate (a) the heat load on the water cooler for the production of 100 kg/h of dry ice, (b) the temperature and quantity of CO_2 liquid produced by venting the inerts to maintain pressure in the condenser if cooled gas at 313 K (40°C) is let down from 200 bar to 40 bar a, (c) the raw gas requirement for 100 kg dry ice production.

Hint: Use critical properties of the gas mixture for finding the correction in heat capacity either by the method given by Lee *et al*[13] or use Fig. 5.3.

[*Ans.* (a) 17.55 kW
(b) 268.75 K (– 4.25°C), 78.2% liquefaction
(c) 301.2 kg]

5.20 Liquid ammonia at 244 K (– 24°C) is transported in an uninsulated tank wagon[63]. The average ambient temperature is 298.15 K (25°C). The inside volume of the tank wagon is 60.663 m³. The wagon is loaded with 32 tonnes of ammonia (total). In transit, the wagon receives the heat from the atmosphere as given by the equation

$$Q = 1.3 \, (T_a - T) + 3.76 \text{ kW}$$

where T_a is the ambient temperature and T is the temperature of ammonia inside the tank wagon in K.

Calculate the time required to attain 256 (– 17°C) in the wagon of ammonia by two methods, (a) the numerical integration approach for each 2 K rise in temperature and (b) use average values of temperature and heat exchange rates.

Table 5.47 Properties of Saturated Ammonia[54]

Temperature K(°C)	Saturation pressure kPa a	Density, kg/m³		Enthalpy, kJ/kg	
		Liquid	Vapour	Liquid	Vapour
244 (−29)	125.48	676.25	1.0844	68.32	1425.06
246 (−27)	138.06	673.50	1.1858	77.25	1427.94
248 (−25)	151.63	671.25	1.2947	86.20	1430.77
250 (−23)	166.24	668.70	1.4114	95.17	1433.55
252 (−21)	181.97	666.15	1.5364	104.17	1436.30
254 (−19)	198.86	663.60	1.6699	113.18	1438.97
256 (−17)	216.97	661.05	1.8124	122.22	1441.61

[*Ans.* (a) 7.319 h, (b) 7.283 h]

5.21 Dry air is transported in 50 mm NB pipe at the rate of 1650 Nm³/h. Air enters the pipe at 463 K (190°C) and is utilised at another end of the pipe which is 150 m away. The pipe is bare and the ambient temperature is 308 K (35°C). The heat loss from such a pipe is given by Fig. 5.23. Assume that the heat capacity of dry air is 1.006 kJ/(kg·K). Calculate the temperature of air at the utilisation point by adopting the numerical integration approach for each 10 K cooling.

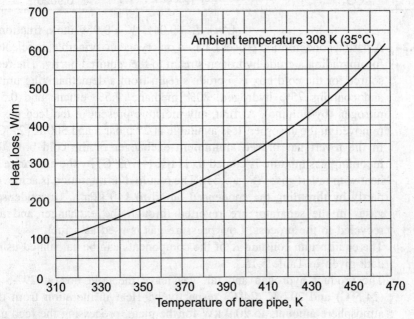

Fig. 5.23 Heat Loss from Bare Pipe of 50 mm NB Size

[*Ans.* 371.4 K (98.4°C)]

5.22 Calculate the bubble point (T_{BB}) and dew point (T_{DP}) of a benzene-toluene mixture having 0.6 mole fraction benzene at 101.325 kPa. Also determine enthalpy of the liquid mixture at T_{BB} and that of the vapour mixture at T_{DP} above 273.15 K (0°C). Compare the enthalpy values with those, read from Fig. 6.1. Assume that the mixture follows ideal behaviour.

[Ans. T_{BB} = 362.75 K (89.75°C), Enthalpy at T_{BB} =13 281 kJ/kmol
T_{DP} = 369.1 K (96.1°C), Enthalpy at T_{DP} = 45 837 kJ/kmol

5.23 Natural gas having the following composition[64] is compressed and cooled to 41.4 bar a and 266.5 K (– 6.5°C). Calculate the liquid and vapour fractions.

Table 5.48 Natural Gas Liquefaction

Component	Mole %	K_i
CH_4	89.57	2.70
C_2H_6	5.26	0.38
C_3H_8	1.97	0.098
$i\text{-}C_4H_{10}$	0.68	0.038
$n\text{-}C_4H_{10}$	0.47	0.024
C_5H_{12}	0.38	0.0075
C_6H_{14}	0.31	0.0019
C_7H_{16}	0.24	0.0007
CO_2	1.12	0.9000

[Ans. L = 0.041, V = 0.959 mole fractions]

5.24 A partial condensation process, based on cryogenic principle, is selected for upgrading a crude hydrogen stream to the required purity. The feed source for the cold box is a crude stream from a demethanizing unit[39] and contains 75% hydrogen, 20% methane, 4.5% ethane and 0.5% nitrogen (by volume). At first, any moisture present in the feed gas is removed in the absorber. It is available at 27.5 bar a and 300 K (27°C). In the revert gas brazed aluminium exchanger of the cold box, the incoming gas mixture is cooled to 111 K (– 163°C) by the exchange of heat with revert gases (Fig. 5.24). The required refrigeration is achieved partly by throttling the condensed liquid to 140 kPa a. Uncondensed gases in the separator are reverted through the exchanger and are recycled to the process. Low pressure gas is used as a fuel.

The equilibrium constant K of the components can be calculated using data given in Table 5.15.

The product hydrogen and tail gas leave the cold box at 297.5 K (24.5°C) and 297 K (24°C) respectively. Heat infiltration from the atmosphere amounts to 20.9 kW for the plant, processing the feed gas at the rate of 18 720 Nm³/h. Supplementary refrigeration is provided in the form of an external refrigeration set. Calculate (a) the recovery of hydrogen defined as kmol hydrogen recycled to that in the feed, (b) the purity of product hydrogen stream in terms of hydrogen and (c) the refrigeration requirement (in kW), using data given in Table 5.49.

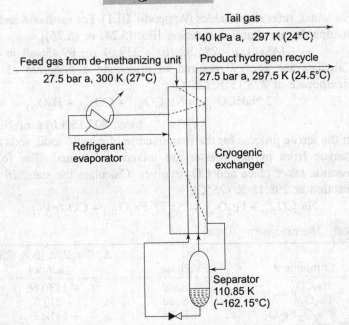

Fig. 5.24 Hydrogen Recovery from Gases from De-methanizing Unit

Table 5.49 Enthalpy of Gases[43]

| Conditions | Enthalpy*, kJ/kg | | | |
	Hydrogen	Methane	Ethane	Nitrogen
27.5 bar a and 300 K (27°C)	4243	– 3569	– 1967	304
27.5 bar a and 297.5 K (24.5°C)	4206	– 3575	– 1973	301
140 kPa a and 297 K (24°C)	4188	– 3550	– 1915	306

*Base Conditions: Enthalpy at 0 kPa a and 0 K = 0 kJ/kg

[*Ans.* (a) 99.4%, (b) 95.1%, (c) 6.67 kW]

5.25 Calculate the heat of formation of the following compounds at 298.15 K (25°C) using the data on heats of combustion.
   (a) Gaseous *n*-heptane
   (b) Gaseous ethyl alcohol
   (c) Liquid 1, 3-butadiene

[*Ans.* (a) – 187.83, (b) – 234.44, (c) + 88.56; all in kJ/mol]

5.26 Calculate the standard heat of formation of the following liquids at 298.15 K (25°C) using the data of standard heat of formation of vapours at 298.15 K (25°C) and the latent heat of vaporization at 298.15 K (25°C).
   (a) Water
   (b) Methanol
   (c) Carbon disulphide

For water, refer steam tables (Appendix III.1). For methanol and carbon disulphide, use Antoine equation [Eq. (5.24) or (5.25)].

[*Ans.* (a) − 285.82 (b) − 239.04 (c) 89.45; all in kJ/mol]

5.27 Calculate the energy required to dissociate a kilogram of sodium bicarbonate at 298.15 K (25°C).

$$2\ NaHCO_{3(s)} = Na_2CO_{3(s)} + CO_{2(g)} + H_2O_{(g)}$$

[*Ans.* 807.15 kJ/kg of $NaHCO_3$]

5.28 In the ferrite process for the manufacture of caustic soda, soda ash and gangue from pyrites roaster are mixed and heated. The following reaction takes place and CO_2 evolves. Calculate the standard heat of reaction at 298.15 K (25°C).

$$Na_2CO_{3(s)} + Fe_2O_{3(s)} = Na_2O \cdot Fe_2O_{3(s)} + CO_2(g)$$

Table 5.50 Thermodynamic Data

Component	Phase	ΔH_f° at 298.15 K (25°C), kJ/mol
Na_2CO_3	Solid	− 1130.68
Fe_2O_3	Solid	− 817.3
$Na_2O.Fe_2O_3$	Solid	− 1412.2
CO_2	Gas	− 393.51

[*Ans.* + 142.27 kJ/mol Na_2CO_3 or kJ/mol Fe_2O_3]

5.29 Refer Exercise 4.15. Make the heat balance and calculate the heat to be added or removed from the system using the absolute enthalpy data given in Table 5.21. [*Ans.* 81 522 kJ (endothermic)]

5.30 Refer Exercises 3.22 and 4.1. Assume heat of formation of coke ($CH_{0.6}$) to be 101.1 kJ/mol at 298.15 K (25°C). Calculate the heat generated during decoking assuming products of combustion as carbon dioxide and water. [*Ans.* 35 kJ]

5.31 Refer Example 4.18. Make heat balance of the plant assuming that air is preheated in the heat exchanger up to 523 K (250°C).

[*Ans.* Heat transfer duty of R I = 4239 kW
Heat transfer duty of R II = 5559.2 kW
Steam generation in boiler = 12 888.2 kg/h
Steam consumption in evaporator = 4011.7 kg/h]

5.32 Obtain an empirical equation for calculating the heat of reaction of temperature T (in K) for the reactions

(a) $CH_{4(g)} + C_2H_{4(g)} = C_3H_{8(g)}$

[*Ans.* $\Delta H_{RT}^\circ = 78\ 154 - 27.598\ T + 49.565 \times 10^{-3}\ T^2$
$- 29.686 \times 10^{-6}\ T^3 + 6.622 \times 10^{-9}\ T^4$]

(b) $CO_{(g)} + H_2O_{(g)} = CO_{2(g)} + H_{2(g)}$

[*Ans.* $\Delta H_{RT}^\circ = - 40\ 198 - 11.544\ T + 34.02 \times 10^{-3}\ T^2$
$- 22.018 \times 10^{-6}\ T^3 + 4.956 \times 10^{-9}\ T^4$]

(c) $CO_{(g)} + 2\ H_{2(g)} = CH_3OH_{(g)}$

[*Ans.* $\Delta H_{RT}^\circ = - 74\ 748 - 61.38\ T + 25.827 \times 10^{-3}\ T^2$
$- 15.76 \times 10^{-6}\ T^3 - 10.49 \times 10^{-9}\ T^4$]

Using the same equation, calculate the heat of reaction at 593 K (320°C) for the reaction (c). [*Ans.* – 100 075 kJ/kmol]

5.33 Enthalpy of a sour gas mixture from a refinery having composition; H_2S: 0.57%, CO_2: 2.46%, N_2: 0.31%, CH_4: 88.41%, C_2H_6: 5.33%, C_3H_8: 2.07% and $n\text{-}C_4H_{10}$: 0.85% (by volume), can be satisfactorily represented by following equation[21] in pressure range of 3000 to 5000 psia (206.4 to 344.7 bar a) and 250 to 350°F (394 to 482 K).

$$H = -34.38 + 0.7209\,t + 7.763 \times 10^{-6}\,t^2 + 1.075 \times 10^5/p$$

where $H =$ Enthalpy, Btu/lb

$t =$ Temperature, °F

$p =$ Pressure, psia

Convert the above equation in SI units.

5.34 Refer Exercise 4.12. Assume that the gaseous mixture enters the reactor at 588 K (315°C). Using the data of C^0_{mp} given in Table 5.1, calculate the outlet temperature of the product gas stream leaving the reactor.

[*Ans.* 671.5 K (398.5°C)]

5.35 Typical compositions of feed gas from various hydrogen production plants to a high temperature shift converter are given in Table 5.51.

Table 5.51 Typical Compositions of Feed Gas to HT Shift Converter

Gas	Partial oxidation of natural gas vol. %	Partial oxidation of fuel oil vol. %	Reforming of natural gas vol. %
CO	37	46	15
H_2	60	48	56
CO_2	2	5	7
N_2	–	–	21.7
Ar	1	1*	0.3
Steam to Gas ratio (x)	1.8		1.2

*Includes sulphur compounds also

Prove that in the temperature range of 618 K (345°C) to 783 K (510°C), the rise in temperature (in K) across the converter will be

$$\Delta T = \frac{12.5\,a}{1 + 1.2\,x}$$

where $a =$ moles of CO reacted per 100 moles of dry inlet gas

and $x =$ steam to dry gas mole ratio at the inlet

Hint: Use the mean heat capacity in the range 618 K (345°C) to 783 K (510°C) and assume that changes in composition due to the reaction does not appreciably affect the mean heat capacity of gas mixture. Also take average heat of reaction between 818 K and 783 K.

5.36 Oxides of nitrogen (NO_x) are the pollutants. The offgases from the dissolution of uranium oxides contain nitrogen, oxygen and nitrogen oxides. In order to eliminate NO_x from the gases, a converter is employed[65] in which Zeolite extrudates (of 1.5 mm diameter) are packed. The offgases are mixed with ammonia and passed through a catalyst bed, thereby reducing NO_x concentration to 50 ppm (v/v). The reaction taking place in the converter is

$$8\,NH_3 + 6\,NO_2 = 7\,N_2 + 12\,H_2O$$

The bed temperature increases significantly during the conversion [up to 1033 K (760°C)], depending on the inlet NO_x concentration] due to the exothermic heat of reaction. The conversion efficiency is nearly 100% when the bed temperature does not exceed about 753 K (480°C). At higher bed temperatures, the conversion efficiency drops to as low as 85% due to cracking of the excess ammonia gas which is needed to drive the reaction to completion. For temperature control, nitrogen is introduced along with the offgases and ammonia, if necessary. To prevent the formation of ammonium nitrate, the bed temperature is not allowed to drop below 588 K (315°C). Figure 5.25 represents the process schematically. Calculate (a) the excess ammonia and (b) the exit temperature of gases.

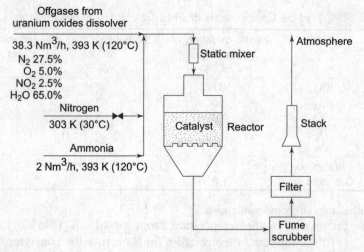

Offgases from
uranium oxides dissolver

38.3 Nm³/h, 393 K (120°C)
N₂ 27.5%
O₂ 5.0%
NO₂ 2.5%
H₂O 65.0%

Nitrogen
303 K (30°C)

Ammonia
2 Nm³/h, 393 K (120°C)

Static mixer

Catalyst Reactor

Atmosphere

Stack

Filter

Fume
scrubber

Fig. 5.25 Elimination of NO_2 from Offgases from Uranium Oxides

[*Ans.* (a) 56.6% (b) 703 K(430°C)]

5.37 Refer Exercise 5.36. Assume that offgases from the dissolver have the composition:

N₂: 26.5%, O₂: 5.0%, NO₂: 3.5% and H₂O: 65.0% (v/v).

Flow rate of offgases and ammonia are kept constant. Calculate the required flow rate of nitrogen for the control to exit temperature at 753 K (480°C).

[*Ans.* 7.31 Nm³/h]

5.38 In the manufacture of benzaldehyde a mixture of dry air and toluene is fed to the converter at a temperature of 448 K (175°C) and 100 kPa g pressure. The mixture passes through the catalyst bed in the converter. The product gas stream leaves the converter at 468 K (195°C). The reaction proceeds as follows:

$$C_6H_5CH_{3(g)} + O_{2(g)} = C_6H_5CHO_{(g)} + H_2O_{(g)}$$

In order to maintain the high yield of benzaldehyde, dry air is supplied in 100% excess. The side reaction taking place is the combustion of toluene to CO_2 and H_2O.

$$C_6H_5CH_{3(g)} + 9\,O_{2(g)} = 7\,CO_{2(g)} + 4\,H_2O_{(g)}$$

Pilot runs indicate that at the above operating conditions, the overall conversion is 13% based on toluene. Approximately 0.5% of the toluene charged burns to CO_2 and H_2O.

Assume that the mean heat capacity of benzaldehyde between 298.15 K (25°C) and 468 K (195°C) is 130 kJ/(kmol·K). Calculate (a) the composition of the wet gas stream leaving the converter and (b) the heat to be removed from or added to the system per kmol toluene fed to the converter.

Assume the standard heat of formation of benzaldehyde at 298.15 K (25°C) to be – 40.04 kJ/mol (ref. 20).

[Ans. (a) C_7H_8: 8.36%; C_6H_5CHO: 1.20%; O_2: 17.59%; N_2: 72.32%; CO_2: 0.34% and H_2O: 0.19 (on mole basis)]
(b) 35 306 kJ heat liberated per kmol toluene fed to the converter

5.39 In the process for manufacture of carbon disulphide (CS_2), natural gas is reacted with sulphur vapours over an activated catalyst according to the equation:

$$CH_{4(g)} + 2\,S_{2(g)} \underset{977\ K(704°C)}{\overset{\text{Activated catalyst}}{=}} CS_{2(g)} + 2\,H_2S_{(g)}$$

Pilot runs indicate that with natural gas containing 60 mole % CH_4 and 40 mole % N_2 reacting with sulphur vapours, S_2, the conversion of sulphur is 80% when 2 moles of natural gas are fed per mole of $S_{2(g)}$. Refer Fig. 5.26.

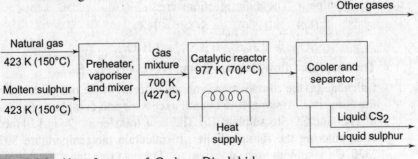

Fig. 5.26 Manufacture of Carbon Disulphide

The temperature in the catalyst reactor is maintained at 977 K (704°C) by supplying heat to the reactor. The gaseous mixture leaving the reactor passes through a cooler and separator where liquid carbon disulphide and liquid sulphur are separated.

Calculate (a) the excess reactant and the percentage excess of the reactant, (b) the kg of CS_2 produced per kmol of $S_{2(g)}$ (c) the analysis, mole %, of the hot gaseous mixture leaving the catalytic reactor, (d) the heat change, kJ per kmol of $S_{2(g)}$ entering the reactor to maintain the temperature at 977 K (704°C) using absolute enthalpies, given in Table 5.21 and (e) the vapour pressure of CS_2 at 298 K (25°C), using the Antoine equation. Absolute enthalpies for S_2 at 700 K and 977 K are + 22 951 and 33 118 kJ/kmol respectively.

[Ans. (a) CH_4 in 140% excess (b) 30.4 kg CS_2 produced per kmol $S_{2(g)}$ feed (c) CH_4: 26.67%; N_2: 26.67%; S_2: 6.67%; CS_2: 13.33%; H_2S: 26.66% (on mole basis) (d) – 2806 kJ/kmol S_2 (exothermic) (e) 48.1 kPa]

Notes: (i) From answer (e) it is clear that liquid carbon disulphide had appreciable vapour pressure of about 48.1 kPa even at 298.15 K. This means that the CS_2 should be cooled to a lower temperature than 298.15 K (25°C) or some other means should be provided for separating out the CS_2, e.g. adsorption on activated carbon, so as to reduce the potentially high losses of CS_2 in waste gas streams.
(ii) Answer (d) indicates that the reaction is slightly exothermic under operating conditions. However, in actual practice, the radiation and convection heat losses will be encountered from the hot shell of the reactor. Hence some heat may have to be supplied to the reactor in actual use.

5.40 The recovery of sulphur from hydrogen sulphide is achieved by the oxidation of H_2S which is available from petroleum refineries when the sour natural gas is purified. The H_2S-rich gaseous stream, also containing some inerts (e.g. N_2) is converted to liquid sulphur by the oxidation process. The two principal equipments in the plant are a furnace boiler where a portion of the H_2S is oxidized to SO_2 to form liquid sulphur. The main reactions are:

$$H_2S_{(g)} + 1.5\,O_{2(g)} = SO_{2(g)} + H_2O_{(g)}$$
$$SO_{2(g)} + 2\,H_2S_{(g)} = 3\,S_{(1)} + 2\,H_2O_{(g)}$$

The simplified flow diagram of the process is Fig. 5.27.

Calculate (a) the composition (volume percent) of the hot gases, leaving the converter. Assume 40% overall excess air and complete conversion of H_2S and SO_2 to sulphur. (b) The heat transfer at Q_1 in kJ/kmol of H_2S, entering the furnace boiler, to maintain the temperature 593 K (320°C), assuming no heat losses. (c) The heat transfer at Q_1 in kW for a production of 9000 kg/h of sulphur.

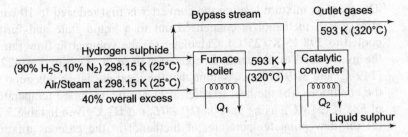

Fig. 5.27 Recovery of Sulphur from Hydrogen Sulphide

> [*Ans.* (a) O_2: 6.11%; N_2: 83.73%; H_2O: 10.16% (on mole basis)
> (b) – 419 370 kJ/kmol H_2S (exothermic)
> (c) Heat evolved at Q_1 is 10 921.1 kW.]

5.41 Methanol can be produced from natural gas at competitive costs. The process may be followed by two overall reactions as shown below, the first for making synthesis gas and the second for converting synthesis gas to methanol.

$$2\,CH_{4(g)} + 3\,H_2O_{(g)} \underset{\text{catalyst}}{\overset{1033\,K\,(760°C)}{=}} CO_{(g)} + CO_{2(g)} + 7\,H_{2(g)}$$

$$CO_{(g)} + 2\,H_{2(g)} \underset{30.9\,MPaa}{\overset{588\,K\,(315°C)}{=}} CH_3OH_{(g)}$$

The simplified flow diagram of the process if Fig. 5.28.

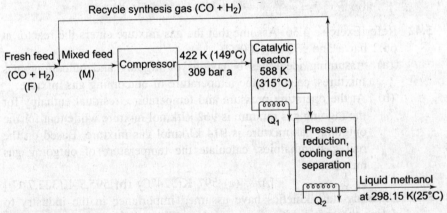

Fig. 5.28 Manufacture of Methanol from Natural Gas

It is desired to produce 1000 t of methanol per day. Fresh synthesis gas enters the system at the theoretical mole ratio of 2 moles of hydrogen per mole of CO. Recycle synthesis gas is added and the compressed mixed feed enters the catalytic converter at 422 K (149°C) and 309 bar a. Heat is exchanged at Q_1, as necessary to maintain the converter at 588 K (315°C). Only 12.5% of the combined feed is converted per pass.

The gaseous mixture leaving the converter is first reduced to 10 bar a, after which methanol is condensed out to a liquid state and further cooled to 298.15 K (25°C). Calculate: (a) the volumetric flow rate of the mixed feed to the catalytic converter in m^3/h, measured at 422 K (149°C) and 30.9 MPa a. Assume that the ideal gas law holds good for the conditions, (b) the heat transfer at Q_1, to maintain the temperature of 588 K (315°C), using data on $(H° - H_0° + \Delta H_{f0}°)$, given in table 5.21, (c) the dew point temperature, of methanol in the gaseous mixture, leaving the catalytic converter after the total pressure has been reduced to 1.0 MPa a, but before any separation has occurred, and (d) the heat to be removed from the methanol to cool 1 kmol of it from gaseous state at 588 K 9315°C) to the liquid at 298.15 K (25°C). Use the Antoine equation.

[*Ans.* (a) 3546.6 m^3/h; (b) + 17 394 kJ/kmol CH_3OH (endothermic) or 6290.8 kW (c) 318.6 K (45.6°C) (d) 39 093 kJ/kmol methanol]

Notes: (i) Since the inlet gas pressure to the reactor is very high the ideal gas law does not hold. Therefore Ans. (a) has only academic significance.

(ii) Since the reaction is taking place at a very high pressure, data of Table 5.21 are not valid. Actual enthalpies of gaseous components at high pressure and high temperature need to be utilised. It was made clear in the text (Example 5.35) that at high pressures the error involved in heat of reaction computation can be substantial.

(iii) Ans. (d) can also be erroneous due to the reasons explained in (ii) above.

5.42 Refer Exercise 4.36. Assume that the gas mixture enters the reactor at 66.2 bar a and 573 K (300°C).

(a) Assuming ideal gas behaviour of ingoing and outcoming gas mixtures, calculate the temperature of outcoming gas mixture.

(b) At the operating pressure and temperature, residual enthalpy for the ingoing gas mixture is 962 kJ/kmol mixture while that for the outgoing gas mixture is 914 kJ/kmol gas mixture. Based on the real gas enthalpies, calculate the temperature of outgoing gas mixture.

[*Ans.* (a) 597 K(324°C) (b) 595.7 K(322.7°C)]

5.43 Unsteady-state kinetics have assumed importance in the industry to define the safe limits of operating conditions of a reactor. Transient material and energy balance calculations together with reaction rate calculations make it possible to identify the runaway conditions which may lead to explosion.

The rate of thermal decomposition of molten salt in a continuous stirred tank reactor (CSTR) is defined as[66]

$$R = \frac{dm}{d\theta} = m \frac{\left\{ e^{(0.080\,73T - 40.1841)} \right\}}{183\,672}$$

where R = Rate of conversion of reactant to gaseous product, kg/s

m = Mass of the reactant in the reactor, kg

T = Temperature of mass, K and

θ = Time, s

The decomposition reaction is exothermic in nature and the heat of reaction is 607 kJ/kg of reactant assuming the reactant in molten condition and the products in gaseous condition. It is nearly constant in the temperature range of 535 K (262°C) to 580 K (307°C). Average heat capacity of the mass in the reactor may be taken as 1.675 kJ/(kg·K).

Assume that the reactor is charged with 250 kg reactant and its temperature is 535 K (262°C). If the feed to the reactor is cut-off and outside cooling is shut-off, the system behaves like a batch reactor. Also assume that the reactor is well insulated. Thus the reactor conditions can be considered adiabatic.

Calculate the rate of reaction, mass of reactant and the reaction temperature after 24 s using iterative calculations.

[*Ans.* 0.029 65 kg/s, 249.3 kg and 536 K(263°C)]

5.44 The heat of solution of $NiSO_4.7H_2O$ at 291.15 K (18°C) is – 17.58 kJ/kmol. Calculate the heat of crystallization of $NiSO_4.7H_2O$ at 291.15 K (18°C) in kJ/kg solute.

[*Ans.* + 62.63 kJ/kg solute (exothermic)]

5.45 Take the standard heat of formation of $CuSO_4$ at 298.15 K (25°C) as – 771.878 kJ/mol. The heat of solution of $CuSO_4.5H_2O$ is – 11.933 kJ/mol solute at 291.15 K (18°C). Assuming that the heat of solution of $CuSO_4.5H_2O$ at 298.15 K (25°C) is same as that of 291.15 K (18°C), calculate the heat of formation of $CuSO_4.5H_2O$ at 298.15 K (25°C).

[*Ans.* – 2213.933 kJ/mol]

5.46 The heat of dilution of one mol $KClO_3$ in 5.56 moles of water at 291.15 K (18°C) is – 37.26 kJ/mol $KClO_3$[67]. Calculate the heat absorbed when 1000 kg solution is to be prepared at 291.15 K (18°C) having the above composition.

[*Ans.* Heat absorbed = 167 290 kJ]

5.47 In Fig. 5.29 an isotherm of $NaClO_3$–H_2O system at 293.15 K (20°C) is given[67]. (a) How much heat is absorbed in dissolving 200 kg $NaClO_3$ to make a 40% solution at 293.15 K (20°C)? (b) How much heat is absorbed in making 500 kg of 30% of $NaClO_3$ solution at 293.15 K (20°C)? (c) A 40% $NaClO_3$ solution is diluted at 293.15 K (20°C). Calculate the heat to be added to or removed from the solution at 293.15 K (20°C).

[*Ans.* (a) 32 160 kJ, (b) 26 445 kJ,
(c) heat added to the solution is 27.6 kJ/kg $NaClO_3$]

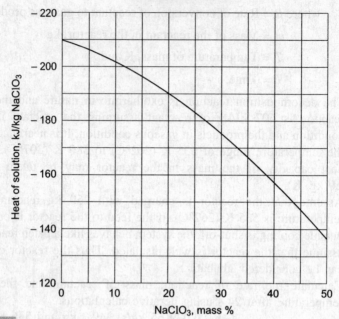

Heat of solution, kJ/kg NaClO₃

NaClO₃, mass %

Fig. 5.29 Integral Heat of Solution of Sodium Chlorate in Water at 293.15 (20°C)

5.48 It is desired to dilute 60% NaOH solution at 373 K (100°C) to 10% strength by adding water at 308 K(35°C). (a) Find the resultant temperature of 10% solution, using Fig. 5.14. (b) Calculate the heat to be removed to cool down the above solution to 298.15 K (25°C) using Figs. 5.14 and 5.4.

[*Ans.* (a) 335 K(63°C), (b) (i) 131.3 kJ/kg; (ii) 141 kJ/kg]

5.49 The endothermic heat of mixing of ethyl alcohol and ethyl acetate at 298.15 K (25°C) are given in Table 5.52. Calculate the integral heat of solution of ethyl acetate in kJ/kg ester for each value given in the table. Plot a graph giving the integral heat of solution on the y-axis and mass fraction of easter on the x-axis.

Table 5.52 Heat of Mixing of Ethanol and Ethyl Acetate[68]

Mole fraction of ethanol	Enthalpy of mixing at 298.15 K (25°C), kJ/kmol
0.05	326.6
0.10	596.1
0.20	1032.3
0.30	1319.8
0.40	1467.0
0.50	1486.1
0.60	1385.8
0.70	1176.3
0.80	859.1
0.90	531.3
0.95	245.8

5.50 The molar excess enthalpy of ethanol-*n*-hexane mixture containing 0.18 mole fraction ethanol at 318 K (45°C) and 101.325 kPa is reported to be 561.4 kJ/kmol (endothermic) mixture. Calculate the enthalpy of the mixture based on reference temperature of 273.15 K (0°C).

[*Ans.* 7513.2 kJ/kmol]

5.51 Calculate the heat of mixing for Exercise 3.14 per 100 kg mixed acid. Assume that both the aqueous acids are available at 303 K (30°C) and the mixed acid temperature should not exceed 313 K (40°C).

[*Ans.* 9369 kJ (exothermic)]

5.52 In an experimental run of 2-methylnaphthalene[69] the spent acid obtained at the end of the run contains 11.3% HNO_3, 44.4% H_2SO_4 and 44.3% H_2O. It is fortified by the addition of 98% H_2SO_4 and 69% HNO_3. The fortified mixed acid has the composition:

HNO_3: 25%, H_2SO_4: 40% and H_2O: 35%

Use Fig. 5.18.

Calculate: (a) The quantities of 98% H_2SO_4 and 69% HNO_3 required to fortify the spent acid and (b) the heat liberated per kg spent acid at 273.15 K (0°C) fortified. All percentages are by mass.

[*Ans.* (a) 22.84 kg 98% H_2SO_4 and 44.11 kg 69% HNO_3

(b) 168.9 kJ/kg spent acid]

5.53 Calculate the heat evolved by mixing anhydrous liquid ammonia at atmospheric pressure [boiling point $\approx$ 239.82 K (– 33.33°C)] and water at 298.15 K (25°C) to produce 100 1 aqueous solution of ammonia having 4.5% (by mass) strength (as NH_3) at 298.15 K (25°C). Use Fig. 5.19 and Table 5.40 for calculations. The specific gravity of 4.5% solution is 0.98 at 298.15 K (25°C).

[*Ans.* (i) 2303 kJ from Fig. 5.19

(ii) 2540.7 kJ from Table 5.40]

5.54 Ammonia liquor having 32.0% (mass) strength is mixed with a dilute solution having 4.5% (mass) strength to produce a solution having final strength of 15.9% (mass). Assume that both the solutions are available at 298.15 K (25°C). Calculate the cooling required to maintain the temperature at 298.15 K (25°C) of 1000 kg of the final 15.9% solution using Table 5.40.

Also calculate the quantities of 32% and 4.5% solutions, required to be mixed using Fig. 5.19.

[*Ans.* 11 546 kJ, 580.6 kg 4.5% solution and 419.4 kg 32% solution]

5.55 Dry gas mixture from a methane-chlorination reactor having the following molar composition enters an absorber at 318 K (45°C).

CH_4: 53.8%, CH_3Cl: 18.3%, CH_2Cl_2: 2.65%, CH_3Cl: 0.65%, CCl_4: 0.15% and HCl: 24.45%

It is scrubbed with water in a falling-film type carbate absorber to remove HCl. Assume that nearly 100% hydrogen chloride gas is removed. Water enters the absorber at 303 K (30°C) and acid-free gases leave the absorber at 6.85 kPa g in saturated conditions at 303 K (30°C). Use Table 5.1 for heat capacity equation constants of the gases.

(a) If the tower is designed for 30% (mass) acid production, calculate the heat to be removed from the system. Assume that 30% acid is to be produced at the bottom at 298.15 K (25°C).

(b) If the tower is designed to produce 5% (mass) acid, calculate the temperature of the 5% acid at the bottom. Assume the heat capacity of aqueous 5% acid to be 4.19 kJ/(kg·K).

Table 5.53 Heat of Formation of Aqueous Hydrochloric Acid Solution[48]

Formula and description	State	Heat of formation at 298.15 K (25°C), ΔH_f°, kJ/mol HCl	Mass % HCl in aqueous solution
HCl, 0 H_2O	gas	− 92.31	100
1 H_2O	aq	− 121.55	67.0
1.5 H_2O	aq	− 132.67	57.5
2 H_2O	aq	− 140.96	50.3
2.5 H_2O	aq	− 145.48	44.8
3 H_2O	aq	− 148.49	40.3
4 H_2O	aq	− 152.92	33.6
5 H_2O	aq	− 155.77	28.9
6 H_2O	aq	− 157.68	25.3
8 H_2O	aq	− 160.00	20.2
10 H_2O	aq	− 161.32	16.9
15 H_2O	aq	− 163.03	11.9
20 H_2O	aq	− 163.85	9.21
25 H_2O	aq	− 164.34	7.50
30 H_2O	aq	− 164.67	6.33
40 H_2O	aq	− 165.10	4.82
50 H_2O	aq	− 165.36	3.90
75 H_2O	aq	− 165.72	2.63

Note: The number in the first column indicates the number of moles of water mixed with one mole of hydrogen chloride.

(Source: National Institute of Standards and Technology, USA)

[*Ans.* (a) 454.8 kW (b) 327.3 K (54.3°C)]

5.56 It is desired to increase the strength of an acid having 19.1% H_2SO_4 by adding oleum having 29.0 mass % free SO_3 (on the basis of 100% acid) both at 291.15 K (18°C) to 53.8% H_2SO_4 concentration. Calculate the heat evolved per kg of the original weak acid, fortified.

Use the data provided in Table 5.42.

[*Ans.* Heat evolved = 556.36 kJ/kg original weak acid]

5.57 Refer Exercise 5.56. What will be the expected rise in temperature? If the above 53.8% H_2SO_4 solution boils at 405 K(132°C), is it possible to achieve the rise in temperature of the solution without cooling? If not, what will happen?

Ans. Rise in temperature works out to 135.3 K Which gives the resultant temperature as 426.3 K (153.3°C). This is not possible as the solution will start boiling at 405 K(132°C).

It should be noted that this answer refers to a case when no heat is removed from the system. However, if the exothermic heat of dilution calculated in Exercise 5.56 is removed by indirect cooling, it is possible to achieve the concentration of 53.8% H_2SO_4.

5.58 It is desired to dilute oleum containing 41.2% free SO_3 with a large volume of water so that the resultant mixture can be considered infinitely dilute. What will be the heat evolution?

[*Ans.* – 1407.8 kJ/kg oleum]

5.59 A flask contains M_0 kmol of a binary mixture of composition x_0 (mole fraction) of a component A at its bubble point. Heat is supplied to the flask at the rate of Q kW. The average latent heat of vaporization of the binary is λ_v kJ/kmol. The relative volatility of the mixture is α. Assuming that (i) the heat of mixing of the binary is negligible, (ii) the variation of the bubble point with the composition is insignificant and (iii) the heat loss to the surroundings is negligible, prove that the mole fraction x of the component A in the liquid mixture at the end of θ h is given by following equation,

$$(1 - K\theta)^{(\alpha - 1)} = \frac{x(1 - x_0)^\alpha}{\left[x_0(1 - x)^\alpha\right]} \quad K\theta < 1$$

where $$K = \frac{Q}{(M_0 \cdot \lambda_v)}$$

Note: When $K\theta = 1$, the complete mixture is boiled off and hence the condition $K\theta > 1$ is non-existent.

5.60 A flask contains 5 kg of a mixture consisting of 50 mole % *n*-heptane and 50 mole % *n*-octane at its bubble point at atmospheric pressure. The flask is supplied heat at the rate of 0.5 kW with the help of an electric mantle. The average relative volatility (α) and average latent heat of vaporization (λ_v) of the mixture can be assumed to be 2.16 and 33 500 kJ/kmol respectively. Assume negligible heat of mixing of the two components. Also, the bubble point variation with the change in composition may be neglected. Calculate (a) the time required to attain a liquid mixture of 30 mole % *n*-heptance in the flask and (b) the composition of the liquid mixture after 15 min from the start to heating. Compute the left-over quantities of the liquid mixture in both the above cases.

[*Ans.* (a) Time: 34.2 min, Quantity: 1.76 kg
(b) Composition: 43.66 mole % *n*-heptane, Quantity: 3.59 kg]

5.61 Refer Exercise 4.40. Calculate the required temperature of superheated ammonia, if (a) preheated air containing 0.016 kg H_2O/kg dry air is introduced to the reactor at 533 K (260°C), (b) the ammonia content of the inlet dry gas mixture is maintained at 10% (v/v), (c) the conversion of ammonia is 100% and (d) the outlet temperature is required to be controlled at 1183 K (910°C).

[*Ans.* 401 K(128°C)]

REFERENCES

1. Himmelblau D. M., *Basic Principles and Calculations in Chemical Engineering*, 5th Ed., Prentice-Hall, Inc., USA, 1987.
2. Smith, J. M., H. C. Van Ness, M. M. Abbott and B. I. Bhatt, *Introduction to Chemical Engineering Thermodynamics*, 6th Ed., Tata McGraw-Hill, New Delhi, 2003.
3. Spencer, H. M., *Ind. Engng. Chem.*, **40** (11), 1948, p. 2152.
4. Thinh, T. P., J. L. Duran, R. S. Ramalho and S. Kaliaguine, *Hydrocarbon Processing*, **50** (1): 1971, p. 98.
5. Yaws, C. L., H. M. Ni and P. Y. Chiang, *Chem. Engng.*, **95** (7), May 9, 1988, p. 91.
6. Reklaitis, G. V. and D. R. Schneider, *Introduction to Material and Energy Balances*, John Wiley & Sons, USA, 1983.
7. Yuan, S. C. and Y. I. Mok, *Hydrocarbon Processing*, **47** (3): 1968, p. 133.
8. Yuan S. C. and Y. I. Mok, *Hydrocarbon Processing*, **47** (7): 1968, p. 153.
9. Duran, J. L., T. P. Thinh, R. S. Ramalho and S. Kaliagunine, *Hydrocarbon Processing*, **55** (8), 1976.
10. Frechette G., J. C. Herbert, T. P. Thinh and T. K. Trong, Central Laboratory, Transport Ministry Government of Quebec, Quebec, Canada (private communication, unpublished results).
11. Yaws, C. L., *Physical Properties*, McGraw-Hill, USA, 1977.
12. Weiss, A. H. and J. Joffee, *Ind. Engng. Chem.*, **49** (1): 1957, p. 120.
13. Lee, B. I. and M. G. Kesler, *AIChE J.*, **21** (3): 1975, p. 510.
14. Reid, R. C., J. M. Prausnitz and B. E. Poling, *The Properties of Gases and Liquids*, 4th Ed., McGraw-Hill, USA, 1987.
15. Thinh T. P., J. L. Duran and R. S. Ramalho, *I&EC Process Design and Development*, **10**: October, 1971, p. 576.
16. Yaws, C. L. and X. Pan, *Chem. Engng.*, **99** (4): 1992, p. 132.
17. A technical manual on *Caustic Soda*, Hooker Chemical Corporation, USA.
18. *Lurgi Atlas on Sulphuric Acid*, Lurgi GmbH, Germany, 1986.
19. A technical manual on *Diphyl-Organic Heat Transfer Media*, Bayer AG, Germany, 1971.

20. Green, D. W. and J. O. Maloney, *Perry's Chemical Engineers' Handbook*, 6th Ed., McGraw-Hill, USA, 1984.
21. Carroll, J. J., *Chem. Engng.*, **108** (10): 2001, p. 91.
22. *API Technical Data Book-Petroleum Refining*, Vols. I and II, 2nd Ed., Published by the American Petroleum Institute, USA, 1970.
23. Boublik, T., V. Fried and E. Hala, *The Vapour Pressures of Pure Substances*, Elsevier Scientific Publishing Co., The Netherlands, 1973.
24. Zwolinski, B. J. and R. C. Wilhoit, *Handbook of Vapour Pressures and Heats of Vaporization of Hydrocarbons and Related Compounds*, API-44-TRC Publication, Thermodynamics Research Centre, USA, 1971.
25. Yaws, C. L., H. C. Yang and W. A. Cawley, *Hydrocarbon Processing*, **69** (6): 1990, p. 87.
26. A technical manual on Dowtherm A, The Dow Chemical Company, USA, 1991.
27. Corpstein R. R. R. A. Dove and D. S. Dickey, *Chem. Engng. Progress*, **75** (2): 1979, p. 66.
28. *ASHRAE Handbook: Fundamentals*, American Society of Heating, Refrigerating and Air-conditioning Engineers, Inc., USA, 1993.
29. Green, R. L., A. H. Larsen and A. C. Pauls, *Chem. Engng.*, **96** (2): 1989, p. 91.
30. Seifert, W. F., *Chem. Engng.*, **96** (2): 1989., p. 99.
31. Sisson. B., *Chem. Engng.*, **84** (4): February 14, 1977, p. 105.
32. Adhia, J. D., *Chem. Age of India*, **26** (10): 1975, p. 749.
33. *Gas Encyclopaedia, L' Air Liquide*, Elsevier Scientific Publishing Co., The Netherlands, 1976.
34. *Pressure-Enthalpy Diagram for Carbon Dioxide*, Published by Büse Anlagenbau GmbH, Germany, 1982.
35. *Tappi*, **47** (10): 1964, p. 197A.
36. *Engineering Data Book*, 9th Ed., Gas Processors Suppliers Association, USA, 1972.
37. Gess, M. A., R. P. Danner and M. Nagrekar, *Thermodynamic Analysis of Vapour-Liquid Equilibria*, American Institute of Chemical Engineers, USA, 1991.
38. Benenati, R. F., *Chem. Engng.*, **84** (6): March 14, 1977, p. 129.
39. *AIChE Student Contest Problem*, 1965.
40. Thinh, T. P. and T. K. Trong, *The Canadian J. of Chem. Engng.*, **54** (8): 1976, p. 344.
41. Yaws, C. L. and P. Y. Chiang, *Chem. Engng.*, **95** (17), Sept. 26, 1988, p. 81.
42. *Physical and Thermodynamic Properties of Elements and Compounds*, United Catalysts. Inc., USA.

43. Canjar, L. N. and F. S. Manning, *Thermodynamic Properties and Reduced Correlations for Gases*, Gulf Publishing Co., USA, 1967.

44. Edmister, W. C., *Hydrocarbon Processing*, **52** (7): 1973, p. 123.

45. Ganapathy, V., *Hydrocarbon Processing*, **72** (2), 1922, p.93.

46. Wolfgang Gerhartz, *Ullmann's Encyclopedia of Industrial Chemistry*, 5th Ed., Vol. A10, VCH Verlagsgesellschaft mbH, Germany, 1987 p. 332.

47. Kroschwitz, J. I., *Kirk-othmer Encyclopaedia of Chemical Technology*, IVth Ed., Vol. 1, John Wiley & Sons, Inc., 1991. p. 1005.

48. Selected Values of Chemical Thermodynamic Properties, Technical Note 270-3 (a Revision of NBS Circular 500), National Bureau of Standards, USA, January, 1968.

49. Bump, T. R. and W. L. Sibbitt, *Ind. Engng. Chem.*, **47**: 1955, p. 1665-1670.

50. Gable, C. M., H. F. Betz and S. H. Maron, *J. of Am. Chem. Soc.*, **72**: 1950, p. 1445-1448.

51. Urbanski, Chemistry and Technology of Explosives, Vol.1 Pergamon Press Ltd., UK, 1964.

52. Albright, K. F., *Chem. Engng.*, **73**: May 9, 1966, p. 161.

53. Landolt and Börnstein, *Values and Functions for Physics, Chemistry, Astronomy, Geophysics and Technics*, 6th Ed., Vol. IV., Part 4, Springer-Verlag, Berlin, Germany, 1972, p. 199.

54. 1993 Fundamentals Handbook (SI), American Society of Heating, Refrigerating and Air-conditioning Engineers, Inc., USA.

55. Walker, J. F., *Formaldehyde*, 3rd Ed., Reinhold Publishing Corporation, UK, 1964.

56. Morgen, R. A., *Ind., Engng.* Chem., **34** (5): 1942, p. 571.

57. *International Data Series (IDS), Series A*, Journal Published by the Thermodynamics Research Centre, USA.

58. *TRC Thermodynamic Tables-Hydrocarbons, and TRC Thermodynamic Tables-Non-Hydrocarbons*, Published by Thermodynamics Research Centre, USA.

59. NBS Tables of Chemical Thermodynamics Properties, *J. Phys. Chem. Ref.* Data, 11, Supplement 2, 1982.

60. Yaws, C.L., *Thermodynamic sand Physical Properties Data*, Gulf Publishing Co., USA, 1993.

61. *International Thermodynamic Tables of the Fluid State by* International Union of Pure and Applied Chemistry (IUPAC), UK.

62. Duecker, W. W. and J. R. West, *The Manufacture of Sulphuric Acid*, Reinhold Publishing Corporation, USA, 1959.

63. Joharapurkar, V. R. and M. Khemani, *Chemical Processing & Engineering*, Annual Issue, 1971, p. 84.

64. Woicik, J. F., *Chem. Engng.*, **83** (17): August 16, 1976, p. 89.

65. Mays, E. B. and M. R. Schwab, *Chem. Engng.*, **84** (4): February 17, 1975, p. 112.
66. Horwitz, B. A., *Chem. Engng.*, **90** (18): Sept. 5, 1983, p. 115.
67. *The Chlorate Manual*, Kerr-McGee Chemical Corporation, USA, 1972.
68. Murti, P. S. and M. V. Winkle, *Ind., Engng. Chem.*, **3**: 1911, p. DS 65.
69. Brink, J. A. and R. N. Shreve, *Ind. Engng. Chem.*, **46** (4): 1954, p. 694.

Chapter 6

Stoichiometry and Unit Operations

6.1 INTRODUCTION

The material and energy balances of chemical reactions as well as simple physical processes such as mixing were discussed in Chapters 4 and 5. However, in chemical engineering, unit operations are as much important as the unit processes. It is therefore desirable to study the stoichiometric aspects of the unit operations in detail.

6.2 DISTILLATION

Distillation or fractionation is an operation in which one or more components of the liquid mixtures of two or more components are separated using thermal energy. Basically, the difference in vapour pressures of different components at the same temperature is responsible for such a separation.

Usually, the throughput to the distillation column with the composition of the feed is known. The desired purities of the components dictate the compositions of overhead and bottom products. These data are sufficient to establish the overall material balance of the column.

Knowing the flow rates of the distillate and bottom products, it is easy to evaluate the thermal loads of the overhead condenser and reboiler.

The following example will demonstrate the material and energy balances of such a column.

Example 6.1 A vapour at 411 K (138°C) and standard atmospheric pressure, containing 0.72 mole fraction benzene and 0.28 mole fraction toluene serves as a feed to a fractionating column in which it is separated into a distillate containing 0.995 mole fraction benzene and bottoms with 0.97 mole fraction toluene. The reflux ratio is desired to be 1.95 kmol/kmol distillate product. For a feed of 100 kmol, compute the overall material and energy balances. Assume that there is no heat loss to the surrounding and the heat of solution is negligible.

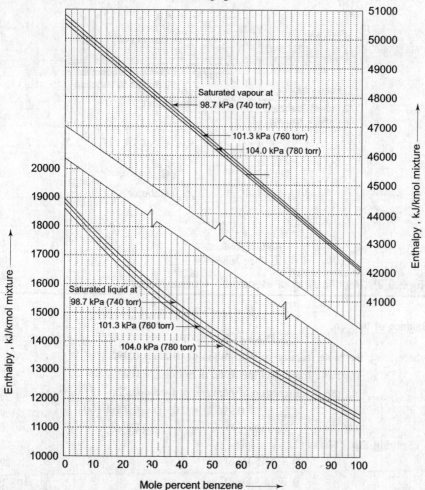

Fig. 6.1 Enthalpies of Benzene - Toluene Mixtures above 273.15 K (0°C)[1]

(Reproduced with permission of the American Chemical Society, USA).

Solution: Basis: 100 kmol feed

A schematic representation of the distillation column is given in Fig. 6.2.

$$\text{Benzene in the feed} = 100 \times 0.72 = 72 \text{ kmol}$$

$$\text{Toluene in the feed} = 100 - 72 = 28 \text{ kmol}$$

Let D be the distillate and B the bottom product in kmol.

Overall material balance;

$$\text{Feed } F = B + D \qquad (6.1)$$

Note: This equation is entirely general. As long as consistent units are used the mass units or mole units can be used.

For the enthalpy data refer to Fig. 6.1.

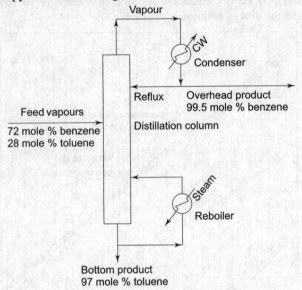

Fig. 6.2 Rectification of Benzene Toluene Mixture

$$B + D = 100 \qquad (1)$$

Balance of benzene,

$$x_D \cdot D + x_B \cdot B = x_F \cdot F \qquad (6.2)$$

where, x_D, the mole fraction of benzene in distillate = 0.995

x_B, the mole fraction of benzene in bottoms = 0.03

x_F, the mole fraction of benzene in feed = 0.72

$$0.995\, D + 0.03\, D = 0.72 \times 100$$
$$= 72 \qquad (2)$$

Solving Eqs. (1) and (2)

$$D = 71.5 \text{ kmol}$$

$$B = 28.5 \text{ kmol} \qquad \qquad Ans.\ (a)$$

Heat load of condenser:

$$\text{Reflux ratio, } R = \frac{\text{Moles of distillate refluxed}}{\text{Mole of distillate removed from the column}}$$

$$= 1.95$$

Total overhead vapours = D (1 + R)

$$= 71.5 \times 2.95 = 210.925 \text{ kmol}$$

Reference temperature, $T_o = 273.15\ (0°C)$

From Fig. 6.1,

Enthalpy of vapours (overhead) = 42 170 kJ/kmol mixture

Enthalpy of liquid (overhead) = 11 370 kJ/kmol mixture

Since the condenser is not expected to subcool the liquid,
the enthalpy removed in the condenser (latent heat duty)

$$= 42\ 170 - 11\ 370 = 30\ 800 \text{ kJ/kmol mixture}$$

Total heat load of condenser = 30 800 × 210.925

$$= 6496\ 490 \text{ kJ} \qquad\qquad Ans. \text{ (b)}$$

Heat load of reboiler:

Enthalpy of distillate product = 11 370 × 71.5 = 812 955 kJ

Enthalpy of bottom product = 18 780 kJ/kmol mixture

Total enthalpy of bottoms = 18 780 × 28.5 = 535 230 kJ

Enthalpy of feed = 44 500 × 100 kJ/kmol mixture

Total enthalpy of feed = 44 500 × 100 = 4450 000 kJ

Heat load of reboiler = enthalpy of distillate

+ heat load of condenser

+ enthalpy of bottoms

− enthalpy of feed

$$= 812\ 955 + 6496\ 490 + 535\ 230 - 4450\ 000$$

$$+ 526\ 310 - 4456\ 700$$

$$= 3394\ 675 \text{ kJ} \qquad\qquad Ans. \text{ (c)}$$

Note: If the feed is liquid at its boiling point (enthalpy = 12 945 kJ/kmol mixture), what will be the heat load of the reboiler?

Ans. 6550 175 kJ

Will there be any change in the heat load of the condenser?

6.3 ABSORPTION AND STRIPPING

Absorption is an unit operation in which a mixture of gases is brought in contact with liquid. A definite component of the gas mixture is dissolved in the liquid. The operation is sometimes also termed as scrubbing. It may be physical absorption only or it may be accompanied by a chemical reaction.

Stripping or desorption is an operation in which a dissolved gas of a solution is stripped off from the liquid using a stripping medium, e.g., steam, air, etc.

In this operation also the overall material balance yields the desired information.

Example 6.2 An absorption tower, packed with Tellerette packings, is used to absorb carbon dioxide in an aqueous monoethanol amine (MEA) solution[2]. The volumetric flow rate of the incoming dry gas mixture is 1000 m^3/h at 318 K (45°C) and 101.3 kPa a (760 torr). The CO_2 content of the gas is 10.4 mole %, while the outgoing gas mixture contains 4.5 mole % CO_2. A 3.2 M MEA solution is introduced at the top of the tower at the rate of 0.625 L/s. Dissolved CO_2 concentration of the entering solution is 0.166 kmol/kmol of MEA. Find the concentration of dissolved CO_2 in the solution leaving the tower.

Solution: Figure 6.3 shows flow process through the absorber.

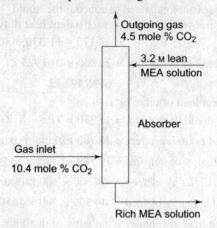

Fig. 6.3   Absorption of CO_2 in Aqueous MEA Solution

Basis: 0.625 L/s of MEA solution

$$\text{Concentration of MEA solution} = 3.2 \text{ M}$$

$$\text{Chemical formula of MEA} = HOCH_2CH_2NH_2$$

$$\text{Molar mass of MEA} = 61$$

$$\text{Concentration of MEA in the solution} = 61 \times 3.2$$

$$= 195.2 \text{ g/L solution}$$

$$\text{Total MEA entering the tower} = 195.2 \times 0.625 \times 3600 \text{ g/h}$$

$$\text{Moles of MEA entering the tower} = 3.2 \times 0.625 \times \frac{3600}{1000}$$

$$= 7.2 \text{ kmol/h}$$

$$\text{Dissolved } CO_2 \text{ in lean MEA} = 0.166 \text{ kmol/kmol MEA}$$

$$CO_2 \text{ in lean MEA} = 0.166 \times 7.2 = 1.1952 \text{ kmol/h}$$

Volumetric flow rate of dry gas mixture = 1000 m^3/h

Specific volume of gas at 318 K (45°C) and

$$101.3 \text{ kPa a}, V = 26.107 \text{ m}^3/\text{kmol} \qquad \text{(Ref. Table 7.8)}$$

$$\text{Molar flow rate of gas } q_v = \frac{1000}{26.107} = 38.3 \text{ kmol/h}$$

$$\text{Moles of } CO_2 \text{ in the inlet gas} = 38.3 \times 0.104 = 3.98 \text{ kmol/h}$$

$$CO_2\text{-free gas} = 38.10 - 3.98 = 34.12 \text{ kmol/h}$$

Outgoing gas contains 4.5 mole % CO_2.

$$\text{Molar flow rate of outgoing gas mixture} = \frac{34.12}{(1 - 0.0455)} = 35.73 \text{ kmol/h}$$

$$CO_2 \text{ absorbed} = 38.10 - 35.73 = 2.37 \text{ kmol/h}$$

Total CO_2 in rich MEA solution $= 1.1952 + 2.37 = 3.5622$ kmol/h

Concentration of CO_2 in rich MEA solution $= \dfrac{3.5622}{7.2}$

$$= 0.495 \text{ kmol/kmol MEA} \qquad Ans.$$

Example 6.3 A gas mixture containing NO_2, N_2O_4 and N_2 enters the bottom of an absorption tower[3]. Caustic soda solution (containing 23.6% by mass NaOH) is introduced at the top of the column. 50 000 m³/h of a gas mixture enters having the composition 5.46% NO_2, 2.14% N_2O_4 and rest N_2 on dry basis. The outgoing gas is found to contain 3.93% NO_2, 0.82% N_2O_4, 0.25% NO and rest N_2 on dry basis. The aqueous solution enters at the rate of 500 L/min. The density of the solution can be taken as 1.25 kg/L. The temperature and pressure of the gas are 295.5 K (22.5°C) and 100 kPa a (750 torr) respectively. Calculate the composition of the aqueous liquor leaving the column. Assume that the gas mixture leaving the tower contains 0.045 kmol water vapour per kmol dry gas mixture.

Solution: Basis: 50 000 m³/h of gas mixture at 295.5 K and 100 kPa a

Specific volume of gas at 295.5 K

$$\text{and } 100 \text{ kPa a, } V = 24.57 \text{ m}^3/\text{kmol}$$

Molar flow rate of incoming gas mixture $= \dfrac{50\,000}{24.57} = 2035$ kmol/h

$$NO_2 \text{ content of the gas} = 2035 \times 0.0546 = 111.11 \text{ kmol/h}$$

$$N_2O_4 \text{ content of the gas} = 2035 \times 0.0214 = 43.55 \text{ kmol/h}$$

$$N_2 \text{ content of the gas} = 2035 - (111.11 + 43.55)$$

$$= 1880.34 \text{ kmol/h}$$

When the mixture passes through the tower, N_2 remains unaffected, i.e., the outgoing gas mixture contains 1880.34 kmol/h of N_2.

The outgoing gas mixture contains 95% N_2.

Molar flow rate of outgoing gas mixture $= \dfrac{1880.34}{0.95} = 1979.3$ kmol/h (dry)

Table 6.1 Composition of Outgoing Gas Mixture

Component	Mole %	kmol/h
NO_2	3.93	77.78
N_2O_4	0.82	16.23
NO	0.25	4.95
N_2	95.00	1880.34
Total	100.00	1979.30

NO_2 removed from the mixture $= 111.11 - 77.78 = 33.33$ kmol/h

N_2O_4 removed from the mixture $= 43.55 - 16.23 = 27.32$ kmol/h

The absorption in the tower is accompanied by the chemical reactions listed below.

$$2\,NO_2 + 2\,NaOH = NaNO_2 + NaNO_3 + H_2O \tag{1}$$

$$N_2O_4 + 2\,NaOH = NaNO_2 + NaNO_3 + H_2O \tag{2}$$

$$3\,NO_2 + 2\,NaOH = 2\,NaNO_3 + H_2O + NO \tag{3}$$

The last reaction is actually the result of two consecutive reactions:

$$3\,NO_2 + H_2O = 2\,HNO_3 + NO \tag{3A}$$

$$2\,HNO_3 + 2\,NaOH = 2\,NaNO_3 + 2\,H_2O \tag{3B}$$

Table 6.2 Molar Masses

Component	Molar mass (rounded values)
NO_2	46
N_2O_4	92
NO	30
$NaOH$	40
$NaNO_2$	69
$NaNO_3$	85
H_2O	18

N_2O_4 absorption (Reaction (2)):

$$NaOH \text{ consumed} = 2 \times 40 \times 27.32 = 2185.8 \text{ kg/h}$$

$$NaNO_2 \text{ produced} = 69 \times 27.32 = 1885.1 \text{ kg/h}$$

$$NaNO_3 \text{ produced} = 85 \times 27.32 = 2322.2 \text{ kg/h}$$

$$H_2O \text{ produced} = 18 \times 27.32 = 491.8 \text{ kg/h}$$

NO production (Reaction (3)):

$$NO_2 \text{ consumed} = 3 \times 4.95 = 14.85 \text{ kmol/h}$$

$$NaOH \text{ consumed} = 2 \times 4.95 \times 40 = 396 \text{ kg/h}$$

$$NaNO_3 \text{ produced} = 2 \times 4.95 \times 85 = 841.5 \text{ kg/h}$$

$$H_2O \text{ produced} = 4.95 \times 18 = 89.1 \text{ kg/h}$$

Thus, out of 32.33 kmol/h of NO_2 absorbed, 14.85 kmol/h are consumed for the production of NO. The rest is absorbed as per Reaction (1).

$$NO_2 \text{ absorbed as per Reaction (1)} = 33.33 - 14.85 = 18.48 \text{ kmol/h}$$

NO_2 absorption (Reaction (1)):

$$NaOH \text{ consumed} = 18.48 \times 40 = 739.2 \text{ kg/h}$$

$$NaNO_2 \text{ produced} = \frac{69 \times 18.48}{2} = 637.6 \text{ kg/h}$$

$$NaNO_3 \text{ produced} = \frac{85 \times 18.48}{2} = 785.4 \text{ kg/h}$$

$$H_2O \text{ produced} = \frac{18 \times 18.48}{2} = 166.3 \text{ kg/h}$$

$$\text{Total } NaNO_2 \text{ produced} = 1885.1 + 637.6 = 2522.7 \text{ kg/h}$$

$$\text{Total NaNO}_3 \text{ produced} = 2322.2 + 841.5 + 785.4 = 3949.1 \text{ kg/h}$$

$$\text{Total H}_2\text{O produced} = 491.8 + 89.1 + 166.3 = 747.2 \text{ kg/h}$$

$$\text{Total NaOH consumed} = 2185.6 + 396 + 739.2 = 3320.8 \text{ kg/h}$$

Material balance of liquid:

$$\text{Flow of liquor} = 500 \text{ L/min} = 625 \text{ kg/min} = 37\,500 \text{ kg/h}$$

$$\text{NaOH in the feed} = 37\,500 \times 0.236 = 8850 \text{ kg/h}$$

Leftover NaOH in the outgoing liquid $= 8850 - 3320.8 = 5529.8$ kg/h

Moisture in the exist gas stream $= 1979.3 \times 0.045$

$$= 89.1 \text{ kmol/h} \equiv 1603.2 \text{ kg/h}$$

Water in the outgoing solution $= 37\,500 - 8850 + 747.2 - 1603.2$

$$= 27\,794 \text{ kg/h}$$

Table 6.3 Composition of Final Liquor

Component	kg/h	Mass %
NaOH	5529.2	13.90
NaNO$_2$	2522.7	6.34
NaNO$_3$	3949.1	9.92
H$_2$O	27794.0	69.84
Total	39795.0	100.00

Ans.

6.4 EXTRACTION AND LEACHING

When a mixture of liquids is not easily separable by distillation, extraction is employed. In this operation, a "solvent" is added to the liquid-liquid mixture. As a result, two immiscible layers are formed, both of which contain varying amounts of different components. These isolated layers are removed as *extract phase* and *reffinate phase* using density difference. Invariably, distillation has to follow extraction for the recovery of the solvent for re-use. For example, furfural is a common solvent in the extraction operations in a petroleum refinery.

Normally the term "extraction" is used for liquid-liquid separation. Leaching is also basically a solid-liquid extraction operation in which a particular component of the solid is leached out with the help of a solvent. A common example of such an operation is the leaching of oil from an oilcake using hexane as a solvent.

Example 6.4 A mixture containing 47.5% acetic acid and 52.5% water (by mass) is being separated by the extraction in a counter-current multistage unit[4]. The operating temperature is 297 K (24°C) and the solvent used is pure *iso*-propyl ether. Using the solvent in the ratio of 1.3 kg/kg feed, the final extraction composition on a solvent free basis is found to be 82% by mass of acetic acid. The raffinate is found to contain 14% by mass of acetic acid on a solvent-free basis. Calculate the percentage of acid of the original feed which remains unextracted.

Solution: Figure 6.4 gives a schematic representation of the extraction column.

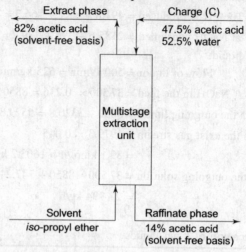

Fig. 6.4 Extraction of Acetic Acid

Basis: 100 kg feed mixture

Let E and R be the masses in kg of the extract phase and raffinate phase respectively.

Overall material balance:

$$\text{Feed } F = E + R \tag{6.1}$$

$$E + R = 100 \tag{1}$$

Balance of acetic acid:

$$x_F \cdot F = x_E \cdot E + x_R \cdot R \tag{6.3}$$

where x_F mass fraction of acetic acid in feed = 0.475

x_E mass fraction of acetic acid in extract = 0.82

x_R mass fraction of acetic acid in raffinate = 0.14

$$0.82\,E + 0.14\,R = 0.475 \times 100 = 47.5 \tag{2}$$

Solving Eqs (1) and (2),

$$E = 49.2 \text{ kg}$$

$$R = 50.8 \text{ kg}$$

Acetic acid leftover in raffinate = $50.8 \times 0.14 = 7.11$ kg

Acetic acid which remained unextracted = $\left(\dfrac{7.11}{47.5}\right)100$

$$= 15\% \qquad \qquad Ans.$$

Example 6.5 A multiple-contract counter-current extractor is employed to extract oil from halibut livers with the help of ethyl ether[4]. The fresh livers are charged to the extractor at the rate of 1000 kg/h and contain 25.7% oil (my mass). Pure ether enters the bottom of the extractor. The overflow from the extractor contains 70% oil (by mass). The underflow rate is 0.23 kg solution/kg of oil-free solids and is known to contain 12.8% oil (by mass). Based on these operating conditions, make the complete material balance and find the flow rate of ether to the extractor. Also, compute the percentage recovery of oil.

Solution: Figure 6.5 gives the schematic representation of the multiple-contact counter-current extractor.

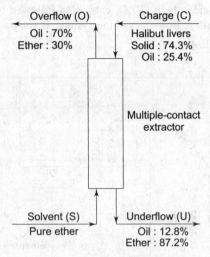

Fig. 6.5 Extraction of Oil from Halibut Liver

Basis: 1000 kg/h halibut livers

$$\text{Oil in the charge} = 1000 \times 0.257 = 257 \text{ kg/h}$$

$$\text{Solids in the charge} = 1000 - 257 = 743 \text{ kg/h}$$

$$\text{Underflow rate (U)} = 0.23 \times 743 = 170.9 \text{ kg/h}$$

$$\text{Oil content of underflow} = 170.9 \times 0.128 = 21.9 \text{ kg/h}$$

$$\text{Ether content of underflow} = 170.9 - 21.9 = 149.0 \text{ kg/h}$$

$$\text{Recovery of oil (in the overflow)} = 257 - 21.9 = 235.1 \text{ kg/h}$$

$$\% \text{ recovery of oil} = \left(\frac{235.1}{257}\right) \times 100 = 91.5 \qquad \textit{Ans.} \text{ (a)}$$

$$\text{Overflow rate, O} = \frac{235.1}{0.7} = 335.9 \text{ kg/h}$$

$$\text{Ether content of overflow} = 335.9 - 235.1 = 100.8 \text{ kg/h}$$

$$\text{Total ether fed to the system} = \text{ether in the underflow}$$

$$+ \text{ether in the overflow}$$

$$= 149 + 100.8 = 249.8 \text{ kg/h} \qquad \textit{Ans.} \text{ (b)}$$

Example 6.6 Recovery of acetic acid from aqueous waste mixtures is of economic importance in a variety of industries such as cellulose acetate manufacture, etc. Study of the vapour-liquid equilibrium data of acetic acid-water reveals low relative volatility (average $\alpha = 1.8$) of the constituents and therefore, a tall column (theoretical stages ≈ 30) and substantial energy are required for the separation. Azeotropic distillation or liquid-liquid extraction followed by distillation are therefore preferred routes for the recovery[5].

In an acetic acid plant, weak acid having 30% acid is obtained. Since the water content of the weak acid is high (70%), extraction followed by distillation is chosen for the recovery of acid. A flowsheet of the system[5] is shown in Fig. 6.6.

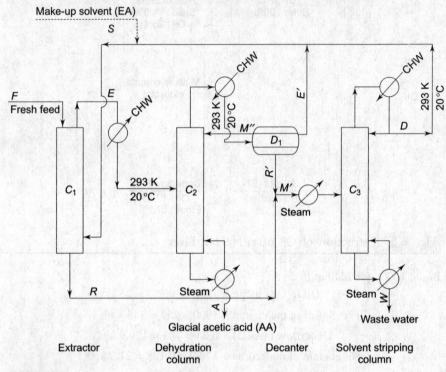

Fig. 6.6 Recovery of Acetic Acid by Ethyl Acetate Extraction

Following operating data are collected from a plant[6].

A.	Stream	Mass % acetic acid (AA)
	Feed to extractor (F)	30
	Extract phase from extractor (E)	21
	Raffinate phase from extractor (R)	5.5
	Bottom layer of decanter (R')	1
	Waste water from solvent stripping column (W)	4

B. Distribution co-efficient[5] (M) in the decanter is 0.89 at 291.5 K(18°C).

C. Overhead product (D) from the solvent stripping column (C_3) is to have azeotropic composition; i.e., ethyl acetate: 76 mole % and water: 24 mole %. Figure 6.7 shows the ternary liquid-liquid equilibrium diagram[5]. Based on the feed rate of 1000 kg/h of weak acid, establish the material balance at each point on the flow sheet.

Solution: Basis: Feed rate, F = 1000 kg/h

In Fig. 6.7, a binodal curve is given. It indicates the change of solubility of ethyl acetate and water-rich phases upon addition of acetic acid. Any mixture outside the curve will be a homogeneous phase. Any mixture underneath the curve, such as M, will form two insoluble, saturated liquid phases of equibilirium compositions, indicated by E (rich in ethyl acetate) and R (rich in water). The line ER joining these equilibrium compositions is a *tie line* which passes through M, representing the mixture as a whole. Other tie lines is $E'R'$ (which passes through M').

At times, there are two binodal curves on a ternary diagram (refer Exercise 6.8). In such a case, liquid mixture between two binodual curves separate in two phases. Mixtures, outside the binodal curves on either side are homogeneous.

Overall Material Balance:

Composition of stream D is given as 0.76 mole fraction ethylacetate and 0.24 mole fraction water. When converted to mass fraction, they are 0.94 and 0.06 respectively. Mark points F, A, W, R, R', and D on the ternary diagram (Fig. 6.7 a and b). Line joining the points A and D gives the distillation boundary. Any mixture on the right side of the line cannot achieve composition of the left side region in a single distillation column. Reverse is also true.

Using line ratio principle (Lever rule),

$$\frac{W}{A} = \frac{AF}{FW} = \frac{15.77 \text{ units}}{5.87 \text{ units}}$$

or

$$\frac{W}{A+W} = \frac{AF}{AW} = \frac{15.77}{(15.77 + 5.87)} = \frac{15.77}{21.64}$$

But

$$A + W = F = 1000$$

$$W = \frac{15.77 \times 1000}{21.64} = 728.7 \text{ kg/h}$$

$$A = 1000 - 728.7 = 271.2 \text{ kg/h}$$

Material balance across C_3:

Feed M' to C_3 is a mixture of R and R' and hence M' lies on line RR'.

M' is a mixture of D and W. Line DW will intersect RR' at M'.

$$R + R' = D + W$$

$$\frac{W}{D} = \frac{DM'}{M'W} = \frac{19.31 \text{ units}}{1.81 \text{ units}}$$

$$D = \frac{1.81}{19.31} \times 728.7 = 68.3 \text{ kg/h}$$

$$M' = D + W = 728.7 + 68.3 = 797.0 \text{ kg/h}$$

$$\frac{R'}{R} = \frac{RM'}{R'M'} = \frac{4.63 \text{ units}}{6.57 \text{ units}}$$

$$\frac{R'}{M'} = \frac{4.63}{(4.63 + 6.57)} = \frac{4.63}{11.2}$$

$$R' = \frac{4.63 \times 793.0}{11.2} = 329.5 \text{ kg/h}$$

$$R = 797.0 - 329.5 = 467.5 \text{ kg/h}$$

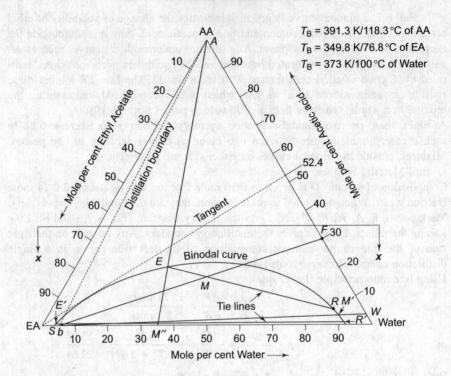

T_B = 391.3 K/118.3 °C of AA
T_B = 349.8 K/76.8 °C of EA
T_B = 373 K/100 °C of Water

Fig. 6.7(a) Ternary Liquid-Liquid Diagram[5] at 293.15 K(20°C)

Material Balance across C2:

Distrbution coefficient (M) is given at 291 K(18°C). Assume that it is same as that at 293 K(20°C).

$$M = \frac{\text{Mass fraction of AA in solvent rich layer}(E')}{\text{Mass fraction of AA in solvent lean layer}(R')} = 0.89$$

Mass fraction of AA in upper layer (E')

$$= 0.89 \times 0.01 = 0.0089$$

Point E' lies on the binodal curve and has 0.0089 mass fraction AA. Mark E' on the diagram. Join E' and R', forming a tie-line.

$$E = A + E' + R'$$

Let $\qquad E' + R' = M''$

$$E = A + M''$$

Thus, point M'' can be located on the diagram by intersecting AE and $E'R'$.

$$\frac{M''}{A} = \frac{EA}{M''E} = \frac{15.6 \text{ units}}{3.97 \text{ units}}$$

$$M'' = \frac{15.6 \times 271.2}{3.97} = 1065.7 \text{ kg/h}$$

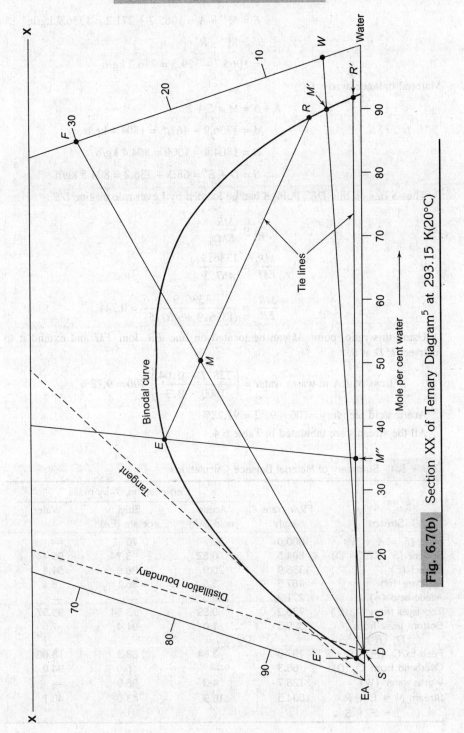

Fig. 6.7(b) Section XX of Ternary Diagram[5] at 293.15 K(20°C)

$$E = M'' + A = 1065.7 + 271.2 = 1336.9 \text{ kg/h}$$

$$E' = M'' - R'$$

$$= 1065.7 - 329.5 = 736.2 \text{ kg/h}$$

Material balance across C_1:

$$F + S = M = E + R$$

$$M = 1336.9 + 467.5 = 1804.4 \text{ kg/h}$$

$$S = 1804.4 - 1000 = 804.4 \text{ kg/h}$$

Also, $\qquad S = D + E' = 68.3 + 736.2 = 804.5 \text{ kg/h}$

Thus S lies on line DE'. Point S can be located by Lever rule on line DE'.

$$\frac{E}{R} = \frac{MR}{EM}$$

$$\frac{MR}{EM} = \frac{1336.9}{467.5}$$

$$\frac{MR}{ER} = \frac{1336.9}{(1336.9 + 467.5)} = 0.741$$

Using this ratio, point M can be located on line ER. Join FM and extend it to intersect $E'D$ at S.

$$\text{Loss of AA in waste water} = \left(\frac{728.7 \times 0.04}{1000 \times 0.3} \right) 100 = 9.72\%$$

Acetic acid recovery $= 100 - 9.72 = 91.28\%$

All the streams are tabulated in Table 6.4.

Table 6.4 Summary of Material Balance Calculations

Stream	Flow rate, kg/h	Composition, % by mass		
		Acetic acid (AA)	Ethyl acetate (EA)	Water
Feed ($F = A + W$)	1000.0	30	70	—
Solvent ($S = E' + D$)	804.5	0.82	3.74	95.44
Extract (E)	1336.9	20.9	28.0	51.1
Raffinate (R)	467.5	5.5	86.1	8.4
Acetic acid (A)	271.2	100.0	—	—
Top layer from D_1 (E')	736.2	0.89	3.54	95.57
Bottom layer from D_1 (R')	329.5	1.0	91.4	7.6
Feed to C_3 ($M' = R + R'$)	797.0	3.64	88.3	8.06
Overhead from C_3 (D)	68.3	—	6.0	94.0
Waste water (W)	728.7	4.0	96.0	—
Stream $M = E + R$ $= F + S$	1804.5	16.9	43.0	40.1

Note: Ternary diagrams are useful in defining the limits of operation. A tangent drawn from the point representing 100% ethyl acetate to the binodal curve will give the maximum limit of extraction (roughly 52 mass % AA). The weak acid of 30% strength can be separated by azeotropic distillation; i.e. with columns C_2 and C_3 only but the entrainer (ethyl acetate) requirement will be quite high (approx. 15.4 kg per kg water). If the waste acid contained less water, probably azeotropic distillation could have been more economical. Also entrainer selection depends on the azeotropic composition. Other entrainers, such as mixture of ethyl acetate and benzene (15 to 20% by vol.), cyclohexanone, methyl cyclohexanone, etc. are also in use, depending on weak acid strength.

6.5 CRYSTALLIZATION

Crystallization is a unit operation in which the dissolved solids of the solution are separated out by solubility differences at different temperatures and/or concentrations of the solution (by evaporation). In this operation, the final mother liquor is always saturated. Solubility data are extensively tabulated in Perry's Chemical Engineer's Handbook [7].

Example 6.7 What will be the yield of Glauber salt ($Na_2SO_4 \cdot 10H_2O$) if a pure 32% solution is cooled to 293.15 K (20°C) without any loss due to evaporation?
Data: Solubility of Na_2SO_4 in water at 293.15 K (20°C) is 19.4 kg per 100 kg water [7].
Solution: Basis: 100 kg free water
   Initial solution is 32% concentrated, i.e., 100 kg original solution contains 32 kg Na_2SO_4 and 68 kg water.
Water associated with Na_2SO_4 = (molar mass of $10H_2O$/molar mass of Na_2SO_4) × 32

$$= \left(\frac{180}{142}\right) \times 32 = 40.56 \text{ kg}$$

$$\text{Free water} = 68 - 40.56 = 27.44 \text{ kg}$$

Glauber salt present in 100 kg free water $= \dfrac{[(32 + 40.56) \times 100]}{27.44} = 264.4 \text{ kg}$

The final mother liquor (at 293.15K) contains 19.4 kg Na_2SO_4 per 100 kg water.

Water associated with Na_2SO_4 in the solution $= \dfrac{(180 \times 19.4)}{142} = 24.6 \text{ kg}$

$$\text{Free water} = 100 - 24.6 = 75.4 \text{ kg}$$

Glauber salt present in 100 kg water $= \left[\dfrac{(19.4 + 24.6)}{75.4}\right] \times \dfrac{1}{100}$

$$= 58.36 \text{ kg}$$

Yield of Glauber salt per 100 kg free water = 264.4 − 58.36

$$= 206.04 \text{ kg Na}_2\text{SO}_4 \cdot 10\text{H}_2\text{O}$$

$$\% \text{ yield of Glauber salt} = \left(\frac{206.04}{264.4}\right) \times 100 = 77.93$$

Note: The same problem can be solved algebraically by assuming x kg yield of crystals per 100 kg original solution and making a material balance of Na$_2$SO$_4$ in the original solution, mother liquor and crystals.

Example 6.8 A saturated solution of MgSO$_4$ at 353 K (80°C) is cooled to 303 K (30°C) in a crystallizer. During cooling, mass equivalent to 4% solution is lost by evaporation of water. Calculate the quantity of the original saturated solution to be fed to the crystallizer per 1000 kg crystals of MgSO$_4$ · 7H$_2$O. Solubilities of MgSO$_4$ at 303 K (30°C) and 353 K (80°C) are 40.8 and 64.2 kg per 100 kg water respectively[7].
Solution: Basis: 100 kg free water in the original solution.

Initial saturated solution is at 353 K.

Associated water in the original solution = (molar mass of 7H$_2$O/molar mass of MgSO$_4$) × 64.2

$$= \left(\frac{128}{120.3}\right) \times 64.2 = 67.24 \text{ kg}$$

Free water = 100 − 67.24 = 32.78 kg

MgSO$_4$ · 7H$_2$O in 100 kg free water = $\dfrac{[(64.20 + 67.24) \times 100]}{32.76}$

$$= 401.2 \text{ kg}$$

It is stated that 4% of the original solution gets evaporated.

Evaporation = (401.2 + 100) × 0.04 = 20.05 kg

In the mother liquor, the free water quantity will be = 100 − 20.05 = 79.95 kg

At 303 K, associated water with MgSO$_4$

in the mother liquor = $\left(\dfrac{126}{120.3}\right) \times 40.8 = 42.73$ kg

Free water in the mother liquor = 100 − 42.73 = 57.27 kg

Crystals of MgSO$_4$ · 7H$_2$O in the mother liquor for

79.95 kg free water = $\dfrac{[(42.73 + 40.80) \times 79.95]}{57.27}$

$$= 116.6 \text{ kg}$$

Yield of crystals = 401.2 − 116.5

$$= 284.6 \text{ kg MgSO}_4 \cdot 7\text{H}_2\text{O}$$

However, it is desired to get 1000 kg crystals.

Quantity of original solution to be fed

$$\text{to the crystallizer} = \frac{(501.2 \times 1000)}{284.6} = 1760.5 \text{ kg} \quad Ans.$$

Alternate Method:

A short-cut to the above calculations can be had with the use of the equation[7] given below:

$$C = R \frac{\left[100W - S(H - E) \right]}{\left[100 - S(R-1) \right]} \qquad (6.4)$$

where C = mass of crystals in the final magma in kg

R = molar mass of hydrated solute/molar mass of anhydrous solute

$$= \frac{246.3}{120.3} = 2.05$$

S = solubility of solute (kg) at the final temperature in 100 kg water

= 40.8 kg

W = mass of anhydrous solute in the original solution

= 64.2

H = total mass of solvent in the batch at the beginning of the process

= 100 kg (basis for calculations)

E = evaporation during the process = $(64.2 + 100) \times 0.04$

= 6.56 kg

Substituting the above values in Eq. (6.4)

$$C = \frac{2.05 \left[(100 \times 64.2) - 40.8 (100 - 6.56) \right]}{\left[100 - 40.80 (2.05 - 1) \right]}$$

= 93.52 kg yield of crystals

For yield of 1000 kg crystals,

$$\text{the charge to the crystallizer} = \frac{(164.2 \times 1000)}{93.52} = 1755.8 \text{ kg} \qquad Ans.$$

Note: Example 6.7 can be solved with the help of the above equation, in which case $E = 0$.

Crystallization is particularly useful for separating inorganic compounds from aqueous solutions be seen from Examples 6.7 and 6.8 above. Organic chemicals are normally purified by distillation. However, in many instances, crystallization is a more attractive method to distillation for reasons, explained in Sec. 6.4, in separating organic compounds. For employing this method, it is important to understand a phase diagram which determines the equilibrium process.

For eutectic systems, crystallization process has a key advantage over distillation as the solid phase separated by cooling is pure. Following examples will be useful in understanding phase diagrams.

Example 6.9 A feed to the crystallizer consists of 70% p-dichlorobenzene (p-DCB) and 30% o-DCB (by mass). It is fed to a crystallizer at 325 K (52°C). Using Fig. 6.8 evaluate the following.

(a) The feed is cooled to 290 K (17°C). Calculate the percentage recovery of p-DCB.

(b) The mixture is further cooled to 255 K (– 18°C) without separating crystals, formed at 290 K(17°C). Calculate the additional recovery of p-DCB.

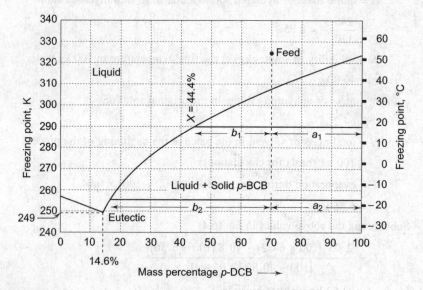

Fig. 6.8 Eutectic diagram of p-DCB and o-DCB[8]

(Reproduced with the permission of Putman Publishing Co., USA)

Solution (a) The feed point, representing 70% p-DCB and 325 K is shown on Fig. 6.8. Cooling of the mixture is represented by a vertical line. A horizontal line at 290 K provides material balance.

$$\text{Solids (p-DCB) separated} = \frac{b_1}{(a_1 + b_1)} \times 100 = \frac{4.91 \times 100}{(4.91 + 5.76)} = 46.0\%$$

Mother liquor at 290 K will contain 44.4% p-DCB.

$$\text{Recovery of p-DCB} = \frac{(46.0 \times 100)}{70} = 65.7\% \qquad \textit{Ans.} (a)$$

(b) At 255 K, solids (p-DCB) separated $= \dfrac{b_2}{(a_2 + b_2)} \times 100 = \dfrac{10.22 \times 100}{(5.76 + 10.22)}$

$$= 64.0\%$$

Mother liquor at 290 K will contain 16.7% p-DCB.

$$\text{Recovery of } p\text{-DCB} = \frac{(64.0 \times 100)}{70} = 91.4\%$$

$$\text{Additional recovery} = 91.4 - 65.7 = 25.7\% \qquad \textit{Ans.} \text{ (b)}$$

Note: It is desirable to separate crystals in a centrifuge at 290 K and only mother liquor (containing 44.4% p-DCB) should further be cooled to achieve additional recovery of 25.7%. Such an operation will result in saving in refrigeration requirement.

Example 6.10 In a batch reaction, a mixture of o- and p-nitrochlorobenzenes (NCB) is produced which is 98% solvent-free. These isomers are to be fractionated into pure products by crystallization. The crystallization section of the plant is shown in Fig. 6.9. The feed, containing 80% p-isomer and 20% o-isomer (mass %), is fed to a simple crystallizer where it is cooled to 289 K (16°C). At this temperature both the isomers form an eutectic mixture, containing 33.1 mole % p-NCB. The liquid mixture, after the removal of crystals of the p-isomer, is taken to an extractive crystallization unit in which p-nitrotoluene is used as a solvent[9]. The operating temperature of the extractive crystallization unit is 278 K (5°C). Isotherms of the ternary system are given in Fig. 6.10. Bottoms from both the crystallization units are collected as p-isomer product. This product is 98% (mass %) pure on a solvent-free basis from the centrifuges. The top product from the extractive unit contains 5% (by mass) solvent.

The solid reflux from the evaporator plays a determining role in the cost of the extraction unit and the empirical relationship between the two parameters is given by

$$C_T = a + R + \frac{1}{R^2}$$

where C_T = cost of extractive crystallization unit

   a = constant

   R = reflux ratio

Based on a feed rate of 5000 kg/h solvent-free product from the reactor, calculate (a) flow rates of products and their purities, and (b) flow rate of the make-up solvent.

Solution   Basis: 5000 kg/h solvent-free mixture (F) to simple crystallization unit

   Molar mass of NCB = 157.5

   p-NCB (B) in the feed = 4000 kg/h = 25.4 kmol/h

   o-NCB (A) in the feed = 1000 kg/h = 6.35 kmol/h

In the simple crystallization unit, the eutectic mixture is formed by cooling it to 289 K (16°C). The mother liquor this unit will contain 33.1 mole % B. The product from the centrifuge will be pure B. Since A does not get crystallized out, it can be used to make the material balance.

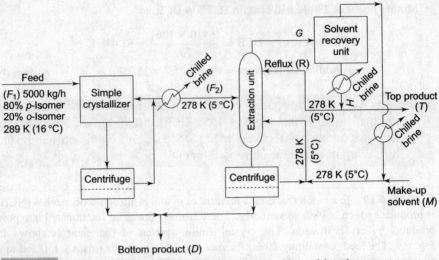

Feed

(F_1) 5000 kg/h
80% p-Isomer
20% o-Isomer
289 K (16 °C)

Simple crystallizer

Chilled brine (F_2)
278 K (5 °C)

Extraction unit

Reflux (R)

Solvent recovery unit

G

278 K (5°C)

Chilled brine

H

Top product (T)

Chilled brine

Make-up solvent (M)

278 K (5°C)

278 K (5°C)

Centrifuge

Centrifuge

Bottom product (D)

Fig. 6.9 Extractive Crystallization of o- and p-Nitrochlorobenzenes

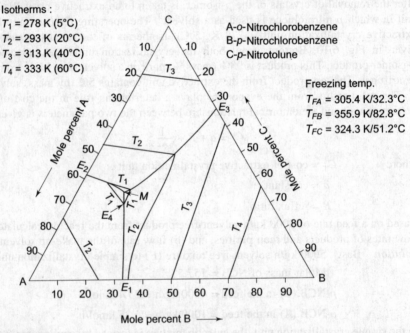

Isotherms :
T_1 = 278 K (5°C)
T_2 = 293 K (20°C)
T_3 = 313 K (40°C)
T_4 = 333 K (60°C)

A-o-Nitrochlorobenzene
B-p-Nitrochlorobenzene
C-p-Nitrotoluene

Freezing temp.
T_{FA} = 305.4 K/32.3°C
T_{FB} = 355.9 K/82.8°C
T_{FC} = 324.3 K/51.2°C

Mole percent A

Mole percent C

Mole percent B →

Fig. 6.10 Ternary Isotherms for Nitrochlorobenzenes and Nitrotoluene[9]

(*Reproduced with the permission of the Indian Institute of Chemical Engineers*)

Total mother liquor entering extractive

$$\text{crystallization unit} = \frac{6.35}{(1 - 0.331)} = 9.49 \text{ kmol/h}$$

B in the mother liquor = 9.49 – 6.35 = 3.14 kmol/h

For optimizing solid reflux,

$$\frac{dC_T}{dR} = 1 - \frac{2}{R^3}$$

$$= 0$$

$$R^3 = 2$$

$$R = 1.26$$

The path of extractive crystallization is shown in Fig. 6.10. Point E_1 represents the eutectic mixture (F_2). Points E_2 and E_3 represent eutectic compositions, containing 42.2 mole % and 67.5 mole % p-nitrotoluene (C) respectively. M is the point representing the ternary eutectic. The molar composition of the ternary eutectic is 48.3% A, 16.5% B and 35.2% C. With the addition of solvent C in F_2, the composition of the ternary mixture follows the path E_1M. Point E_4 lies on the isotherm of 278 K (5°C) and hence it represents the composition of the mother liquor.

Table 6.5 Composition of Mother Liquor from Extractive Crystallization Unit

Component	Composition of E_4 mixture	
	mole %	mass %
o-nitrochlorobenzene (A)	51	53.1
p-nitrochlorobenzene (B)	19	19.8
p-nitrotoluene (C)	30	27.1

Let T and D be the flow rates of the top product from extraction unit and bottom product from both units together respectively and x be the mass fraction of the B in T. Overall material balance:

p-isomer (B):

$$0.98\, D + xT = 4000 \qquad (1)$$

o-isomer (A):

$$0.02\, D + (1 - 0.05 - x)\, T = 1000 \qquad (2)$$

Material balance around solvent recovery unit:

p-isomer (B):

$$2.26\, Tx = 0.198\, G = xH \qquad (3)$$

o-isomer (A):

$$2.26\, T\,(0.95 - x) = 0.531\, G \qquad (4)$$

Solving Eqs. (1) to (4),

$$T = 1337.6 \text{ kg/h}$$

$$D = 3729.5 \text{ kg/h}$$

$$G = 3939.0 \text{ kg/h}$$

$$x = 0.258$$

Table 6.6 Composition of Various Streams

Component	T		D		G	H
	kg/h	mass %	kg/h	mass %	kg/h	kg/h
A	925.6	69.2	74.6	2.0	2091.9	2091.9
B	345.1	25.8	3654.9	98.0	779.9	779.9
C	66.9	5.0	Nil	—	1067.2	151.2
Total	1337.6	100.0	3729.5	100.0	3939.0	3023.0

Purity of top product = 69.2% A, Purity of bottom product = 98.0% B   *Ans.* (a)

Loss of solvent in T = Make-up solvent = 66.9 kg/h   *Ans.* (b)

Compositions of H, T and R are same.

6.6 PSYCHROMETRY

Psychrometry is the subject which deals with the properties of gas-vapour mixtures. In this type of operation, the gas is brought into contact with a pure liquid in which the gas is essentially insoluble. As a consequence, the liquid can evaporate and the gas becomes saturated with respect to the liquid. Alternatively, by cooling the gas, condensation of the liquid can take place. It is not necessary that the gas is saturated with respect to the liquid in each case. Unsaturation of the gas is expressed in different ways.

6.6.1 Humidification Operations

One of the most important psychrometric operations is the air-water contact operation. These operations are also referred to as humidification operations. In fact, humidification operations are so often encountered in day-to-day practice that whenever reference is made to a psychrometric operation, it is understood to be a humidification operation, unless clarified. Humidification operations also involve dehumidification.

Terminology

The common terminologies used for air-water contact operations are listed below.

(i) *Dry-bulb temperature* (*DB*)

The temperature of the vapour-gas mixture, recorded by the immersion of a thermometer in the mixture, is termed as dry-bulb temperature (*DB*).

(ii) *Absolute humidity* (*H*):

The mass of water vapour, present in a unit mass of dry air is termed as absolute humidity (*H*). It follows, therefore, that the units of H are g water vapour/kg dry air, or kg water vapour/kg dry air. Note that commonly used symbol in literature for humidity and enthalpy is same; i.e. H.

In some books, absolute molar humidity (H_m) is referred to. This is expressed as kmol water vapour/kmol dry air.

According to Dalton's law of partial pressure (see Chapter 2), each constituent, in a mixture of perfect gases exerts the same pressure as if it alone were present in the space occupied by the mixture at the temperature of the mixture. Total pressure of the gases is the sum of their partial pressures and the volume of the mixture of gases is the same as the volume occupied by each gas at its partial pressure.

$$p = \text{total pressure of the system} = p_w + p_a \qquad (6.5)$$

In humidification operation, usually p is the standard atmospheric pressure (101.325 kPa or 760 torr).

$$p_w = \text{partial pressure of water vapours in the mixture, kPa}$$

$$p_a = \text{partial pressure of air in the mixture, kPa}$$

If n_w are the number of moles water vapour present in n_a moles of dry air,

$$H_m = \frac{n_w}{n_a} \tag{6.6}$$

$$n_w = \frac{p_w \cdot V}{RT}$$

$$\text{and } n_a = \frac{p_a \cdot V}{RT}$$

$$H_m = \frac{p_w}{p_a}$$

$$= \frac{p_w}{p - p_w} \tag{6.7}$$

Thus, molar humidity is the ratio of partial pressure of water vapours to the partial pressure of air.

Absolute humidity can be expressed as

$$H = \frac{H_m \cdot M_w}{M_a} \tag{6.8}$$

where $M_w = \text{Molar mass of water} = 18.0153 \text{ kg/kmol}$

$$M_a = \text{Molar mass of air} = 28.9697 \text{ kg/kmol}$$

$$H = \frac{18.0153}{28.9697} H_m = 0.622\, H_m \tag{6.9}$$

$$= 0.622 \frac{p_w}{(p - p_w)} \tag{6.10}$$

When $p_w = p_s$, the vapour pressure of water at DB, the air is fully saturated. The absolute humidity at 100% saturation is called saturation humidity (H_s).

$$H_s = 0.622 \frac{p_s}{(p - p_s)} \tag{6.11}$$

(iii) *Percentage humidity or percentage absolute humidity or percentage saturation*:

Percentage humidity is defined as the ratio of the actual absolute humidity to the saturation humidity.

$$\text{Percentage humidity} = \left(\frac{H}{H_s} \right) \times 100$$

$$= \frac{p_w (p - p_s)}{p_s (p - p_w)} \times 100 \tag{6.12}$$

(iv) *Relative humidity or percentage relative humidity or relative saturation (RH)*

Relative humidity is defined as the ratio of the partial pressure of water vapour in air to the vapour pressure of water at the dry bulb temperature (*DB*).

$$RH = \left(\frac{p_w}{p_s}\right) \times 100 \qquad (6.13)$$

Use of Eq. (6.5) to (6.13) requires the vapour pressure data. Table 6.7 gives the pressure of aqueous vapour over ice for temperature from 175 K (− 98°C) to 273 K (0°C). The vapour pressure of water between 273 K (0°C) and 374.9 K (101.9°C) is given in Table 6.8.

(v) *Humid heat* (C_H):

Humid heat is defined as the heat capacity of 1 kg dry air and the moisture contained in it.

$$C_H = 1.006 + 1.84\,H \text{ kJ/(kg dry air} \cdot \text{K)} \qquad (6.14)$$

Insignificant error (less than 0.5%) will be realised by the use of Eq. (6.14) in the temperature range 233 K to 353 K (− 40°C to 80°C).

(vi) *Humid volume* (V_H)

Humid volume is the volume of a mixture of air and accompanying water vapour per kg of dry air. This is also known as *psychrometric volume*.

$$V_H = \frac{RT}{p_w \cdot M_w} \qquad (6.15)$$

$$V_{Hs} = \frac{RT}{p_s \cdot M_w} \qquad (6.16)$$

$$R = \text{Universal gas constant}$$

$$= 8.314\,51 \text{ m}^3 \cdot \text{kPa/(kmol} \cdot \text{K)}$$

Table 6.7 Vapour Pressure of Ice[10]

Temperature		Vapour pressure, Pa				
°C	K	Tiemperature interval, K				
		0	2	4	6	8
− 90	183.15	0.0093	0.0064	0.0044	0.0029	0.002
− 80	193.15	0.0533	0.0387	0.0267	0.0187	0.0133
− 70	203.15	0.2586	0.1907	0.14	0.1027	0.0747
− 60	213.15	1.077	0.8186	0.6186	0.4653	0.348
− 50	223.15	3.94	3.066	2.373	1.84	1.413
− 40	233.15	12.879	10.239	8.119	6.413	5.04
− 30	243.15	38.12	30.90	24.97	20.09	16.12

(Contd.)

Table 6.7 (Contd.)

Temperature		Vapour pressure, Pa				
°C	K	Tiemperature interval, K				
		0.0	0.2	0.4	0.6	0.8
– 29	244.15	42.26	41.46	40.53	39.73	38.93
– 28	245.15	46.8	45.86	44.93	44	43.2
– 27	246.15	51.86	50.8	49.86	48.8	47.86
– 26	247.15	57.33	56.26	55.2	54	52.93
– 25	248.15	63.46	62.26	60.93	59.73	58.53
– 24	249.15	70.13	68.66	67.33	65.99	64.79
– 23	250.15	77.33	75.86	74.39	72.93	71.46
– 22	251.15	85.33	83.59	81.99	80.39	78.93
– 21	252.15	93.99	92.13	90.39	88.66	86.93
– 20	253.15	103.5	101.5	99.59	97.73	95.86
– 19	254.15	113.9	111.7	109.6	107.5	105.5
– 18	255.15	125.2	122.8	120.5	118.3	116
– 17	256.15	137.5	134.9	132.4	130	127.5
– 16	257.15	150.9	148.1	145.5	142.7	140.1
– 15	258.15	165.5	162.5	159.5	156.7	153.7
– 14	259.15	181.5	178.1	174.9	171.7	168.5
– 13	260.15	198.7	195.2	191.6	188.1	184.8
– 12	261.15	217.6	213.6	209.8	206.1	202.4
– 11	262.15	238	233.7	229.6	225.4	221.4
– 10	263.15	260	255.4	251	246.5	242.2
– 9	264.15	284.1	279	274.2	269.4	264.6
– 8	265.15	310.1	304.6	299.4	294.2	289
– 7	266.15	338.2	332.4	326.6	321	315.6
– 6	267.15	368.6	362.4	356.2	350.1	344.1
– 5	268.15	401.7	394.9	388.2	381.6	375
– 4	269.15	437.3	430	422.8	415.6	408.6
– 3	270.15	475.7	467.8	460.1	452.4	444.8
– 2	271.15	517.3	508.8	500.4	492.1	484
– 1	272.15	562.2	552.9	543.3	534.9	526.1
– 0	273.15	610.8	600.5	590.8	581.2	571.6
+ 0.01*	273.16	611.2				

*Triple point of water (basis of Steam Tables)
(*Reproduced with permission of CRC Press Inc, USA from Handbook of Chemistry and Physics, 64th Ed.*)

(vii) *Dew point* (*DP*):

Dew point is the temperature at which the air-water vapour mixture becomes saturated when the mixture is cooled at constant total pressure in the absence of liquid water. During measurement of *DP*, air-water vapour mixture is cooled and temperature corresponding to first dew is measured and hence it is termed as dew point. This means that the partial pressure of water vapour in the mixture equals the vapour pressure of water at *DP*. Dew point is always lower or equal to the dry bulb temperature.

(viii) *Wet bulb temperature* (*WB*):

If a thermometer, having the bulb covered with a wet wick, is kept in air-water vapour mixture, it will read a steady value after a few seconds. This

Table 6.8 Vapour Pressure of Water

Temperature		Vapour Pressure, kPa — Temperature Interval, K or °C									
t °C	T K	0	0.1	0.2	0.3	0.4	0.5	0.6	0.7	0.8	0.9
0	273.15	0.6108	0.615	0.6195	0.6241	0.6286	0.6333	0.6379	0.6426	0.6473	0.6519
1	274.15	0.6566	0.6615	0.6663	0.6711	0.6759	0.6809	0.6858	0.6907	0.6958	0.7007
2	275.15	0.7055	0.7109	0.7159	0.721	0.7262	0.7314	0.7366	0.7419	0.7473	0.7526
3	276.15	0.7575	0.7633	0.7687	0.7742	0.7797	0.7851	0.7907	0.7963	0.8019	0.8077
4	277.15	0.8129	0.8191	0.8249	0.8306	0.8365	0.8423	0.8483	0.8543	0.8603	0.8663
5	278.15	0.8718	0.8785	0.8846	0.8907	0.9033	0.9095	0.9158	0.9222	0.9286	
6	279.15	0.9345	0.9415	0.9481	0.9546	0.9611	0.9678	0.9745	0.9813	0.9881	0.9949
7	280.15	1.0012	1.0086	1.0155	1.0224	1.0295	1.0366	1.0436	1.0508	1.0580	1.0652
8	281.15	1.072	1.0799	1.0872	1.0947	1.1022	1.1096	1.1172	1.1248	1.1324	1.14
9	282.15	1.1472	1.1556	1.1635	1.1714	1.1792	1.1872	1.1952	1.2032	1.2114	1.2195
10	283.15	1.227	1.2294	1.2443	1.2526	1.261	1.2694	1.2779	1.2864	1.2951	1.3038
11	284.15	1.3116	1.3212	1.33	1.3388	1.3478	1.3567	1.3658	1.3748	1.3839	1.3931
12	285.15	1.4014	1.4116	1.421	1.4303	1.4397	1.4492	1.4587	1.4683	1.4779	1.4876
13	286.15	1.4965	1.5072	1.5171	1.5269	1.5369	1.5471	1.5572	1.5673	1.5776	1.5879
14	287.15	1.5973	1.6085	1.6191	1.6296	1.6401	1.6508	1.6615	1.6723	1.6831	1.694
15	288.15	1.7039	1.7159	1.7269	1.7381	1.7493	1.7605	1.7719	1.7832	1.7947	1.8061
16	289.15	1.8168	1.8293	1.841	1.8529	1.8648	1.8766	1.8886	1.9006	1.9128	1.9249
17	290.15	1.9362	1.9494	1.9618	1.9744	1.9869	1.9994	2.0121	2.0249	2.0377	2.0505
18	291.15	2.0624	2.0765	2.0896	2.1028	2.116	2.1293	2.1426	2.156	2.1694	2.183
19	292.15	2.1957	2.2106	2.2245	2.2383	2.2523	2.2663	2.2805	2.2947	2.309	2.3234
20	293.15	2.3366	2.3523	2.3668	2.3815	2.3963	2.4111	2.4261	2.441	2.4561	2.4713
21	294.15	2.4853	2.5018	2.5171	2.5326	2.5482	2.5639	2.5797	2.5955	2.6144	2.6274
22	295.15	2.6422	2.6595	2.6758	2.6922	2.7086	2.7251	2.7418	2.7584	2.7751	2.7919
23	296.15	2.8076	2.8259	2.843	2.8602	2.8775	2.895	2.9124	2.93	2.9478	2.9655
24	297.15	2.9821	3.0014	3.0195	3.0378	3.056	3.0744	3.0928	3.1113	3.1299	3.1485

(Contd.)

Table 6.8 Contd.

| Temperature | | Vapour Pressure, kPa | | | | | | | | | |
| t °C | T K | Temperature Interval, K or °C | | | | | | | | | |
		0	0.1	0.2	0.3	0.4	0.5	0.6	0.7	0.8	0.9
25	298.15	3.166	3.186	3.205	3.224	3.2432	3.2625	3.282	3.3016	3.3213	3.3411
26	299.15	3.3597	3.3809	3.4009	3.4211	3.4413	3.4616	3.482	3.5025	3.5232	3.544
27	300.15	3.5636	3.586	3.607	3.6282	3.6496	3.671	3.6925	3.7141	3.7358	3.7577
28	301.15	3.7782	3.8016	3.8237	3.846	3.8683	3.8909	3.9135	3.9363	3.9593	3.9823
29	302.15	4.004	4.0286	4.0519	4.0754	4.099	4.1227	4.1466	4.1705	4.1945	4.2186
30	303.15	4.2415	4.2673	4.2918	4.3164	4.3411	4.3659	4.3908	4.4159	4.4412	4.4667
31	304.15	4.4911	4.518	4.5439	4.5698	4.5958	4.6219	4.6482	4.6746	4.7011	4.7279
32	305.15	4.7534	4.7816	4.8087	4.8359	4.8632	4.8907	4.9184	4.9461	4.974	5.002
33	306.15	5.0288	5.0585	5.0869	5.1154	5.1441	5.173	5.202	5.2312	5.2605	5.2898
34	307.15	5.318	5.349	5.3788	5.4088	5.439	5.4693	5.4997	5.5302	5.5609	5.5918
35	308.15	5.6216	5.6541	5.6854	5.7168	5.7485	5.7802	5.8122	5.8443	5.8766	5.9088
36	309.15	5.94	5.9739	6.0067	6.0396	6.0727	6.106	6.1395	6.1731	6.207	6.241
37	310.15	6.2739	6.3093	6.3437	6.3783	6.4131	6.448	6.4831	6.5183	6.5537	6.5893
38	311.15	6.624	6.6609	6.6969	6.733	6.7693	6.8058	6.8425	6.8794	6.9166	6.9541
39	312.15	6.9908	7.0294	7.0673	7.1053	7.1434	7.1817	7.2202	7.2589	7.2977	7.3367
40	313.15	7.375	7.414	7.454	7.494	7.534	7.574	7.614	7.654	7.695	7.737
41	314.15	7.777	7.819	7.861	7.902	7.943	7.986	8.029	8.071	8.114	8.157
42	315.15	8.199	8.242	8.285	8.329	8.373	8.417	8.461	8.505	8.549	8.594
43	316.15	8.639	8.685	8.73	8.775	8.821	8.867	8.914	8.961	9.007	9.054
44	317.15	9.1	9.147	9.195	9.243	9.291	9.339	9.387	9.435	9.485	9.534
45	318.15	9.582	9.633	9.682	9.731	9.781	9.831	9.882	9.933	9.983	10.034
46	319.15	10.086	10.138	10.19	10.242	10.294	10.346	10.399	10.452	10.506	10.559
47	320.15	10.612	10.666	10.72	10.775	10.83	10.884	10.939	10.994	11.048	11.104
48	321.15	11.162	11.216	11.274	11.331	11.388	11.446	11.503	11.56	11.618	11.676
49	322.15	11.736	11.794	11.852	11.911	11.971	12.031	12.091	12.151	12.211	12.272

(Contd.)

Table 6.8 Contd.

| Temperature | | Vapour Pressure, kPa Temperature Interval, K or °C | | | | | | | | | |
| t | T | | | | | | | | | | |
°C	K	0	1	2	3	4	5	6	7	8	9
50	323.15	12.335	12.961	13.613	14.293	15.002	15.741	16.511	17.313	18.147	19.016
60	333.15	19.92	20.861	21.838	22.855	23.921	25.009	26.15	27.334	28.563	29.838
70	343.15	31.162	32.535	33.958	35.434	36.964	38.549	40.191	41.891	43.652	45.474
80	353.15	47.36	49.311	51.329	53.416	55.573	57.803	60.108	62.489	64.948	67.487

| Temperature | | Vapour Pressure, kPa Temperature Interval, K or °C | | | | | | | | | |
| t | T | | | | | | | | | | |
°C	K	0	0.1	0.2	0.3	0.4	0.5	0.6	0.7	0.8	0.9
90	363.15	70.109	70.362	70.63	70.898	71.167	71.437	71.709	71.981	72.254	72.527
91	364.15	72.815	73.075	73.351	73.629	73.907	74.186	74.465	74.746	75.027	75.31
92	365.15	75.608	75.876	76.162	76.447	76.734	77.022	77.31	77.599	77.89	78.182
93	366.15	78.489	78.767	79.06	79.355	79.651	79.948	80.245	80.544	80.844	81.145
94	367.15	81.461	81.749	82.052	82.356	82.661	82.968	83.275	83.583	83.892	84.202
95	368.15	84.526	84.825	85.138	85.452	85.766	86.082	86.4	86.717	87.036	87.356
96	369.15	87.686	67.997	88.319	88.643	88.967	89.293	89.619	89.947	90.275	90.618
97	370.15	90.944	91.266	91.598	91.931	92.266	92.602	92.939	93.276	93.615	93.954
98	371.15	94.301	94.636	94.979	95.323	95.667	96.012	96.359	96.707	97.056	97.407
99	372.15	97.761	98.109	98.463	98.816	99.171	99.528	99.885	100.244	100.602	100.964
100	**373.15**	**101.325**	101.688	102.052	102.417	101.782	103.15	103.517	103.887	104.258	104.629
101	374.15	105.001	105.374	105.749	106.125	106.501	106.879	107.258	107.638	108.019	108.402

(Reproduced from (I) Perry's Chemical Engineers Handbook, 6th Edition, McGraw.Hill, USA, 1984 and (ii) 1980 JSME Steam Tables in SI, The Japan Society of Mechanical Engineers, Japan with permissions.)

temperature is called the wet bulb temperature (*WB*). It represents the dynamic equilibrium of the heat transfer by convection to the surface and the mass transfer to the surroundings from the surface.

When wet bulb temperature is measured, errors due to the effects of radiation, convection, conduction and diffusion are expected. It is therefore recommended that air velocity of the order of 2.5 – 10.0 m/s is achieved over the long wet wick (extending well up the thermometer stem) for true measurement of the wet bulb temperature. For this purpose, a whirling psychrometer is normally preferred.

Wet bulb temperature is always lower than or equal to dry bulb temperature.

At 100% saturation, *DB* = *DP* = *WB*

This is an important property of psychrometry.

(ix) *Adiabatic saturation temperature (AST)*:

Adiabatic process is the one in which no heat flows into or out of the system but during which thermal changes usually occur within the system. When a definite quantity of water is allowed to evaporate in a stream of air adiabatically, the dry bulb temperature of air drops and the humidity of air increases. The final temperature of the intimately-mixed stream is termed as adiabatic saturation temperature (*AST*).

For air-water systems, *WB* and *AST* are practically same. This is because the latent heat of vaporization of water is quite high in comparison to the sensible heat content of air-water mixture. However, for any other gas vapour system, two temperatures may differ appreciably.

Carrier[11] presented following equation which is very useful in correlating most psychrometric properties of air-water vapour mixtures, known as *DBT*, *WBT* and the barometric (total) pressure.

$$p_W = p_{WB} - \left(\frac{(p - p_{WB})(T_{DB} - T_{WB})}{1546 - 1.44(T_{WB} - 273.15)} \right) \tag{6.17}$$

where p_W = actual partial pressure of water vapour at *DP*, kPa

p_{WB} = vapour pressure of water vapour at wet bulb temperature, kPa

p = total pressure, kPa

T_{DB} = dry bulb temperature, K

T_{WB} = wet bulb temperature, K

(x) *Enthalpy of humid air*:

Enthalpy of air-water mixture is the sum of the enthalpies of each constituent at its partial pressure and common (dry bulb) temperature.

$$i_a = 1.006(T_{DB} - 273.15) + H \cdot i_w \text{ kJ/kg dry air} \tag{6.18}$$

where i_w = total enthalpy of water vapour at T_{DB}, kJ/kg

At saturation,

$$i_{as} = 1.006(T_{DP} - 273.15) + H_s \cdot i_{ws} \text{ kJ/kg dry air} \tag{6.19}$$

Values of i_w and i_{ws} can be had from Steam Tables (Appendix III).

$$d = i_{as} - i_a \tag{6.20}$$

Thus d is the difference in enthalpy of air-water vapour mixture at T_{DB} and enthalpy of saturated air on adiabatic saturation. This is also known as *enthalpy deviation*. Note that for differentiation in nomenclature, enthalpy is denoted by i.

Psychrometric Chart for Air-water System

The psychrometric properties of the air-water system, as described in the above section, can be conveniently plotted in a chart form which is known as a psychrometric chart. Such a chart is more convenient for determining the properties of moist air and is useful for delineating the various humidification processes.

Fig. 6.11 is a psychrometric chart for the normal temperature range of 263 K (– 10°C) to 328 K (55°C) at 101.325 kPa. Similarly Fig. 6.12 is the high temperature psychrometric chart for the temperature range of 293 K (20°C) to 393 K (120°C) at 101.325 kPa. Table 6.9 gives the correction factors for different barometric pressures. These factors are to be applied to the values read from Fig. 6.11 and 6.12 when the barometric pressure is other than 101.325 kPa.

Table 6.9 Corrections in Psychrometric Properties of Air Due to Change in Barometric Pressure[12]

Barometric Pressures, kPa a (torr)	Humid (Specific) Volume	Humidity	Enthalpy
101.3 (760)	1.000	1.000	1.000
100.0 (750)	1.013	1.016	1.008
98.7 (740)	1.027	1.030	1.018
97.3 (730)	1.041	1.045	1.026
96.0 (720)	1.055	1.062	1.040
94.7 (710)	1.070	1.077	1.054
93.3 (700)	1.085	1.094	1.070
92.0 (690)	1.101	1.110	1.081
90.7 (680)	1.117	1.126	1.093
89.3 (670)	1.134	1.142	1.105
88.0 (660)	1.150	1.160	1.117
86.7 (650)	1.169	1.180	1.130

In both the psychrometric charts, dry bulb temperatures are plotted on the abscissa (*x*-axis). Right ordinate (*y*-axis) represents the absolute humidity in a g moisture per kg dry air for Fig. 6.11 and kg moisture/kg dry air for Fig. 6.12. In addition, constant humid volume lines, wet bulb lines and enthalpy deviation [d – refer Eq. (6.20)] are plotted on the graph. Enthalpy value at saturation are given on the left. Enthalpy of an unsaturated air-water vapour mixture is obtained by adding enthalpy deviation algebraically to the saturation enthalpy. It may be noted on the charts that *DB* and *WB* lines meet at one point on the saturation line which is called dew point (*DP*).

The use of psychrometric charts eliminates the input of physical properties in heat and mass balance calculations. In absence of this chart, Eq. (6.17) can be used to correlate various properties.

Example 6.11 Air at 7 bar g and 313 K (40°C) is used for pneumatic instruments. If its dew point is measured to be 233.15 K (– 40°C) at atmospheric pressure (i.e., 101.325 kPa) with the help of a dew point instrument, calculate the dew point of air under line pressure.

Solution

$$H_{\text{m}} = \left(\frac{p_w}{p_1 - p_w}\right) \qquad \text{Eq. (6.7)}$$

p_{w_1} = Vapour pressure of ice at 233.15 K

$\qquad$ = 12.879 Pa $\qquad\qquad$ (Table 6.7)

p_1 = 101.325 kPa

$$H_{\text{m}} = \frac{12.879}{(101\,325 - 12.879)} = 0.000\,1271 \text{ kmol/ kmol dry air}$$

At p_2 = 7 bar g = 801.325 kPa a

$$\frac{p_2}{p_2 - p_{w_2}} = 0.000\,1271$$

or $\qquad\qquad\qquad p_{w_2}$ = 101.835 kPa

From Table 6.7, $\quad$ dew point = 252.9 K (– 20.2°C) $\qquad\qquad$ *Ans.*

Note: From the above calculation, it is clear that the dew point of a gas is independent of its molar mass. Further, dew point under pressure is higher than at atmospheric pressure.

Example 6.12 The dry bulb temperature and dew point of ambient air were found to be 302 K (29°C) and 291 K (18°C) respectively. The barometer reads 100.0 kPa a (750 torr).

Compute (a) the absolute molar humidity, (b) the absolute humidity, (c) the % *RH*, (d) the % saturation, (e) the humid heat and (f) the humid volume. Also read these values from the psychrometric chart (Fig. 6.11) and evaluate enthalpy of air.

Solution $\quad$ Partial pressure of water in air = vapour pressure of water at *DP*

$$p_w = 2.0624 \text{ kPa} \qquad\qquad \text{(Table 6.8)}$$

$$p = 100.0 \text{ kPa a}$$

$$H_{\text{m}} = \frac{p_w}{(p - p_w)}$$

$$= \frac{2.0624}{(100.0 - 2.0624)}$$

$$= 0.021\,06 \text{ kmol water vapour/kmol dry air} \quad \textit{Ans. (a)}$$

$$H = 0.622\, H_m$$

$$= 0.622 \times 0.021\,06$$

$$= 0.0131 \text{ kg moisture/kg dry air} \qquad \textit{Ans. (b - i)}$$

At saturation,

$$DB = WB = DP$$

Vapour pressure at saturation

(i.e., at 302 K), $p_s = 4.004$ kPa

$$\% \, RH = \frac{p_w}{p_s} \times 100$$

$$= \left(\frac{2.0624}{4.004}\right) \times 100 = 51.51 \qquad \textit{Ans. (c - i)}$$

$$H_s = \left[\frac{p_s}{(p - p_s)}\right] 0.622$$

$$= 0.622 \times \frac{4.004}{(100.0 - 4.004)}$$

$$= 0.025\,94 \text{ kg/kg dry air}$$

$$\% \text{ Saturation} = \left(\frac{H}{H_s}\right) \times 100$$

$$= \left(\frac{0.0131}{0.025\,94}\right) \times 100 = 50.49 \qquad \textit{Ans. (d)}$$

$$C_H = 1.006 + 1.84\, H$$

$$= 1.006 + 1.84\,(0.0131)$$

$$= 1.03 \text{ kJ/(kg dry air} \cdot \text{K)} \qquad \textit{Ans. (e)}$$

$$\text{Humid volume } V_H = \left[\left(\frac{H}{M_A}\right) + \left(\frac{1}{M_B}\right)\right] 22.4136$$

$$\times \left[\frac{DB}{273}\right] \times \left(\frac{101.325}{p}\right)$$

$$= (0.000\,73 + 0.034\,48)\,(22.4136)\,(1.1062)\,(1.0133)$$

$$= 0.8846 \text{ m}^3\text{/kg dry air} \qquad \textit{Ans. (f - i)}$$

The above results can be had from the psychrometric chart (Fig. 6.11) and by applying correction factor from Table 6.9.

$$H = 0.0013 \text{ kg moisture/kg dry air at 101.3 kPa a}$$

$$= 0.0132 \text{ kg moisture/kg dry air at 100.0 kPa a } \textit{Ans. (b - ii)}$$

$$\% \, RH = 51.5 \qquad \textit{Ans. (c - ii)}$$

$$V_H = 0.8844 \text{ m}^3\text{/kg dry air} \qquad \textit{Ans. (f - ii)}$$

From Fig. 6.11, $WB = 294.4$ K (21.4°C)

$$i_{as} = 62.75 \text{ kJ/kg dry air and}$$

$$d = -0.28 \text{ kJ/kg dry air}$$

Hence enthalpy of ambient air-water mixture

$$i_a = 62.75 - 0.28$$

$$= 62.47 \text{ kJ/kg dry air} \qquad\qquad Ans. \text{ (g)}$$

Example 6.13 In a textile industry located in Ahmedabad, it is desired to maintain 80% *RH* in the weaving department. For this reason, fresh air is first saturated and then heated to obtain 80% *RH*. Fresh air enters the spray chamber (air-washer) at 314 K (41°C) *DB* and 297 K (24°C) *WB*. Air comes out from the air-washer at 95% *RH* which is subsequently heated indirectly to attain 80% *RH* with the help of saturated steam at 300 kPa a pressure.

Compute (a) the moisture added to the air during the above operation, (b) the *DB* and *WB* temperatures of the final air and (c) the heating load of the steam coil per kg dry air. (d) If the fresh air rate is 25 000 m³/h, calculate the steam consumption in kg/h.

Solution Basis: 1 kg dry air entering the air-washer

The two operations (i.e., saturation and heating) are shown schematically in Fig. 6.13. Both the paths of operation are indicated on the psychrometric chart in Fig. 6.14.

Let H_1 and H_2 be the absolute humidities of air before and after saturation respectively. Further the heating operation is performed at constant humidity and hence the absolute humidity of air before and after heating remains constant.

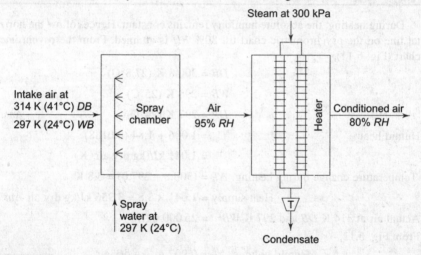

Fig. 6.13 Humidification of Air

From the psychrometric chart (Fig. 6.11), $H_1 = 11.8$ g/kg dry air. During saturation, the path of operation is the same as the wet bulb temperature line (or adiabatic saturation line). Travel on this line till 95% *RH* is attained.

At 297 K *WB* and 95% *RH*,

$$H_2 = 18.8 \text{ g/kg dry air}$$

Moisture added to the air during the saturation,

$$H = H_2 - H_1$$

$$= 18.8 - 11.8 = 7.0 \text{ g/kg dry air} \qquad\qquad Ans. \text{ (a)}$$

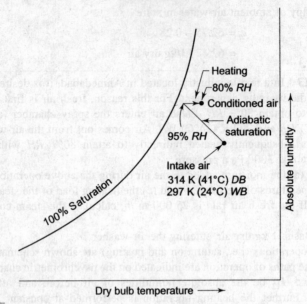

Fig. 6.14 Psychrometric Path for Humidification of Air

During heating, the absolute humidity remains constant. Hence follow the horizontal line on the psychrometric chart till 80% *RH* is attained. From the psychrometric chart (Fig. 6.11),

$$DB = 300.8 \text{ K } (27.8°C)$$

$$WB = 298 \text{ K } (25°C)$$

$$DP = 297 \text{ K } (24°C) \qquad \textit{Ans. (b)}$$

Humid heat

$$C_H = 1.006 + 1.84 \,(0.0188)$$

$$= 1.041 \text{ kJ/(kg dry air} \cdot \text{K)}$$

Temperature change during heating, $\Delta T = (300.8 - 297.0) = 3.8$ K

Heat supply $= 1.041 \times 3.8 = 3.956$ kJ/kg dry air *Ans. (c)*

Actual air at 314 K *DB* and 297 K *WB* $= 25\,000$ m³/h

From Fig. 6.11,

Humid volume, $V_H = 0.907$ m³/kg dry air

Mass flow rate of air, $q_m = \dfrac{25\,000}{0.907} = 27\,563.4$ kg dry air/h

Total heat load on heater, $\phi = 27\,563.4 \times 3.956 = 109\,035$ kJ/h

$$\equiv 30.29 \text{ kW}$$

At steam pressure $p = 300$ kPa a

Latent heat of evaporation, $\lambda_v = 2163.2$ kJ/kg   (See Appendix - III.2)

Steam consumption at the heater $= \dfrac{109\,035}{2163.2} = 50.4$ kg/h   *Ans. (d)*

Alternative calculations:

From Fig. 6.11, the enthalpy of air after saturation,

$$i_{a2} = 72.4 \text{ kJ/kg dry air}$$

Enthalpy of air after heating $i_{a3} = 76.4 - 0.1 = 76.3$ kJ/kg dry air

Change in enthalpies $= 76.3 - 72.4 = 3.9$ kJ/kg dry air *Ans.* (e)

Total heat load of heater $\doteq 3.9 \times 27\,563.4 = 107\,497$ kJ/h $\equiv 29.86$ kW

$$\text{Steam consumption} = \frac{107.49}{2163.2} = 49.7 \text{ kg/h} \qquad Ans. (f)$$

Note: In the heater, it is assumed that only latent heat of steam is given up and no subcooling takes place. Why?

Example 6.14 A waste heat recovery unit is installed on a stentering machine (drying machine) in a textile industry. It is basically a packed tower consisting of Pall rings. In the tower, hot air at 393 K (120°C) *DB* and 330 K (57°C) *WB* enters at the bottom and water is sprayed at the rate of 1.167 L/s at 305 K (32°C). Saturated air leaves the top at 313 K (40°C) while the hot water comes out at 323 K (50°C) from the bottom of the tower. The hot air rate is measured to be 2000 kg/h. Calculate (a) the heat loss rate from the hot air in the bed and (b) the percentage heat recovery in hot water, based on heat loss from the air.

Solution: Basis: 1 kg dry air fed to the tower

From Fig. 6.12, the following figures are read.

Absolute humidity of air at 393 K *DB*, 330 K *WB*, $H_1 = 0.0972$ kg/kg dry air

$$DP \text{ of the above air} = 325 \text{ K (52°C)}$$

Absolute humidity of saturated air at 313 K, $H_2 = 0.0492$ kg/kg dry air

Moisture condensed in the tower, $H = H_1 - H_2$

$$= 0.0972 - 0.0492$$
$$= 0.048 \text{ kg/kg dry air}$$

Humid heat of air at 393 K *DB* and 330 K *WB*,

$$C_{H_1} = 1.006 + 1.84 (0.0972)$$
$$= 1.185 \text{ kJ/(kg dry air} \cdot \text{K)}$$

Humid heat of saturated air at 313 K,

$$C_{H_2} = 1.1006 + 1.84 (0.0492)$$
$$= 1.0965 \text{ kJ/(kg dry air} \cdot \text{K)}$$

Enthalpy of entering air,

$$i_{a_1} = 1.006 (325 - 273) + 0.0972 \times 2596 + 1.185 (393 - 325)$$
$$= 52.31 + 252.33 + 80.58$$
$$= 385.22 \text{ kJ/kg dry air}$$

From Fig. 6.12,

$$i'_{a_1} = (393.8 - 7.5) = 386.3 \text{ kJ/kg dry air}$$

Enthalpy of outgoing air,

$$i_{a_2} = 1.006 \,(313 - 273) + 0.0492 \times 2574.4$$
$$= 166.9 \text{ kJ/kg dry air}$$

From Fig. 6.12,

$$i'_{a_2} = 166.6 \text{ kJ/kg dry air}$$

Total heat removed from the air (based on Fig. 6.12),

$$i = (i'_{a_1} - i'_{a_2})$$
$$= 386.3 - 166.6 = 219.7 \text{ kJ/kg dry air}$$

Mass flow rate of dry air, $q_m = \dfrac{2000}{(1 + 0.0972)} = 1822.82 \text{ kg/h}$

Heat loss rate from air, $\phi_1 = 219.7 \times 1822.82$

$$= 400\,474 \text{ kJ/h} \equiv 111.24 \text{ kW} \qquad\qquad \textit{Ans. (a)}$$

Heat gained by water, $\phi_2 = 1.167 \times 3600 \times 4.1868\,(323 - 305)$

$$= 316\,613 \text{ kJ/h} \equiv 87.95 \text{ kW}$$

$$\% \text{ Heat recovery} = \frac{(87.95 \times 100)}{111.24} = 79.06 \qquad\qquad \textit{Ans. (b)}$$

6.6.2 Psychrometric Operations Other Than Air-water Contact Operations

In Sec. 6.6.1, air-water contact operations were studied in detail. The terminology outlined in the section can be extended to any liquid-gas contact operation, such as the water-gas system, nitrogen-acetone system, carbon disulphide-hydrogen system, benzene-nitrogen system, etc. Psychrometric charts can also be constructed for these systems. The use of a computer is essential for generating the data necessary to construct these charts. However, in normal practice, these charts are not in day-to-day use and hence the calculations outlined in Sec. 6.6.1 can be used for these systems.

Example 6.15   It is desired to absorb 600 kg/h of carbon disulphide (CS_2) vapours on activated carbon from a stream of CS_2 in gaseous hydrogen. The CS_2-rich hydrogen stream enters the adsorber at a temperature of 293 K (20°C), total pressure of 106.7 kPa a (800 torr) and dew point of 273 K (0°C). CS_2-lean stream leaves with a dew point of 253 K (– 20°C). The exhausted activated carbon is regenerated by passing superheated steam through the adsorbent. The entering (regenerated) activated carbon has a CS_2 content of 0.04 kg CS_2 per kg of bone-dry (BD) activated carbon and that leaving has a CS_2 content of 0.32 kg CS_2 per kg of BD activated carbon.

The flow diagram is shown in Fig. 6.15.

Calculate (a) the volumetric flow rate of the entering CS_2–H_2 mixture, (b) the requirement of inlet activated carbon in kg/h and (c) the temperature to which the CS_2–H_2 mixture entering the system would have to be cooled after compression to 405 kPa a to remove as much CS_2 by condensation as done by adsorption. Use Eq. (5.24) and the data contained in Table 5.4.

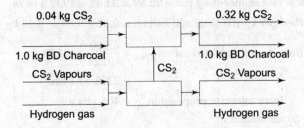

Fig. 6.15 Recovery of Carbon Disulphide by Adsorption

Solution: Basis: 800 kmol of inlet $CS_2 - H_2$ mixture

$$CS_2 \text{ entering with } H_2 = (p_{CS_2}) \times n/p$$

where p_{CS_2} is the partial pressure

of CS_2 in the inlet mixture = vapour pressure of CS_2 at dew point

= 16.93 kPa at 273.15 K (0°C)   [Eq. (5.24)]

p is the total pressure = 106.7 kPa a

n is the total number of moles of mixture = 800 kmol

$$CS_2 \text{ entering with } H_2 = \left(\frac{16.93}{106.7}\right) \times 800 = 126.9 \text{ kmol}$$

Hydrogen in the mixture = 800 – 126.9 = 673.1 kmol

$$CS_2 \text{ leaving the adsorber} = \left[\frac{p_{CS_2}}{(p - p_{CS_2})}\right] \times n_{H_2}$$

where p_{CS_2} is the vapour pressure of CS_2 at dew point in

outlet mixture = 6.194 kPa at 253 K (– 20°C)   [Eq. 5.24)]

p is the total pressure = 101.325 kPa

n_{H_2} = no. of moles of H_2 = 673.1 kmol

$$CS_2 \text{ leaving the adsorber} = \left[\frac{6.194}{(101.325 - 6.194)}\right] \times 673.1 = 43.83 \text{ kmol}$$

CS_2 adsorbed on activated carbon = 126.9 – 43.83 = 83.07 kmol

mass of CS_2 adsorbed = 83.07 × 76.143 = 6325.2

The design adsorption rate of CS_2 is 600 kg/h.

$$\text{Molar flow rate of inlet gas mixture} = \left(\frac{800}{6325.2}\right) \times 600$$

= 75.89 kmol/h

Specific volume of an ideal gas at 106.7 kPa and 293 K,

$$V = \frac{RT}{p} = 8.314 \times \frac{293}{106.7}$$

$$= 22.83 \text{ m}^3/\text{kmol}$$

Volumetric flow rate of incoming gas = $75.89 \times 22.83 = 1732.5 \ m^3/h$ *Ans.* (a)

    CS_2 absorbed per kg BD activated carbon = $0.32 - 0.04 = 0.28$ kg

      Mass flow rate of activated carbon, $q_m = \left(\dfrac{600}{0.28}\right) \times 1.04$

$$= 2228.57 \ kg/h \qquad \textit{Ans. (b)}$$

In an alternate proposition, $p = 405$ kPa a

Final desired concentration of

$$\text{the outlet } CS_2 - H_2 \text{ mixture} = \frac{43.83}{673.1} \ kmol \ CS_2/kmol \ H_2$$

$$= \frac{p_{CS_2}}{\left(p - p_{CS_2}\right)}$$

$$= \frac{p_{CS_2}}{\left(405 - p_{CS_2}\right)}$$

Solving the equation, $p_{CS_2} = 24.763$ kPa

By trial and error, the saturation temperature of CS_2 corresponding to the vapour pressure of 24.763 kPa is calculated to be 281.7 K (8.7°C) with the help of Eq. (5.24). Hence it can be concluded that the original CS_2–H_2 mixture must be cooled to 281.7 K at 405 kPa a for achieving the same concentration of the outlet CS_2–H_2 mixture with adsorption.

> **Note:** This example also covers the material balance of another unit operation known as "adsorption".

Example 6.16 A plant employing Hooker-type diaphragm cells produces caustic soda at the rate of 4000 kg/h. Chlorine produced in this plant is first scrubbed in water and later cooled in a Trombone cooler with the help of chilled water to remove the water contained in chlorine. It leaves the cooler saturated at 291.15 K (18°C) and enters an adsorption tower to remove the last traces of water. Concentrated sulphuric acid (90% by mass) is sprayed at the top of the tower. The acid leaving the bottom of the tower is made-up in concentration by adding the required quantity of 98% (by mass) sulphuric acid and is then recirculated. The quantity of acid circulated is so large that hardly any change in its temperature or concentration takes place. The heat of dilution of 1 kmol of 100% sulphuric acid with liquid water can be approximated by the formula[13],

$$Q = \frac{74\,780\,n}{(n + 1.7983)} \ kJ/kmol \ H_2SO_4$$

$$\text{(at 101.325 kPa and 291.15 K)}$$

where n = kmol of H_2O/kmol of H_2SO_4

Find the heat liberation rate in the tower.

Solution: Basis: 4000 kg/h of NaOH produced

The reactions taking place in the Hooker cell are as follows:

$$2 \ NaCl \rightarrow 2 \ Na^+ + 2 \ Cl^-$$

$$2\ Cl \rightarrow Cl_2 \qquad \text{(At anode)}$$

$$2\ Na^+ + H_2O \rightarrow 2\ NaOH + 2\ H^+$$

$$2\ H^+ \rightarrow H_2 \qquad \text{(At cathode)}$$

From the above reaction, it can be seen that when two moles of NaOH are produced, one mole of Cl_2 is produced.

$$2\ kmol\ NaOH = 1\ kmol\ Cl_2$$

$$\text{Chlorine produced} = \left(\frac{71}{80}\right) \times 4000 = 3550\ kg/h$$

$$\text{Molar rate of } Cl_2 = \frac{3550}{71} = 50\ kmol/h$$

Chlorine leaves the Trombone cooler saturated at 291 K.

Total pressure of system, $p = 101.325\ kPa$

Partial pressure of water, $p_w = 2.0624\ kPa$ at 291 K

$$\text{Moisture in chlorine} = \left[\frac{2.0624}{(101.325 - 2.0624)}\right] \times \left(\frac{18.0154}{70.906}\right)$$

$$= 0.005\ 279\ kg\ water/kg\ dry\ Cl_2$$

Total water in saturated $Cl_2 = 3550 \times 0.005\ 279 = 18.74\ kg/h$

Now, heat liberated in the absorption tower,

$$Q = \frac{74780n}{(n+1.7983)} \ kJ/kmol\ H_2SO_4 \qquad (1)$$

In order to obtain the heat of dilution per kmol water absorbed, it is necessary to differentiate Eq. (1) with respect to n.

$$\frac{dQ}{dn} = Q'$$

$$= \frac{134477}{(n+1.7983)^2} \ kJ/kmol\ H_2O \qquad (2)$$

For 90% concentration of acid,

$$n = \left[\frac{10}{18.0153}\right] \bigg/ \left[\frac{98.0776}{90}\right]$$

$$= 0.6049\ kmol\ H_2O/kmol\ acid$$

$$Q' = \frac{134477}{(0.6049 + 1.7983)^2}$$

$$= 23\ 285\ kJ/kmol\ H_2O \equiv 1292.5\ kJ/kg\ H_2O$$

In addition to the heat of dilution, latent heat of vaporization is also given up by water vapour when it condenses.

$$\lambda_v = 2459.0\ kJ/kg\ \text{at 291 K} \quad \text{Ref.A III.1}$$

$$\text{Total heat load} = Q' + \lambda_v$$

$$= 1292.5 + 2459.0 = 3751.5\ kJ/kg$$

Total heat liberated, $\phi = 3751.5 \times 18.74$

$$= 70\ 303 \text{ kJ/h} \equiv 19.53 \text{ kW} \qquad \textit{Ans.}$$

Example 6.17 Feed purge gas (dry) from the ammonia synthesis loop contains N_2: 20.6%, H_2: 62.0%, Ar: 4.1%, CH_4: 11.1% and NH_3: 2.2% (mole %). Feed gas is available at 50 bar g and 263 K (– 10°C). It is heated to 283 K (10°C) by exchanging heat with demineralised water, available at 307 K (34°C). Pressure drop in the heat exchanger is 50 kPa. Cooled water is sprayed at the top of the absorber and aqueous ammonium hydroxide solution containing 4% NH_3 (mass) is produced. Assume that: (i) the gas leaves the absorber at saturated conditions at the feed water temperature, (ii) ammonia slip from the absorber is 50 ppm (v/v) and (iii) pressure drop in the absorber is negligible. Refer Fig. 6.16 for the process flow. Calculate (a) the temperature of feed water to absorber and (b) the temperature of the aqueous ammonia solution leaving the absorber.

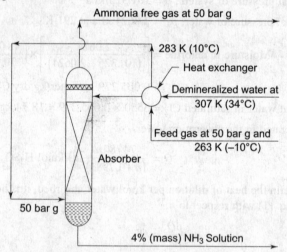

Fig. 6.16 Absorption of Ammonia from Purge Gas

Solution: Basis: 100 kmol feed gas

Assume that heat capacity constants of Table 5.1 are valid at high pressure.

Heat capacity constants:

$$\Sigma n_i \cdot a_i = 20.6 \times 29.5909 + 62 \times 28.6150 + 4.1 \times 20.7723$$
$$+ 11.1 \times 19.2494 + 2.2 \times 25.6503$$
$$= 609.573 + 1773.851 + 85.166 + 213.668 + 56.431$$
$$= 2738.689$$

$$(\Sigma n_i \cdot b_i) \times 10^3 = 20.6 \times (- 5.141) + 62 \times 1.0194$$
$$+ 11.1 \times 52.1135 + 2.2 \times 33.4806$$
$$= - 105.905 + 63.203 + 578.46 + 73.657$$
$$= 609.415$$

$$(\Sigma n_i \cdot c_i) \times 10^6 = 20.6 \times 13.1829 + 62 \times (- 0.1476)$$
$$+ 11.1 \times 11.973 + 2.2 \times 0.3518$$

$$= 271.568 - 9.151 + 132.9 + 0.774$$
$$= 396.091$$

$(\Sigma\, n_i \cdot d_i) \times 10^9 = 20.6 \times (-4.968) + 62 \times 0.769$
$$+ 11.1 \times (-11.3173) + 2.2 \times (-3.0832)$$
$$= -102.341 + 47.678 - 125.622 - 6.783$$
$$= -187.068$$

Heat gained by gas mixture $= 2738.689\,(283 - 263)$

$$+ 609.415 \times 10^{-3}\, \frac{(283^2 - 263^2)}{2}$$

$$+ 396.091 \times 10^{-6}\, \frac{(283^3 - 263^3)}{3}$$

$$- 187.068 \times 10^{-9}\, \frac{(283^4 - 263^4)}{4}$$

$$= 54\,773.8 + 3327.4 + 590.7 - 76.2$$
$$= 58\,615.7 \text{ kJ}$$

Heat gained by ammonia alone $= 1533.8$ kJ

Ammonia in feed gas $= 2.2$ kmol

Ammonia-free feed gas $= 97.8$ kmol

Average $\Sigma\,(n_i \cdot C^{\circ}_{mpi})$ for 97.8 kmol

$$\text{ammonia free gas mixture} = \frac{(58\,615.7 - 1533.8)}{20}$$

$$= 2854.1 \text{ kJ/(K} \cdot 97.8 \text{ kmol gas)}$$

In the outgoing gas mixture from the absorber,

ammonia-free gas $= 99.995\%$ (mole basis)

$$\text{Outgoing gas mixture} = \frac{97.8}{0.999\,95} = 97.805 \text{ kmol}$$

Ammonia absorbed $= 2.2 - 0.005 = 2.195$ kmol $\equiv 37.382$ kg

$$\text{Flow rate of 4\% ammonia solution} = \frac{37.382}{0.04} = 934.55 \text{ kg}$$

Water content of solution $= 934.55 - 37.382 = 897.168$ kg

Assume at first that the water outgoing with the gas mixture from the absorber is negligible.

$$\text{Fall in water temperature} = \frac{58\,615.7}{(897.168 \times 4.1868)} = 15.6 \text{ K}$$

Temperature of water

leaving the heat exchanger $= 307 - 15.6 = 291.4$ K (18.4°C) *Ans.* (a)

Vapour pressure of water at 291.4 K $= 2.116$ kPa (Table 6.8)

Total pressure $= 50$ bar g $= 5101.325$ kPa a

Assuming ideal gas behaviour, moisture content of the gas mixture

$$= \frac{97.805 \times 2.116}{(5101.325 - 2.116)}$$

$$= 0.0406 \text{ kmol} \equiv 0.73 \text{ kg}$$

Total demineralised water requirement $= 897.17 + 0.73 = 897.9$ kg

Actual fall in temperature of water in heat exchanger

$$= \frac{58\,615}{(897.9 \times 4.1868)} = 15.59 \text{ K}$$

This figure is quite close to 15.6 K, calculated earlier.

Now from Table 5.40,

$$\Delta H_f^\circ \text{ of 4\% solution} = -80.093 \text{ kJ/mol NH}_3$$

and $\qquad \Delta H_f^\circ$ of pure $NH_3 = -45.94$ kJ/mol NH_3

Heat of solution of 4% NH_3 solution $= -80.093 - (-45.94)$

$$= -34.153 \text{ kJ/kmol NH}_3$$

Total heat evolved $= 34\,153 \times 2.195 = 74\,996$ kJ

In the absorber, gas is further heated form 283 K to 291.4 K.

Heat picked up by the ammonia-free gas mixture (97.8 kmol)

$$= 2854.1 \,(291.4 - 283) = 23\,974.4 \text{ kJ}$$

Heat picked up by the ammonia solution

$$= 74\,996 - 23\,974.4 = 50\,991.6 \text{ kJ}$$

Assuming heat capacity of 4% NH_3 solution to be same as that of water, i.e., 4.1868 kJ/(kg · K),

$$\text{Rise in temperature} = \frac{50\,991.6}{934.55 \times 4.1868} = 13.0 \text{ K}$$

Temperature of aqueous ammonia solution leaving the absorber

$$= 291.4 + 13$$

$$= 304.4 \text{ K } (31.4°\text{C}) \qquad\qquad \textit{Ans. (b).}$$

> **Note:** It is assumed that the heat of solution calculated at 298.15 K(25°C) remains unchanged for all practical purpose. Reader may try heat load calculations by applying pressure correction to C_{mpi}°, using Fig. 5.3.

6.7 DRYING

Drying is an unit operation in which the solvent is evaporated with the help of heat and the final product is normally in the solid form. In most of the drying operations, the heat is provided by hot air or any other gas in which the solvent evaporates. The balance of bone-dry solids (tie material) helps in calculating the evaporation of the solvent. Similarly, the solvent contents of the incoming and outgoing gas allow the calculations of the volumetric or mass flow rate of gas.

In many of the drying operations, water is the solvent which is evaporated in air. The air-water mixture is exhausted out of the atmosphere via a once-through system. Recently, there has been increasing interest in evaporating organic solvents which must be recovered for both economic and environmental reasons. The required system design is a "closed loop" with a provision for solvent recovery. The design (material and energy balance) calculations for closed-cycle dryers to evaporate solvents differ from once-through units to evaporate water in three major respects:

(i)   The solvent must be recovered rather than discharged to the atmosphere.
(ii) Air cannot be used as the drying medium in most cases due to safety reasons. The drying gas is usually nitrogen. Properties of both are practically the same.
(iii) The properties of solvents are very different from that of water and from each other.

The first of the above differences indicates that the system is a closed loop and the solvent is recovered usually by adsorption/desorption followed by a scrubber/condenser with its recycle cooled by water or a refrigerant. The drying gas is returned from the condenser, reheated and recycled. Exercise 8.18 is a typical example in which *n*-hexane is used as a solvent.

The need for reliable and accurate physical properties data was adequately stressed in Chapter 5. In drying calculations, the effect that physical properties have on design factors has been studied extensively[14]. The percentage change in results caused by a + 1% change in properties of a simulated solvent at the dryer inlet temperature of 422 K (149°C) and dryer outlet temperature of 333 K (60°C) are given in Table 6.10. For the simulated solvent, properties considered were; the latent heat of vaporization of 465 kJ/kg, molar mass of 100 and heat capacities of liquid and vapour to be 1.884 and 1.465 kJ/(kg·K) respectively.

Table 6.10   Effect of + 1% Change in Physical Properties on the Final Results While Drying a Simulated Solvent[14]

Physical property	% Change in final results of	
	Volumetric flow rate	Head load
Latent heat of vaporization	0.76	0.77
Boiling point	0.09 to 0.52	0.05
Molar mass	− 0.05 to 0.20	Nil
Heat capacity of liquid	0.19	0.20
Heat capacity of vapour	− 0.06 to − 0.14	− 0.06

The following example relates to the drying of cloth in which water is the solvent.

Example 6.18   In a textile mill, wet cloth passes through a hot air dryer. The cloth enters with 90% moisture regain and leaves at 6% moisture regain at a speed of 1.15 m/s. The width of the cloth is 120 cm and its specific density on bone-dry basis is 0.095 kg/m^2. The temperature of the cloth leaving the dryer is 368 K (95°C). The ambient air enters the dryer at 303 K (30°C) *DB* and 298 K (25°C) *WB* while the hot air leaves the dryer at 393 K (120°C) *DB* and 328 K (55°C) *WB*. Saturated steam is used at 8 bar a and consumption rate is measured to be 885 kg/h. The heat capacity of cloth is 1.256 kJ/(kg · K).

(i) Calculate: (a) the bone-dry production of the dryer, (b) the evaporation taking place in the dryer and (c) the air circulation rate.

(ii) Make the complete heat balance of the dryer.

Solution: Basis: Cloth speed = 1.15 m/s

Production of bone-dry cloth = $1.15 \times 1.20 \times 3600 \times 0.095$

$$= 471.96 \text{ kg/h} \qquad \text{Ans. (i-a)}$$

Moisture regain of the cloth is defined as the kg moisture per kg bone-dry cloth.

Inlet moisture of the cloth = 0.90 kg moisture/kg bone-dry cloth

Outlet moisture of the cloth = 0.06 kg moisture/kg bone-dry cloth

Evaporation = $471.96 (0.9 - 0.06)$

$$= 396.45 \text{ kg/h} \qquad \text{Ans. (i-b)}$$

From Fig. 6.11 and Fig. 6.12,

Humidity of inlet air, $H_1 = 0.018\,05$ kg moisture/kg dry

air at 303 K *DB* and 298 K *WB*

Humidity of outlet air, $H_2 = 0.0832$ kg moisture/kg dry air

at 393 K *DB* and 328 K *WB*

Rise in humidity of circulating air = $H_2 - H_1$

$$= 0.0832 - 0.01805$$

$$= 0.065\,15 \text{ kg moisture/kg dry air}$$

$$\text{Fresh air rate, } q_{m_1} = \frac{396.45}{0.06515} = 6085.2 \text{ kg dry air/h}$$

Thus, the fresh air (or exhaust) rate should not be misunderstood as the recirculation rate of air. Usually, the air recirculation rate is five to ten times the fresh air entry. Humid volume of air at 303 K *DB* and 298 K *WB*,

$$V_H = 0.8837 \text{ m}^3/\text{kg dry air}$$

Volumetric flow rate of incoming air, $q_v = 6085.2 \times 0.8837 = 5377.5$ m^3/h *Ans.* (i-c)

Heat balance of the dryer:

DP of ambient air = 296.5 K

Latent heat of evaporation of water at 296.5 K, $\lambda_{v_1} = 2446.4$ kJ/kg

DP of exhaust air = 322.5 K

Latent heat of evaporation of water at 322.5 K, $\lambda_{v_2} = 2384.1$ kJ/kg

Reference temperature, $T_0 = 273.15$ K

Heat picked up by cloth, $i_1 = 471.96 \times 1.256 (368 - 303)$

$$+ 471.96 \times 0.06 (368 - 303) \times 4.1868$$

$$= 46\,237.2 \text{ kJ/h} \equiv 12.844 \text{ kW}$$

It will be assumed that the evaporation takes place at *DP* of the exhaust air, i.e., 322.5 K

Heat utilised for evaporation, $i_2 = 396.45 (322.5 - 303)$

$$+ 396.45 \times 2384.1$$

$$= 977\,544 \text{ kJ/h} \equiv 271.54 \text{ kW}$$

Enthalpy of ambient air over 273 K,

$$i_{a_1} = 1.006 (303 - 273.15) + 2556.4 \times 0.018\,05$$
$$= 76.32 \text{ kJ/kg dry air}$$

From Fig. 6.11, $\qquad i'_{a_1} = 76.4 - 0.2 = 76.2$ kJ/kg dry air

Enthalpy of exhaust air over 273 K, $DP = 322.8$ K (49.8°C)

$$i_{a_2} = 1.006 (322.8 - 273.15) + 2591.5 \times 0.0832$$
$$\qquad + (1.006 + 1.84 \times 0.0832)(393 - 328.8)$$
$$= 50.1 + 215.61 + 81.36$$
$$= 347.07 \text{ kJ/kg dry air}$$

From Fig. 6.12,

$$i'_{a_2} = 354.8 - 7.0 = 346.8 \text{ kJ/kg dry air}$$

$$\text{Enthalpy lost in air} = 346.8 - 76.2 = 270.6 \text{ kJ/kg dry air}$$
$$= 1646\,655 \text{ kJ/h} \equiv 457.404 \text{ kW}$$

This enthalpy also takes into account the heat lost due to evaporation.

Heat lost in exhaust air (sensible heat part) = 457.404 − 271.54 = 185.864 kW

At 8 bar a from Appendix A III·2,

$$h = 720.94 \text{ kJ/kg}$$
$$\lambda_v = 2046.5 \text{ kJ/kg}$$
$$\text{Total input by steam} = (720.94 + 2046.5)\,885$$
$$= 2449\,238 \text{ kJ/h} \equiv 680.344 \text{ kW}$$

It will be assumed that only the latent heat of steam is useful in heating the air and thus the condensate leaves at saturation temperature, having the sensible heat.

$$\text{Heat lost in condensate} = 720.94 \times 885$$
$$= 638\,032 \text{ kJ/h} \equiv 177.231 \text{ kW}$$

$$\text{Specific steam consumption, } q_{m_2} = \frac{885}{396.45}$$
$$= 2.232 \text{ kg/kg evaporation}$$

Table 6.11 Heat Balance of Dryer

	kW	%
Input: Steam	680.344	100.00
Output:		
Sensible heat of cloth	12.844	1.89
Heat utilised for evaporation	271.540	39.91
Heat lost in exhaust air	185.864	27.32
Heat lost in condensate	177.231	26.05
Unaccounted heat loss (by difference)	32.864	4.83
Total	680.344	100.00

Ans. (ii)

6.8 EVAPORATION

Evaporation is basically a similar operation to drying except that the final product is in the liquid form. This operation is usually carried out in a closed equipment (an exception is the open pan evaporator) and air is not used for the evaporation.

The energy crisis has led to a reconsideration of the evaporation systems. Multiple-effect evaporation is not the only answer for reducing the energy input. Mechanical vapour recompression, thermal recompression, use of flash steam, etc. are also considered as additional economy measures. However, each plant or operation must be evaluated from various considerations and the final choice must be made only after that. For example, the steam condensate purity can be lost in the case of thermal recompression, prohibiting the return of the condensate for use as the boiler feed make-up water.

Multiple effect evaporators have gained popularity in concentrating effluents in chemical industries. Vapours from the evaporators are partially utilised for evaporation by recompression. Balance vapours are condensed and used as boiler feed make-up or cooling tower make-up water.

Example 6.19 A quadruple-effect evaporator is fed with 1060 kg/h of 4% (by mass) caustic soda solution in a textile mill[15]. It is concentrated to 25% (by mass) lye. The saturated steam at 7 bar g is fed to the first effect. The cold feed also enters the first effect at 303 K (30°C). The final effect operates at 50.60 kPa a (vacuum of 380 torr). The operating pressure in first, second and third effects are observed to be 3.7, 2.35 and 0.8 bar g respectively. Neglect the boiling point elevation effects and assume that no heat loss due to radiation takes place from the evaporator bodies.

Table 6.12 Heat Capacity Data

Solution	Heat Capacity kJ/(kg · K)
Feed (C_{1F})	4.04
Solution leaving first effect (C_{11})	3.977
Solution leaving second effect (C_{12})	3.936
Solution leaving third effect (C_{13})	3.894
Solution leaving fourth effect (C_{14})	3.873

Evaluate the thermal performance of the system.
Solution: Basis: Weak liquor flow rate = 1060 kg/h
The flow patterns of the liquid and vapours are shown in Fig. 6.17.

$$\text{Solids in the weak liquor} = 1060 \times 0.04 = 42.4 \text{ kg/h}$$

$$\text{Concentrated liquor, leaving the fourth effect} = \frac{42.4}{0.25} = 169.6 \text{ kg/h}$$

$$\text{Total evaporation in all four effects} = 1060 - 169.6 = 890.4 \text{ kg/h}$$

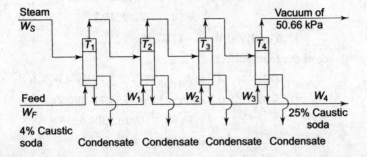

Fig. 6.17 Quadruple Effect Forward Feed Evaporator

Table 6.13 Operating Conditions in the Evaporator Stages

Effect number	Pressure, kPa g	Saturation temperature, K(°C)	Latent heat of evaporation of steam, λ_v kJ/kg
First	370	422.6 (149.6)	2114.4 (λ_{v_1})
Second	235	410.5 (137.5)	2151.5 (λ_{v_2})
Third	80	390.3 (117.2)	2210.2 (λ_{v_3})
Fourth	– 50.66	354.7 (81.7)	2304.6 (λ_{v_4})

Latent heat of steam at 700 kPa g, $\lambda_{vs} = 2046.3$ kJ/kg

Let

W_F be the feed flow rate = 1060 kg/h
W_S be the feed flow of steam to the first effect in kg/h
W_1 be the feed flow of liquor, leaving the first effect in kg/h
W_2 be the feed flow of liquor, leaving the second effect in kg/h
W_3 be the feed flow of liquor, leaving the third effect in kg/h
W_4 be the feed flow of liquor, leaving the last effect = 169.6 kg/h

Enthalpy balance of the first effect:

$$W_s\, \lambda_s = W_F\, C_{1F}\, (T_1 - T_F) + (W_F - W_1)\, \lambda_{v_1}$$

$$W_s \times 2046.3 = 1060 \times 4.04\,(422.6 - 303)$$

$$+ (1060 - W_1)\, 2114.4$$

$$W_s = 1345.57 - 1.033\, W_1 \qquad\qquad (1)$$

Enthalpy balance of the second effect:

$$(W_F - W_1)\, \lambda v_1 = W_1 \cdot c_{11}\, (T_2 - T_1) + (W_1 - W_2)\, \lambda_{v_2}$$

$$(1060 - W_1)\, 2114.4 = W_1 \times 3.977\,(410.5 - 422.6)$$

$$+ (W_1 - W_2)\, 2151.4$$

$$W_1 = 531.38 + 0.510\, W_2 \qquad\qquad (2)$$

Enthalpy balance of the third effect:

$$(W_1 - W_2)\, \lambda_{v_2} = W_2 \cdot c_{12}\, (T_3 - T_2) + (W_2 - W_3)\, \lambda_{v_3}$$

$$(W_1 - W_2)\, 2151.5 = W_2 \times 3.936\,(390.2 - 410.5)$$
$$+ (W_2 - W_3)\, 2210.2$$
$$W_1 - 1.990\, W_2 = -1.027\, W_3 \tag{3}$$

Enthalpy balance of the fourth effect:

$$(W_2 - W_3)\, \lambda_{v_3} = W_3 \cdot c_{13}\,(T_4 - T_3) + (W_3 - W_4)\, \lambda_{v_4}$$
$$(W_2 - W_3)\, 2210.2 = W_3 \times 3.894\,(354.7 - 390.2)$$
$$+ (W_3 - 169.6)\, 2304.6$$
$$W_2 - 1.98\, W_3 = -176.84 \tag{4}$$

Solving the above four equations algebraically,

$$W_3 = 416.7 \text{ kg/h}$$
$$W_2 = 648.2 \text{ kg/h}$$
$$W_1 = 862 \text{ kg/h}$$

Steam consumption, $\qquad W_s = 455.2$ kg/h

Mathcad solution gives the same values.

$$\text{Steam economy} = \frac{890.4}{455.2}$$
$$= 1.956 \text{ kg evaporation/kg steam}$$
$$\text{Specific steam consumption} = \frac{1}{1.956}$$
$$= 0.511 \text{ kg steam/kg evaporation} \qquad Ans.$$

Note: The above problem is quite simplified for calculation purposes. However, the actual enthalpies of the solutions are different from that of water and the boiling point elevations are quite significant. The reader may try the solution of the above problem with the actual enthalpies in Fig. 5.14.

6.9 LESS CONVENTIONAL OPERATIONS

In the preceding sections, the more commonly-encountered operations were discussed. Reverse osmosis, dialysis, thickening, etc. are less conventional operations. A few examples, relationg to reverse osmosis, were dealt in Chapter 3. The following illustration will deal with the thickening operation.

Example 6.20 A four-compartment washing thickener is employed in the recausticizing system of a kraft mill for washing of the white mud to recover soda values[16]. The unit is operated with the top two trays and the bottom two trays in parallel as shown in Fig. 6.18. The top two trays are operated in a counter-current fashion with respect to the bottom two rays. The entering white mud, M_2 is mixed with the overflow from the bottom two trays, O_1 and fed to the feedbox of the top two trays. The underflow from the top two trays, M_1 is mixed with the effluent from the water scrubber from a calcining kiln, W and fed to the feedbox of the bottom two rays. The overflow from the top two trays, O_2 passes onto the weak wash storage where it is employed for dissolving the smelt from the recovery furnances. The underflow from the bottom two trays, M_o is considered washed white mud and is pumped to the white mud storage tank. Later, it is filtered and the cake is calcined in a rotary kiln to CaO. The average of several samples taken over a 24-hour period shows the following results:

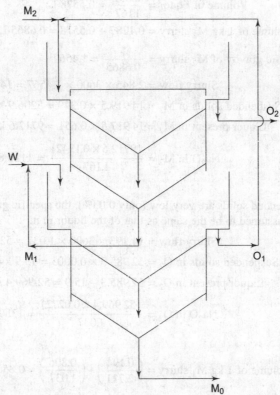

Fig. 6.18 Four Compartment Washing Thickener

Table 6.14 Operating Data of Thickener

Stream	Suspended solids, mass %	Na$_2$O concen-tration, kg/L of liquor	Specific gravity	Slurry, L/s
M_2	34.90	0.1342	1.167	2.845
O_2	0.03	0.0272	1.037	14.193
M_1	19.40	0.0252	1.034	–
W	3.70	0.0024	1.000	14.977
O_1	0.02	0.0096	1.014	–
M_o	40.20	0.0162	1.022	3.627

Assuming that the liquor contains only caustic soda and the suspended solids are calcium carbonate (specific gravity = 2.711), make a material balance on all streams of the slurry, suspended solids, liquor and Na$_2$O.

Solution: The material balance of each stream will be considered individually.

Stream M_2:

1 kg M_2 contains 0.349 kg $CaCO_3$ and 0.651 kg liquor.

$$\text{Volume of } CaCO_3 = \frac{349}{2.711} = 0.1287 \text{ L}$$

$$\text{Volume of liquor} = \frac{0.651}{1.167} = 0.5578 \text{ L}$$

$$\text{Total volume of 1 kg } M_2 \text{ slurry} = 0.1287 + 0.5578 = 0.6865 \text{ L}$$

$$\text{Specific gravity of } M_2 \text{ slurry} = \frac{1}{0.6865} = 1.4567$$

$$\text{Slurry flow} = 2.845 \times 3600 \times 1.4567 = 14\,919.5 \text{ kg/h}$$

$$\text{Suspended solids in } M_2 = 14\,919.5 \times 0.349 = 5206.9 \text{ kg/h}$$

$$\text{Liquor present in } M_2 = 14\,917.5 \times 0.651 = 9712.6 \text{ kg/h}$$

$$Na_2O \text{ in } M_2 = \frac{(9712.6 \times 0.1342)}{1.167} = 1116.8 \text{ kg/h}$$

Stream O_2:

Since the suspended solids are very low (only 0.03%), the specific gravity of the slurry will be assumed to be the same as that of the liquor in it.

$$\text{Slurry flow} = 14.193 \times 3600 \times 1.037 = 52\,985.3 \text{ kg/h}$$

$$\text{Suspended solids in } O_2 = 52\,985.3 \times 0.0003 = 15.9 \text{ kg/h}$$

$$\text{Liquor present in } O_2 = 52\,985.3 - 15.9 = 52\,969.4 \text{ kg/h}$$

$$Na_2O \text{ in } O_2 = \frac{(52\,969.4 \times 0.0272)}{1.037} = 1389.4 \text{ kg/h}$$

Stream M_1:

$$\text{Total volume of 1 kg } M_1 \text{ slurry} = \left(\frac{0.194}{2.711}\right) + \left(\frac{0.806}{1.037}\right) = 0.8511 \text{ L}$$

$$\text{Specific gravity of slurry} = \frac{1}{0.8511} = 1.175$$

Assume that all the suspended solids in M_2 are recovered in M_1

$$\text{Slurry flow in } M_1 = \frac{5206.9}{0.194} = 26\,839.7 \text{ kg/h}$$

$$\text{Liquor flow in } M_1 = 26\,839.7 - 5206.9 = 21\,632.8 \text{ kg/h}$$

$$Na_2O \text{ in } M_1 = \frac{(21\,632.8 \times 0.0252)}{1.034} = 527.2 \text{ kg/h}$$

Stream O_1:

In this stream also the specific gravity of the slurry will be assumed to be the same as that of the liquor, since suspended solids are negligible.

$$\text{Slurry flow in } O_1 = \text{slurry flow in } O_2 + \text{slurry flow in } M_1 - \text{slurry flow in } M_2$$

$$= 52\,985.3 + 26\,839.7 - 14\,919.5$$

$$= 64\,905.5 \text{ kg/h}$$

$$\text{Solids in O}_1 = 64\,905.5 \times 0.0002 = 13.0 \text{ kg/h}$$

$$\text{Liquor present in O}_1 = 64\,905.5 - 13.0 = 64\,892.5 \text{ kg/h}$$

$$\text{Na}_2\text{O in O}_1 = \frac{(64\,892.5 \times 0.0096)}{1.014} = 614.4 \text{ kg/h}$$

Stream W:

$$\text{Total volume of 1 kg W slurry} = \left(\frac{0.037}{2.711}\right) + \left(\frac{0.963}{1}\right)$$

$$= 0.9766 \text{ L}$$

$$\text{Specific gravity of W slurry} = \frac{1}{0.9766} = 1.024$$

$$\text{Slurry flow in W} = 14.977 \times 3600 \times 1.024 = 55\,211.2 \text{ kg/h}$$

$$\text{Solids in W} = 55\,211.2 \times 0.037 = 2042.8 \text{ kg/h}$$

$$\text{Liquor present in } W = 55\,211.2 - 2042.8 = 53\,168.4 \text{ kg/h}$$

$$\text{Na}_2\text{O in W} = \frac{(53\,168.4 \times 0.0024)}{1.000}$$

$$= 127.6 \text{ kg/h}$$

Stream M_0:

$$\text{Total volume of 1 kg M}_\text{o} \text{ slurry} = \left(\frac{0.402}{2.711}\right) + \left(\frac{0.598}{1.022}\right)$$

$$= 0.7334 \text{ L}$$

$$\text{Specific gravity of M}_0 \text{ slurry} = \frac{1}{0.7334} = 1.3635$$

$$\text{Slurry flow in M}_0 = 3.627 \times 3600 \times 1.3635 = 17\,803.5 \text{ kg/h}$$

$$\text{Solids in M}_0 = 17\,803.5 \times 0.402 = 7157.0 \text{ kg/h}$$

$$\text{Liquor present in M}_0 = 17\,803.5 - 7157 = 106\,46.5 \text{ kg/h}$$

$$\text{Na}_2\text{O in M}_0 = \frac{(10\,646.5 \times 0.0162)}{1.022} = 168.8 \text{ kg/h}$$

The material balance calculations are summarized in Table 6.15.

Table 6.15 Material Balance of Thickener

Item	Stream, kg/h					
	M_2	O_2	M_1	O_1	W	M_0
Slurry	14 919.5	52 985.3	26 839.7	64 905.5	55 211.2	17 803.5
Suspended solids	5 206.9	15.9	5 206.9	13.0	2 042.8	7 157.0
Liquor	9 712.6	52 969.4	21 632.8	64 892.5	53 168.4	10 646.5
Na_2O	1 116.9	1 389.4	527.2	614.4	127.6	168.8

EXERCISES

6.1 A solution of ethyl alcohol containing 8.6% alcohol is fed at the rate of 1000 kg/h to a continuous distillation column. The product (distillate) is a solution containing 95.5% alcohol. The waste solution from the column carries 0.1% of alcohol. All percentages are by mass. Calculate (a) the mass flow rates of top and bottom products in kg/h and (b) the percentage loss of alcohol.

[*Ans.* (a) Distillate product: 89.2 kg/h
Bottoms product: 910.8 kg/h
(b) Percent loss of Alcohol: 1.06]

6.2 A 50:50 mixture (by mass) of diethanolamine-triethanolamine is distilled in a packed tower to produce a 99.0% (by mass) DEA distillate product and 95.0% (by mass) TEA bottom product. To preclude the thermal degradation of the amine solution, the absolute pressure in the reboiler must be limited to 1.33 kPa (10 torr). The reflux ratio is 0.8 kmol/kmol distillate product. Compute the overall material and energy balances for 10 000 kg/h feed, assuming (i) no heat loss to the surroundings and (ii) negligible heat of mixing.

Table 6.16 Data on DEA and TEA

	Phase	mass % DEA	Temperature K(°C)	Enthalpy kJ/kg
Distillate	Liquid	99.0	420 (147)	372.2
Distillate	Vapour	99.0	420 (147)	1572.6
Feed	Liquid	50.0	430 (157)	418.7
Bottoms	Liquid	5.0	467 (194)	558.1

[*Ans.* Distillate product = 4787.2 kg/h
Bottoms product = 5212.8 kg/h
Enthalpy removed in the condenser = 2873.29 kW
Heat load of reboiler = 3013.3 kW]

6.3 A feed consisting of 50 : 50 (by mass) of toluene and methylcyclohexane (MCH) is fed to an extractive distillation column[17] at the rate of 10 000 kg/h. The distillation operation is shown in Fig. 6.19. It is desired to recover 95% of toluene as 99% pure product (free from solvent) from the solvent recovery tower. The ratio of the recycled solvent to the fresh feed is kept at 3.3. The recycled solvent contains 99.1% phenol and 0.9% toluene. The overhead product from the extractive distillation column should not contain more than 0.2% phenol. All the percentages are expressed on mass basic. Compute (a) feed rate F_2 and its composition, (b) overhead product rate from the extractive distillation column and its composition and (c) make-up phenol rate.

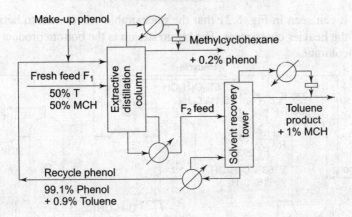

Fig. 6.19 Extractive Distillation of Toluene with Methylcyclohexane

[*Ans.* (a) and (b) see Table 6.17]

Table 6.17 Material Balance of Extractive Distillation Column

	Feed F_2	Overhead product from extractive distillation column
Rate, kg/h	37 798	5212.4
Composition, mass %		
Toluene	13.35	4.8
MCH	0.13	95.0
Phenol	86.52	0.2

(c) Make-up phenol rate = 10.4 kg/h]

6.4 Azeotropic distillation is a known technique for separation of ethanol from ethanol-water azeotrope. In this process, benzene is added as an entrainer which forms a ternary azeotrope at 101.3 kPa (760 torr) and 338 K (65°C) having composition of 22.8% C_2H_5OH, 53.9% C_6H_6 and 23.3% H_2O on mole basis. As shown in Fig. 6.20, the fresh feed of ethanol and water containing 96% (mass) ethanol is fed to the azeotropic column.

A separator separates a phase richer in benzene at 293 K (20°C) which is refluxed back to the distillation column. Benzene is recovered in the second column while water is removed in the third column. Calculate (a) the recycle rate of ethanol-water mixture from the third column per 100 kg of fresh feed and (b) composition of reflux (R) to the first column C_1.

[*Ans.* (a) 6.65 kg per 100 kg fresh feed
(b) 9.1% C_2H_5OH and 90.9% C_6H_6 (mass)]

6.5 Purge distillation columns are often used to purge undesirable components[18] from a reactor recycle stream. Typical systems are shown in Fig. 6.21 and Fig. 6.22.

(a) It can seen in Fig. 6.21 that the undesirable component to be purged is the heavier component. The purge stream is the bottom product from the column.

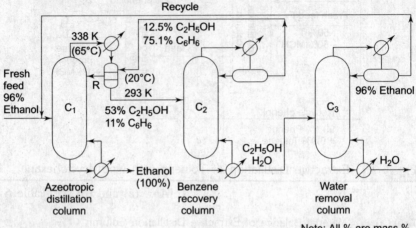

Fig. 6.20 Separation of Ethanol and Water Using Benzene

(i) Prove that recycle composition is independent of the feed (F_P) to the purge distillation column.

(ii) Develop an equation for the minimum possible feed rate (F_{pm}) to the purge distillation column.

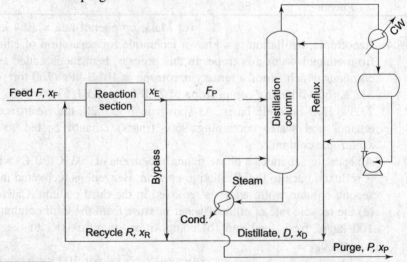

Fig. 6.21 Purge Distillation Column with Purge of Heavier Component

(b) In Fig. 6.22, the undesirable component to be purged is the lighter component. The purge stream is the overhead distillate product. Prove that the minimum feed rate (F_{pm}) to the purge column is related as

$$F_{pm} = P \cdot x_p / x_E$$

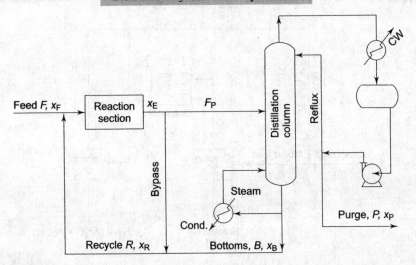

Fig. 6.22 Purge Distillation Column with Purge of Lighter Component

6.6 In the manufacture of aqueous hydrochloric acid, the gas obtained from the burner contains 35% HCl (by volume) and balance N_2. The gas is passed through an absorption tower where 96% of HCl is absorbed in water. The gas enters the absorption tower at 318 K (45°C) and 100 kPa (750 torr) and leaves it at 303 K (30°C) and 98 kPa (735 torr). Water enters at 308 K (35°C) and 3.9% (by mass) HCl solution leaves the tower. If the volumetric flow rate of the feed gas is 100 m^3/h, calculate (a) the volumetric flow rate of the gas mixture leaving the column, (b) the % HCl (by volume) in the outgoing gas mixture and (c) the temperature of the outgoing solution. Use the data given in Table 5.53 and assume heat capacity of 3.9% solution as 4.19 kJ/(kg · K).

> [*Ans.* (a) 68.16 m^3/h
> (b) 2.1% HCl (by volume)
> (c) 325.2 K(52.2°C)]

6.7 Isothermal and isobaric absorption of SO_2 is carried out in a packed tower containing Raschig rings[19]. The gases enter the bottom of the tower containing 14.8% SO_2 by volume. Water is distributed at the top of the column at the rate of 16.5 L/s. The total volume of the gas handled at 101.3 kPa (760 torr) and 303 K (30°C) is 1425 m^3/h. The gases leaving the tower are found to contain 1% SO_2 by volume. Calculate the % SO_2 by mass in the outlet water.

> [*Ans.* 0.99% SO_2 by mass]

6.8 It is desired to purify branched nine carbon atom alkane (C9) from a mixture of C9, acetic acid (AcOH) and acetic anhydride (Ac_2O). A process flow diagram of the recovery system and the ternary diagram[20] at 303 K (30°C) are given in Fig. 6.23 and Fig. 6.24 respectively. Fresh feed at 303 K (30°C) to the system contains 76% C9, 18% AcOH and balance Ac_2O. Using the ternary diagram, make complete material

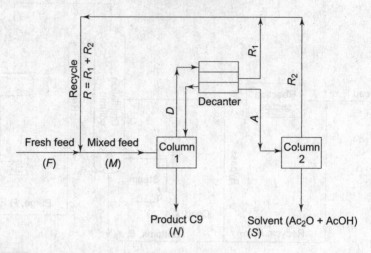

Fig. 6.23 Process Flowsheet for C9 Recovery

balance calculations for the entire system for the production rate of 1000 kg/h of C9 (stream N) from Column-1.

[*Ans.* See Table 6.18]

Table 6.18 Material Balance of C9 Purification System

Stream	Flow rate kg/h	Composition, % by mass		
		AcOH	Ac$_2$O	C9
N	1000	—	—	100.0
R_1	1023.7	37.2	7.2	55.9
R_2	78.9	64.0	—	36.0
F	1315.8	18.0	6.0	76.0
M	2418.4	27.6	6.3	66.1
A	394.7	72.8	20.0	7.2
D	1418.4	47.0	10.8	42.2
S	315.8	75.0	25.0	—

6.9 Raw hydrogen is prepared in a catalytic reformer by reacting naphtha and steam. The analysis of gases from the reformer yields 16.5% CO_2, 78% H_2 and the rest N_2 (by volume). The volumetric flow rate of the gas at 300 K (27°C) and 101.3 kPa is 6500 m^3/h in terms of 100% H_2. In order to remove CO_2, the gas is passed through perforated plate-type scrubber in which triethanolamine [$N(CH_2CH_2OH)_3$ - TEA] is sprayed at the top of the tower[21]. The gases enter the bottom of the tower at 16 bar g. The outgoing gases from the scrubber contain 0.5% CO_2 (by volume). Aqueous solution of 50% by mass TEA is circulated at the rate of 15 L/s (density - 1.05 kg/L). The solution enters the tower at 336 K (63°C) and has the concentration of CO_2 equivalent to 2420 ml per litre of solution at 101.3 kPa (760 torr) and 300 K (27°C). It leaves the tower at 350 K (77°C) and goes to another regenerating system in

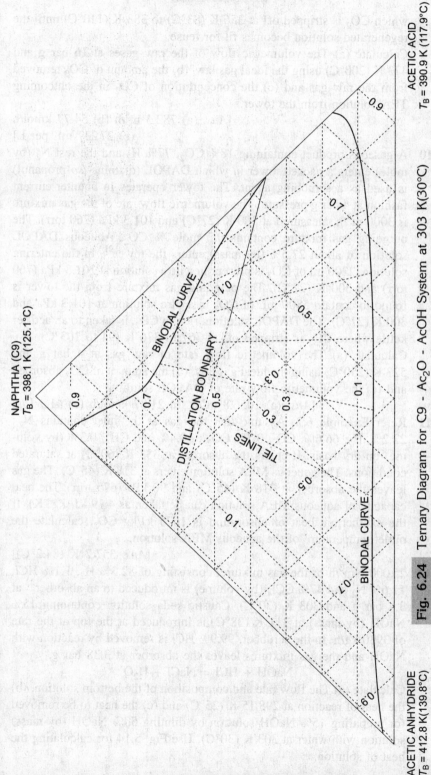

Fig. 6.24 Ternary Diagram for C9 - Ac₂O - AcOH System at 303 K(30°C)

(Courtesy: Eastman Chemical Company, USA.)

which CO_2 is stripped off at 356 K (83°C) to 383 K (110°C) until the regenerated solution becomes fit for reuse.

Calculate (a) The volumetric flow of the raw gases at 16 bar g and 473 K (200°C) using the ideal gas law, (b) the amount of CO_2 removed from the raw gas and (c) the concentration of CO_2 in the outcoming TEA solution from the tower.

[*Ans.* (a) 782.3 m^3/h (b) 54.77 kmol/h
(c) 27 237 mL per L]

6.10 A gaseous product containing 18% CO_2, 77% H_2 and the rest N_2 (by mole) enters a packed tower in which DAPOL (diamine-*iso*-propanol) is used as a scrubbing agent. The tower operates in counter-current fashion at 4 bar g pressure. The volumetric flow rate of the gas mixture is 3000 m^3/h, measured at 300 K (27°C) and 101.3 kPa (760 torr). The outgoing gas mixture contains 0.2 mole % CO_2. Aqueous DAPOL solution of about 27.5% (by mass) enters the tower[21]. In the entering solution, 2200 ml of CO_2 is present in a litre solution at 101.3 kPa (760 torr) and 300 K (27°C). The outgoing gas mixture from the tower is found to contain 5800 mL of CO_2 in a litre solution at 101.3 kPa and 300 K (27°C). The DAPOL solution, rich in CO_2, is taken to an actifier kettle where CO_2 is stripped off at 367 to 376 K (94 to 103°C).

Calculate (a) The volumetric flow rate of raw gas at 4 bar g and 523 K (250°C) using the ideal gas law, (b) the amount of CO_2 absorbed and (c) the volumetric flow rate of DAPOL solution.

[*Ans.* (a) 1056.8 m^3/h (b) 21.87 kmol/h (c) 41.3 L/s]

6.11 Refer Example 6.2. Assume that the gas at the inlet contains N_2 : 22.2%, H_2: 66.6%, CO : 0.5% CO_2 : 10.4% and CH_4: 0.3% (by volume) on dry basis. It enters the absorber at 333 K (60°C) at saturated conditions. The aqueous MEA solution enters at 318 K (45°C). The gas leaves the absorber at 318 K (45°C) and 90 kPa (675 torr). The heat capacity of aqueous MEA solution can be taken as 4.19 kJ/(kg · K). If the exothermic heat of absorption is 1675 kJ/kg CO_2, calculate the outlet temperature of the aqueous MEA solution.

[*Ans.* 357.2 K (84.2°C)]

6.12 25 000 Nm^3/h of the gas mixture, consisting of 82.3% H_2, 1.1% HCl, 11.6% N_2 and 47% CCl_4 (by volume) is introduced to an absorber[22] at 3.4 bar g and 303 K (30°C). Caustic soda solution containing 15% NaOH (by mass) at 311 K (38°C) is introduced at the top at the rate of 3930 kg/h. In the scrubber, 99.9% HCl is removed by reaction with NaOH and the gas mixtures leaves the absorber at 3.38 bar g.

$$NaOH + HCl = NaCl + H_2O$$

Calculate (a) The flow rate and composition of the bottom solution, (b) the heat of reaction at 298.15 K (25°C) and (c) the heat to be removed for preparing 15% NaOH solution by diluting 50% NaOH (by mass) solution with water at 303 K (30°C). Use Fig. 5.14 for calculating the heat of solution.

[*Ans.* (a) 3896 kg/h containing 18.45% NaCl,
2.51% NaOH and 79.04% H_2O (by mass)
(b) $\Delta H_R^0 = -446.13$ kW (c) 75 kW]

6.13 Refer Exercise 4.40 and Exercise 5.61. The gas mixture and secondary air enter the absorber at 1.5 bar g and 313 K (40°C). The tail gas leaves the absorber at 10 kPa g and 323 K (50°C). Demineralised water is introduced at 298 K (25°C) and final 58% HNO_3 (mass) is withdrawn from the bottom at 313 K (40°C). The cooling water enters the cooling coil located in the absorber at 303 K (30°C) and the rise in its temperature is recorded to be 8 K.

The data on standard heat of formation of aqueous nitric acid are given in Table 6.19.

Calculate the cooling water flow rate in the cooling coil.

Table 6.19 Standard Heat of Formation of Aqueous Nitric Acid Solution[23]

Formula and description	State	Heat of formation at 298.15 K (25°C), ΔH_f°, kJ/mol HNO_3	Mass % HNO_3 in solution
HNO_3, 0 H_2O	1	-174.2	100
1 H_2O	aq	-187.63	77.8
2 H_2O	aq	-194.56	63.6
3 H_2O	aq	-198.68	53.8
4 H_2O	aq	-201.10	46.7
5 H_2O	aq	-202.77	41.2

(*Source: National Institute of Standards and Technology, USA.*)

[*Ans.* 382.6 m³/h]

Note: The number in the first column indicates the number of moles of water mixed with one mole of nitric acid.

6.14 Oil is to be extracted from meal by a continuous counter-current extractor. The unit is charged with 1000 kg/h meal based on oil-free solids. Untreated meal contains 0.4 kg oil and 0.025 kg benzene per kg oil-free meal. Fresh solvent is benzene containing 1.5% oil (mass %). The ratio of the fresh solvent to the oil-fresh meal is kept at 0.065 kg/kg. The solid meal retains 0.507 kg solution per kg solid. The solution retained by the meal contains 11.83% oil (by mass). Make a complete material balance and find the composition and the amount of overflow from the extractor[4].

The process is shown in Fig. 6.25.

[*Ans.* Overflow rate = 583 kg/h containing 60% Oil]

6.15 A crystallizer is charged with 7500 kg of an aqueous solution at 377 K (104°C), 29.6% (by mass) of which is anhydrous sodium sulphate. The solution is cooled. During the cooling operation, 5% of the initial water is lost by evaporation. As a result, crystals of $Na_2SO_4 \cdot 10H_2O$ crysta-

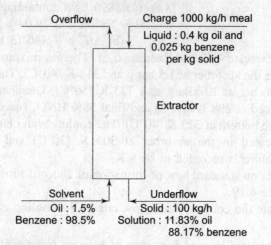

Fig. 6.25 Extraction of Oil from Meal

llize out. If the mother liquor is found to contain 18.3% (by mass) anhydrous Na_2SO_4, calculate the yield of crystals and the quantity of mother liquor.

[*Ans.* Yield of crystals = 3472.1 kg

Final mother liquor = 3763.9 kg]

6.16 Copperas (crude ferrous sulphate) is purified by dissolving it in water and recrystallizing it in a crystallizer. First, copperas is dissolved in pure water to give a solution containing 28% $FeSO_4$ (by mass). The solution is cooled to 283 K (10°C) to give out the crystals of $FeSO_4$. $7H_2O$. The loss of water due to evaporation during the cooling operation is 5% on the basis of total solution, charged to the crystallizer. It is desired to yield 0.5 t of $FeSO_4$. $7H_2O$ crystals. The original copperas contains 96% $FeSO_4$.$7H_2O$ (by mass). Find the quantity of copperas charged to the crystallizer. The solubility of $FeSO_4$ at 283 K (10°C) is 20.51 g per 100 g water[7]. Assume that the solubility of $FeSO_4$ at 283 K (10°C) is unaffected by the impurities present in copperas.

[*Ans.* 719.7 kg copperas]

6.17 An aqueous solution containing 58% $NaNO_3$ (by mass) from an evaporator is crystallized to yield the crystals containing 4% water (by mass). The crystals are removed from the crystallizer which carry off 4% water. The mother liquor containing 0.5 kg $NaNO_3$ per kg water is recycled to the evaporator with 1000 kg/h feed containing 20% $NaNO_3$ (by mass). Find (a) the yield of crystals, (b) the recycled mass flow rate of the mother liquor, (c) the total feed rate to the evaporator, and (d) the feed composition.

[*Ans.* (a) 208.3 kg/h (wet crystals)

(b) 321 kg/h (c) 1321 kg/h

(d) 23.2% $NaNO_3$ (by mass)]

6.18 Liquid paraffin wax is crystallized in a continuous crystallizer which is essentially a scrapped-surface heat exchanger. The test results on a particular crystallizer are as follows:

Product rate of liquid paraffin wax = 675 kg/h

Temperature, in = 332 K (59°C)

Temperature, out = 320 K (47°C)

Mean heat capacity, C_1 = 2.93 kJ/(kg · K)

Latent heat of crystallization, λ_f = 168.7 kJ/kg

Crystallization temperature = 320 K (47°C)

Power input at shaft = 17 kW

Jacket water flow = 1.92 L/s

Rise in Jacket water temperature = 5.8 K

Assuming no radiation loss, calculate the mass flow rate of the crystals and the percentage crystallization taking place in the heat exchanger.

[*Ans.* 491.5 kg/h, 72.8%]

Note: The scrapped-surface heat exchanger provides a high ratio of heat-transfer surface to a relatively small material volume, coupled with continuous product film removal and vigorous agitation, using a rotor inside the heat exchanger.

6.19 Feed to a vacuum crystallizer contains 82% urea, 0.5% biuret and 17.5% water by mass. In the crystallizer, 50% water is evaporated at 323 K (50°C) at which temperature the solubility of urea is 205 g per 100 g water. If the mother liquor is found to contain 1.6% biuret, find the yield of urea crystals and its biuret content.

[*Ans.* 78.12% yield and 0.11% biuret content (mass)]

6.20 A 1000 kg mixture of NaCl and NH_4Cl is to be separated by the fractional crystallization. It contains 40% NaCl by mass. It is dissolved in pure water at 323 K (50°C).

(a) If stoichiometric quantity of water is used for dissolution, calculate the quantity of the component remaining undissolved and also the quantity of the saturated solution.

(b) If the saturated solution at 323 K (50°C) mentioned in (a) above is cooled to 283 K (10°C), calculate the additional quantity of the original mixture which can be dissolved and also the total quantity of the component remaining out of the solution.

(c) If the saturated solution at 323 K (50°C) mentioned in (a) above is heated to 373 K (100°C), calculate the additional quantity of the original mixture which can be dissolved and also the total quantity of the component remaining out of the solution.

Table 6.20 Solubility Data of NaCl-NH$_4$Cl System

Temperature	Solubility, g/100 g water	
K (°C)	NaCl	NH$_4$Cl
283 (10)	18.25	12.49
323 (50)	14.26	22.50
373 (100)	10.77	33.98

[*Ans.* (a) 3647 kg saturated solution, 19.7 kg NaCl remains undissolved
(b) 266 kg mixture can be treated, 426.5 kg NH$_4$Cl is separated
(c) 510.2 kg mixture can be treated, 297.2 kg NaCl is separated]

6.21 Nitrogen gas containing 5 ppm (v/v) of moisture (max.) is required for deriming a cold box of a cryogenic plant.
Calculate: (a) The dew point of nitrogen when measured with the dew point apparatus at atmospheric pressure and (b) the dew point at 8 bar a when measured with the help of an on-line instrument.

[*Ans.* (a) 207.5 K (– 65.5°C)
(b) 223 K (– 50°C)]

6.22 On a particular day in Mumbai, a newspaper reported the weather conditions of the previous day as 308 K (35°C) *DB*, 80% *RH* and barometric pressure of 100 kPa (750 torr). Calculate (a) The absolute humidity, (b) the dew point, (c) the percentage saturation, (d) the humid heat and (e) the enthalpy over 273.15 K (0°C).

[*Ans.* (a) 0.0292 kg/kg dry air
(b) 304 K (31°C).
(c) 79%, (d) 1.06 kg/(kg dry air·K)
(e) 108 kJ/kg dry air]

6.23 A textile mill situated in Mumbai considers 307 K (34°C) *DB* and 300.5 K (27.5°C) *WB* temperatures as design intake-air temperatures for an air-conditioning system. It is desired to bring down the *RH* to 50% for the supply to the spinning department. Although this is possible by heating the air, the temperature of the final air is considered high for the comfort of the workers. It is, therefore desired to chill the air with chilled water at 288 K (15°C) and make it cold saturated air. Later, the cold air is to be heated so that the final conditions of air are 303 K (30°C) and 50% *RH*. The air rate for design is 60 000 m^3/h. Refer Figs 6.26 and 6.27 for the process paths. (a) Find the cooling load, (b) Compute the heating load and steam consum-ption in the heater, if the saturated steam is fed to it at 400 kPa a.

[*Ans.* (a) Cooling load = 676.3 kW
(b) Heating load = 225.32 kW, Steam consumption = 380.3 kg/h]

6.24 A saturated CO$_2$-water vapour mixture comes out from a spray cooler at 117.3 kPa a (880 torr) and 313 K (40°C) before its compression. Find the absolute humidity in the mixture.

[*Ans.* 0.0275 kg/kg dry CO$_2$]

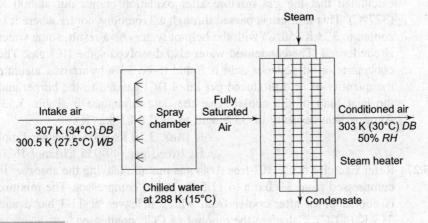

Fig. 6.26 Dehumidification of Air

(b) Heating load = 225.32 kW
Steam consumption = 380.3 kg/h

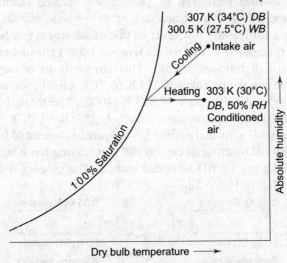

Fig. 6.27 Psychromatic Path for Dehumidification of Air

6.25 In a process for bleaching the jute, chlorine is used as a bleaching agent. The jute is bleached in a chlorine atmosphere containing some moisture. In a particular experiment, the *DP* was measured to be 291 K (18°C) while the total pressure in the system is 101.3 kPa a (760 torr). Find the moisture content of chlorine in (a) kg/kg dry chlorine and (b) ppm (mass).

[*Ans.* (a) 0.005 279 kg/kg dry Cl_2
(b) 5171 ppm]

6.26 In Example 5.36, oxidation of HCl gas to chlorine is referred to. It is calculated that the gas mixture after oxidation comes out at 600 K (327°C). This mixture is passed through a Trombone cooler where it is cooled to 323 K (50°C) with the help of water. As a result, some water is condensed. The condensed water also dissolved some HCl gas. The concentration of aqueous acid is found to be 33% by mass. Calculate the quantity of acid produced per kmol HCl gas fed to the burner and the heat load of the cooler. Use the data contained in Table 5.53. Assume heat capacity of 33% acid to be 2.6 kJ/(kg · K).

[*Ans.* 3.39 kg 33% acid per kmol
HCl feed gas, 49 935 kJ/kmol HCl]

6.27 Refer Exercise 6.12. HCl-free (0%) gas mixture leaving the absorber is compressed from 3.3 bar a to 11.5 bar a in a compressor. The mixture is cooled in an after cooler from which it leaves at 11.3 bar a and 313 K (40°C). Calculate the amount of CCl_4 condensed.

[*Ans.* 3927 kg/h]

6.28 Activated charcoal, a regenerative adsorbent, is employed industrially to remove organic vapours (VOC) from inert gases. The absorbed vapour is then recovered by passing superheated steam through the adsorbent till the partial pressure of the organic vapour in the steam falls to a sufficiently low level so that of adsorbent can be recirculated to the process. It is desired to remove 1000 kg/h of benzene from a benzene-rich nitrogen stream. This stream is to be supplied to the adsorber at a temperature of 333 K (60°C), a total pressure of 104 kPa (780 torr) and a dew point of 313 K (40°C). The sream leaves at 101.3 kPa (760 torr) and a dew point of 283 K (10°C). The entering (regenerated) activated carbon has a benzene content of 0.05 kg per kg bone-dry (BD) activated carbon and that leaving has a benzene content of 0.35 kg per kg BD activated carbon. The process is schematically represented in Fig. 6.28.

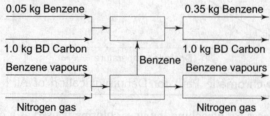

Fig. 6.28 Removal of Benzene by Adsorption on Activated Carbon

Calculate (a) The mass flow rate of nitrogen on bone-dry basis in kg/h, (b) the requirement of inlet activated carbon on bone-dry basis in kg/h and (c) the pressure to which the benzne-nitrogen inlet stream would have to be compressed at a constant temperature of 333 K (60°C) to achieve the same removal of benzene as with the activated carbon under the process conditions outlined above. Use Eq. (5.24) and the data contained in Table 5.4.

[*Ans.* (a) 1480.2 kg/h (b) 3333 kg/h (c) 870.9 kPa a]

6.29 In industrial practice, *n*-hexane is used to extract the oil from soybean flakes. In a process of this type, the soybean flakes leaving the extraction unit are reduced in solvent content by a stream of nitrogen which vaporizes the hexane. The reduction is from 0.61 kg hexame per kg bone-dry (BD) flakes to 0.025 kg hexane per kg BD flakes. The entering nitrogen leaves at 343 K (70°C) with a relative saturation of 65%. The pressure in the desolventizer is 101.325 kPa (760 torr) and 25 000 kg/h of BD flakes pass through the disolventizer. The processes are shown in Fig. 6.29.

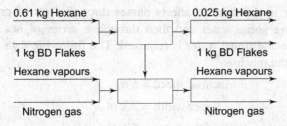

Fig. 6.29 Hexane Recovery

Calculate (a) The kmol of wet gases (i.e., nitrogen plus hexane) leaving the disolventizer per kg of soyabean flakes (BD basis) processed and (b) the volumetric flow rate of wet gases, leaving the desolventizer. (c) The nitrogen leaving the desolventizer is compressed and cooled to 293 K (20°C), thus condensing out the hexane picked up in the desolventizer. What must be the pressure in the condenser if the gas is to have a dew point of 283 K (10°C) at the pressure of desolventizer? Use Eq. (5.24) and the data contained in Table 5.4.

[*Ans.* (a) 0.0106 kmol/kg BD flakes
(b) 7458.2 m³/h (c) 162.3 kPa]

6.30 It is desired to dry a solid organic pigment in a continuous counter-current adibatic dryer. The drying air enters at 373 K (100°C) and 114 kPa (855 torr) with a saturation temperature (i.e., *DP*) of 294 K (21°C). The wet pigment is fed at the rate of 100 kg/h containing 50% water and is to be dried to 30% water (by mass). Under these conditions, 2.08 kg of water is evaporated per 100 m³ of the entering air. The air leaves at a total pressure of 108 kPa a (810 torr). Refer to Fig. 6.30 for the process flow diagram.

Calculate (a) The kmol of bone-dry air per kg of water evaporated from the pigment, (b) the *DP* of outgoing air and (c) the volumetric flow rate of the entering air.

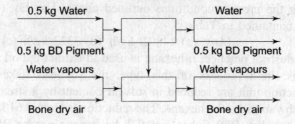

Fig. 6.30 Pigment Drying

[*Ans.* (a) 1.7289 kmol/kg moisture removed
(b) *DP* = 308 K (35°C) (c) 2329.3 m³/h]

6.31 Paper in the form of sheets passes through a set of pressure rolls to remove some water and then through a series of hot surface dryers where additional water is removed. The following data were collected rom the machine[24].

Machine speed = 5 m/s

Paper width = 3.8 m

Moisture leaving the dryer = 5% (by mass)

Moisture leaving the presses = 60% (by mass)

Specific density of paper = 0.081 kg/m² (on bone-dry basis)

Filler clay present = 20% of total solids

Assuming that the filler clay and fibre are the only solids present and that none is lost in the drying section, calculate (a) the bone-dry paper production, (b) the amount of fibre, water and filler leaving the dryers and (c) the water lost in the drying section.

[*Ans.* (a) 133 t/d on bone-dry basis
(b) Water in the paper = 277.0 kg/h
Filler in the paper = 1052.9 kg/h
Fibre in the paper = 4211.7 kg/h
(c) Evaporation = 7620 kg/h]

6.32 A thin black liquor from the digesters in a kraft pulp mill is concentrated by passing it through a sextuple-effect evaporator system[25]. The flow of the thin liquor is 50 L/s and a solid content of 15% (by mass). The concentrated liquor leaves the system at 55% solids (by mass). The density of the thin liquor can be assumed to be 1.08 kg/L. Saturated steam at 300 kPa a is consumed at the rate of 28 500 kg/h. Calculate (a) The total evaporation taking place in the system and (b) the steam economy of the system.

[*Ans.* (a) 141 382 kg/h
(b) 4.961 kg evaporation/kg steam]

6.33 A sulphite paper mill concentrates spent cooking liquor from 10% to 50% (by mass) dissolved solids in a quadruple-effect evaporator system[24]. Saturated steam is available at 103 kPa g and a vaccum of 660 torr is maintained in the fourth effect. The feed to the evaporator is 8.85 L/s in the forward direction at a specify gravity of 1.05 and 313 K (40°C). The liquor can be assumed to have a negligible elevation in the boiling point and its heat capacity can be assumed to be 4.1868 kJ/(kg · K) at all concentrations. It can also be assumed that no salt or other solids separate on evaporation and that the heat of dilution is negligible. The condensate leaves the steam chests at the saturation temperature of steam. Radiation can be neglected. All the evaporator bodies are to be of the same size (75.84 m^2 per effect). The operating data of the system are given in Table 6.21.

Table 6.21 Operating Conditions of Forward Feed Evaporator

Effect	Temperature, K (°C)	Overall heat transfer coefficient, kW/(m^2 · K)
First	376 (103.0)	4.14
Second	367 (94.0)	5.62
Third	353.5 (80.5)	4.08
Fourth	324.6 (51.6)	1.99

Evaluate the thermal performance of the system.

[*Ans.* Total evaporation = 26 712 kg/h
Steam consumption = 10 191.6 kg/h
Steam economy = 2.621 kg evaporation/kg steam]

6.34 The evaporator system described in Exercise 6.33 is operated in the backward feed manner. The operating conditions are described in Table 6.22.

Table 6.22 Operation Conditions of Backward Feed Evaporator

Effect	Temperature, K (°C)	Overall heat transfer coefficient, kW/(m^2 · K)
First	362 (89.0)	1.99
Second	347.5 (74.5)	4.08
Third	337.5 (64.5)	5.62
Fourth	324.6 (51.6)	4.14

Evaluate the thermal performance of the system.

[*Ans.* Steam consumption = 8294 kg/h
Steam economy = 3.221 kg evaporation/kg steam]

6.35 A two-stage washer is employed in a neutral sulphite semi-chemical pulp mill for washing the cooking liquor from the pump discharged from a continuous digester[25]. This washer is actually a drum-type filter, but for purposes of analysis, it can be considered as two distinct contacting stages in which the pulp mat is washed by a counter-currently moving stream of wash liquor. The pulp slurry fed to this system contains 1.5% suspended pulp solids and 9.25% dissolved salts (by mass) which are to be recovered. The specific gravity of the liquor in which the pulp is suspended is 1.30. Fresh wash water containing no dissolved salts enters the second stage at the rate of 9.85 L/s and the washed pulp leaving this stage has a solids content of 18% (by mass), suspended in a liquor of 1.03 specific gravity. This specific gravity corresponds to 1.63% dissolved salts (by mass). The washing system handles 175 t/d of oven dry pulp. Assuming that the wash liquor leaving a given contacting stage is in equilibrium with the liquor associated with the pulp leaving the same stage, calculate the efficiency for each stage and the overall efficiency.

[*Ans.* First stage efficiency = 97.97%
Second stage efficiency = 26.51%
Overall efficiency = 98.51%]

6.36 A fractionating column is designed to separate water from an aqueous solution containing methylene chloride (1.68 mass %) and methanol (2.02 mass %). The fractionation is achieved by blowing live steam (available at 3.5 bar g) in the column as shown in Fig. 6.31. The bottom product (W) from the column is pure water, practically free from any impurity. The overhead vapours are taken to a condenser where the vapours are condensed. The condensed liquid flows to a decanter where it separates into two layers. The compositions[26] of which are given in Table 6.23.

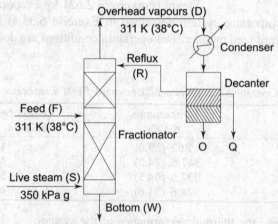

Fig. 6.31 Recovery of Methylene Chloride and Methanol from Aqueous Solution by Fractionation

Table 6.23 Composition of Immiscible Layers in Decanter

Component	Mass %	
	Upper Layer (Q or R)	Lower Layer (O)
Methylene chloride	7.63	90.70
Methanol	16.06	9.30
Water	76.31	Nil

A part of the upper layer is withdrawn as a product (Q) while the rest is recycled back to the tower (R). The reflux ratio of 0.5 kmol/kmol of the overhead product drawn can be taken for calculations. Assume that the tower operates at nearly atmospheric pressure and the temperature of the overhead vapours is 311 K (38°C).

Radiation losses can be assumed to be 2%. Based on fresh feed rate of 10 000 kg/h, compute (a) the flow rate of streams Q and O, (b) the steam input rate and (c) the bottom product rate.

Use Eq. (5.24) and the data contained in Table 5.4.

[*Ans.* (a) Flow rate of Q = 1209.4 kg/h,
Flow rate of O = 83.5 kg/h (b) Steam input = 2576 kg/h
(c) Bottom product rate, W = 11 283.4 kg/h]

REFERENCES

1. Griswold, J. and P. B. Stewart, *Ind. Engng. Chem.*, **39**(6): 1947, p. 758.
2. Teller, A. J. and H. E. Ford, *Ind. Engng. Chem.*, **50**(8): 1958, p. 1201.
3. Chambers, F. S. and T. K. Sherwood, *Ind. Engng. Chem.*, **29**(12): 1937, p. 1415.
4. Ellis, S. R. M., *Chem. Engng.* **63**: Sep. 1956, p. 185.
5. Eaglesfield, P., B. K. Kelly and J. F. Short, *The Industrial Chemist*, June, 1953, p. 147 and p. 243.
6. Brown, W. V., *Chem. Engng. Progress,* **59**(10): 1963, p. 65.
7. Green, D. W. and J. O. Malonev, *Perry's Chemical Engineers Handbook*, 6th Ed., McGraw-Hill, New York, USA, 1984.
8. Meyer, D. W., *Chemical Processing*, **53**(1): Jan. 1990, p. 50.
9. Khare, B. M. and M. R. Chivate, *Indian Chemical Engineer, Transactions* **XVI** (4): 1974, p. 25.
10. Weast, R. C., *Handbook of Chemistry and Physics*, 64th Ed., CRC Press Inc., USA, 1983-84.
11. Carpenter, J.H., *Fundamentals of Psychrometics (SI Units)*, Carrier Corporation, Publication No. T 300 - 20, USA, 1983.
12. Private communication with Anhydro A/S, Denmark.

13. *Tappi*, **47**(7): 1964, p. 171A.
14. Cook, E. M., *Chem. Engg. Progress*, **74**(4): 1978, p. 75.
15. Bhatt, B. I., S. P. Deshpande and K. Subrahmaniyam, *Chemical Age of India*, **20**(12): 1970, p. 1135.
16. *Tappi*, **48**(3): 1965, p. 170A.
17. Smith, B. D., *Design of Equilibrium Stage Processes*, McGraw-Hill, USA, 1963, p. 424.
18. Luyben, W. L., *Chem Engng. Progress*, **77**(10): 1981, p. 78.
19. *Tappi*, **47**(8): 1964, p. 114A.
20. Partin, L. R., *Chem Engng Progress*, **89**(1): 1993, p. 43.
21. Gregory, L. B. and W. G. Scharmann. *Ind. Engng Chem.*, **29**(5): 1937, p. 514.
22. *AIChE Student Contest Problem*, 1961.
23. *Selected Values of Chemical Thermodynamic Properties*, Technical Note 270-3 (a revision of NBS Circular 500), National Bureau of Standards, USA, January, 1968.
24. *Chemical Engng. Problems in the Pulp and Paper Industry*, Technical Association of the Pulp and Paper Industry (*Tappi*), USA.
25. *Tappi*, **47**(3): 1964, p. 136A.
26. Drew, J. W., *Chem. Engng. Progress*, **71**(2): 1975, p. 95.

Chapter 7

Combustion

7.1 INTRODUCTION

Fuels are burnt with oxygen to supply energy to the process industry. Excluding the use of electrical energy for the supply of thermal energy is isolated cases, fuels are extensively used to supply thermal energy. Nuclear energy and solar energy are also used to supply thermal energy in specific cases. Considering the important role of fuels in the process industry, this chapter will be exclusively devoted to combustion.

Combustion is an unit process in which the oxidation reaction takes place. However, all oxidation reactions are not termed as combustion, e.g. the oxidation of toluene to benzaldehyde, oxidation of hydrogen chloride to chlorine etc., are not normally termed as combustion processes. Broadly, the union of carbon, hydrogen and sulphur with oxygen is termed as combustion. If the products of combustion are carbon dioxide, water and sulphur dioxide respectively from the above three elements, the combustion is termed as a complete combustion. If carbon monoxide appears in the product gases, the combustion is termed *incomplete* or *partial combustion* because CO can further combine with oxygen to produce CO_2. Although SO_2 can be further oxidized so SO_3 it is customary to regard the union as a complete union for stoichiometric calculations. However, the complete union of S and O_2 yields SO_3 which requires specific conditions for the union.

7.2 FUELS

Fuels can be broadly classified as follows:

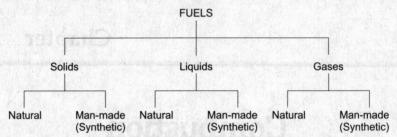

The classical fossil fuel (natural) is coal. Lignite is also found in nature. It is an earthy-brown fuel, generally low in mineral-matter content. Wood is used as a solid fuel in many instances. Coke, bagasse, rice husk, saw dust, etc. are other examples of synthetic solid fuels.

Crude oil obtained from sub-soil drilling is a natural liquid fuel. Gasoline (petrol), diesel oil, alcohols, kerosene, fuel oils and other organic liquids are man-made liquid fuels. Manufacture of biocrude from organic waste using high pressure steam is a reality on a pilot scale. Biodiesel, obtained from catalytic transesterification of vegetable oils, is emerging as a substitute for the traditional diesel fuel.

Natural gas (and associated gas) is an important natural gaseous fuel. Coke oven gas, producer gas, blast-furnace gas, liquefied petroleum gas (LPG) and refinery gas are examples of synthetic gaseous fuels. Dimethyl ether (DME) is gaining popularity as a synthetic gaseous fuel.

The combustibles in the fuel should be known for stoichiometric calculations. The analyses of various fuels must be known for this reason. It will now be seen how the analyses of each of the fuels are represented. In particular, the interpretation of coal analysis requires a clear understanding of the subject.

7.3 CALORIFIC VALUES OF FUELS

The *calorific value* of a fuel is nothing but the heat of combustion of the fuel. It is defined as the total heat produced when a unit mass of fuel is completely burnt with pure oxygen. It is also said to be the *heating value* of the fuel.

As discussed earlier, when a fuel is burnt, hydrogen combines with oxygen and gets converted into water. When water vapour is present in the flue gases, the latent heat of vaporization is lost. Hence this quantity of heat is not available for any useful purpose. Therefore, when the calorific value of a fuel is determined, considering that the water is present in the vapour form, it is said to be *net calorific value* (NCV) or *net heating value* (NHV) or *lower heating value* (LHV).

If the above vapours are condensed, the latent heat of water vapour can be made available for useful purposes. Thus, if this part of heat is added to the net calorific value, *gross calorific value* (GCV) or *gross heating value* (GHV) or *higher heating value* (HHV) is obtained.

Usually, NCV and GCV of the fuels are reported at 298.15 K (25°C). Appendix IV.2 at the end of the text gives the NCV and GCV of various compounds. Normally, NCV and GCV are reported in kJ/kg or kJ/mol units, kJ/m^3 (for gaseous fuels) units are also used occasionally, depending on the convenience. It is customary to specify the abbreviations NCV or GCV when the calorific values are reported, as the case may be. However, if no mention is made, the reported calorific value is taken as GCV.

The calorific value of a fuel is determined in a calorimeter in which the fuel is burnt with pure oxygen and the heat liberated is absorbed in water. The rise in temperature of water gives the calorific value of the fuel.

$$NCV = GCV - (\text{mass \% hydrogen}) \ (9) \ (\lambda_v) \ \text{kJ/kg} \qquad (7.1)$$

In this equation λ_v is the latent heat of water vapour at the reference temperature. Normally 298.15 K (25°C) is considered to be the reference temperature at which $\lambda_v = 2442.5$ kJ/kg.

7.4 COAL

Coal is the most important fossil fuel. In India, although the coal reserves are abundant, most of the collieries are situated in Madhya Pradesh, West Bengal, Bihar and the banks of river Godavari. As a result, the transportation of coal to other parts of the country is quite expensive. In addition, the best grade coal is limited in quantity as compared to *steam coal*. Hence, the best quality coal is reserved for the manufacture of steel.

Two different analyses of coal are reported, namely *proximate analysis* and *ultimate analysis*. Both of them will now be separately studied.

7.4.1 Proximate Analysis

Normally, the proximate analysis of *air-dried coal* is reported as follows. An *air-dried* coal sample is one which is exposed to the atmosphere of a laboratory to bring it in equilibrium with the humidity conditions of the laboratory so that the sample does not gain or loose mass during analysis.

Moisture: Water expelled in its various forms when tested under specified conditions.

Volatile matter (VM): Total loss in weight minus the moisture in coal when coal is heated under specified conditions.

Mineral matter: Inorganic residue left over when coal or coke is incinerated in air to constant mass under specified conditions. It is ordinarily referred to as *ash*.

Fixed Carbon (FC): Obtained by subtracting from 100, the sum of the percentages by mass of moisture, VM and mineral matter.

Ordinarily, percentage sulphur (by mass) does not form a part of the proximate analysis. However, due to the harmful effects of sulphur dioxide and sulphur trioxide produced by burning sulphur to the environment, percentage sulphur (by mass) is also included when only proximate analysis is to be specified.

IS: 1350 (Part-I) gives the methods of test for coal/coke/lignite relating to proximate analysis.

IS: 1350 (Part-II) relates to determination of the calorific value of coal/coke/lignite.

IS: 1350 (Part-III) relates to the determination of sulphur in coal/coke/lignite.

7.4.2 Forms and Conditions of Moisture in Coal/Lignite

(i) Total moisture

Coal that is exposed to water in the seam or in a washery, or the coal wetted by rain, can carry free moisture. This moisture plus the moisture within the material is known as the total moisture.

(ii) Moisture at 313 K (40°C) and 60% *RH*

The moisture present in coal which is equilibrated at 313 K (40°C) at 60% relative humidity (*RH*) is sometimes reported.

(iii) Moisture at 313 K (40°C) and 96% *RH*

This is also termed as the near saturation moisture or bed moisture. It is the moisture present in coal which is equilibrated at 313 K (40°C) and 96% *RH* and is exclusive of free visible moisture.

(iv) Free moisture

It represents the visible wetness of coal only.

(v) Moisture in air-dried sample

This is the moisture content of coal when it is equilibrated with the ambient conditions of the laboratory.

7.4.3 Tests for Proximate Analysis

The general procedures for the analysis relating to proximate analysis is described below as per IS: 1350 (Part-I). For full details, the original standard may be referred to.

(i) Moisture

The moisture in the sample is determined by drying the known mass of the coal at 381 K ± 2 K (108°C ± 2°C).

(ii) Volatile Matter (VM)

The method for the determination of VM consists of heating a weighed quantity of air-dried sample at a temperature of 1173 K ± 10 K (900°C ± 10°C) for a period of seven minutes. Oxidation has to be avoided as far as possible. VM is the loss in mass other than that due to moisture.

(iii) Mineral Matter (Ash)

In this determination, the sample is heated in air up to 773 K (500°C) for 30 min from 773 K to 1088 K (500°C to 815°C) for a further 30 to 60 min and maintained at this temperature until the sample mass becomes constant.

(iv) FC

    As explained earlier, FC is determined by deducting the moisture, VM and mineral matter (as mass %) from 100.

7.4.4 Ultimate Analysis of Coal

The ultimate analysis of coal gives the constituent elements, namely; carbon, hydrogen, nitrogen and sulphur. The percentage carbon given in the ultimate analysis should not be confused with FC, the latter being always lower than the former. The oxygen content of the coal is obtained by finding the difference of 100 and the sum of other constituent elements. IS: 1350 gives the test methods for the ultimate analysis of coal.

    For the ultimate analysis, the coal sample is burnt in a current of oxygen. As a result, the hydrogen, carbon and sulphur get oxidized to water, carbon dioxide and sulphur dioxide respectively. Water and carbon dioxide are absorbed in suitable solvents and the constituents are determined gravimetrically. Sulphur products are retained by lead chromate. Precautions have to be taken to eliminate the oxides of nitrogen which can form during combustion. The nitrogen in the coal is determined by the Kjeldahl method.

    The hydrogen determined by the above procedure includes the hydrogen content of organic matter of VM and the hydrogen of the moisture present in the coal. The actual hydrogen burnt during combustion is calculated by subtracting 11.2% of the mass percentage moisture content of the air-dried sample of the coal from the total hydrogen determined by above process.

    The classification of coal is done on the basis of proximate analysis. A technologically significant grading system adopted in India is given in Table 7.1

Table 7.1 Classification of Bituminous Coal[1]

S.No.	Class	Grade	Specifications
1.	Non-coking coal, produced in all states—other than Assam, Meghalaya, Arunachal Pradesh and Nagaland	A	HU* exceeding 25 960 kJ/kg or 6200 kcal/kg
		B	HU exceeding 23 450 kJ/kg or 5600 kcal/kg but not exceeding 25 960 kJ/kg or 6200 kcal/kg
		C	HU exceeding 20 680 kJ/kg or 4940 kcal/kg but not exceeding 23 450 kJ/kg or 5600 kcal/kg
		D	HU exceeding 17 580 kJ/kg or 4200 kcal/kg but not exceeding 20 680 kJ/kg or 4940 kcal/kg
		E	HU exceeding 14 070 kJ/kg or 3360 kcal/kg but not exceeding 17 580 kJ/kg or 4200 kcal/kg
		F	HU exceeding 10 050 kJ/kg or 2400 kcal/kg but not exceeding 14 070 kJ/kg or 3360 kcal/kg

(Contd)

Table 7.1 (Contd.)

S.No.	Class	Grade	Specifications
		G	HU exceeding 5440 kJ/kg or 1300 kcal/kg but not exceeding 10 050 kJ/kg or 2400 kcal/kg
2.	Non-coking coal, produced in Assam, Meghalaya, Arunachal Predesh and Nagaland		Not graded
3.	Coking coal	Steel grade I	Ash content not exceeding 15%
		Steel grade II	Ash content exceeding 15% but not exceeding 18%
		Washery grade I	Ash content exceeding 18% but not exceeding 21%
		Washery grade II	Ash content exceeding 21% but not exceeding 24%
		Washery grade III	Ash content exceeding 24% but not exceeding 28%
		Washery grade IV	Ash content exceeding 28% but not exceeding 35%
4.	Semi-coking and weakly coking coal	Semi-coking I	Ash plus moisture content not exceeding 19%
		Semi-coking II	Ash plus moisture content exceeding 19% but not exceeding 24%
5.	Hard coke	By product premium	Ash content exceeding 25%
		By product ordinary	Ash content exceeding 25% but not exceeding 30%
		Beehive premium	Ash content not exceeding 27%
		Beehive superior	Ash content exceeding 27% but not exceeding 31%
		Beehive ordinary	Ash content exceeding 31% but not exceeding 36%

*HU = Useful heat value

= 8900 − 138 (Ash + Moisture) kcal/kg

= 37 262.5 − 577.8 (Ash + Moisture) kJ/kg

Notes: 1. In the case of coal having moisture less than 2% and VM content less than 19%, the HU shall be the value arrived at as above reduced by 628 kJ/kg (150 kcal/kg) for each 1% reduction in VM content below 15%.

2. Moisture at 313 K (40°C) and 60% *RH* [Sec. 7.4.2 (ii)] shall be used in evaluation of HU.

Another classification of coals and lignites is recommended in IS: 770 which depends on (i) the nature, rank and combustible matter of fuel, (ii) the nature and quantities of the impurities, present in the fuel and (iii) the size of the fuel.

Attempts have been made to correlate the ultimate analysis of a fuel with its calorific value. One of the most commonly used relationships is that given by Dülong.

GCV of coal in kJ/kg of fuel

$$= 33\,950\,C + 144\,200\left[H - \left(\frac{O}{8}\right)\right] + 9400\,S \qquad (7.2)$$

where   C = mass fraction of carbon

S = mass fraction of sulphur

H – (O/8) = mass fraction of net hydrogen

= total hydrogen – 1/8 (oxygen)

The above equation assumes that the calorific value of a fuel is the algebraic sum of heating values of the constituents, which is not entirely correct. Hence, the equation can be taken as a rough estimate only. Calorimetric data are always preferred to empirical equations.

A Calderwood equation[2] is useful in finding the total carbon content of the coal if the proximate analysis and the GCV of it are known.

mass % carbon = 5.88 + 0.00 512 (B – 40.5 S)

$$\pm\,0.0053\left[80 - 100\left(\frac{VM}{FC}\right)\right]^{1.55} \qquad (7.3)$$

where   B = GCV in Btu/lb

S = mass % sulphur

if 100 (VM/FC) > 80, the sign outside the main parentheses is negative and *vice versa*.

Example 7.1 A sample from Godavari colliery has the following proximate and ultimate analyses.

Table 7.2 Analysis of Coal from Godavari Colliery

Air dried coal				As received analysis	
Proximate analysis	mass %	Ultimate analysis	mass %	Ultimate analysis	mass %
Moisture	7.0	Carbon	54.0	Carbon	50.22
Volatile matter	26.0	Hydrogen	3.0	Hydrogen	2.79
Fixed carbon	46.0	Sulphur	0.4	Sulphur	0.37
Ash	21.0	Nitrogen	2.2	Nitrogen	2.05
		Ash	21.0	Ash	19.53
		Oxygen (by diff.)	19.4	Oxygen	18.04
				Moisture	7.00
Total	100.0		100.0		100.00

The gross calorific value (as analysed on dry ash-free) = 23 392 kJ/kg at 298.15 K (25°C). Calculate (a) The net hydrogen in the coal, (b) the combined water in the coal, (c) GCV based on the Dülong formula, (d) NCV (actual) of the coal, (e) the carbon content of coal, using Calderwood equation and (f) the moisture-free and ash-free proximate analyses of coal.

Solution:

Basis 100 kg as received coal

$$\text{Oxygen in the coal} = 18.04 \text{ kg} = 0.564 \text{ kmol}$$

Equivalent hydrogen (to combine

$$\text{with oxygen present in the coal)} = 2 \times 0.564 = 1.128 \text{ kmol} \equiv 2.255 \text{ kg}$$

$$\text{Net hydrogen} = 2.79 - 2.255 = 0.535 \text{ kg or mass \%} \quad \textit{Ans. (a)}$$

$$\text{Total water produced by burning } H_2 = 1.128 \text{ kmol} = 20.304 \text{ kg}$$

$$\text{Moisture in coal} = 7\% \text{ or kg}$$

$$\text{Combined water} = 20.304 - 7.0$$

$$= 13.304 \text{ kg or mass \%} \quad \textit{Ans. (b)}$$

$$\text{From Dülong's formula, GCV} = 33\,950\, C + 144\,200 \left[H - \left(\frac{O}{8} \right) \right] + 9400\, S$$

$$= 33\,900 \times (50.22/100) + 144\,200 \times$$

$$\left(\frac{0.535}{100} \right) + 9400 \times \left(\frac{0.37}{100} \right)$$

$$= 17\,024.6 + 771.5 + 34.5$$

$$= 17\,830.9 \text{ kJ/kg} \quad \textit{Ans. (c)}$$

$$\text{Total hydrogen in the fuel} = 2.79\% \text{ or kg} = 1.395 \text{ kmol}$$

$$\text{Total water vapour in the product gas stream} = 1.395 \times 18 + 7 = 32.02 \text{ kg}$$

$$\text{Total heat of vaporization} = \frac{2442.5 \times 32.02}{100} = 782.1 \text{ kJ/kg fuel}$$

$$\text{Reported GCV on dry ash-free basis} = 23\,392 \text{ kJ/kg}$$

To convert the GCV to as-received coal basis, correction factor

$$= (1 - \text{Moisture} - \text{Ash})$$

$$= 1 - 0.21 - 0.07 = 0.72$$

$$\text{GCV of as-received coal} = 23\,392 \times 0.72 = 16\,842.2 \text{ kJ/kg}$$

Thus, Dülong's formula has given about 5.87% higher GCV.

$$\text{NCV of the fuel} = 16\,842.2 - 782.1$$

$$= 16\,060.1 \text{ kJ/kg coal on}$$

$$\text{as-received basis} \quad \textit{Ans. (d)}$$

Calderwood Equation

$$\text{Total carbon} = 5.88 + 0.005\,12\, (B - 40.5\, S)$$

$$\pm 0.0053 \left[80 - \left(100 \frac{VM}{FC} \right) \right]^{1.55}$$

$$100 \left(\frac{VM}{FC} \right) = \frac{100 \times 26}{46} = 56.52; \ i.e. < 80$$

$$B = 16\,842.2 \ kJ/kg = 7240.8 \ Btu/lb$$

Total carbon $= 5.88 + 0512 \ (7240.8 - 40.5 \times 0.37)$

$$+ 0.0053 \ (80 - 56.52)^{1.55}$$

$$= 5.88 + 37.00 + 0.71 = 43.59 \qquad Ans. \ (e)$$

Table 7.3 Proximate Analysis of Ash-free and Moisture-free Coal

	kg	mass %
Volatile matter	26	36.11
Fixed carbon	46	63.89
Total	72	100.00

Ans. (f)

7.5 LIQUID FUELS

All liquid fuels are organic in nature. The ultimate analyses of liquid fuels are reported as indicated in the case of coal. Usually liquid fuels contain negligible water. Mostly carbon, hydrogen, oxygen and sulphur are the constituents of the fuel. The gross calorific value is normally reported with the ultimate analysis.

Table 7.4 reports typical analyses of crude oils of different origins in India. Table 7.5 gives typical characteristics of other liquid fuels, marketed in India.

In Chapter 2, it was mentioned that specific gravity of petroleum fractions (expressed in °API) is an important property. Approximate GCV and NCV of the petroleum derivatives are plotted as a function of °API in Fig. 7.1.

Example 7.2 Crude oil is found to contain 87.1% carbon, 12.5% hydrogen and 0.4% Sulphur (by mass). Its GCV at 298.15 K (25°C) is measured to be 45 071 kJ/kg oil. Calculate its NCV at 298.15 K (25°C).

Solution: Basis: 1 kg crude oil

$$\text{Hydrogen burnt} = 0.125 \ kg$$

$$\text{Water formed} = \left(\frac{0.125}{2} \right) \times 18 = 1.125 \ kg$$

Latent heat of water vapour

$$\text{at } 298.15 \ K \ (25°C) = 1.125 \times 2442.5 = 2747.8 \ kJ$$

$$NCV = GCV - \text{latent heat of water vapours}$$

$$= 45\,071 - 2747.8$$

$$= 42\,323.2 \ kJ/kg \ oil \qquad Ans.$$

Table 7.4 Typical Characteristic Data of Some Indian Crude Oils

Property	Crude from					
	Bassein Ankaleshwar	Bombay High	Cauvery High	Basin	Gandhar	Heera
API gravity	46.9	38.4	39.4	46.4	46.9	36.3
Specific gravity at 288.7 K (15.55°C)	0.793	0.833	0.828	0.795	0.793	0.842
Asphaltenes, mass %	ND	0.14	0.28	0.16	0.06	0.26
Characteristic factor, KUOP	ND	11.85	11.7	11.6	12.15	11.98
Pour point, K (°C)	298 + (15+)	306 + (33+)	303 + (30+)	303 + (27+)	300+	306 + (33+)
Reid vapour pressure at 310.8 K (37.8°C), kPa	46.1	22.6	33.3	26.5	40.2	18.6
Salt Content, g/m^3	8.6	42.8	31.4	< 2.8	22.8	17.1
Sulphur, mass %	0.05	0.15	0.17	0.06	0.041	0.24
Kinematic viscosity, mm^2/s	1.90 at 311 K (37.8°C)	4.25 at 311 K (37.8°C)	3.28 at 313 K (40°C)	1.14 at 313 K (40°C)	2.21 at 311 K (40°C)	5.24 at 311 K (37.8°C)
Wax content, mass %	4.0	11.5	10.6	10.6	8.9	14.6

(Contd.)

Table 7.4 (Contd.)

Property	Crude from					
	Lakwa	Moran	Nahorkatiya	Narianam	North Gujarat Mix	Ratna
API gravity	26.5	34.9	31.3	47.1	26.8	35.2
Specific gravity at 288.7 K 15.15°C	0.896	0.850	0.869	0.792	0.893	0.849
Asphaltenes, mass %	ND	ND	ND	0.12	0.45	0.53
characteristic factor, KUOP	ND	11.35	11.4	11.90	12.0	12.0
Pour point, K (°C)	300 + (27+)	303 + (30+)	303 + (30+)	273 (0)	294 + (21+)	309 + (36+)
Reid vapour pressure at 310.8 K (37.8*C), kPa	12.7	50.0	35.3	53.9	4.3	14.7
Salt Content g/m^3	ND	ND	ND	82.7	74.2	496.4
Sulphur, Mass %	0.26	0.25	0.25	0.085	0.17	0.26
Kinematic viscosity, mm^2/s	8.82 at 311 K (37.8°C)	4.2 at 311 K (37.8°C)	4.88 at 311 K (37.8°C)	1.50 at 313 K (40°C)	63.44 at 311 K (37.8°C)	9.52 at 311 K (37.8°C)
Wax content, mass %	8.5	13.47	10.1	2.8	6.8	20.0

(*Source: Indian Institute of Petroleum, Dehradun, Uttaranchal*)

Table 7.5 Characteristic Data of Liquid Fuels

Characteristic	Diesel Fuel (IS: 1460–1974) - as amended up to Oct. 1985		Motor gasolene IS: 2769 1971) IInd Revision		Fuel oils (IS: 1593–1983) IInd Revision	
	HSD	LDO	87 Octane	93 Octane	Grade MV2	Grade HV
Flash point (min.), K (°C)	305 (32)	339 (66)	ND	ND	339 (66)	339 (66)
Pour point (max.) K (°C)	279 (6)	285 (12)- winter 291 (18)- summer	ND	ND	–	–
Kinematic viscosity, mm²/s	2.0 - 7.5 at 311 K (38°C)	2.5 - 15.7 at 311 K (38°C)	ND	ND	180 at 323 K (50°C)	370 at 323 K (50°C)
API gravity (typical)	40.7 – 42.8	35 - 37	63.9	57.9	19	19
Special gravity at 288.7 K (15.55°C)	0.822 – 0.812	0.85 - 0.84	0.724	0.747	0.94	0.94
Distillation	90% (min.) recovery at 639 K (306°C)	–	FBP (max.) = 488 K (215°C)	FBP (max.) = 488 K (215°C)	ND	ND
Reid vapour pressure, at 311 K (37.8°C), (max.), kPa	ND	ND	68.6	68.6	Negligible	Negligible
Water content (max.), mass %	0.05	0.10	ND	ND	1.0	1.0
Sulphur content, (max) mass % as S	1.0	1.8	0.25	0.40	4.0	4.0
Lead (max.), g/L	–	–	0.56	0.80	–	–
Sediments, (max.) mass %	1.0	0.10	ND	ND	0.25	4.0
Estimated C/H ratio (mass)	6.2 - 6.3	6.35 - 6.5	5.6	5.8	7.0 - 7.5	7.0 - 7.5
Gross calorific value, kJ/kg (normal/typical)	46 050 – 46 470	45 550 – 45 680	47 270	47 020	41 870/44 170	41 870/44 170
Additional requirement						Ash max. 01% (by mass)

Table 7.5 (Contd)

Characteristic	Kerosene (IS:1459 - 1974) IInd Revision Amendment No. 2, Nov. 1984	Low Sulphur Heavy Stock (LSHS) or Heavy Petroleum Stock (HPS)	Aviation Turbine Fuel (Kerosene type) (IS:1571-1982) 4th Revision	Naphtha Low Aromatic (LAN)	Naphtha High Aromatic (HAN)
Flash point (min.), K (°C)	308 (35)	366 (93)	311 (38)	298 (15)	298 (15)
Pour point (max.), K (°C)	–	345 + (72+)	ND	–	–
Kinematic Viscosity, mm²/s	ND	500 at 323 K (50°C) 100 at 373 K (100°C)	8 at 253 K (– 20°C)	ND	ND
API gravity (typical)	45.4	16-20	51-39	76.6-61.8	86-70.6
Specific gravity at 288.7 K (15.55°C)	0.8	0.96-0.93	0.775-0.930	0.68-0.732	0.65-0.7
Distillation	FBP (max.) = 573 K (300°C)	ND	FBP (max.) = 561 K (288°C)	FBP (max.) = 453 K (180°C)	FBP (max.) = 453 K (180°C)
Reid vapour pressure, at 311K (37.8°C), (max.), kPa	ND	Negligible	ND	68.7	68.7
Water content (max.), mass %	ND	1.0	Nil	–	–
Sulphur content(max.), mass % as S	0.25	1.0	0.2	0.25	0.25
Lead (max.), g/L	–	–	–	0.002	0.002
Sediments, (max.) mass %	ND	ND	ND	–	–
Estimated C/H ratio (mass)	5.8	7.3-7.6	6.0	5.3-5.8	–
Gross calorific value, kJ/kg normal/typical	47 020	41 030-43 540	46 980	42 710 (min.)	42 710 (min.)
Additional requirement	–	Ash: 0.1% (max. by mass)	Freezing point: 223 K (– 50°C) (max.)	Aromatics = 15% (v/v) (max.)	Aromatics = 15 – 25% (v/v)

(*Courtesy: Indian Oil Corporation Ltd.*)

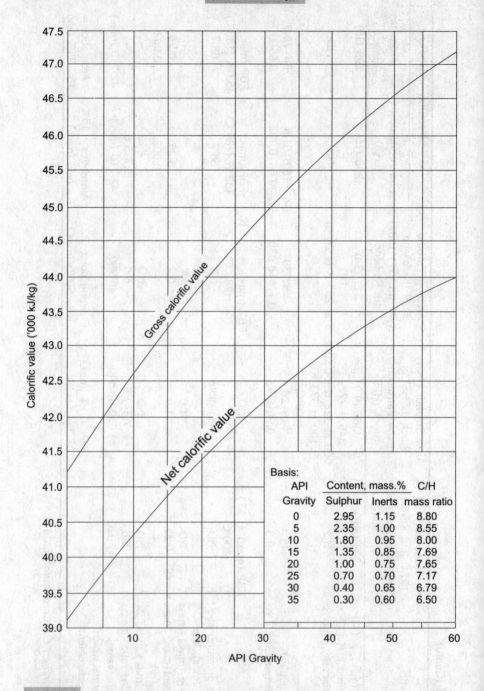

Fig. 7.1 Calorific Values of Petroleum Derivatives

All organic liquids (exceptions being carbon tetrachloride, fluorocarbon compounds etc.) are combustibles. Methanol, ethanol, acetone, etc., can be used as fuels. There is a recent interest in utilizing methanol and ethanol mixed fuels to avoid environmental hazards due to presence of pollutants in flue gases.

7.6 GASEOUS FUELS

Gaseous fuels are ideal from the standpoint of complete combustion. The air to be supplied for complete combustion easily diffuses with the fuel and ensures complete combustion. In comparison to all the three types of fuels, gaseous fuels of petroleum origin offer higher heating values.

Methane, ethane, propane, butane and other gaseous hydrocarbons can be used as gaseous fuels. Natural gas (and associated gas) essentially consists of methane with small quantities of higher hydrocarbons. Coal gas, sewage (bio -) gas, etc., are also used as fuels which are lean in nature. Liquefied petroleum gas (LPG) contains chiefly propane and butane. It is a fuel with a high heating value. Dimethyl ether (DME) is also a high heating value fuel for auto vehicles, power generators, boilers, etc.

In addition, various industrial waste gases can also be used as fuels. The major sources of industrial waste gases are from the iron and steel industry, power plants, fertilizer industry and non-ferrous industry. The waste gases of the iron and steel industry are the coke-oven gas and the blast furnace gas. Of late, addition to the list of recoverable byproduct waste gases in the steel industry is the gas produced during the converter steel production. Waste gases are also collected from other installations, such as carbide furnaces, phosphorous smelting furnaces, aluminium reduction furnaces, off gases in carbon black plant, etc. Hydrogen, carbon monoxide, nitrogen, carbon dioxide, methane, ethylene and other hydrocarbons are the main constituents of industrial waste gases. Purge (tail) gas streams in chemical process industry are normally utilised as fuel in industry. Constituents, such as hydrogen and carbon monoxide have economical significance as base materials for chemical processes. Therefore, the use of these gases as fuel cannot be fully justified considering the potential for their utilization. Cryogenics, pressure swing or vacuum swing adsorption, membraned diffusion and other methods are developed for the economic recovery of a constituent (such as hydrogen) from a gas mixture. Tail gas stream from such a separation plant is used as a fuel.

Table 7.6 lists the gaseous fuels of industrial importance.

Example 7.3 The GHV of gaseous propane is 2219.71 kJ/mol at 298.15 K (25°C). Calculate its NHV.

Solution: Basis: 1 mol gaseous propane (formula: C_3H_8)

The combustion reaction is

$$C_3H_8 + 5\ O_2 = 3\ CO_2 + 4\ H_2O$$

Thus, when 1 mole of propane is burnt, 4 moles of water are produced.

Mass of water produced = $4 \times 18.0153 = 72.06$ g

$$NHV = 2219.71 - \frac{(72.06 \times 2442.5)}{1000} = 2043.7 \text{ kJ/mol} \qquad Ans.$$

Table 7.6 Properties of Gaseous Fuels[3] of Industrial Importance

Fuel	Source	Average composition (by volume)	GCV, kJ/m^3	Remarks
Blast furnace gas	Byproduct of iron making	58% N_2, 27% CO, 12% CO_2 2% H_2 and CH_4	3350-3770	Good fuel when clean. Used mainly at source.
Butane	Byproduct of gasoline making	C_4H_{10} (usually has some butylene: C_4H_8 and propane: C_3H_8)	119 330-79 550	Liquefies under slight pressure, sold as liquid (cylinder gas).
Casing-head gas	Oil wells	Varies, mostly butane, propane	44 800-75 360	Used mostly in oil fields.
Carburetted water gas	Manufactured from coal, enriched with oil vapour	34% H_2, 32% CO, 16% CH_4, 7% N_2, 5% C_2H_4, 4% CO_2, 2% C_6H_6	18 630-22 360	Good fuel but usually costly — part of most city gas.
Coke oven gas	Byproduct from coke-ovens	48% H_2, 32% CH_4, 8% N_2, 6% CO, 3% C_2H_4, 2% CO_2 and 1% O_2	18 630-22 360	Good fuel when clean, often used at source.
Liquefied petroleum gas (LPG)	Refineries and NG processing plants	26% C_3H_8, 24% i-butane, 50% n-butane		Good domestic fuel. Also used in gas engines for power generation. Costly.
Natural gas or associated gas	Gas wells	Varies, mostly CH_4, C_2H_6, C_3H_8	35 380-42 910	Ideal fuel, piped to point of use.
Offgas	Carbon black plant	15% H_2, 18% CO, 0.5% CH_4, 4% CO_2, 0.5% C_2H_2 and 62% N_2	4200-4500	Good fuel, requires cleaning. Captive consumption.
Oil gas	Manufactured from petroleum	54% H_2, 27% CH_4, 10% CO, 3% N_2, 3% CO_2, 3% C_2H_4	18 630-20 528	Good fuel, often mixed with coke-oven gas.

(Contd.)

Table 7.6 (Contd.)

Fuel	Source	Average composition (by volume)	GCV, kJ/m^3	Remarks
Producer gas	Manufactured from coal, coke, wood, etc.	51% N_2, 25% CO, 16% H_2, 6% CO_2, 2% CH_4	5020-6180	Requires cleaning.
Propane	Byproduct of gasoline	C_3H_8	93 160	Similar to butane.
Refinery gas	Byproduct of petroleum processing	Varies; mostly butane and propane	44 800-75 360	Used mainly at refineries, sold as liquefied fuel (cylinder gas).
Sewage gas	Sewage disposal plants	65% CH_4, 30% CO_2, 2% H_2, 3% N_2, traces of O_2, CO and H_2S	22 400-26 170	Good fuel.
Gas	Distillery spent wash	55 to 65% CH_4, 1 to 2% H_2S and rest CO_2	20 680-24 440	Good fuel.

* 1 Sm^3 means value occupied by and ideal gas at 101.325 kPa a and 288.7 K (15.6°C) or 60 °F.

(*Part of table reproduced with the permission of McGraw-Hill Book Company, New York, USA. Further updated with industrial information.*)

Example 7.4 Calculate the gross and net calorific values of the natural gas 298.15 K (25°C) which has the following molal composition:

CH_4: 89.4%, C_2H_6: 5.0%, C_3H_6: 1.9%, iso-C_4H_{10}: 0.4%
n-C_4H_{10}: 0.6%, CO_2: 0.7% and N_2: 2.0%

Solution Basis: 1 mol natural gas

In a mixture of gases, the heating value of the mixture is made up of the heating values of individual gases present in it.

Table 7.7 Heating Values of Natural Gas

Component	mol n_i	Molar mass M_i	kg $n_i \cdot M_i$	Heating value* kJ/mol		Total heating value kJ	
				GCV	NCV	$n \cdot GCV$	$n \cdot NCV$
CH_4	0.894	16.0425	14.342	890.65	802.62	796.24	717.54
C_2H_6	0.050	30.069	1.503	1560.69	1428.64	78.03	71.43
C_3H_8	0.019	44.0956	0.838	2219.17	2043.11	42.16	38.82
iso-C_4H_{10}	0.004	58.1222	0.232	2868.20	2648.12	11.47	10.59
n-C_4H_{10}	0.006	58.1222	0.349	2877.40	2657.32	17.26	15.94
CO_2	0.007	44.0095	0.308	–	–	–	–
N_2	0.020	28.0134	0.560	–	–	–	–
Total	1.000		18.132			945.16	855.32

* See Appendix IV.2

Alternate calculations for NCV:

Combustion reactions are:

$$CH_4 + 2\,O_2 = CO_2 + 2\,H_2O$$
$$C_2H_6 + 3.5\,O_2 = 2\,CO_2 + 3\,H_2O$$
$$C_3H_8 + 5\,O_2 = 3\,CO_2 + 4\,H_2O$$
$$C_4H_{10} + 6.5\,O_2 = 4\,CO_2 + 5\,H_2O$$

Total of water formed $= 2 \times 0.894 + 3 \times 0.05 + 4 \times 0.019$
$$+ 5\,(0.004 + 0.006) = 2.064 \text{ mol}$$
$$\equiv 37.184 \text{ g}$$

Heat lost due to vaporization of water $= \dfrac{(37.184 \times 2442.5)}{1000} = 90.83$ kJ/mol fuel

$$NCV = 945.16 - 90.83 = 854.33 \text{ kJ/mol}$$

Average molar mass of the natural gas $= 18.132$

$$GCV = \frac{(945.16 \times 1000)}{18.132} = 52\,126.6 \text{ kJ/kg}$$

$$NCV = \frac{(855.32 \times 1000)}{18.132} = 47\,171.9 \text{ kJ/kg}$$

Specific volume at 101.3 kPa
and 298.15 K (25°C) = 24.465 m^3/kmol   (Table 7.8)

$$GCV = \frac{(945.16 \times 1000)}{24.465} = 38\,633.1 \text{ kJ/m}^3$$

$$NCV = \frac{(855.32 \times 1000)}{24.465} = 34\,920 \text{ kJ/m}^3 \qquad Ans.$$

Note: In this example, the heating values are expressed in three different units.

7.7 AIR REQUIREMENT AND FLUE GASES

For any combustion reaction, oxygen is a must which will combine with carbon, hydrogen and sulphur. Pure oxygen is an expensive proposition and is ruled out for burning a fuel in normal practice. Air is the cheapest source of oxygen for combustion which contains about 21 mole % oxygen. However, one drawback of air utilization is the presence of nitrogen during combustion which amounts to about 79 mole % of air. Nitrogen reduces the flame temperature considerably and also accounts for high heat loss to the stack.

The *theoretical* or *stoichiometric* amount of air is the minimum air required to burn the fuel completely so that carbon, hydrogen and sulphur are converted to CO_2, H_2O and SO_2 respectively. Consider the following combustion reactions:

Combustion reaction	Ignition temperature[2]
$C + O_2 = CO_2$	680 K (407°C)
$H_2 + \frac{1}{2}O_2 = H_2O$	855 K (582°C)
$S + O_2 = SO_2$	516 K (243°C)

This shows that each atom of carbon and sulphur requires one mole of oxygen (each) for complete combustion. One mole of hydrogen requires half a mole of oxygen. From the first two reactions, it follows that methane requires two moles of oxygen for complete combustion. Similarly, it is easy to calculate the theoretical oxygen demand of a fuel.

$$\text{Theoretical air demand in moles} = \frac{\text{theoretical oxygen demand in moles}}{0.21} \quad (7.4)$$

In actual practice, theoretical air is not sufficient to get complete combustion. Two obvious phenomena of incomplete or partial combustion are carbon monoxide formation and carbon appearance in the flue gases. *Excess air* supply (or, in other words, excess oxygen supply) is a must for complete combustion. It is defined as follows:

$$\% \text{ Excess air} = \frac{(\text{actual air supply} - \text{theoretical air demand}) \times 100}{\text{theoretical air demand}} \quad (7.5)$$

The actual percentage excess air depends on the fuel used for combustion. Normally gaseous fuels require very less excess air. Liquid and solid fuels require somewhat more excess air than gaseous fuels depending on their combustion. Current designs of combustion equipments permit gaseous fuels to be burnt with 5 to 15% excess air while liquid and solid fuels require 10 to 50% excess air.

The effect of excess air is to reduce the flame temperature and to increase the heat losses through the flue gases.

Air is usually supplied at ambient conditions. Some moisture (depending on the humidity of air) enters the combustion chamber with the air.

The theoretical as well as actual air requirements are expressed in either kg/kg fuel or m^3/kg fuel units, depending on the convenience. For converting moles of air into mass, the average molar mass of air can be taken as 29. For converting moles of air into volume units, the ideal gas law can be used. For ready reference, Table 7.8 gives the specific volume of air at different ambient conditions. Normally 101.3 kPa a (760 torr) and 288.7 K (15.56° C or 60°F) are considered standard conditions (STP). In India, NTP [101.325 kPa a and 273.15 K(0°C)] conditions are common for specifying air requirements.

Flue gases are the product gases which are produced by burning a fuel. Normally flue gases contain CO_2, CO, H_2O, O_2, SO_2, (SO_3) and N_2. SO_3 is usually in very low concentration in the flue gases.

The flue gases are analyzed with the help of an instrument called the *Orsat analyzer*. Since the water of the flue gases interferes with the analysis, it is removed by sampling the gas through a strong sulphuric acid container. The dry gases are collected in a measuring tube. CO_2 and SO_2 are absorbed in aqueous K_2CO_3 solution from the gas. The reduction in the volume of the sample gas gives the volume % (or mole %) of (CO_2 + SO_2), expressed as CO_2. Pyrogalol is used for O_2 measurement while the solution of Cu_2Cl_2 is used for CO determination. By subtracting the sum of CO_2, O_2 and CO from 100, the mole % of N_2 can be calculated. Thus, with an Orsat apparatus, the molar analysis of dry flue gases can be obtained. Excess air can be conveniently read from a monograph (Fig. 7.2) if the dry flue gas analysis is known. The Orsat test is manually performed test and has a number of disadvantages. It is slow, involves tedious labour and has relatively poor accuracy. A Fyrite apparatus is available for quick manual determination of CO_2 and O_2 in dry flue gas which also works on chemical absorption principle. Both these instruments have a serious disadvantage that there is no mechanism to provide an output signal for a recorder or control system.

For measurement of oxygen in flue gas on a continuous basis there are three common methods, the paramagnetic sensor, the wet electrochemical cell and the zirconium oxide ceramic cell. Out of the three methods, the zirconium oxide cell is the most preferred oxygen sensor for continuous monitoring of oxygen is hot dirty gases without sample conditioning. While Orsat apparatus and Fyrite apparatus give flue gas analysis on dry basis, the zirconium oxide cell gives oxygen content on wet basis. In addition to continuous oxygen monitoring across-the stack, CO, SO_2 and NO_x analyzers are also available. While CO

Table 7.8 Specific Volume of Ideal Gas at Various Temperatures and Pressures

Specific volume, m^3/kmol

Absolute pressure kPa (Torr)	Temperature K (°C)											
	273 (0)	278 (5)	283 (10)	288 (15)	288.7 (15.6)	293 (20)	298 (25)	303 (30)	308 (35)	313 (40)	318 (45)	323 (50)
98.7 (740)	23.020	23.441	23.867	24.284	24.330	24.705	25.127	25.548	25.969	26.391	26.812	27.234
99.3 (745)	22.865	23.284	23.702	24.121	24.167	24.539	24.958	25.377	25.795	26.214	26.632	27.051
100.0 (750)	22.711	23.129	23.595	23.960	24.006	24.376	24.792	25.207	25.623	26.039	26.455	26.870
100.7 (755)	22.562	22.975	23.388	23.801	23.847	24.214	24.627	25.040	25.453	25.866	26.279	26.692
101.3 (760)	**22.414**	22.824	23.235	23.645	**23.690**	24.055	24.465	24.876	25.286	25.696	26.107	26.517
102.0 (765)	22.268	22.675	23.086	23.490	23.535	23.898	24.306	24.713	25.121	25.528	25.936	26.343
102.7 (770)	22.123	22.528	22.933	23.338	23.382	23.743	24.148	24.553	24.958	25.363	25.768	26.173

analysis provide useful data on leftover combustibles in the flue gas, monitoring of SO_2 and NO_x has assumed importance due to their pollution effects in the environment. For continuous monitoring of O_2 and CO, the reader is advised to refer Ref. 5.

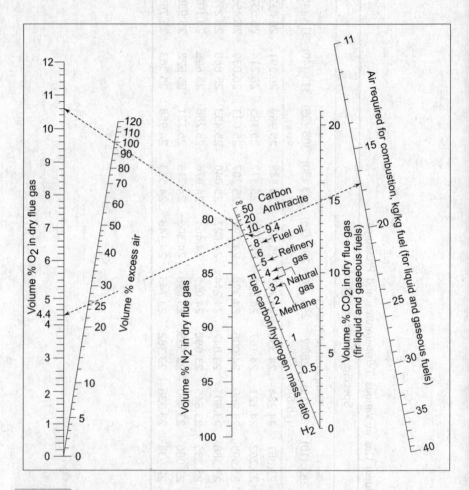

Fig. 7.2 Combustion Air Requirements for Fuels[4]

(*Reproduced with permission of McGraw-Hill, Inc., USA*)

The water vapour, present in the superheated form in flue gases, comes from the following three sources:

(i) The water vapour produced by the combustible hydrogen present in the fuel.

(ii) The moisture of the fuel gets evaporated during combustion. Solid fuels have usually considerable moisture but liquid and natural gaseous fuels contain negligible moisture.

(iii) The water vapour accompanying the air enters the combustion chamber.

The water vapour present in the flue gases reduces the availability of heat from the flue gases. This was discussed in detail in Sec. 7.3 while discussing the concept of NCV.

One of the important determinations in combustion calculations is the *dew point* (*DP*) of the flue gases. The greater the moisture present in the flue gases, the higher is the dew point. Usually in a boiler house, the excess heat of flue gases from a steam generator is recovered in an economizer (where the incoming water is preheated) or in an air preheater (where the incoming air is preheated). In either case, if the temperature of the incoming water/air is less than *DP* of the flue gases, condensation of water vapour takes place. In these droplets of water, CO_2 and SO_2 are dissolved (forming H_2CO_3 and H_2SO_3 respectively). These acids are corrosive and effect the tubes. Therefore it is necessary to introduce water/air into the economizer/air preheater at a temperature higher than the *DP* of flue gases and hence the importance of *DP* evaluation.

For calculating the *DP*, the method outlined in Chapter 6 is recommended. First calculate the partial pressure of the water vapour in flue gases and then obtain the *DP* from a table on the vapour pressure of water (Table 6.8).

The above dew point DP, should not be confused with (*sulphuric*) *acid dew point*. The latter requires special attention when an oil containing sulphur compounds is burnt. Most of the sulphur compounds in the oil are oxidized in the combustion to form SO_2. The conversion of SO_2 to SO_3 depends on the sulphur content of the fuel and flame temperature. This conversion is not very dependent on excess air. Research in combustion engineering has demonstrated that a very small amount of SO_2 is converted to SO_3 in the furnace, slightly more across the high temperature superheater. Most of the SO_3 is catalytically generated in the lower temperature zone of the boiler, where gas temperature is in the range of 875 to 1025 K (602 to 752°C). This happens to be the ideal temperature for vandium oxides in oil-ash deposits and iron oxides on metal surfaces to act as catalysts in the presence of sufficient oxygen for conversion of SO_2 to SO_3. Although SO_3 exists at temperatures above the acid dew point, H_2SO_4 is formed by condensation at the cold end of the boiler as the gases encounter cooler metal temperatures. Dry SO_3 is non-corrosive but condensed acid is highly corrosive. Condensation of sulphuric acid creates extensive corrosion in the heater, economizer, gas ducts, induced draft fans and metal chimney. Therefore, while designing an oil-fired boiler, particularly one with high sulphur content, such as furnace oil (IS: 1593), care should be taken to avoid the acid dew point. Fig. 7.3 can be used for prediction of the acid dew point of the flue gas. The graph is based on (a) carbon fraction and sulphur content of the fuel, (b) excess air and (c) chemical equilibrium of the two sulphur oxides. For the assumptions underlying in preparation of the graph, the reader is requested to refer Ref. 6.

Empirical equations are available for predicting acid dew points due to condensation of sulphurous acid (H_2SO_3), sulphuric acid (H_2SO_4), hydrochloric acid (HCl) etc. Reader is advised to refer Ref. 7 for these equations.

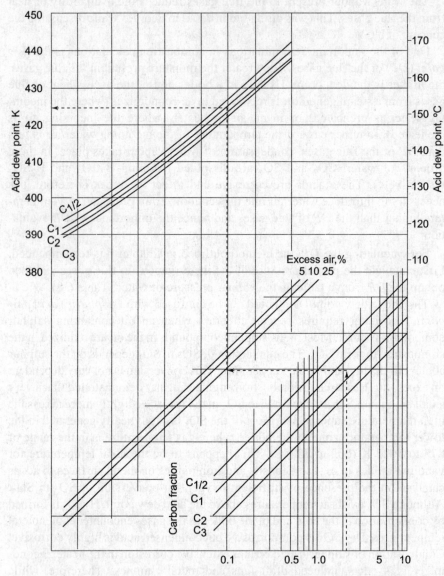

Fig. 7.3 Prediction of Acid Dew Point of Flue Gas[6]

(Reproduced with the permission of Gulf Publishing Co., USA).

Air emission regulations globally have added to design challenges. Low initial investment and low operating costs are no longer the only criteria to select a combustion equipment. Design of such equipment is also required to limit the emissions of CO, NO_x, SO_x and particulates. Of these objectionable pollutants, NO_x has drawn significant attention. NO_x generation is a function of temperature, oxygen and residence time of gases in high temperature zones. Reduction of flue gas temperature from 1480°C to 1260°C is claimed to reduce NO_x generation by a factor of 10. Excess air level of 15 to 20% results in lower CO emissions without excess NO_x generation.

A new innovative approach to combustion of gaseous fuels is introduced. Flue gases, leaving the furnace after air preheating section, are partially recycled and mixed with the gaseous fuel being fired. Flue gas circulation in the range of 30 - 35% has been found to limit the NO_x emission below 10 ppm (v/v). Such a recirculation calls for total review of design of fire-side hardware. Flue gas recirculation is found to be less effective with oil-firing.

Exercise 7.22 gives a case study of flue gas recirculation and its effect on flame temperature.

Selection of fuel also plays an important role in emissions. Ethanol mixed gasoline (petrol), DME, methanol, hydrogen etc. are gaining prominence in light of lower emissions. Catalytic converters are developed for auto vehicles to reduce pollutants' emissions.

Example 7.5 The coal specified in Example 7.1 is burnt with 100% excess air. Calculate (a) The theoretical oxygen requirement per unit mass of coal, (b) the theoretical dry air requirement per unit mass of fuel and (c) the wet and Orsat analyses of flue gases when the coal is burnt with 100% excess dry air.
Solution: Basis: 100 kg coal as-received

Table 7.9 Oxygen Requirement of Coal

Constituent	Mass kg	kmol	O_2 requirement for complete combustion kmol
Carbon	50.22	4.185	+ 4.185
Hydrogen	2.79	1.395	+ 0.698
Sulphur	0.37	0.012	+ 0.012
Oxygen	18.04	0.564	− 0.564
Total	71.42	6.156	4.331

Stoichiometric O_2 requirement = 4.331 kmol = 138.6 kg

Theoretical O_2 requirement to fuel ratio = $\dfrac{138.6}{100}$

$$= 1.386 \text{ kg } O_2/\text{kg coal} \qquad Ans. (1)$$

The above O_2 is fed in the form of air. Therefore, N_2 also enters with O_2.

$$N_2 \text{ entering with } O_2 = \left(\frac{79}{21}\right) \times 4.331 = 16.293 \text{ kmol}$$

Total theoretical dry air requirement

for complete combustion = 4.331 × 32 + 16.293 × 28

= 138.6 + 456.2 = 594.8 kg

Average molar mass value of 29 for air yields theoretical dry air requirement of 598.1 kg.

$$\text{Ratio,} \quad \frac{\text{Theoretical air requirement}}{\text{Fuel}} = \frac{594.8}{100} = 5.948 \text{ kg/kg coal} \qquad \textit{Ans. (b)}$$

$$\text{Actual air supply} = 5.948 \times 2 = 11.896 \text{ kg/kg coal}$$

$$\text{Actual O}_2 \text{ supply} = 4.331 \times 2 = 8.662 \text{ kmol}$$

$$\text{N}_2 \text{ accompanying O}_2 = \left(\frac{79}{21}\right) \times 8.662 = 32.586 \text{ kmol}$$

$$\text{or} \qquad = 2 \times 16.293 = 32.586 \text{ kmol}$$

$$\text{N}_2 \text{ in the coal} = \frac{2.05}{28} = 0.073 \text{ kmol}$$

$$\text{Total N}_2 \text{ in the flue gas} = 32.586 + 0.073 = 32.659 \text{ kmol}$$

$$\text{Total moisture in the flue gas} = 1.395 + \left(\frac{7.00}{2}\right) = 4.895 \text{ kmol}$$

Table 7.10 Composition of Flue Gases

Component	kmol	Wet analysis, mole%	Dry analysis considering SO$_2$ as CO$_2$ (Orsat analysis), mole%
CO$_2$	4.185	9.08	10.19
SO$_2$	0.012	0.03	–
O$_2$	4.331	9.40	10.52
N$_2$	32.659	70.87	79.29
H$_2$O	4.895	10.62	–
Total	46.082	100.00	100.00

Ans. (c)

$$\frac{C}{H} = \frac{50.22}{2.79} = 18$$

For C/H = 18 and excess air = 100%, volume % O$_2$ and N$_2$ in dry flue gas can be read from Fig. 7.2 as 10.6% and 80.3% respectively.

Example 7.6 The ultimate analysis of a residual fuel oil (RFO) sample is given below:

C: 88.4%, H: 9.4% and S: 2.2% (mass)

It is used as a fuel in a power-generating boiler with 25% excess air. Air is available at 303 K (30°C) *DB* and 293 K (20°C) *WB* temperatures. Find (a) the theoretical dry air requirement, (b) the actual dry air supplied, (c) the Orsat composition of flue gases, (d) the concentration of SO$_2$ in ppm (mass) and in ppm (v/v) in the flue gas, (e) the concentration of SO$_2$ in mg/m^3 in the gases if the gases are discharged at 523 K (250°C) and 100.7 kPa a (755 torr) and (f) acid dew point of the flue gas.
Solution: Basis: 100 kg RFO

$$\text{Theoretical O}_2 \text{ requirement} = 9.79 \text{ kmol}$$

$$\text{Theoretical N}_2 \text{ requirement} = \left(\frac{79}{21}\right) \times 9.79 = 36.83 \text{ kmol}$$

Table 7.11 Oxygen Requirement of RFO

Constituent	Mass, kg	kmol	O_2 requirement for complete combustion, kmol
Carbon	88.4	7.37	7.37
Hydrogen	9.4	4.70	2.35
Sulphur	2.2	0.07	0.07
Total	100.0	12.14	9.79

Total dry air requirement (theoretical) = 9.79 + 36.83 = 46.62 kmol ≡ 1352 kg

$$\frac{\text{Theoretical } O_2 \text{ requirement}}{\text{Fuel}} = \frac{1352}{100}$$

$$= 13.52 \text{ kg dry air/kg RFO} \qquad \textit{Ans. (a)}$$

$$\text{Actual air supply} = 46.62 \times 1.25 = 58.275 \text{ kmol}$$

$$\text{mass of actual air supply} = 58.275 \times 29 = 1690 \text{ kg}$$

$$\text{Ratio,} \frac{\text{Actual air supply}}{\text{Fuel}} = \frac{1690}{100} = 16.9 \text{ kg dry air/kg RDO}$$

$$\textit{Ans. (b)}$$

Table 7.12 Composition of Dry Flue Gases

Constituent	Molar mass	kmol	Mass, kg	Orsat, analysis
CO_2	44	7.37	324.28	13.30
SO_2	64	0.07	4.48	—
O_2	32	2.45	78.4	4.38
N_2	28	46.035	1288.98	82.32
Total		55.925	1696.4	100.00

$$\frac{C}{H} = \frac{88.4}{9.4} = 9.4$$

From Fig. 7.2, for C/H = 9.4 and excess air = 25%,

Volume % O_2 in dry flue gas = 4.4

Volume % N_2 in dry flue gas = 82.0

Combustion air requirement = 16.75 kg/kg fuel

Humidity of air

at 303 K *DB* and 293 K *WB* = 0.0106 kg/kg dry air

Moisture entering with air = 0.0106 × 1690 = 17.914 kg

≡ 0.995 kmol

Water formed by combustion = 4.7 kmol

Total water vapour present in the flue gases = 4.7 + 0.995

$$= 5.695 \text{ kmol} \equiv 102.51 \text{ kg}$$

$$\text{Mole fraction of } SO_2 = \frac{0.07}{(55.925 + 5.695)} = 0.001\,136$$

The mole fraction represents kmol of SO_2 per kmol of wet gases. Volumetric relationship follows the same pattern.

$$\text{ppm by volume/volume} = 0.001\,136 \times 10^6 = 1136 \qquad \textit{Ans. (d-i)}$$

$$\text{Concentration by mass of } SO_2 = \frac{4.48 \times 10^6}{(1696.14 + 102.51)}$$
$$\text{(ppm by mass)}$$
$$= 2490.8 \text{ mg/kg (wet basis)} \qquad \textit{Ans. (d-ii)}$$

Volume of wet flue gases at 523 K (250°C) and 100.7 kPa a

$$V = \frac{[(55.925 + 5.695) \times 8.314 \times 523]}{100.7}$$

$$= 2660.7 \text{ m}^3$$

$$\text{Concentration of } SO_2 = \frac{(4.48 \times 10^6)}{2660.7} = 1683.8 \text{ mg/m}^3 \qquad \textit{Ans. (e)}$$

$$\text{For the given RFO analysis, C/H mole ratio} = \frac{7.37}{4.70} = 1.57$$

$$\text{S content} = 2.2 \text{ mass \%}$$

From Fig. 7.3, for 25% excess air, acid dew point = 424.4 K (151.4°C)

$$\textit{Ans. (f)}$$

Note: SO_2 is considered as a pollutant in the flue gases. Since its concentration is usually low, it is customary to represent the concentration of it in either ppm (mass or v/v) or mg/m³. The case with the CO or NO_x content of the flue gases is similar. Since the flue gas temperature (523 K) is above the acid dew point (424.4 K), corrosion problem is not envisaged. Reader may calculate sulphurous acid (H_2SO_3) dew point using formula, given in Exercise 7.26.

Example 7.7 The Orsat analysis of the flue gases from a boiler house chimney gives CO_2: 11.4%, O_2: 4.2 % and N_2: 84.4% (mole %). Assuming that complete combustion has taken place, (a) calculate the % excess air, and (b) find the C : H ratio in the fuel.

Solution: Basis: 100 kmol dry flue gases

$$O_2 \text{ accounted} = O_2 \text{ in } CO_2 + O_2 \text{ as such} = 11.4 + 4.2 = 15.6 \text{ kmol}$$

For the calculations of the actual supply of O_2, nitrogen is a tie component which provides the clue as it comes from air.

$$O_2 \text{ available from air} = \left(\frac{21}{79}\right) \times 84.4 = 22.435 \text{ kmol}$$

$$\text{Excess } O_2 = 4.2 \text{ kmol}$$

$$O_2 \text{ unaccounted} = 22.435 - 15.6 = 6.835 \text{ kmol}$$

This O_2 must have been utilized for the burning of hydrogen.

Hydrogen burnt = 2 × 6.835 = 13.67 kmol

Theoretical oxygen requirement = 11.4 + 6.835 = 18.235 kmol

or = 22.435 − 4.2 = 18.235 kmol

$$\% \text{ excess air} = \frac{(4.2 \times 100)}{18.235} = 23.03 \qquad Ans. \text{ (a)}$$

Mass of hydrogen burnt = 13.67 × 2 = 27.34 kg

Mass of carbon burnt = 11.4 × 12 = 136.8. kg

$$\text{Carbon/hydrogen (mass) ratio in the fuel} = \frac{136.8}{27.34} = 5.00 \qquad Ans. \text{ (b)}$$

7.8 COMBUSTION CALCULATIONS

In the above sections, fuels were classified and the air requirements of various fuels were studied. In industries, the fuels are fired in boilers, producing steam, hot water or hot oil. In various furnaces, the fuels are burnt to provide the heat for the chemical reaction or for the phase change. For example, in a primary reformer of a fertilizer plant, the combustion of fuel provides the heat for endothermic reforming reactions. In foundries, the metal is melted by burning the fuel.

In all the above cases, the firing rate of the fuel is known. There is no direct measurement of the air input. However, the Orsat analysis of the flue gases, leaving the chimney of a furnace, is made available. The analysis of the fuel can be had from the laboratory. Various temperatures can be measured at different points on the combustion side.

The useful heat gain can be calculated by knowing the total steam generated and its conditions. The feed water temperature is an important parameter.

In furnaces, the heat gain can be calculated easily, based on the methods outlined in Chapter 5.

The thermal efficiency of boiler or a furnace is calculated, using the following equation:

$$\text{Thermal efficiency} = \left(\frac{\text{useful heat gain}}{\text{total heat input}} \right) \times 100 \qquad (7.6)$$

Usually, thermal efficiencies (i.e., total heat inputs) are defined on the GCV basis of the fuels. However, in many cases NCV is specified for thermal efficiency calculations.

The common heat losses of the combustion side are mentioned below.

(i) The heat is lost in the flue gases which leave the chimney at a high temperature. Usually, the flue gases leave at around 475 K (202°C). Boilers, fired with biofuels, such as rice husk, saw dust, etc. can be designed to have lower fuel gas temperature (below 425 K) as they have no sulphur.

(ii) The heat is lost in the refuse which remains at the end of combustion. In the refuse, some combustibles are always left over which account for the heat loss. When coal is fired, the refuse is called *cinder*. When liquid fuel is burnt, carbon deposition in the furnace can take place. Gaseous fuels normally do not leave any refuse.

(iii) The solid fuels contain considerable moisture. This and the moisture produced by the burning of net hydrogen have to be evaporated. For this, latent heat is expended which accounts for the heat loss. Liquid and gaseous fuels contain very low moisture.

(iv) The blow-down heat loss in steam boilers.

(v) The radiation loss from the surfaces of the furnace or boiler. Usually this heat loss is difficult to calculate, if not impossible. In practice, the total useful heat gain and above four heat losses are added together and deducted from 100 to get the radiation loss.

Considering the various heat losses mentioned above, one would like to minimize them in order that the available useful heat is maximized.

The heat loss in the refuse and in the moisture of coal can be minimized by selecting the "better" coal. Very often, the choice may not exist for a buyer in India and hence there is a limited scope in the reduction of these heat losses.

The radiation heat loss can be kept to a minimum by properly lagging the surfaces while the blow-down losses can be reduced by feeding better quality water in the steam boilers. IS: 10 392 gives the requirements of feed water and boiler water for low and medium pressure boilers. Both these measures have assumed considerable importance in the process industry due to the energy crisis.

There are two aspects to the problem of heat loss through the flue gases:

(i) Reduce the temperature of the outlet flue gas to the chimney to maximum "possible" level by using the economizer and/or air preheater. Although, in many boiler plants a possibility exists, it is not always possible to reduce the temperature below a certain limits such as the one dictated by the acid dew point.

(ii) Minimize the use of excess air. This can be controlled by checking the Orsat analysis of the flue gases. High CO_2 content and low O_2 content of the flue gases are desired, but too low excess air may result in CO and carbon formation, which indicate incomplete combustion. Therefore, excess air is supplied to ensure complete combustion.

When a fuel is burnt, based on enthalpy balance, it is possible to calculate the adiabatic reaction temperature which is termed as *adiabatic flame temperature* or simply, *flame temperature* in combustion. This can be calculated based on the methods outlined in Chapter 5. Usually, adiabatic flame temperatures are not obtained in practice due to radiation losses. Hence actual flame temperatures are lower than adiabatic flame temperatures.

The greater the adiabatic flame temperature (AFT), the higher is the rate of heat transfer because of increased temperature differences. For this reason also, excess air should be limited to the bare minimum. However higher AFT is found responsible for higher NO_x emission.

In many furnaces, e.g., where heat treatment is carried out, the flame temperature in the furnace is a controlling variable in the process. In another case, sulphur is not accepted in the fuel due to possible sulphur pick-up by the product in the furnace. Where such controls are necessary, the selection of the fuel is critical.

Steam generating units are tested in accordance with several codes. Among these, Power Test Code (PTC) 4.1 for stationary steam generating units, published by the Americans Society of Mechanical Engineers (ASME) and British Standard BS: 2885 are popular. These codes also give the computational methods of evaluation of the boiler efficiency. In Table 7.13, simplified boiler heat balance calculations are enumerated.

Table 7.13 Boiler Heat Balance Calculations

Basis: 1 kg fuel

Heat Input:

1. H_1 = Gross calorific value, kJ
2. Heat of input fuel
$$H_2 = C_s (T_f - T_o) \text{ kJ} \tag{7.7}$$
Where T_f is the temperature of fuel (K), T_o is the reference temperature (K) and C_s is the heat capacity of fuel, [kJ/(kg·K)]
3. Heat of input air,
$$H_3 = W_a C_H (T_a - T_o) \text{ kJ} \tag{7.8}$$
Where W_a is the input dry air (kg/kg fuel), T_a is the temperature of incoming air (K) and C_s C_H is the humid heat of air, [kJ/(kg dry air · K)]
$$C_H = 1.006 + 1.84 \, H \text{ and}$$
H is the humidity of air (kg/kg dry air)
Total heat input,
$$H_1 = H_1 + H_2 + H_3 \text{ kJ} \tag{7.9}$$

Heat Output:

1. Heat gain in steam generation:
   (a) Economizer:
$$H_4 = W_f (h_{ew} - h_{fw}) \text{ kJ} \tag{7.10}$$
where W_f is the water fed (kg/kg fuel), h_{ew} is the enthalpy of the outlet water from the economizer (kJ/kg) and h_{fw} the enthalpy of he feed water (kJ/kg).
   (b) Boiler (steam generator):
$$H_5 = W_s (H_{bs} - h_{ew}) \text{ kJ} \tag{7.11}$$
where W_s is the steam generated (kg/kg fuel) and H_{bs} is the enthalpy of saturated steam (kJ/kg).
   (c) Superheater:
$$H_6 = W_s (H_{ss} - H_{bs}) \text{ kJ} \tag{7.12}$$
where H_{ss} is the enthalpy of superheated steam (kJ/kg).
2. Heat lost in flue gases:
Approximate calculations:
$$H_7 = w_{fg} \cdot C_{mpf} (T_{fg} - T_o) \text{ kJ} \tag{7.13a}$$
where w_{fg} is the mass of the dry flue gas (kg/kg), T_{fg} is the temperature of flue gases, entering the chimney (K) and C_{mpf} is the humid heat of flue gases [kJ/(kg dry gas · K)]

Accurate calculations:

$$H_7 = (\Sigma\, n_i \cdot C^\circ_{mpi})\,(T_{fg} - 298.15)\ \text{kJ} \tag{7.13b}$$

where n_i is the number of kmol of the ith component, present in the flue gas mixture per kg of fuel and C°_{mpi} is the mean heat capacity at T_{fg}, [kJ/(kmol · K)] (Refer Table 7.14 for C°_{mpm} values.)

3. Heat loss due to evaporation:

Heat loss due to evaporation of moisture, formed by burning hydrogen of the fuel:

$$H_8 = W_{mf} \cdot \lambda_v\ \text{kJ} \tag{7.14}$$

where W_{mf} is the mass of moisture formed by burning hydrogen (kg/kg coal) and λ_v is the latent heat of vaporization of water at the dew point of flue gases (kJ/kg)

$$H_9 = W_{mfr} \cdot \lambda_v\ \text{kJ} \tag{7.15}$$

where W_{mfr} is the mass of moisture (of fuel) evaporated.

4. Loss due to incomplete combustion of Carbon as Carbon Monoxide:

$$H_{10} = \left[\frac{CO}{(CO + CO_2)}\right] C\ (23\,560)\ \text{kJ} \tag{7.16}$$

where CO is the % by volume of carbon monoxide in dry flue gases, CO_2 is the % by volume of carbon dioxide in dry flue gases and C is the burnt carbon (kg/kg fuel).

5. Loss due to unconsumed Carbon in refuse:

$$H_{11} = W_c\ (32\,762)\ \text{kJ} \tag{7.17}$$

where W_c is the mass of the unburnt carbon in the refuse (kg/kg fuel).

6. Loss due to blow-down:

$$H_{12} = W_{bl}\,(h_{bw} - H_{fw})\ \text{kJ} \tag{7.18}$$

where W_{bl} is the mass of the water blown down (kg/kg) fuel and h_{bw} is the enthalpy of the boiler water (kJ/kg)

$$W_f = W_s + W_{bl} \tag{7.19}$$

7. Balance unaccounted loss:

$$H_{13} = H_1 - \sum_{i=4}^{i=12} H_i \tag{7.20}$$

Notes:

(i) The reference temperature T_o can be taken as 298.15 K (25°C) or the ambient air temperature, depending on the convenience.

(ii) λ_v is the latent heat of vaporization of water at the dew point temperature. However, if dew point calculations are to be avoided, it may be taken as 2490 kJ/kg which is a good approximation.

(iii) The unaccounted heat loss (H_{13}) accounts for radiation, grit, emission, etc.

Calculation of heat loss in flue gas involving polynomial heat capacity equation (Ref. Table 5.1) is quite laborious. Also the humid heat equation (Eq. 6.14) when applied to the flue gas gives gross error in the heat loss value. It is therefore suggested to use mean heat capacity (C°_{mpm}) data given in the Table 7.14 for heat loss calculations in Eq. (7.13b). Refer Sec. 5.13 for discussion on mean heat capacity.

Table 7.14 Mean Heat Capacity Data for Combustion Gases

Temperature	Mean heat capacity over 298.15 K (25°C) C^o_{mpm}, kJ/(kmol · K) at 101.325 kPa a (760 torr)					
	Gas component					
K (°C)	CO_2	O_2	N_2	CO	H_2O	H_2
350 (77)	39.24	26.35	28.60	28.60	33.17	28.95
400 (127)	39.92	26.60	28.75	28.77	33.46	28.98
425 (152)	40.26	29.72	28.83	28.86	33.61	29.00
450 (177)	40.60	29.84	28.91	28.95	33.75	29.01
475 (202)	40.94	29.96	28.98	29.03	33.90	29.03
500 (227)	41.28	30.09	29.06	29.12	34.04	29.05
525 (252)	41.62	30.21	29.14	29.21	34.19	29.06
550 (277)	41.96	30.33	29.21	29.30	34.34	29.08
575 (302)	42.30	30.45	29.29	29.38	34.48	29.09
600 (327)	42.64	30.57	29.36	29.47	34.63	29.11
625 (352)	42.98	30.70	29.44	29.56	34.78	29.13
650 (377)	43.32	30.82	29.52	29.65	34.92	29.15
675 (402)	43.66	30.94	29.59	29.73	35.07	29.16
700 (427)	44.00	31.06	29.67	29.82	35.22	29.18
725 (452)	44.34	31.18	29.75	29.91	35.36	29.19
750 (477)	44.68	31.31	29.82	30.00	35.51	29.21
775 (502)	45.02	31.43	29.90	30.08	35.66	29.23
800 (527)	45.36	31.55	29.97	30.17	35.80	29.24

Different methods for performance evaluation of a furnace are compared by Fehr[8]. A designer may be concerned with maximum extraction of heat from a fuel on its way through the installation. On the other hand, an engineer involved in energy audit may be concerned with the best utilization of available heat. For example, the audit engineer normally subdivides the heat utilization into subsections, tries to find faults by sections and points out the steps for correction. Dr. Fehr had defined a number of efficiencies for performance evaluation. He has also stressed the importance of reference temperature, reliable data on calorific values of fuels and measurement of correct operating parameters for evaluation of the performance.

Example 7.8 A boiler in a sugar factory is burnt with bagasse having the following composition[9].
Proximate analysis (mass %):

Moisture	:	52.0%
Volatile matter	:	40.2%
Fixed carbon	:	6.1%
Ash	:	1.7%

Ultimate analysis (mass %)

Carbon	: 23.4%
Hydrogen (net)	: 2.8%
Sulphur	: Traces
Nitrogen	: Traces
Oxygen	: 20.1%
Moisture	: 52.0%
Ash	: 1.7%

The GCV of bagasse is measured to be 10 300 kJ/kg (moist basis, i.e. as-received basis). In a typical run of the boiler, the following test data were collected.

Orsat analysis of flue gases: 15.65% CO_2 on volume basis

Air supply for combustion: 100.0 kPa a (750 torr), 308 K (35°C) *DB* and 296 K (23°C) *WB*.

Water is fed to the economizer at 343 K (70°C).

Flue gases leave the chimney at 433 K (160°C) and 99.3 kPa a (745 torr).

Steam is produced at 21.5 bar a and 643 K (370°C).

Rate of steam generation = 2.6 kg/kg fuel

Calculate (a) the theoretical air requirement, (b) the actual air supply as % excess air, (c) the dew point of flue gases, (d) the thermal efficiency of the boiler, (e) the heat balance of the boiler and (f) the adiabatic flame temperature.

Assume that the refuse does not contain any combustibles and complete combustion of bagasse takes place.

Solution: Basis: 100 kg bagasse fired in the boiler

Table 7.15   Oxygen Requirement of Bagasse

Constituent	kg	kmol	O_2 requirement, kmol
Carbon	23.4	1.95	+ 1.95
Hydrogen	2.8	1.40	+ 0.70
Oxygen	20.1	0.63	− 0.63
Total	46.3	3.98	2.02

Theoretical oxygen requirement = 2.02 kmol = 64.64 kg

$$N_2 \text{ entering with } O_2 \text{ through air} = \left(\frac{79}{21}\right) \times 2.02 = 7.6 \text{ kmol} \equiv 212.8 \text{ kg}$$

Total theoretical air = 64.64 + 212.80 = 277.44 kg

$$\text{Theoretical air/fuel ratio} = \frac{277.44}{100} = 2.77 \text{ kg dry air/kg fuel} \quad Ans. \text{ (a)}$$

CO_2 produced = 1.95 kmol

Dry flue gases contain 15.65% CO_2.

$$\text{Total dry flue gases} = \frac{1.95}{0.1565} = 12.46 \text{ kmol}$$

Let x be the excess O_2 in the flue gases.

Excess O_2 + nitrogen from air = 12.46 − 1.95 = 10.51 kmol

Total O_2 entering the furnace = $(2.02 + x)$ kmol

Total N_2 entering through air = $\left(\dfrac{79}{21}\right) \times (2.02 + x)$

$$= (7.6 + 3.76\, x)\ \text{kmol}$$

$$x + 7.6 + 3.76\, x = 10.51$$

$$x = 0.61\ \text{kmol}$$

$$\% \text{ Excess air} = \left(\dfrac{0.61}{2.02}\right) \times 100 = 30.26 \qquad\qquad Ans.\ (b)$$

Moisture in flue gases:

Moisture produced by the combustion

of net hydrogen of the fuel = 1.4 kmol

Free moisture in bagasse = 52.0 kg = 2.889 kmol

Moisture of air:

Absolute humidity of air at 308 K

DB and 296 K WB at 101.325 kPa = 12.8 g/kg dry air   (Fig. 6.11)

$$= 0.0206\ \text{kmol/kmol dry air}$$

Molar humidity at 100.0 kPa = 13.0 kg/kg dry air

$$= 0.020\ 95\ \text{kmol/kmol dry air (Ref. Table 6.9)}$$

Moisture entering with air = $\left[\dfrac{(2.02 + 0.61)}{0.21}\right] 0.020\ 95 = 0.262$ kmol

Total moisture in the flue gases = 1.4 + 2.889 + 0.262 = 4.551 kmol

Table 7.16 Composition of Flue Gases

Component	Molar mass	kmol	mole % (wet basis)	kg
CO_2	44	1.95	11.47	85.80
O_2	32	0.61	3.59	19.52
N_2	28	9.89	58.17	276.92
H_2O	18	4.551	26.77	81.92
Total		17.001	100.00	464.16

$$\text{Average molar mass of flue gases} = \dfrac{464.16}{17.001} = 27.3^*$$

---

* *Note*: Average molar mass of lean fuels like bagasse, lignite, rice husk, saw dust etc. is lower than normal average molar mass of the flue gas, i.e., approximately 29.

Partial pressure of water vapour in flue gases = $100 \times 0.2677 = 26.77$ kPa

Dew point of flue gases = 339.7 K (66.7°C) (Ref. Table 6.8)

Ans. (c)

$$\text{Absolute humidity of flue gases} = \frac{81.92}{(464.16 - 81.92)}$$

$$= 0.2143 \text{ kg/kg dry flue gas}$$

For approximate calculations, the average heat capacity (humid heat) equation [Eq. (6.14)] can be used.

$$C_{Hf} = 1.006 + 1.84 \times 0.2143 = 1.4 \text{ kJ/(kg dry gas} \cdot \text{K)}$$

Latent heat of water at 339.7 K = 2343.6 kJ/kg

Heat balance:

For the heat balance calculations, assume $T_o = 298.15$ K (25°C)

$$\text{Heat lost in flue gases, } H_7 = W_{fg}, C_{Hf} (T_{fg} - T_o)$$

$$= (464.16 - 81.92) \times 1.4 (433 - 298.15)$$

$$= 72\,243 \text{ kJ}$$

Table 7.17 Mean Heat Capacity Data

Compounds	n_i kmol	$C°_{mpm}$, kJ/(kmol·K) between 298.15 – 433 K (Refer Table 7.14)	$n_i \cdot C°_{mpmi}$, kJ/K
CO_2	1.95	40.366	78.714
O_2	0.61	29.759	18.153
N_2	9.89	28.854	285.366
H_2O	4.551	33.652	153.150
Total	17.001		535.383

Heat lost in flue gases, $H_7 = 535.383 (433 - 298.15) = 72\,277$ kJ

For computing the heat loss in the moisture evaporated during combustion, the latent heat value at the dew point (i.e., 2343.6 kJ/kg at 339.7 K) needs to be considered.

Heat loss due to evaporation of free moisture,

present in bagasse, $H_9 = 52 \times 2343.6 = 121\,867$ kJ

Heat loss due to evaporation moisture, produced by burning of

net hydrogen of the fuel, $H_8 = 1.4 \times 18 \times 2343.6 = 59\,059$ kJ

Heat gain:

Water enters the economizer at 343 K (70°C) (which is above the *DP* of flue gases). From Appendix III.3,

Enthalpy of feed water at 343 K, $h_{fw} = 292.97$ kJ/kg

Enthalpy of superheated steam at

21.5 bar a and 643 K, $H_{ss} = 3180.15$ kJ/kg

Net heat gained by water

in steam raising = $3180.15 - 292.97 = 2887.18$ kJ/kg

Total heat gained by water, $H_6 = 2.6 \times 2887.18 \times 100 = 750\,667$ kJ

Heat input:

Heat supplied by fuel, $H_1 = 100 \times 10\,300 = 1030\,000$ kJ

Overall thermal efficiency of the

$$\text{boiler (on GCV basis)} = \left(\frac{750\,667}{1030\,000}\right) \times 100 = 72.88 \qquad Ans.\ (d)$$

Heat input by air:

$$C_{Ha} = 1.006 + 1.84\,(0.013) = 1.03 \text{ kJ (kg dry air} \cdot \text{K)}$$

$$\text{Heat input by air, } H_3 = (9.89 \times 28 + 2.63 \times 32) \times 1.03 \times (308 - 298.15)$$

$$= 3719 \text{ kJ}$$

Table 7.18 Heat Balance of Bagasse Fired Boiler

	Heat in kJ	%
Input:		
Burning of fuel	1030 000	99.64
Air	3 719	0.36
Total	1033 719	100.00
Output:		
Steam raising	750 667	72.62
Heat lost in flue gases	72 243	6.99
Heat loss due to evaporation:		
(i) Free moisture of fuel	121 867	11.79
(ii) Moisture produced by burning net hydrogen of fuel	59 059	5.71
Unaccounted heat loss by difference (due to radiation, blow-down, etc.)	29 883	2.89
Total	1033 719	100.00

Ans. (e)

In Table 7.18, the sensible heat of bagasse is neglected.

Figure 7.4 gives the split-up of the heat supply. It is known as a *heat-flow diagram*.

The boiler capacity is usually rated from and at (F&A) 373.15 K (100°C) and 101.325 kPa.

At these conditions, water needs to be supplied with the latent heat of vaporisation (2256.9 kJ/kg) only to generate saturated steam.

Evaporation of boiler capacity

$$\text{from and at (F\&A) 373.15 K (100°C)} = \frac{750\,667}{(2256.9 \times 100)} = 3.327 \text{ kg/kg fuel}$$

Boiler rating at F&A 373.15 K(100°C) get reduced by 21.85% for actual steam generation at 21.5 bar a and 643 K (370°C).

Now in combustion calculations, adiabatic flame temperatures are likely to exceed 1500 K (1227°C) in furnaces. Particularly when a fuel is fired with air close to stoichiometric requirements, these temperatures are quite high and therefore equations valid in the high temperature range (> 1500 K) should be utilised. In furnaces fired with bagasse, lignite and other poor quality coals, adiabatic flame temperatures could be around 1500 K (1227°C) or less.

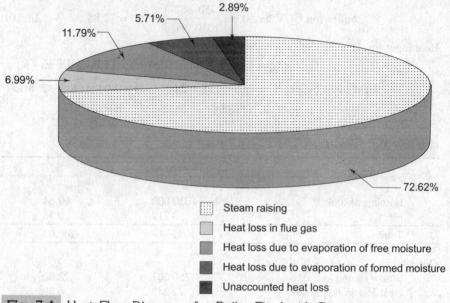

2.89%

5.71%

11.79%

6.99%

72.62%

:::: Steam raising

   Heat loss in flue gas

   Heat loss due to evaporation of free moisture

   Heat loss due to evaporation of formed moisture

   Unaccounted heat loss

Fig. 7.4   Heat Flow Diagram of a Boiler Fired with Bagasse

Keeping the above facts in mind, empirical constants of the heat capacity equation for the correct temperature range should be utilised. In Table 5.1 data for CO_2, H_2O, N_2 and O_2 are available for temperature up to 4000 K. SO_2 content of flue gas is normally low and hence the SO_2 content can be combined with the CO_2 content (as is the case with Orsat analysis) and data for CO_2 can be used for the combined concentration.

Actual flame temperatures will be lower than adiabatic flame temperatures and the difference depends on the design of the furnace.

Adiabatic flame temperature (AFT):

For the evaluation of AFT, NCV of the fuel must be considered. This is because moisture is present in the vapour form in the flue gases.

$$\text{NCV of fuel (at 298.15 K)} = 10\,300 - \left[\frac{(52 + 1.4 \times 18)}{100} \right] \times 2442.5$$

$$= 8514.4 \text{ kJ/kg}$$

Heat input based on NCV, $H_1' = 8514.4 \times 100$

$$= 851\,440 \text{ kJ}$$

$T_0 = 298.15$ K and $T =$ adiabatic flame temperature

Enthalpy of flue gas up to 1500 K,

$$H_2' = 504.626\,(1500 - 298.15) + 64.149 \times 10^{-3} \frac{\left(1500^2 - 298.15^2\right)}{2}$$

Table 7.19 Heat Capacity Equation Constants for Flue Gas of Bagasse Fired Boiler

Heat capacity equation constants	Component				
	CO_2	O_2	N_2	H_2O	Total
n_i kmol	1.95	0.61	9.89	4.551	17.001
$(n_i \cdot a_i)_1{}^*$	41.662	15.875	292.751	154.338	504.626
$(n_i \cdot a_i)_2{}^*$	72.489	11.224	307.759	114.496	505.988
$(n_i \cdot b_i)_1 \times 10^3$	125.354	7.171	– 54.657	– 13.719	64.149
$(n_i \cdot b_i)_2 \times 10^3$	45.312	13.248	31.617	98.853	187.03
$(n_i \cdot c_i)_1 \times 10^6$	– 80.051	– 1.430	137.059	69.166	124.744
$(n_i \cdot c_i)_2 \times 10^6$	– 14.389	– 5.066	– 4.007	– 24.302	– 47.764
$(n_i \cdot d_i)_1 \times 10^9$	19.113	0.342	– 52.173	– 22.103	– 54.821
$(n_i \cdot d_i)_2 \times 10^9$	1.602	0.705	0.023	2.196	4.526

* 1 and 2 refer to heat capacity data for temperature ranges 298.15–1500 K and 1500–4000 K, respectively.

$$+ 124.744 \times 10^{-6} \frac{\left(1500^3 - 298.15^3\right)}{3} - 54.821 \times 10^{-9} \frac{\left(1500^4 - 298.15^4\right)}{4}$$

$$= 606\,560 + 69\,319 + 139\,237 - 69\,275 = 745\,841 \text{ kJ}$$

Enthalpy of flue gas above 1500 K,

$$H'_3 = H'_1 - H'_2$$

$$= 851\,440 - 745\,841 = 105\,559 \text{ kJ}$$

$$= 505.988\,(T - 1500) + 187.03 \times 10^{-3} \frac{\left(T^2 - 1500^2\right)}{2}$$

$$- 47.764 \times 10^{-6} \frac{\left(T^3 - 1500^3\right)}{3} + 4.526 \times 10^{-9} \frac{\left(T^4 - 1500^4\right)}{4}$$

$$= 505.988\,T + 93.515 \times 10^{-3}\,T^2 - 15.921 \times 10^{-6}\,T^3$$

$$+ 1.132 \times 10^{-9}\,T^4 - 921\,384$$

$$1.132 \times 10^{-9}\,T^4 - 15.921 \times 10^{-6}\,T^3 + 93.515 \times 10^{-3}\,T^2 + 505.899\,T = 1026\,943$$

Mathcad solution: $f(T) := 1.132 \times 10^{-9}\,T^4 = 15.921 \times 10^{-6}\,T^3 + 93.515 \times 10^{-3}\,T^2$

$$+ 505.988\,T - 1026\,943$$

$$T = 1600 \text{ K}$$

$$\text{soln} := \text{root}\,(f(T), T)$$

$$\text{soln} = 1651 \text{ K}$$

or $$T = 1651 \text{ K } (1377°C) \qquad\qquad Ans.\ (f)$$

Example 7.9 A stocker-fired water-tube boiler is fired with coal at the rate of 3.9 t/h[10]. The proximate analysis of the fuel indicates ash 12.68% and moisture 7.91% (by mass). The GCV of the coal is measured to be 26 170 kJ/kg. The boiler produces steam at 30 bar a and 703 K (430°C) at the rate of 29 t/h. The Orsat analysis of the flue gases indicated CO_2: 12.8%, O_2: 6.5% and the rest N_2 (volume basis). The combustibles (essentially carbon) present in cinder as a percentage of the coal supplied were found to be 2.7% (by mass). The feed water temperature was measured to be 363 K (90°C). Flue gases leave the economizer at 423 K (150°C) and 100.7 kPa a (755 torr). Air enters the burner at 303 K (30°C) *DB* and 295 K (22°C) *WB* temperatures. Assume that negligible oxygen and sulphur were present in the coal. Evaluate the boiler performance.

Solution: Basis: 100 kmol dry flue gases

$$N_2 \text{ in the flue gases} = 100 - 12.8 - 6.5 = 80.7 \text{ kmol}$$

$$O_2 \text{ supply from air} = \left(\frac{21}{79}\right) 80.7 = 21.45 \text{ kmol}$$

$$\text{Oxygen accounted for} = 12.8 + 6.5 = 19.3 \text{ kmol}$$

O_2 utilized for hydrogen burning

$$\text{(i.e., unaccounted } O_2) = 21.45 - 19.3 = 2.15 \text{ kmol}$$

$$\text{Hydrogen burnt} = 2.15 \times 2 = 4.3 \text{ kmol}$$

$$\text{Water produced} = 4.3 \text{ kmol}$$

$$\text{Carbon retained in the cinder} = \frac{(2.7 \times 3.9 \times 1000)}{100} = 105.3 \text{ kg/h}$$

$$\equiv 8.775 \text{ kmol/h}$$

$$\text{(FC + VM) in coal} = 100 - 12.68 - 7.91 = 79.41\%$$

$$\frac{\text{Carbon unburnt}}{\text{(FC + VM - unburnt C)}} \text{ ratio} = \frac{2.7}{(79.41 - 2.7)} = 0.0352$$

$$\text{Carbon in the flue gasses} = 12.8 \text{ kmol} = 153.6 \text{ kg}$$

$$\text{Hydrogen in the flue gases} = 4.3 \times 2 = 8.6 \text{ kg}$$

$$\text{Total burnt combustibles} = 153.6 + 8.6 = 162.2 \text{ kg}$$

Total unburnt for 100 kmol

$$\text{dry flue gas} = 0.0352 \times 162.2$$

$$= 5.71 \text{ kg} \equiv 0.48 \text{ kmol}$$

$$O_2 \text{ required to burn the unburnt carbon} = 0.48 \text{ kmol}$$

$$\text{Excess } O_2 = 6.5 - 0.48 = 6.02 \text{ kmol}$$

Total theoretical O_2 required

$$\text{for complete combustion} = 12.8 + 0.48 + 2.15 = 15.43 \text{ kmol}$$

$$\text{Excess air} = \left(\frac{6.02}{15.43}\right) \times 100 = 39.0\%$$

$$\text{Free moisture entering with coal} = 7.91\%$$

Now for 79.71 kg combustion of coal, free moisture entering the boiler is 7.91 kg. For 162.2 kg combustibles of coal, free moisture

$$\text{appearing in the flue gases} = \left(\frac{7.91}{79.41}\right) \times 162.2 = 16.16 \text{ kg} \equiv 0.898 \text{ kmol}$$

Humidity of air at 303 K *DB*

and 295 K *WB* at 101.3 kPa a = 0.0134 kg/kg dry air   (Fig. 6.11)

$$= 0.0216 \text{ kmol/kmol dry air}$$

Humidity at 100.7 kPa a = $1.008 \times 0.0134 = 0.0135$ kg/kg dry air

$$\equiv 0.0218 \text{ kmol/kmol dry air}$$

Total moisture of air entering

the combustion zone = $0.0218 (21.45 + 80.7) = 2.227$ kmol

Total moisture in the flue gases = $4.30 + 0.898 + 2.227 = 7.425$ kmol

Table 7.20 Composition of Flue Gases

Component	kmol	kg (dry gas)	mole % (wet basis)	Orsat analysis, %
CO_2	12.8	563.2	11.92	12.8
O_2	6.5	208.0	6.05	6.5
N_2	80.7	2259.6	75.12	80.7
H_2O	7.425	–	6.91	—
Total	107.425	3030.8	100.00	100.00

Average molar mass of dry flue gas = 30.3

$$\text{Moisture in flue gas} = \frac{7.425 \times 18}{(100 \times 30.3)} = 0.04 \text{ kg/kg dry gas}$$

Partial pressure of water

vapour in the flue gases = $100.7 \times 0.0691 = 6.96$ kPa

DP of the flue gases = 312.9 K (39.9°C)

Latent heat of water at 312.9 K = 2407.6 kJ/kg

Heat balance:

Reference temperature, T_o = 298.15 (25°C)

Enthalphy of water at 363 K (90°C), h_{fw} = 376.94 kJ/kg

Enthalpy of steam at 30 bar a

and 703 K, h_{ss} = 3299.9 kJ/kg

Heat gained by water in the

boiler (i.e. in the economizer,

boiler and superheater) = $3299.9 - 376.94 = 2922.96$ kJ/kg

Total hear gained, $\phi_6 = 2922.96 \times 29\,000$

$$= 84\,765\,840 \text{ kJ/h} \equiv 23\,546.07 \text{ kW}$$

Calorific value of carbon

GCV (= NCV) = 393 510 kJ/kmol

Heat lost in the combustibles, = $8.775 \times 393\,510$

$$= 3453\,050 \text{ kJ/h} \equiv 959.18 \text{ kW}$$

Total free moisture

evaporated from coal = $\left(\dfrac{16.1}{162.2}\right) \times 3900 \times 0.7971 = 308.6$ kg/h

Heat loss due to evaporation

of free moisture, $\phi_9 = 308.6 \times 2407.6$

$$= 742\,985 \text{ kJ/h} \equiv 206.38 \text{ kW}$$

Moisture formed due to combustion

of the net hydrogen of the coal $= \left(\dfrac{4.3}{162.2} \right) \times 3900 \times 0.7971$

$$= 82.413 \text{ kmol/h}$$

Heat loss due to evaporation of

the moisture due to combustion, $\phi_8 = 82.413 \times 18 \times 2407.6$

$$= 3571\,516 \text{ kJ/h} \equiv 992.09 \text{ kW}$$

Heat capacity of flue gas, $C_{Hf} = 1.006 + 1.84 \times 0.046$

$$= 1.091 \text{ kJ/(kg dry gas} \cdot \text{K)}$$

Heat lost in flue gases $H_7 = 1.091 \times 100 \times 30.3 \,(423 - 298.15)$

$$= 413\,216 \text{ kJ (approximate)}$$

Alternate calculations:

Table 7.21 Mean Heat Capacity Data

Component	n_i kmol	C^0_{mpmi} between 298 K and 423 K, kJ/(kmol $\cdot$ K)	$n_i \cdot C^0_{mpmi}$ kJ/K
CO_2	12.8	40.23	514.944
O_2	6.5	29.71	193.115
H_2O	80.7	33.59	249.406
N_2	7.425	28.82	2325.774
Total	107.425	—	3283.239

For 100 kmol dry flue gas, heat

lost in the flue gases $H'_7 = 3283.239\,(423 - 298.15) = 410\,405 \text{ kJ}$

H_7 and H'_7 differ by only 0.68%.

Total heat loss in flue gases

for 3.9 t/h fuel firing rate, $\phi_7 = 410\,405 \times (3900/162.2) \times 0.7941$

$$= 7836\,129 \text{ kJ/h} \equiv 2176.70 \text{ kW}$$

Heat of fuel burning, $\phi_1 = 3.9 \times 1000 \times 26\,170$

$$= 102\,063\,000 \text{ kJ/h}$$

$$\equiv 28\,350.83 \text{ kW}$$

Neglect the heat input of air which is at 303 K (30°C).

Overall thermal efficiency of the boiler = 83.05% (Refer Table 7.22)　　　*Ans.*

Figure 7.5 gives the split-up of the heat losses.

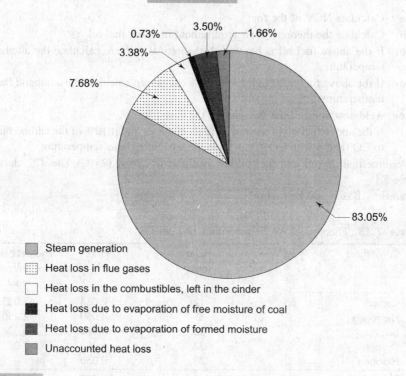

- Steam generation
- Heat loss in flue gases
- Heat loss in the combustibles, left in the cinder
- Heat loss due to evaporation of free moisture of coal
- Heat loss due to evaporation of formed moisture
- Unaccounted heat loss

Fig. 7.5   Heat Flow Diagram of a Water Tube Boiler

Table 7.22   Heat Balance of a Coal Fired Water-tube Boiler

	Heat flow, kW	%
Input:		
Fuel firing	28 350.83	100.00
Output:		
(a) Steam generation	23 546.07	83.05
(b) Heat loss in flue gases	2 176.70	7.68
(c) Heat loss in the combustibles, left in the cinder	959.18	3.38
(d) Heal loss due to evaporation:		
(i) Of free moisture of coal	206.38	0.73
(ii) Of moisture produced by burning of net H_2 of coal	992.09	3.50
(e) Unaccounted heat loss (by difference)	470.41	1.66
Total	28 350.83	100.00

Example 7.10   Fuel oil having the following ultimate analysis is desired to be fired in a boiler:

Carbon 85%, hydrogen 9%, sulphur 3%, oxygen 2% and nitrogen 1% (by mass). Assume negligible steam requirement for atomization of fuel oil. GCV of the fuel oil is measured to be 43 540 kJ/kg at 298.15 K(25°C).

(a) Calculate NCV of the fuel.

(b) Calculate the theoretical air requirement in kg/kg fuel oil.

(c) If the above fuel oil is burnt with theoretical oxygen, calculate the adiabatic temperature.

(d) If the above fuel oil is burnt with 30% excess air, calculate the adiabatic flame temperature.

(e) Acid dew point of the flue gas for the case (d).

(f) If the above fuel oil is burnt with inadequate air and if 10% of the carbon burns to CO (and rest to CO_2), calculate the adiabatic flame temperature.

Assume that dry air and fuel oil are available at 298 K (25°C). Use C°_{mp} data of Table 5.1.

Solution: Basis: 100 kg fuel oil

Table 7.23 Theoretical Air Requirement of Fuel Oil

Constituent	kg	Molar mass	kmol	Theoretical O_2 requirement, kmol
Carbon	85	12	7.083	7.083
Hydrogen	9	2	4.500	2.250
Sulphur	3	32	0.094	0.094
Oxygen	2	32	0.063	– 0.063
Nitrogen	1	28	0.036	—
Total	100		11.776	9.364

Theoretical O_2 requirement for complete combustion

$$= 9.364 \text{ kmol}$$

$$N_2 \text{ entering with } O_2 \text{ through air} = \left(\frac{79}{21}\right) \times 9.364 = 35.226 \text{ kmol}$$

$$\text{Total } N_2 \text{ in the flue gases} = 35.226 + 0.036 = 35.262 \text{ kmol}$$

$$\text{Total air} = 9.364 \times 32 + 35.226 \times 28 = 1286 \text{ kg}$$

$$\text{Dry air required (stoichiometric)/fuel oil ratio} = \frac{1286}{100} = 12.86 \text{ kg/kg } Ans.(b)$$

$$\text{Water vapour formed} = 4.5 \text{ kmol} = 81 \text{ kg}$$

Latent heat of water at 298.15 K (25°C) = 2442.8 kJ/kg

$$\text{Latent heat loss in water vapour} = 2442.8 \times 81 = 197\,867 \text{ kJ/100 kg fuel}$$

$$\text{NCV} = 43\,540 - 1978.67$$

$$= 41\,561.33 \text{ kJ/kg at 298.15 K}$$

Total heat liberated by complete combustion (assuming that formed moisture is in vapour form), $H_1 = 100 \times 41\,561.33 = 4156\,133$ kJ

Table 7.24 Composition of Flue Gases without Excess Air

Component	kmol	Mole % (wet basis)	Orsat analysis mole %
CO_2	7.083	15.09	16.91
H_2O	4.500	9.59	—
SO_2	0.094	0.20	—
N_2	35.262	75.12	83.09
Total	49.939	100.00	100.00

Note: It may be noted that maximum CO_2 content of dry flue gas can be maximum 17% (v/v) for fuel oil conforming to IS:1593. Also theoretical air requirement is approximately 13 kg/kg fuel oil.

Use C°_{mpi} data from Table 5.1.

$T_0 = 298.15$ K and T = adiabatic flame temperature (AFT)

Table 7.25 Heat Capacity Equation Constants for Flue Gas

Heat capacity equation constant	Component			
	CO_2	N_2	H_2O	Total
n_i, kmol	7.177	35.262	4.500	49.939
$(n_i \cdot a_i)_1$*	153.338	1043.779	152.609	1349.726
$(n_i \cdot a_i)_2$*	266.798	1097.29	113.213	1477.301
$(n_i \cdot b_i)_1 \times 10^3$	461.367	− 194.878	− 13.565	252.924
$(n_i \cdot b_i)_2 \times 10^3$	166.773	112.729	95.768	375.270
$(n_i \cdot c_i)_1 \times 10^6$	− 294.627	488.672	63.391	257.436
$(n_i \cdot c_i)_2 \times 10^6$	− 52.958	− 14.288	− 24.03	− 91.276
$(n_i \cdot d_i)_1 \times 10^9$	70.343	− 186.02	− 21.855	− 137.532
$(n_i \cdot d_i)_2 \times 10^9$	5.894	0.081	2.171	8.146

* 1 and 2 refer to heat capacity data for temperature ranges 298.15–1500 K and 1500–4000 K, respectively.

Enthalpy of flue gas up to 1500 K,

$$H_7' = 1349.726 \,(1500 - 298.15) + 252.924 \times 10^{-3} \frac{\left(1500^2 - 298.15^2\right)}{2}$$

$$+ \, 257.436 \times 10^{-6} \frac{\left(1500^3 - 298.15^3\right)}{3} - 137.532 \times 10^{-9} \frac{\left(1500^4 - 298.15^4\right)}{4}$$

$$= 1622\,371 + 273\,309 + 287\,341 - 174\,064 = 2008\,960 \text{ kJ}$$

Enthalpy of flue gas above 1500 K,

$$H_7'' = H_1 - H_7'$$

$$= 4156\,133 - 2008\,980 = 2147\,173 \text{ kJ}$$

$$= 1477.301 \,(T - 1500) + 375.270 \times 10^{-3} \frac{\left(T^2 - 1500^2\right)}{2}$$

$$- \, 91.276 \times 10^{-6} \frac{\left(T^3 - 1500^3\right)}{3} + 8.146 \times 10^{-9} \frac{\left(T^4 - 1500^4\right)}{4}$$

$$= 1477.301 \, T + 187.635 \times 10^{-3} \, T^2 - 30.425 \times 10^{-6} \, T^3$$

$$+ \, 2.037 \times 10^{-9} \, T^4 - 2340\,386$$

$2.037 \times 10^{-9} \, T^4 - 30.425 \times 10^{-6} \, T^3 + 187.635 \times 10^{-3} \, T^2 + 1477.301 \, T = 4487 \, 559$

Mathcad Solution:

$$T = 2509 \text{ K } (2236°C)$$

Note: Maximum flame temperature can thus be 2509 K (2236°C) for fuel oil, conforming to IS: 1593.

Combustion with 30% excess air:

$$\text{Actual } O_2 \text{ supply} = 9.364 \times 1.30 = 12.173 \text{ kmol}$$

$$\text{Excess } O_2 = 12.173 - 9.364 = 2.809 \text{ kmol}$$

$$N_2 \text{ entering with } O_2 \text{ through air} = \left(\frac{79}{21}\right) \times 12.173 = 45.794 \text{ kmol}$$

$$\text{Total } N_2 \text{ in the flue gases} = 45.794 + 0.036 = 45.83 \text{ kmol}$$

Table 7.26 Composition of Flue Gases with 30% Excess Air

Component	kmol	Mole % (wet basis)	Orsat analysis (mole %)
CO_2	7.083	11.74	12.86
H_2O	4.500	7.46	—
O_2	2.809	4.66	5.03
N_2	45.830	75.98	82.11
SO_2	0.094	0.16	—
Total	60.316	100.00	100.00

Table 7.27 Heat Capacity Constants for Flue Gases with 30% Excess Air

Heat capacity equation constant	Component				
	CO_2	O_2	N_2	H_2O	Total
n_i, kmol	7.177	2.809	45.830	4.500	60.316
$(n_i . a_i)_1$*	153.338	73.105	1356.599	152.609	1735.651
$(n_i . a_i)_2$*	266.798	51.779	1426.147	113.213	1857.937
$(ni . b_i)_1 \times 10^3$	461.367	33.024	− 253.283	− 13.565	227.543
$(ni . b_i)_2 \times 10^3$	166.773	61.004	146.514	95.768	470.059
$(ni . c_i)_1 \times 10^6$	− 294.627	− 6.586	635.126	68.391	402.304
$(ni . c_i)_2 \times 10^6$	− 52.958	− 23.328	− 18.570	− 24.03	− 118.886
$(ni . d_i)_1 \times 10^9$	70.343	− 1.576	− 241.77	− 21.855	− 194.858
$(n_i . d_i)_2 \times 10^9$	5.894	3.247	0.105	2.171	11.417

*1 and 2 refer to heat capacity data for temperature ranges 298.15–1500 K and 1500–4000 K respectively.

$$T_0 = 298.15 \text{ K and } T = \text{AFT}$$

Enthalpy of flue gas up to 1500 K,

$$H'_7 = 1735.651 \, (1500 - 298.15) + 227.543 \times 10^{-3} \frac{(1500^2 - 298.15^2)}{2}$$

$$+ 402.304 \times 10^{-6} \frac{\left(1500^3 - 298.15^3\right)}{3} - 194.858 \times 10^{-9} \frac{\left(1500^4 - 298.15^4\right)}{4}$$

$$= 2086\,253 + 245\,883 + 449\,043 - 246\,233 = 2534\,946 \text{ kJ}$$

Enthalpy of flue gas above 1500 K,

$$H_7'' = H_1 - H_7'$$

$$= 4156\,133 - 2534\,946 = 1621\,187 \text{ kJ}$$

$$= 1857.937\,(T - 1500) + 470.059 \times 10^{-3} \frac{\left(T^2 - 1500^2\right)}{2}$$

$$- 118.886 \times 10^{-6} \frac{\left(T^3 - 1500^3\right)}{3} + 11.417 \times 10^{-9} \frac{\left(T^4 - 1500^4\right)}{4}$$

$$= 1857.937\,T + 235.03 \times 10^{-3}\,T^2 - 39.629 \times 10^{-6}\,T^3$$

$$+ 2.854 \times 10^{-9}\,T^4 - 3196\,424$$

$$2.854 \times 10^{-9}\,T^4 - 39.629 \times 10^{-6}\,T^3 + 235.03 \times 10^{-3}\,T^2 + 1857.937\,T = 4817\,611$$

Mathcad solution:

$$T = 2179 \text{ K } (1906°C) \qquad\qquad\qquad Ans.\ (d)$$

For $\dfrac{C}{H} = 1.574$ (mole ratio) and excess air = 30%,

from Fig. 7.3, acid dew point = 429 K (156°C)   *Ans.* (e)

At times, carbon monoxide appears in the flue gas if inadequate air is supplied.

Total carbon burnt = 7.083 kmol

Carbon burnt to CO = 0.708 kmol

Carbon burnt to CO_2 = 6.375 kmol

$$O_2 \text{ for combustion of carbon} = 6.375 + \left(\frac{0.708}{2}\right) = 6.729 \text{ kmol}$$

$$O_2 \text{ supplied} = 6.729 + 2.250 + 0.094 - 0.063$$

$$= 9.01 \text{ kmol}$$

$$N_2 \text{ entering with } O_2 \text{ through air} = \left(\frac{79}{21}\right) \times 9.01 = 33.895 \text{ kmol}$$

Total N_2 in the flue gases = 33.895 + 0.036 = 33.931 kmol

Table 7.28 Composition of Flue Gases with Inadequate Air

Component	kmol	Mole % (wet basis)	Orsat analysis (mole %)
CO_2	6.375	13.98	15.74
CO	0.708	1.55	1.72
H_2O	4.500	9.87	—
N_2	33.931	74.40	82.54
SO_2	0.094	0.20	—
Total	45.608	100.00	100.00

Heat of combustion of CO to CO_2 = 282 980 kJ/kmol

Unavailable heat due to CO formation = 282 980 × 0.708

$$= 200\ 350\ \text{kJ}$$

Actual heat liberated (based on NCV), $H_1' = 4156\ 133 - 200\ 350$

$$= 3955\ 783\ \text{kJ}$$

Table 7.29   Heat Capacity Equation Constants for Flue Gas with Inadequate Air

Heat capacity equation constant	Component				
	CO_2	CO	N_2	H_2O	Total
n_i, kmol	6.469	0.708	33.931	4.500	45.608
$(n_i \cdot a_i)_1$*	138.212	20.551	1004.381	152.609	1315.753
$(n_i \cdot a_i)_2$*	270.479	19.411	1055.872	113.213	1458.975
$(n_i \cdot b_i)_1 \times 10^3$	415.854	− 1.995	− 187.522	− 13.565	212.772
$(n_i \cdot b_i)_2 \times 10^3$	150.321	6.102	108.474	95.768	360.665
$(n_i \cdot c_i)_1 \times 10^6$	− 265.563	8.258	470.226	68.391	281.312
$(n_i \cdot c_i)_2 \times 10^6$	− 47.733	− 1.915	− 13.749	− 24.03	− 87.427
$(n_i \cdot d_i)_1 \times 10^9$	63.405	− 3.335	− 178.999	− 21.855	− 140.784
$(n_i \cdot d_i)_2 \times 10^9$	5.313	0.215	0.078	2.171	7.777

*1 and 2 refer to heat capacity data for temperature ranges 298.15–1500 K and 1500–4000 K respectively.

$$T_0 = 298.15\ \text{K and } T = \text{AFT}$$

Enthalpy of flue gas up to 1500 K,

$$H'_7 = 1315.753\ (1500 - 298.15) + 212.772 \times 10^{-3}\ \frac{\left(1500^2 - 298.15^2\right)}{2}$$

$$+ 281.312 \times 10^{-6}\ \frac{\left(1500^3 - 298.15^3\right)}{3} - 140.784 \times 10^{-9}\ \frac{\left(1500^4 - 298.15^4\right)}{4}$$

$$= 1581\ 533 + 229\ 921 + 313\ 914 - 177\ 902 = 1947\ 548\ \text{kJ}$$

Enthalpy of flue gas above 1500 K,

$$H''_7 = H'_1 - H'_7$$

$$= 3955\ 783 - 1947\ 548 = 2008\ 235\ \text{kJ}$$

$$= 1458.975\ (T - 1500) + 360.665 \times 10^{-3}\ \frac{\left(T^2 - 1500^2\right)}{2}$$

$$- 87.427 \times 10^{-6}\ \frac{\left(T^3 - 1500^3\right)}{3} + 7.777 \times 10^{-9}\ \frac{\left(T^4 - 1500^4\right)}{4}$$

$$= 1458.975\ T + 180.333 \times 10^{-3}\ T^2 - 29.142 \times 10^{-6}\ T^3$$

$$+ 1.944 \times 10^{-9}\ T^4 - 1890\ 909$$

$$1.994 \times 10^{-9}\ T^4 - 29.142 \times 10^{-6}\ T^3 + 180.33 \times 10^{-3}\ T^2 + 1458.975\ T = 3899\ 144$$

Mathcad solution:

$$T = 2242\ \text{K } (1969°\text{C}) \qquad\qquad\qquad Ans.\ \text{(d)}$$

Note: This example is cited to illustrate the influence of excess/inadequate air on: (i) the theoretical flame temperature and (ii) the total moles of flue gases. The flame temperature has a strong effect on: (i) furnace design and (ii) furnace performance.

Example 7.11 A water-tube boiler is fired with heavy fuel oil having the ultimate analysis, C: 85.1%, H: 10.9%, S: 1.5%, O: 2.5% (by mass). The ash content and free moisture content of the fuel oil can be assumed to be negligible. Also assume negligible steam requirement for atomization. The test run data of the boiler are given below.

Steam generated at 16 bar a (saturated) = 4365 kg/h

Fuel oil-firing rate = 400 kg/h

GCV of the fuel = 42 260 kJ/kg at 298.15 K (25°C)

Orsat analysis of the dry flue gases, CO_2: 7.01%, O_2: 11.94% and N_2: 81.05% (volume basis)

Air supply: *DB* 308 K (35°C), *WB* 300.5 K (27.5°C), 100.7 kPa a (755 torr)

Average temperature of the flue gases = 563 K (290°C)

Pressure at the bottom of the stack = 99.3 kPa a (745 torr)

Temperature of the water fed to the boiler = 316 K (43°C)

Assume that fuel oil is fired at 353 K (80°C) and the heat capacity of the fuel oil is 1.758 kJ/(kg · K)

Evaluate the thermal performance of the boiler.

Solution: Basis: 100 kg fuel oil

Table 7.30 Oxygen Requirement of Fuel Oil

Constituent	mass, kg	kmol	Theoretical O_2 requirement, kmol
Carbon	85.1	7.092	7.092
Hydrogen	10.9	5.450	2.725
Sulphur	1.5	0.047	0.047
Oxygen	2.5	0.078	− 0.078
Total	100.0	12.667	9.786

Material balance of carbon:

Moles of CO_2 appearing in the flue

gases (including the moles of SO_2) = 7.092 + 0.047 = 7.139 kmol

Since the flue gases contain 7.01

mole % CO_2, N_2 in the flue gas = $\dfrac{(7.139 \times 81.05)}{7.01}$ = 82.541 kmol

O_2 in the flue gas = $\dfrac{(11.94 \times 7.139)}{7.01}$ = 12.16 kmol

Total dry flue gas = 101.84 kmol

Material balance of oxygen:

Moles of O_2 from air = $\left(\dfrac{21}{79}\right) \times 82.541 = 21.941$ kmol

Moles of dry air entering the boiler = 82.541 + 21.941 = 104.482 kmol

Total O_2 entering the burner = 21.941 + 0.078 = 22.019 kmol

Excess O_2 = 22.019 − 9.864 = 12.155 kmol

This excess O_2 tallies with O_2 present in the flue gas.

$$\% \text{ Excess air} = \left(\frac{12.155}{9.786}\right) \times 100 = 124.21$$

Material balance of water vapour:

Moisture formed due to combustion of (net) hydrogen of the fuel

= 5.45 kmol

Absolute humidity of at 101.3 kPa a = 0.0204 kg/kg dry air (Fig. 6.11)

= 0.0329 kmol/kmol dry air

Corrected humidity at 100.7 kPa a = 0.0205 kg/kg dry air (Ref. Table 6.9)

= 0.0331 kmol/kmol dry air

Moisture from air = 0.0331 × 104.482 = 3.458 kmol

Total moisture is the flue gases = 5.45 + 3.458 = 8.908 kmol

Table 7.31 Composition of Flue Gases

Component	kmol	kg (dry gas)	Mole % (wet basis)	Orsat analysis, %
CO_2	7.092	312.0	6.40	7.01
SO_2	0.047	3.0	0.04	—
O_2	12.155	389.0	10.98	11.94
N_2	82.541	2311.1	74.53	81.05
H_2O	8.908	–	8.04	—
Total	110.743	3015.1	100.00	100.00

$$\text{Average molar mass of dry flue gas} = \frac{3015.1}{101.835} = 29.61$$

Partial pressure at water vapour

in the flue gases, p_w = 99.3 × 0.0804 = 7.984 kPa

Dew point = 314.4 K (41.4°C) (Ref. Table 6.8)

Heat loss in flue gases:

$$\text{Humid heat of flue gas, } C_{\text{Hf}} = 1.006 + 1.84 \times \left[\frac{8.908 \times 18.015}{(101.835 \times 29.61)}\right]$$

= 1.1039 kJ/(kg dry gas · K)

Total heat lost in flue gas H_7 = (110.743 − 8.908) × 29.61 × 1.1039

(563 − 298.15)

= 882 086 kJ

Alternate calculations:

Table 7.32 Sensible Heat Calculations of Flue Gases

Component	n_i, kmol	$C^°_{mpmi}$, kJ/(kmol · K) 298.15 – 563 K	$n_i · C^°_{mpmi}$, kJ/K
CO_2	7.092	42.134	298.814
SO_2	0.047	42.628	2.004
O_2	12.155	30.393	369.427
N_2	82.541	29.251	2414.407
H_2O	8.908	34.413	306.551
Total	110.743		3391.203

Total heat lost in flue gases, H'_7, = 3391.203 (563 – 298.15) = 898 669 kJ

H_7 and H'_7 differ by 1.85%.

However, the fuel firing rate is 400 kg/h.

$$\text{Total heat lost in the flue gases } \phi_7 = 898\,669 \times \left(\frac{400}{100}\right)$$

$$= 3594\,676 \text{ kJ/h} \equiv 998.52 \text{ kW}$$

Heat gain in boiler:

Inlet temperature of water = 316 K

Enthalpy of water = 179.99 kJ/kg

Steam pressure = 16 bar a

From seam tables (Appendix AIII.2),

$$T_s = 474.52 \text{ K } (201.37°C)$$

$h = 858.56$ kJ/kg $\lambda_v = 1933.2$ kJ/kg $H = 2791.7$ kJ/kg

Total heat supplied in the boiler = 2791.7 – 179.99 = 2611.71 kJ/kg

Total heat utilized for steam generation, ϕ_5= 2611.71 × 4365

$$= 11400\,114 \text{ kJ/h} \cong 3166.70 \text{ kW}$$

Heat loss due to evaporation of moisture:

Latent heat of vaporization of water at 314.4 K = 2402.8 kJ/kg

$$\text{Heat loss due to evaporation of moisture, } \phi_8 = 5.45 \times 18 \times \left(\frac{400}{100}\right) \times 2402.8$$

$$= 948\,051 \text{ kJ/h} \cong 263.35 \text{ kW}$$

Heat input by fuel combustion:

GCV of the fuel oil = 42260 kJ/kg

Heat input, ϕ_1 = 400 × 42260

$$= 16\,904\,000 \text{ kJ/h} \cong 4695.56 \text{ kW}$$

Heat input by air:

Average humid heat of air, C_H = 1.006 + 1.84 × 0.0205

$$= 1.0437 \text{ kJ/(kg dry air · K)}$$

$$\text{Total dry air rate} = \frac{(104.48 \times 29)\,400}{100} = 11\,120 \text{ kg/h}$$

Sensible heat of incoming air, $\phi_3 = 12\,120 \times 1.0437\,(308 - 298.15)$

$$= 126\,499 \text{ kJ/h} \cong 35.14 \text{ kW}$$

Sensible heat of fuel oil:

Sensible heat input of fuel oil, $\phi_2 = 400 \times 1.758\,(353 - 298.15)$

$$= 38\,676 \text{ kJ/h} \cong 10.74 \text{ kW}$$

Table 7.33 Heat Balance of Boiler

	Heat flow, kW	%
Input:		
Heat of combustion	4695.56	99.03
Heat of moist air	35.14	0.74
Heat of fuel oil	10.74	0.23
Total	4741.44	100.00
Output:		
Heat utilised for steam generation	3166.70	66.77
Heat lost in flue gases	998.52	21.05
Heat lost due to evaporation of formed moisture	263.35	5.56
Unaccounted heat loss (by difference)	312.87	6.62
Total	4741.44	100.00

Figure 7.6 is the heat flow diagram of the boiler fired with heavy fuel oil. Overall thermal efficiency of the

$$\text{boiler based on GCV of the fuel} = \frac{(3166.70 \times 100)}{4695.56} = 67.43\%$$

$$\text{NCV of the fuel} = 42\,260 - \left(\frac{18.015}{2.016}\right) \times 0.109 \times 2442.8$$

$$= 39\,880 \text{ kJ/kg}$$

Overall thermal efficiency of the

$$\text{boiler, based on NCV of the fuel} = \frac{(11\,400\,114 \times 100)}{(400 \times 39\,880)} = 71.61\%$$

Both thermal efficiencies indicate poor performance of the boiler on account of very high excess air and relatively high flue gas temperature.

$$\text{Steam to fuel ratio} = \frac{4365}{400} = 10.91$$

$$\text{Boiler capacity from and at 373.15 K} = \frac{11\,400\,114}{2256.9} = 5051.2 \text{ kg/h}$$

$$\text{Air flow rate at 100.7 kPa a and at 308 K} = (104.48 + 3.34) + \left(\frac{400}{100}\right) \times 25.453$$

$$= 10\,977.4 \text{ m}^3/\text{h}$$

Volumetric flow rate of flue gases, $q_v = \dfrac{nRT}{p}$

$$= 110.628 \times \left(\frac{4000}{100}\right) \times 8.3145$$

$$\times \left(\frac{563}{99.3}\right) \times 101.325$$

$$= 21\ 137\ \text{m}^3/\text{h} \qquad\qquad Ans.$$

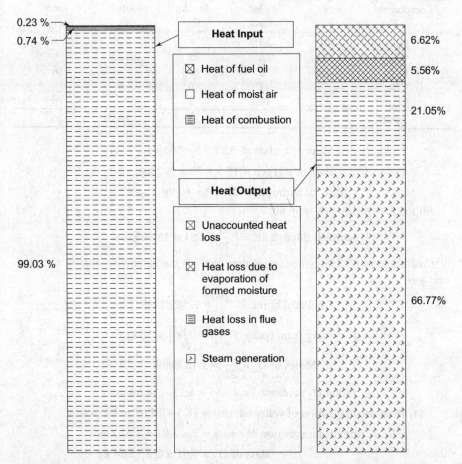

Fig. 7.6 Stacked Bar Diagram for a Boiler Fired with Heavy Fuel Oil

---

Example 7.12 A coal having the ultimate analysis, C: 67.2%, H: 5.5%, S: 0.4%, O: 6.1% and ash 20.8% (by mass) is used for gassifying. Free moisture in the coal is found to be 2.6% (by mass). The producer gas obtained from the coal has the molar composition N_2: 51.0%, CO: 25% H_2: 16%, CO_2: 6% and CH_4: 2% (on dry basis; SO_2 neglected). The dew point of the producer gas is measured to be 295 K (22°C) at 100.7 kPa a (755 torr).

Compute (a) Nm^3 of the producer gas obtained per kg coal used, (b) Nm^3 of air supplied per kg coal gassified and (c) quantity of steam supplied per kg coal used.

Solution: Producer gas is made for use in industrial furnaces by passing air plus a small quantity of steam through a thick fuel bed in which the fuel is burnt partially.

Basis: 100 kmol dry producer gas

Table 7.34 Material Balance of Producer Gas Generator

Component	kmol	Molar mass	kmol C	kmol O_2	kmol H_2
N_2	51	28	–	–	–
CO	25	28	25	12.5	–
H_2	16	2	–	–	16
CO_2	6	44	6	6	–
CH_4	2	16	2	–	4
Total	100		33	18.5	20

$$\text{Mass of carbon} = 33 \times 12 = 396 \text{ kg}$$

$$\text{Mass of oxygen} = 18.5 \times 32 = 592 \text{ kg}$$

$$\text{Mass of hydrogen} = 20 \times 2 = 40 \text{ kg}$$

All the nitrogen comes from air.

$$O_2 \text{ supplied through air} = \left(\frac{21}{79}\right) \times 51 = 13.56 \text{ kmol}$$

Coal contains 67.2% carbon. Assuming that all the carbon appears in the producer gas,

$$\text{Total coal burnt} = \frac{396}{0.672} = 589.3 \text{ kg}$$

$$O_2 \text{ coming from coal} = 589.3 \times 0.061 = 36 \text{ kg}$$

$$\text{Moles of } O_2 = \frac{36}{32} = 1.13 \text{ kmol}$$

$$\text{Total } O_2 \text{ accounted} = 13.56 + 1.13 = 14.69 \text{ kmol}$$

$$O_2 \text{ from decomposition of water (steam)} = 18.5 - 14.69 = 3.81 \text{ kmol}$$

$$H_2 \text{ from decomposition of steam} = 2 \times 3.81 = 7.62 \text{ kmol}$$

$$\text{Mass of } H_2 = 7.62 \times 2 = 15.24 \text{ kg}$$

$$\text{Moles of steam decomposed} = 7.62 \text{ kmol}$$

$$H_2 \text{ from fuel} = 20.0 - 7.62 = 12.38 \text{ kmol}$$

$$\frac{\text{Dry producer gas}}{\text{coal}} \text{ ratio} = \frac{100}{589.3} = 0.1697 \text{ kmol/kg coal}$$

$$\equiv 3.803 \text{ Nm}^3/\text{kg coal} \qquad \textit{Ans.} \text{ (a-i)}$$

The vapour pressure of water at 295 K, $p_w = 2.642$ kPa   (Refer Table 6.8)

$$\text{Absolute humidity} = \frac{2.642}{(100.7 - 2.642)}$$

$$= 0.027 \text{ kmol/kmol dry gas}$$

$$\text{Water vapour in the producer gas} = 0.027 \times 100 = 2.7 \text{ kmol}$$

$$\frac{\text{Moist producer gas}}{\text{coal ratio}} = \frac{102.7}{589.3} = 0.1743 \text{ kmol/kg coal}$$

$$\equiv 3.906 \text{ Nm}^3/\text{kg coal} \qquad Ans. \text{ (a–ii)}$$

$$\text{Dry air supplied} = 51 + 13.56 = 64.56 \text{ kmol}$$

$$\text{Mass of dry air} = 51.0 \times 28 + 13.56 \times 32 = 1862 \text{ kg}$$

$$\frac{\text{Dry air}}{\text{coal ratio}} = \frac{1862}{589.3} = 3.16 \text{ kg/kg coal}$$

$$\frac{\text{Volume of dry air}}{\text{coal ratio}} = \left(\frac{3.16}{29}\right) \times 22.414 = 2.442 \text{ Nm}^3/\text{kg coal}$$

$$Ans. \text{ (b)}$$

$$\text{Total steam supplied} = 7.62 + 2.7 - \left(\frac{589.3 \times 0.026}{18}\right)$$

$$= 9.47 \text{ kmol}$$

$$\frac{\text{steam}}{\text{coal ratio}} = \frac{(9.47 \times 18)}{589.3} = 0.29 \text{ kg/kg coal} \qquad Ans. \text{ (c)}$$

Example 7.13 A gas producer generates the gas having the following molar composition on dry basis:

$$\text{CO: } 25\%, \text{ H}_2\text{: } 8\%, \text{ CO}_2\text{: } 5\% \text{ and N}_2\text{: } 62.0\%$$

Based on the dew point measurements, the gas is found to contain 0.056 kg water vapour per kg dry producer gas. It is available at 1073 K (800°C).

The above gas is used as a fuel in an open hearth steel furnace at the rate of 27 650 kg/h (on dry basis) with air at 308 K (35°C) *DB* and 295 K (22°C) *WB*. The furnace is capable of taking a 75 t charge. On an average the total heat gained by the charge is calculated to be 9400 kW. The flue gases leave the furnace at 833 K (560°C) and enter the waste heat boiler. The temperature of the outgoing flue gases from the boiler plant is 478 K (205°C). In the waste heat boiler, the steam is generated at 12.5 bar a and 573 K (300°C) at the rate of 7.1 t/h. The Orsat analysis of the flue gases indicate 16.9% CO_2, 2.8% O_2 and 80.3% N_2 (by volume). The inlet and oulet temperatures of water to and from the economizer are 338 K (65°C) and 433 K (160°C) respectively. Flue gases leave the chimney at 100.0 kPa a (750 torr).

Evaluate the thermal performance of the furnace and the waste heat boiler.

Solution: The flow diagram of the above operations is given in Fig. 7.7.

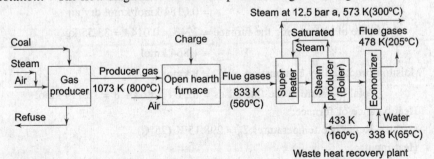

Fig. 7.7 Producer Gas Utilization and Waste Heat Recovery

Basis: 100 kmol dry producer gas

Water vapour in the producer gas = 2672 × 0.056 = 149.63 kg

$$\equiv 8.31 \text{ kmol}$$

Table 7.35 Oxygen Requirement of Producer Gas

Constituent	kmol	Molar mass	kg	Theoretical O_2 requirement for complete combustion, kmol
CO	25	28	700	12.5
H_2	8	2	16	4.0
CO_2	5	44	220	–
N_2	62	28	1736	–
Total	100	100	2672	16.5

Total wet producer gas = 108.31 kmol

Total CO_2 produced after combustion = 25 + 5 = 30 kmol

The flue gas contain 16.9% CO_2 by volume.

$$\text{Moles of flue gases} = \frac{30}{0.169} = 177.51 \text{ kmol}$$

$$\text{Excess } O_2 \text{ in the flue gases} = 177.51 \times 0.028 = 4.97 \text{ kmol}$$

$$N_2 \text{ in the flue gases} = 177.51 \times 0.803 = 142.54 \text{ kmol}$$

$$N_2 \text{ entering with air} = 142.54 - 62 = 80.54 \text{ kmol}$$

$$O_2 \text{ supplied through air} = \frac{(21 \times 80.54)}{79} = 21.41 \text{ kmol}$$

$$\text{Excess } O_2 = 21.41 - 16.5 = 4.91 \text{ kmol}$$

$$\text{Excess air} = \left(\frac{4.91}{16.5}\right) \times 100 = 29.76\%$$

Total dry air entering = 21.41 × 32 + 80.64 × 28 = 2943 kg

Absolute humidity of air at

308 K *DB* and 295 K *WB* = 11.4 g/kg dry air

$$= 0.0184 \text{ kmol/kmol dry air}$$

Moisture of air entering the furnace = 2943 × 0.0144 = 33.55 kg

$$\equiv 1.864 \text{ kmol}$$

Moisture produced by combustion of H_2 = 8 kmol

Total moisture in the flue gases = 8.31 + 1.864 + 8 = 18.174 kmol

Heat balance of furnace:

Reference temperature: $T_0 = 298.15$ K (25°C)

Heat input:

$$T_1 = 1073 \text{ K } (800°C)$$

Table 7.36 Composition of Flue Gases

Constituent	kmol	Mole % (wet basis)	Orsat analysis, %
CO_2	30.00	15.34	16.91
O_2	4.91	2.51	2.77
N_2	142.54	72.86	80.33
H_2O	18.174	9.29	–
Total	195.624	100.00	100.00

Table 7.37 Heat Capacity Equation Constants for Producer Gas

Component	n_i, kmol	Heat capacity equation constants			
		$n_i \cdot a_i$	$n_i \cdot b_i \times 10^3$	$n_i \cdot c_i \times 10^6$	$n_i \cdot d_i \times 10^9$
CO	25	725.6925	– 70.4125	291.0925	– 117.6575
H_2	8	228.884	8.1552	– 1.1808	6.152
CO_2	5	106.8275	312.4205	– 205.253	48.9995
N_2	62	1834.6358	– 318.742	817.3398	– 308.016
H_2O	8.31	270.0094	0.6615	109.7809	– 37.7889
Total	108.31	3166.0492	– 58.9173	1011.7794	– 408.3109

$$H_2' = \int_{T_0}^{T_1} (\Sigma n_i \cdot C^\circ_{mpi}) \, dT$$

$$= 3166.0492 \, (T_1 - T_0) - (58.9173 \times 10^{-3}) \frac{(T_1^2 - T_0^2)}{2}$$

$$+ (1011.7794 \times 10^{-6}) \frac{(T_1^3 - T_0^2)}{3} - (408.3109 \times 10^{-9}) \frac{(T_1^2 - T_0^2)}{2}$$

$$= 2453\,688 - 31300 + 407\,717.6 - 134\,505$$

$$= 2695\,600 \text{ kJ}$$

For the dry producer gas @ 2672 kg, H_2' equals 2695 600 kJ.
Actual rate of dry producer gas is 27 650 kg/h.

$$\phi_2 = \left(\frac{27\,650}{2672}\right) \times 2695\,600$$

$$= 27\,894\,215 \text{ kJ/h} \equiv 7748.39 \text{ kW}$$

Sensible heat of air:

Humid heat $C_H = 1.006 + 1.84 \times 0.0114$

$$= 1.027 \text{ kJ/(kg dry air} \cdot \text{K)}$$

$$H_3 = 1.027 \times 2943 \times (308 - 298.15) = 30\,225 \text{ kJ}$$

$$\phi_3 = \left(\frac{27650}{2672}\right) \times 30225$$

$$= 312\,766 \text{ kJ/h} \equiv 86.88 \text{ kW}$$

Heat of combustion:

$$GCV \text{ of } H_2 = 285\,830 \text{ kJ/kmol}$$

$$CV \text{ of } CO = 282\,980 \text{ kJ/kmol}$$

Total heat liberated by the combustion of H_2 and CO

$$H'_1 = 25 \times 282\,980 + 8 \times 285\,830 = 9366\,140 \text{ kJ}$$

$$\phi_1 = \left(\frac{27650}{2672}\right) \times 9366\,140$$

$$= 96\,921\,321 \text{ kJ/h} = 26\,922.59 \text{ kW}$$

Heat output:
Useful heat gain by the charge

in the furnace, $\phi_4 = 9400$ kW

Partial pressure of water

vapour in the flue gases, $p_w = 0.0929 \times 100 = 9.29$ kPa

DP of the flue gas mixture = 317.6 K (44.6°C)

Latent heat of water at DP = 2396.3 kJ/kg

Heat loss due to evaporation of moisture, produced by burning

the hydrogen of the fuel, $\phi_8 = 8 \times 18 \times 2396.3 \times \left(\frac{27650}{2672}\right)$

$$= 3570\,774 \text{ kJ/h} \cong 991.88 \text{ kW}$$

Heat loss in the outgoing flue gases:

Moisture in the flue gas $= \dfrac{18.174 \times 18}{\left[(195.624 - 18.174)\,29\right]}$

$$= 0.0636 \text{ kg/kg dry gas}$$

Humid heat of flue gas = $1.006 + 1.84 \times 0.0636$

$$= 1.123 \text{ kJ/(kg dry gas} \cdot \text{K)}$$

Heat loss, $\phi'_7 = (195.624 - 18.174) \times 1.123$

$$\times 29\,(833 - 298.15) \times \left(\frac{27650}{2672}\right)$$

$$= 31\,993\,829 \text{ kJ/h} \equiv 8887.17 \text{ kW (approximate)}$$

Alternate calculations:

Table 7.38 Mean Heat Capacity of Flue Gas

Component	n_i, kmol	C°_{mpm1} 298.15-833 K	$n_i \cdot C^\circ_{mpm1}$ kJ/K	C°_{mpm2} 298.15-478 K	$n_i \cdot C^\circ_{mpm2}$ kJ/K
CO_2	30.00	45.81	1374.30	40.94	1228.20
O_2	4.91	31.72	155.75	29.97	147.15
N_2	142.54	30.07	4286.18	29.00	4133.66
H_2O	18.174	35.85	651.54	33.92	616.46
Total	195.624		6467.77		6125.47

$$\text{Heat loss in flue gas, } \phi_7 = 6467.77 \, (833 - 298.15) \times \left(\frac{27\,650}{2672}\right)$$

$$= 36\,806\,925 \text{ kJ/h} \equiv 9946.37 \text{ kW}$$

Note: Approximate heat loss (ϕ_7) differs significantly (by 10.65%) as compared to ϕ_7' as the flue gas temperature (833 K) is quite high and high CO_2 content.

Table 7.39 Heat Balance of Open Hearth Furnace

	kW	%
Heat input:		
Heat of combustion	26 922.59	77.46
Sensible heat of fuel	7 748.39	22.29
Sensible heat of air	86.88	0.25
Total	34 757.86	100.00
Heat output:		
Useful heat gain in furnace	9 400.00	27.04
Heat loss due to evaporation of moisture formed by the combustion of H_2	991.88	2.85
Sensible heat loss in flue gases	9 946.37	28.61
Unaccounted heat loss	14 419.61	41.50
Total	34 757.86	100.00

Heat balance of boiler:

Total heat entering the waste heat boiler, $\phi_7 = 9946.37$ kW

Heat output: Basis: 1 kg steam

Refer Appendix III.2 and III.3.

Economizer: Heat load, $H_4 = 675.47 - 272.03 = 403.44$ kJ/kg

Boiler: At 12.5 bar a

$T_s = 463$ K (181.8°C) $h = 806.69$ kJ/kg

$\lambda_v = 1977.4$ kJ/kg $H_{ss} = 2784.1$ kJ/kg

Heat load, $H_5 = 2784.1 - 675.47 = 2108.83$ kJ/kg

At 12.5 bar a and 573 K,

total heat of superheated steam = 3045.6 kJ/kg

Heat load of the superheater, $H_6 = 3045.6 - 2784.1 = 261.5$ kJ/kg

Total heat load of economizer,

$$\phi_4' = 403.44 \times 7100$$

$$= 2864\,424 \text{ kJ/h} \equiv 795.67 \text{ kW}$$

Total heat load of boiler, $\phi_5' = (2784.1 - 675.47)\,7100$

$$= 14\,971\,273 \text{ kJ/h} \equiv 4158.69 \text{ kW}$$

Total heat load of superheater,

$$\phi_6' = 261.5 \times 7100$$

$$= 1856\,650 \text{ kJ/h} \equiv 515.74 \text{ kW}$$

Total useful heat recovery, $\phi_4' + \phi_5' + \phi_6' = 5470.1$ kW

Boiler capacity from and at 373.15 K = $\dfrac{5470.1 \times 3600}{2256.9}$ = 8725.4 kg/h

Heat loss in flue gase; ϕ'_8 = 177.45 × 29 × 1.123

$$(478 - 298.15)\,(27\,650 - 2672)$$

$$= 10\,764\,279 \text{ kJ/h} = 2900.08 \text{ kW}$$

(approximate)

Alternate calculations: (Refer Table 7.38)

Heat loss in flue gases, ϕ'_8 = 6125.47 (478 − 298.15) (27 650/2672)

$$= 11\,409\,605 \text{ kJ/h}$$

$$\equiv 3169.33 \text{ kW}$$

Table 7.40 Heat Balance of Waste Heat Boiler

	kW	%
Heat output:		
Steam raising:		
Economizer	795.67	8.00
Steam generator	4158.69	41.81
Superheater	515.74	5.19
Heat lost in flue gases	3169.33	31.86
Unaccounted heat loss	1306.94	13.14
Total	9946.37	100.00

The heat flow diagrams for the furnace as well as the waste heat boiler are combined in Fig. 7.8.

EXERCISES

7.1 The proximate analysis of a Chirimiri coal sample shows moisture 5.3%, VM 24.6%, FC 49.8% and ash 20.3%. The sulphur content of the coal is found to be 0.7%. Calorimetric tests give the gross-calorific value of the coal on dry ash-free basis as 24 070 kJ/kg. Using the Calderwood equation, find the carbon per cent of the coal.

[*Ans.* 46.21% carbon]

7.2 A coal sample from Chirmiri colliery has following proximate and ultimate analyses.

Gross calorific value = 27 235 kJ/kg on dry ash-free basis

Calculate (a) the net hydrogen available for combustion, (b) the combined water, (c) the gross calorific value, using the Dulong's formula, (d) the carbon content, using the Calderwood equation, (e) the analysis of coal on ash-free and moisture-free basis, (f) theoretical air requirement in kmol per kg coal and (g) the analysis of flue gases, if the coal is burnt with 60% excess air.

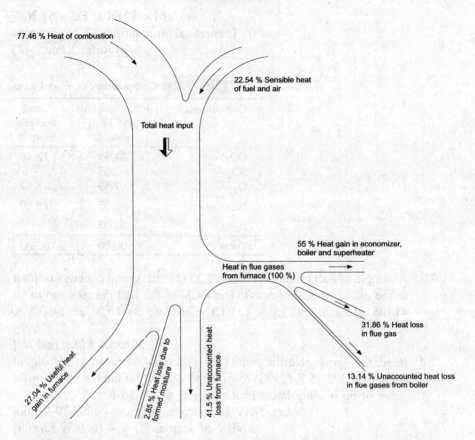

Fig. 7.8 Heat Flow Diagram of a Furnace Accompanied by a Steam Generator

Table 7.41 Analysis of Coal

Proximate analysis		Ultimate analysis	
	mass %		mass %
Moisture	4.0	Carbon	61.5
VM	26.7	Hydrogen	3.5
FC	55.1	Sulphur	0.4
Ash	14.2	Ash	14.2
		Nitrogen	1.8
Oxygen (by diff.)	18.6		
Total	100.0	Total	100.0

[*Ans.* (a) Net H_2 = 1.18%
(b) Combined water = 16.92%
(c) GCV from Dulong's formula = 21 778 kJ/kg
(d) Calderwood equation, carbon = 55.96%

(e) VM = 32.64%, FC = 67.36%
(f) Theoretical air required = 7.2 kg/kg coal
(g) Refer Table 7.42]

Table 7.42	Composition of Flue Gases	
Component	Actual analysis (wet basis) mole %	Orsat analysis mole %
CO_2	11.95	12.48
SO_2	0.03	–
O_2	7.59	7.92
N2	76.35	79.60
H_2	4.03	–
Total	100.00	100.00

7.3 A sample of fuel oil has C/H ratio 9.33 (by mass) and contains sulphur to the extent of 1.3% (mass). The GCV of the fuel is measured to be 41785 kJ/kg at 298.15 K (25°C). Calculate its NCV at 298.15 K (25°C).

[*Ans*. 39685.4 kJ/kg fuel oil]

7.4 Read the gross calorific values of gaseous *n*-propanol and liquid acetone at 298.15 K (25°C) from Appendix IV.2. Find the net calorific value of each using latent heat of water at 298.15 K (25°C).

[*Ans*. NHV of *n*-propanol (g) = – 1892.79 kJ/mol
NHV of acetone (l) = – 1660.39 kJ/mol]

7.5 Refer Example 5.26. It is decided to mix 10% ethanol (by mass) in the motor spirit for improving its octane number. Calculate average NCV of the blend and prove that it will emit nearly same greenhouse gas (i.e. CO_2) into the atmosphere as that with motor spirit when compared on heat values.

[*Ans*. NCV of blend = 42 326.8 kJ/kg]

7.6 Calculate the GHV and NHV at 298.15 K (25°C) of the associated gas having the composition, CH_4: 74.4%, C_2H_6: 8.4%, C_3H_8: 7.4%, *i*-C_4H_{10}: 1.7%, *n*-C_4H_{10}: 2.0%, *i*-C_5H_{12}: 0.5%, *n*-C_5H_{12}: 0.4%, N_2: 4.3% and CO_2: 0.9% (on volume basis).

[*Ans*. GHV: 49 537 kJ/kg or 44 801 kJ/m^3
NHV: 44 801 kJ/kg or 40 708 kJ/m^3
(at 298.15 K and 101.3 kPa)]

7.7 A sample of refinery gas is found to contain, H_2: 74.0%, CH_4: 13.5%, C_2H_6: 7.4%, C_3H_8: 3.6%, *n*-C_4H_{10}: 1.2% and *n*-C_5H_{12}: 0.3% (mole basis). Calculate the GCV and NCV at 298.15 K (25°C) of refinery gas.

Ans. **Table 7.43** GCV and NCV of Refinery Gas

GCV	NCV
572.288 kJ/mol	508.275 kJ/mol
23 392 kJ/m^3	20 776 kJ/m^3
68 488 kJ/kg	60 828 kJ/kg

7.8 The purge gas obtained from ammonia synthesis loop has the composition[11], H_2: 69.0%, N_2: 23.0%, Ar: 2.7% and CH_4: 5.3% (mole basis). It is burnt with 20% excess air. Calculate (a) the GCV and NCV at 298.15 K (25°C) of the purge gas, (b) theoretical air required, and (c) the molar composition of the dry flue gases.

[*Ans.* (a) GCV = 25 075 kJ/kg, NCV = 21 493 kJ/kg
(b) Theoretical air required = 6.39 kg/kg purge gas
(c) Flue gas composition: CO_2: 2.18%,
Ar: 1.11%, N_2: 93.01%, O_2: 3.7% (on dry volume basis)]

7.9 Synthetic natural gas (SNG from a US-based plant) has the molar composition, CH_4: 96.59%, H_2: 1.29%, CO: 0.22% and CO_2: 1.90%. Calculate the GCV and NCV at NTP.

Ans. **Table 7.44** Heating Values of SNG

GCV	NCV
864 589 kJ/kmol	778 993 kJ/kmol
52 649 kJ/kg	47 437 kJ/kg
38 574 kJ/Nm^3	34 755 kJ/Nm^3

7.10 Refer Example 4.18. Calculate GCV and NCV at 298.15 K (25°C) of wet tail gas, leaving absorber of the formaldehyde plant in kJ/Nm^3.

[*Ans.* GCV = 19 358 kJ/Nm^3
NCV = 17 513 kJ/Nm^3]

7.11 A sample of coal is found to contain 65% carbon and 12.7% ash (by mass). The refuse obtained after burning the fuel is found to have 8.6% carbon. Assume that negligible oxygen is present in the coal. Flue gas analysis showed CO_2: 10.6%, O_2: 8.7% and N_2: 80.7% (by volume). Calculate (a) the actual mass of (dry) air used to burn the coal, (b) the actual mass of flue gases produced by burning the coal and (c) the amount of combustible hydrogen present in the fuel.

[*Ans.* (a) 14.86 kg/kg fuel (b) 15.46 kg (wet)/kg fuel
(c) 4.32% (by mass)]

7.12 A furnace is fired with fuel oil. The Orsat analysis of the flue gases indicates 10.6% CO_2, 6.0% O_2 and rest N_2 (by volume). Find (a) the percentage excess air and (b) the C : H ratio in the fuel oil, assuming that fuel oil does not contain nitrogen.

[*Ans.* (a) 37.10% (b) C : H ratio = 5.71 : 1 (mass)]

7.13 A fuel gas constitutes of CO_2: 3.4%, C_2H_4: 3.7%, C_6H_6: 1.5%, O_2: 0.3%, CO: 17.4%, H_2: 36.8%, CH_4: 24.9% and N_2: 12.0% (on mole basis). It is burnt with air in a furnace. The Fyrite analyzer indicated 10.0 mole % CO_2 (on dry basis) in the flue gases. Find (a) the percent excess air used and (b) the complete Orsat analysis.

[*Ans.* (a) 37.07%
(b) CO_2: 10.0%, O_2: 5.9%, N_2: 84.1%]

7.14 The Orsat analysis of the flue gases shows CO_2: 12.4%, CO_2: 3.1%, O_2: 5.4% and N_2: 79.1% (by volume). All the hydrogen but only 85% of the carbon in the fuel appears in the flue gases. Calculate the per cent excess air used. Assume that negligible oxygen and nitrogen are present in the fuel.

[*Ans.* 5.6%]

7.15 Bottled gas [Liquefied Petroleum Gas (LPG)], conforming to IS: 4576, is found to contain 1.2% ethane, 25.2% propane, 23.9% *i*-butane and 49.7% *n*-butane (on mole basis). It is available at Rs. 20 per kg. Associated gas, having the molar composition CH_4: 86.6%, C_2H_6: 8.6%, C_3H_8: 3.9%, n-C_4H_{10}: 0.7%, i-C_4H_{10}: 0.2%, is available at Rs. 9/Nm^3.

A fuel is to be selected from the above two for curing a refractory lined furnace. Which is cheaper?

[*Ans.* Cost of energy:
Bottled gas: Rs 435.6 per GJ (LCV basis)
Associated gas: Rs 218.9 per GJ (LCV basis)]

7.16 Blast furnace gas is used as a fuel for steel manufacture. A sample of blast furnace gas is found to contain H_2: 3.2%, CO: 26.2%, CO_2: 13.0%, N_2: 57.6% (mole %). The gas is made available at 333 K (60°C). The air for combustion is available at 298.15 K (25°C) *DB*, 291 K (18°C) *WB* and 100.0 kPa (750 torr). The gas is desired to be burnt with 20% excess air. Compute (a) the theoretical requirement of air per kg fuel, (b) the molar composition of flue gases (wet basis) and (c) the adiabatic flame temperature.

[*Ans.* (a) 0.7 kg/kg fuel
(b) CO_2: 22.96%, O_2 1.73%
H_2O: 2.68%, rest N_2 (by volume)
(c) 3052.7 K (2779.7°C)]

7.17 The coal mentioned in Exercise 7.1 is fired in a battery of three water tube Babcock and Wilcox boilers. The operating data on a particular date are given below.

Fuel firing rate = 2500 kg/h
Excess moisture sprinkled on coal over the moisture in the coal as fired = 5%
Air is supplied at 307 K (34°C) *DB*, 297 K (24°C) *WB* and 100.0 kPa (750 torr). Orsat analysis of flue gases indicates CO_2: 8.8%, O_2: 9.2% and rest N_2 (volume basis).

Flue gas temperature entering the economizer = 543 K (270°C)

Flue gas temperature leaving the economizer = 463 K (190°C)

Draft at the base of chimney = 0.2 kPa g

Temperature of water entering the economizer = 311 K (38°C)

Temperature of water leaving the economizer = 368 K (95°C)

Steam:
Pressure: 9 bar g
Temperature: 473 K (200°C)
Steam generation = 12 150 kg/h under pressure
The cinder (refuse) contains 5.9% combustibles. Assume that coal contains negligible nitrogen and the combustibles in the refuse are carbon. Use the mean heat capacity data provided in Table 7.14. Evaluate the boiler performance.

[*Ans.* Excess air = 32%
Dew point of flue gases = 319 K (comments?)
Volumetric flow rate of moist air = 29 834 m³/h
Volumetric flow rate of flue gases = 47 093 m³/h
Overall thermal efficiency of the boiler = 72.4%]

Table 7.45 Heat Balance of Water-Tube Boilers

Heat input by burning the coal*	12436.11 kW	100%
Heat output	kW	%
1. Useful heat gain		
Economizer	805.44	6.48
Boiler	8026.80	64.54
Superheater	169.76	1.37
2. Heat lost in flue gases	1722.37	13.85
3. Heat lost in refuse	289.85	2.33
4. Heat lost due to evaporation of moisture of coal and water produced by burning H_2	1150.87	9.25
5. Unaccounted heat loss	271.02	2.18
Total	12436.11	100.00

* Enthalpy of combustion air is neglected.

7.18 A vertical cross-tube boiler is fitted with a low air pressure burner, firing furnace oil[12]. The boiler pressure was 7 bar g, carbon dioxide content in the flue gases was 6.5% (by volume) and the temperature of the flue gases was 643 K (370°C) on an average. The pressure of the flue gases at the base of chimney was 100.7 kPa (755 torr). Air enters at 298.15 K (25°C) *DB* and 295 K (22°C) *WB*.
The ultimate analysis of the furnace oil indicates:

C: 84.0%, H: 12.7%, O: 1.2%, S: 0.4% and N: 1.7% (by mass).
GCV of the oil at 298.15 K (25°C) = 43 730 kJ/kg
Determine (a) the mass of air theoretically required to burn one kg of fuel oil, (b) the volume of dry and wet flue gases per kg of furnace oil at NTP when burnt with theoretical air, (c) theoretical percentage of CO_2 in the dry flue gases, (d) actual volume of the flue gases per kg of fuel oil burnt and percent excess air, (e) the dew point of flue gases, (f) heat loss due to hot flue gases leaving the chimney per kg of oil and (g) heat loss due to evaporation of moisture produced due to the burning of the furnace oil.

[*Ans.* (a) 14.02 kg
(b) Dry flue gases = 10.14 m³/kg oil
Wet flue gases = 11.84 m³/kg oil
(c) 15.5% CO_2
(d) Volume of flue gases = 62.03 m³/kg oil
Excess air = 129.24%
(e) 314.2 K (41.2°C) (f) 12 531.4 kJ/kg oil over 298.25 K
(g) 2747.2 kJ/kg oil over 298.15 K]

7.19 In an oil mill, there are two water tube boilers each with an evaporation capacity of 20 000 kg/h at a rated pressure of 16 bar g. Each boiler is fitted with an economizer and a superheater. At a time, only one boiler is on load and the other is standby. The boilers are fired with furnace oil. A trial was conducted to assess the performance of the boiler. Observation were taken every 15 min and average readings obtained during the trial are given as follows.

Duration of trials	= 6 h 15 min
No. of boilers on load	= One
Oil consumption during the trial	= 6630 kg
Ambient air: *DB* 308 K (35°C), *WB* 302.5 K (29.5°C)	
Steam sent to the factory as recorded by the meter	= 76.2 t
Average steam temperature	= 553 K (280°C)
Average steam pressure	= 14 bar g
Average oil inlet temperature	= 350 K (77°C)
Average draft at the base of the chimney	= 0.12 kPa g
Average temperature of the water, entering the economizer	= 355 K (82°C)
Average temperature of the water, leaving the economizer	= 388 K (115°C)
Average CO_2 in the flue gases before the economizer	= 11.5% (v/v)

Average temperature of gases before the economizer = 634 K (361°C)

Average temperature of gases, leaving the economizer = 550 K (277°C)

There is a continuous blowdown of 1000 kg/h from the boiler.
Barometer reading = 100 kPa (750 torr)
Ultimate analysis of furnace oil: C: 85.65%, H: 11.35%, S: 3.0% (mass)
GCV of furnace oil at 298.15 K (25°C) = 43 040 kJ

Specific gravity of oil = 0.95

Mean heat capacity of furnace oil = 1.675 kJ/(kg · K)

Evaluate the thermal performance of the boiler.

[*Ans.* Excess air = 37.06%

Dew point of the flue gases = 321.7 K (48.7°C)

Thermal efficiency of boiler (based on GCV) = 70.77%

Air supply to the burner = 18 561.3 m^3/h

Volumetric flowrate of flue gases = 34 563 m^3/h]

Table 7.46 Heat Balance of Boiler

Reference temperature = 298.15 K (25°C)

	kW	%
Input:		
Total gross heat input by burning the fuel	12 682.45	99.34
enthalpy of air	59.00	0.46
enthalpy of fuel oil	25.67	0.20
Total	12 767.12	100.00
Output:		
Heat gain		
in economizer	471.39	3.69
in steam generator	7 814.73	61.21
in superheater	689.86	5.40
Heat loss due to blowdown	139.27	1.09
sensible heat loss in flue gases	1 609.08	12.60
Heat loss due to evaporation of	719.29	5.64
moisture formed by burning of H$_2$ of fuel		
unaccounted heat loss	1 323.50	10.37
Total	12 767.12	100.00

7.20 Methanol is burnt as a fuel in a high-powered racing engine.
(a) Calculate the theoretical dry air requirement per kg of methanol
burnt. (b) If the fuel is burnt with 40% excess air and if it is assumed

that the combustion is complete, calculate the adiabatic flame temperature, using the data on C°_{mp} provided in Table 5.1.

Assume the availability of methanol and dry air at 298.15 K (25°C).

[*Ans*. (a) 6.47 kg dry air/kg fuel (b) 2845.1 K (2581.1°C)]

7.21 SNG, described in Exercise 7.9, is to be burnt with 10% excess air in
a boiler; both at 298.15 K (25°C). Steam is to be generated at 65 bar
a and 673 K (400°C) in the boiler using water at 373 K (100°C).
Assume 83% thermal efficiency of the boiler, based on GCV. Calculate

  (a) the steam generation per hour ii the fuel firing rate can be allowed
to be 3000 Nm³/h,

  (b) combustion air requirement, and

  (c) adiabatic flame temperature.

Data: Moisture content of combustion air = 0.018 kmol/kmol dry air

[*Ans*. (a) 33.64 t/h,

(b) 10.341 kmol wet air/kmol fuel,

(c) 2155 K (1882°C)]

7.22 At high adiabatic temperatures, NO_x content of flue gas is measured to
be high which is an objectionable pollutant. Special treatment of flue
gas such as selective catalytic reaction is thus necessary which is a
costly proposition. In a newly developed COOLFuel® technology [13] for
gas fired furnaces a part of flue gas is recycled and mixed with the fuel
gas, upstream of the burner as shown in Fig. 7.9.

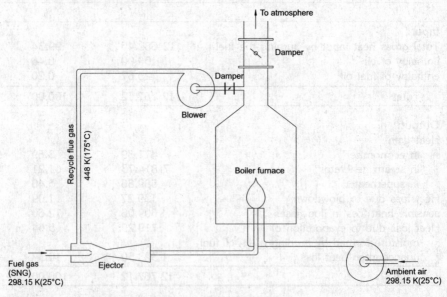

Fig. 7.9 COOLFuel Technology for Gas Firing

For this purpose, an ejector is used in which fuel gas is used as a motive
fuel to draw partially recycled flue gas. For the SNG firing, described

in Exercise 7.21, recycled flue gas [at 448 K (175°C)] flowrate is fixed in such a way that GCV of mixed gas is 288200 kJ/kmol mixture. Such firing results in lower adiabatic flame temperature, thereby achieving low NO_x emission (~ 30 ppm by v/v) and no costly treatment of flue gas becomes necessary. Calculate:

(a) recycle ratio of flue gas, defined as kmol recycled/kmol total flue gases from furnace.
(b) combustion air requirement, and
(c) adiabatic flame temperature for the revised conditions.

[*Ans.* (a) 0.1518
(b) 10.187 kmol wet air/kmol SNG,
(c) 1936 K (1663°C)]

7.23 Water gas is produced by blowing steam and air alternatively over a red-hot bed of coal. A coal with proximate analysis, moisture: 2.7%, VM: 26.9%, FC: 52.9% and ash: 17.5% (by mass) is used for the purpose. The refuse collected after gassification contained 19% combustibles (as carbon). The dry water gas (blue gas) contained H_2: 48.5%, CO: 44.2%, CO_2: 2.3%, N_2: 2.4%, O_2: 1.0% and CH_4: 1.6% (by volume).

Assume that coal contains negligible quantities of sulphur, oxygen and nitrogen. Compute

(a) kmol of dry blue gas produced per 100 kg coal used,
(b) mass of steam decomposed per kg coal used and
(c) mass % carbon and net hydrogen in coal.

[*Ans.* (a) 13.02 (b) 1.16 kg
(c) C: 79.23%, H (net): 0.57%]

7.24 In a carburetted water gas plant, blue water gas and the finished carburetted water gas have the compositions shown in Table 7.47.

Table 7.47 Composition of Gases

| | Composition, % by volume (on dry basis) | |
Component	Blue water gas	Carburetted water gas
H_2	49.0	37.0
CH_4	0.8	14.0
CO	41.0	30.5
C_3H_6	–	7.0
CO_2	4.7	5.6
O_2	–	0.4
N_2	4.5	5.5
Total	100.0	100.0

For carburetting the water gas, furnace oil having the composition 87% carbon and 13% hydrogen (by mass) is used. After carburetion, the tar

(uncarburized material) removed from the gas contained 20% of all the carbon and 10% of all the hydrogen present in the oil. Calculate
- (a) the mass of fuel oil in kg used for carburetion of one kmol blue gas,
- (b) the total kmol of the dry carburetted water gas produced per kmol dry blue water gas, and
- (c) the amount of steam decomposed (in kg) during the carburetion process per kmol dry carburetion process per kmol dry carburetted water gas.

[*Ans.* (a) 13.48 (b) 1.75 (c) 2.20]

7.25 A sample of coal is found to contain the followings:
C: 62.0%, H: 3.6%, S: 0.6%, N: 6.0%, O: 9.3% and ash: 18.5% (by mass). GCV of the fuel = 27 800 kJ/kg at 298.15 K (25°C) on dry ash-free basis. The above coal is used to generate the producer gas having the molar composition, H_2: 10.5%, CH_4: 2.1%, C_2H_4: 0.4%, CO:22.0%, CO: 7.7%, N_2: 57.3% (on dry basis; SO_2 neglected). The dew point of the gas is measured to be 298.15 K (25°C) at 106.7 kPa (800 torr). The gas is obtained at 1200 K (927°C).

The refuse from the gassifying oven contained 6.2% combustibles (reported as carbon). Air is available at 311 K (38°C) *DB* and 299 K (26°C) *WB*. Steam is introduced at 4 bar a and 623 K (350°C).

Compute:
- (a) the mass of the producer gas generated per kg coal used,
- (b) the mass of moist air used per kg coal used,
- (c) the amount of steam decomposed in gassifying oven per kg coal, and
- (d) the complete heat balance of the generator for 100 kmol dry producer gas.

[*Ans.* (a) 4.16 kg moist producer gas per kg coal
(b) 3.223 kg moist air per kg coal
(c) 0.144 kg steam decomposed per kg coal
(d) Refer Table 7.48]

Table 7.48 Heat Balance of Producer Gas Generator

Reference temperature: 298.15 K (25°C)	Heat, in kJ	%
Input:		
GCV of coal	14 582 951	97.91
Steam	284 144	1.91
Air	27 492	0.18
Total	14 894 587	100.00
Output:		
GCV of producer gas	11 668 808	78.34
Sensible heat of gas at 1200 K	784 472	5.27
Heat lost in evaporation of formed moisture of coal	508 298	3.41
Unaccounted heat loss	1 933 009	12.98
Total	14 894 587	100.00

7.26 Waste liquor from a cellulose industry has the following ultimate analysis. C: 7.5%, H: 0.5%, S: 5.7%, H_2O: 58.8% and balance inorganics (majority sodium compounds) on mass basis.

NCV at 298.15 K (25°C) = 3520 kJ/kg of waste liquor

The above waste liquor is incinerated in a steam generator along with natural gas as the stabilizing fuel. Composition of natural gas may be assumed of Example 7.4. Design of the boiler is based on 15% excess air. The adiabatic flame temperature in the boiler is not permitted to exceed 1200 K (927°C) due to various reasons such as high temperature corrosion due to high sulphur content of the waste liquor, possible thermal decomposition of the organic substances at high temperatures, adhesion of inorganic salts at high temperature on heat transfer surfaces, etc.

Saturated steam is generated at 15 bar g from the boiler. Assume (i) flue gas temperature to be 475 K (202°C), (ii) boiler feed water availability at 350 K (77°C), (iii) availability of both fuels at 298.15 K (25°C), (iv) furnace pressure of 103.5 kPa (776 torr) and (v) overall boiler efficiency to be 85% on NCV basis.

Calculate (a) the natural gas requirement and waste liquor firing rates and (b) the water dew point, sulphurous acid (H_2SO_3) dew point and (sulphuric) acid dew point. For evaluation of H_2SO_3 dew point, use the following formula[7].

$$\frac{1000}{T_{DP}} = 3.5752 - 0.1845\ A - 9.33 \times 10^{-4}\ B - 9.13 \times 10^{-4}\ (A \cdot B)$$

where T_{DP} = dew point of H_2SO_3, K

$A = \ln(p_{H_2O})$

$B = \ln(p_{SO_2})$

[*Hint*: Use absolute enthalpies, listed in Table 5.21.]

[*Ans.* (a) 4969.5 kg/h waste liquor
373.8 Nm³/h natural gas
(b) Water dew point = 348.7 K (75.7°C)
H_2SO_3 dew point = 345.6 K (72.6°C)
H_2SO_4 dew point = 426 K (153°C)]

7.27 A fuel having composition C_nH_m and no inerts is fired in a furnace. If the mole fraction of oxygen in flue gas is α on dry basis (measured with the help of Fyrite apparatus), prove[14] that

$$\% \text{ Excess air} = \left[\frac{100\ \alpha}{1 - 4.762\ \alpha}\right]\left[\frac{19.048 + 3.762\ r}{4 + r}\right]$$

where $r = \dfrac{m}{n} = \dfrac{\text{atoms of hydrogen}}{\text{atoms of carbon}}$

In a furnace, fired with pure methane, the oxygen content of flue gas is found to be 5% O_2 (by volume) on dry basis. Calculate the % excess air.

[*Ans.* 27.97%]

7.28 Assume that the mole fraction of inerts (N_2, Ar, etc.) of the fuel, considered in Exercise 7.27, is 'a'. Prove that:

$$\% \text{ Excess air} = \left[\frac{100\,\alpha}{1 - 4.762\,\alpha}\right]\left[\frac{19.048 + 3.762\,r}{4 + r} + c_f\right]$$

where
$$c_f = \frac{4\alpha}{[n(1-a)(4+r)]}$$

In Exercise 7.27, consider that the fuel (methane) contains 5% inerts. Calculate the % excess air.

[*Ans.* 28.14%]

7.29 Consider a combination-type firing in which (i) fuels are mixed having compositions $C_{n1}H_{m1}$, $C_{n2}H_{m2}$, ... $C_{ni}H_{mi}$ (without having inerts). If the mole fraction of oxygen in flue gases is α on dry basis, prove that:

$$\% \text{ Excess air} = \left[\frac{100\,\alpha}{1 - 4.762\,\alpha}\right]\left[\frac{19.048 + 3.762\,r_m}{4 + r_m}\right]$$

where
$$r_m = \frac{\displaystyle\sum_{j=1}^{i} x_j\,n_j\,r_j}{\displaystyle\sum_{j=1}^{i} x_j\,n_j}$$

$$r_j = \frac{m_j}{n_j}$$

x_j = mole fraction of the fuel having $C_{nj}H_{mj}$ composition

7.30 Assume that mole fraction of inerts (N_2, Ar, etc.) of the fuels considered in Exercise 7.29 are a_1, a_2, ..., a_i. Prove that:

$$\% \text{ Excess air} = \left[\frac{100\,\alpha}{1 - 4.762\,\alpha}\right]\left[\frac{19.048 + 3.762\,r_m}{4 + r_m} + c_{fm}\right]$$

where
$$c_{fm} = \frac{\displaystyle\sum_{j=1}^{i} 4\,x_j\,a_j}{\left[\displaystyle\sum_{j=1}^{i}\{x_j\,n_j\,(1-a_j)(4+r_j)\}\right]}$$

a_j = mole fraction of the fuel having $C_{nj}H_{mj}$ composition

$$\text{and} \qquad r_{\mathrm{m}} = \left(\frac{\left[\sum\limits_{j=1}^{i} (1 - a_{j})\, x_{j}\, n_{j}\, r_{j} \right]}{\left(\sum\limits_{j=1}^{i} (1 - a_{j})\, x_{j} n_{j} \right)} \right)$$

REFERENCES

1. The *Gazette of India* (*Extraordinary*) No. 688, December 30., 1988.
2. Culp, A. W. Jr., *Principles of Energy Conversion*, 2nd Ed., McGraw-Hill, Inc., USA, 1991, p. 56 and 59.
3. Elonka, S. M. and Kohan, A. L, *Standard Boiler Operator's Questions and Answers*, Tata McGraw-Hill Publishing Co. Ltd., New Delhi, 1969, p. 177.
4. Tan, S. H., *Chem. Engng.*, **86** (18), Aug. 27, 1979, p. 117.
5. *Flue Gas Measurement*, AMETEK Inc., USA. 1988.
6. Badger, B. V., *Hydrocarbon Processing*, **67** (7), 1987, p. 53.
7. Ganapathy, V., *Hydrocarbon Processing*, **72**. (2), 1993, p. 93.
8. Fehr, M., *Hydrocarbon Processing*, **67** (11), 1988, p. 93.
9. Gupta, S. C., S. L. Saxena, S. K. Ghosh and P. N. R. Rao, *Steam and Fuel Users Journal*, **17** (1): 1967, p. 25.
10. Kumaran, N. C., *Steam and Fuel Users Journal*, **17** (1): 1967, p. 41.
11. Charlesworth, P. L., *The Chemical Engineer*, April 1965, p. CE 87.
12. *Liquid Fuels and Steam Utilization*, National Productivity Council, New Delhi, 1969, p. 41.
13. *Chem. Engng.*, **108** (6): 2001, p. 19.
14. Michael Antony, S., *Chem. Engng.*, **88** (25): Dec. 14. 1981, p. 107.

Chapter 8

Stoichiometry and Industrial Problems

8.1 INTRODUCTION

In the previous seven chapters an attempt was made to put forward the principles of chemical processes in a graded manner. Although many industrial problems have been included in the earlier chapters, this chapter is exclusively devoted to process design problems of industrial nature. Most of them are drawn from industrial practice and hence one should find them interesting.

Example 8.1 PuraSiv S® process utilizes molecular sieve unit for removal of sulphur dioxide gas from sulphuric acid plant's tail gas[1]. Two adsorbers, packed with molecular sieve, are normally installed. While one bed is in service the other one is being regenerated. Normal cycle time is 4 hours. Regeneration of the bed is carried out with dry air and SO_2-rich air is recycled back to the sulphur burner exit gas mixture thereby increasing the productivity of the sulphur acid plant. Fig. 8.1 is the process flow diagram of the adsorption system.

In a sulphuric acid plant of 180 t/d capacity, adsorption system, based on PuraSiv S process, is installed. On a particular day, the plant was being operated at 145 t/d capacity. Tail gas is passed through an adsorber. Data on SO_2 concentration at the inlet and outlet of the adsorber during the service cycle period are presented in Table 8.1.

Table 8.1 Adsorption Data for SO_2

Time min.	SO_2 concentration at inlet to adsorber, ppm (v/v)	SO_2 concentration at outlet from adsorber, ppm (v/v)
0	4680	0
10	4660	3
20	4640	5
30	4640	8
40	4660	14
50	4680	19
60	4780	28
70	5010	48
80	5200	59
90	5100	68
100	5200	72
110	5140	78
120	4960	84
130	5000	91
140	5020	100
150	4680	106
160	4480	115
170	4440	120
180	4320	124
190	4320	129
200	4300	134
210	4160	142
220	4160	145
230	4120	150
240	4110	155

Plot the graphs of inlet and outlet SO_2 concentrations with respect of time and calculate the following.

(a) Average inlet concentration of SO_2 during the service cycle.
(b) Average emission rate from the adsorption unit.
(c) Percentage recovery of SO_2 by adsorption
(d) Assume (i) constant flow rate of incoming tail gas at 11 200 Nm³/h, (ii) 100% recycle of the adsorbed SO_2 and (iii) 100% utilization of recovered SO_2 to produce sulphuric acid. Calculate the increased production per day.
(e) Emission from PuraSiv S® plant in kg SO_2/t H_2SO_4 produced.

Solution: In Fig. 8.2, inlet and outlet SO_2 concentrations are plotted against time.

Area under the SO_2 inlet curve, A_1 = 56 007.8 square units

Scale: 100 square units = 10 min × 200 ppm

= 2000 ppm · min

Total time of adsorption = 4 h = 240 min

Average concentration of SO_2 at inlet = $\dfrac{56\,007.8 \times 2000}{100 \times 240}$

= 4667.3 ppm (v/v)　　　*Ans.* (a)

Area under the SO_2 outlet curve, A_2 = 19 106 square units

Scale: 100 square units = 10 min × 10 ppm

= 100 ppm · min

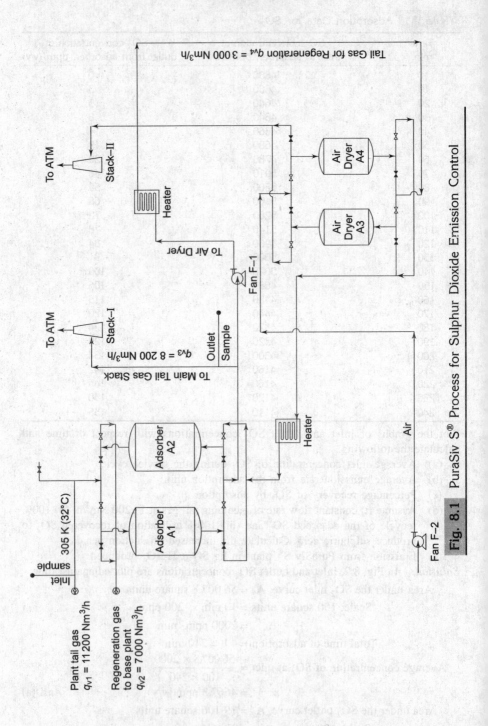

Fig. 8.1 PuraSiv S® Process for Sulphur Dioxide Emission Control

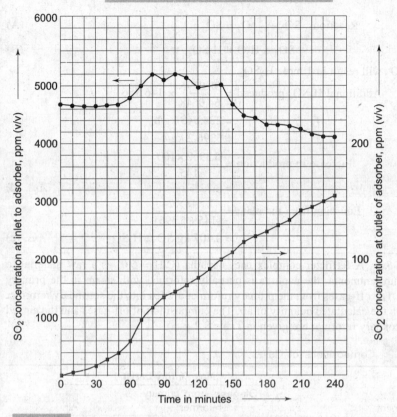

Fig. 8.2 Adsorption/Desorption data for SO_2

$$\text{Average emission rate} = \frac{19\,106 \times 100}{100 \times 240}$$

$$= 79.6 \text{ ppm (v/v)} \qquad \textit{Ans. (b)}$$

Flow rate of tail gas mixture, ingoing to adsorber = 11 200 Nm^3/h

$$\text{Inflow of } SO_2 = 11\,200 \, \frac{Nm^3}{h} \times 4667.3 \times 10^{-6}$$

$$\frac{Nm^3 \, SO_2}{Nm^3 \, \text{tail gas}} \times \frac{1}{22.4136} \frac{kmol}{Nm^3}$$

$$\times 64.0648 \, \frac{kg \, SO_2}{kmol}$$

$$= 149.414 \text{ kg/h}$$

$$\text{Outflow of } SO_2 = 11200 \times 79.6 \times 10^{-6} \times 64.0648/22.4136$$

$$= 2.548 \text{ kg/h}$$

SO_2 adsorbed (or recycled during regeneration)

$$= 149.414 - 2.548$$

$$= 146.856 \text{ kg/h}$$

$$\% \, SO_2 \text{ recovery} = \frac{146.856 \times 100}{149.414}$$

$$= 98.29 \qquad \textit{Ans. (c)}$$

Reactions: $SO_2 + \frac{1}{2} O_2 = SO_3$ (A)

$SO_3 + H_2O = H_2SO_4$ (B)

1 mole SO_2 will result in 1 mole H_2SO_4.

Additional H_2SO_4 produced $= \dfrac{98.0795}{64.0648} \times 146.856$

$= 224.843$ kg/h

$\equiv 5396.2$ kg/d

Increase in production $= \dfrac{5.3962 \times 100}{145}$

$= 3.72\%$ *Ans. (d)*

Emission from the plant $= \dfrac{2.548 \times 24}{(145 + 5.396)}$

$= 0.407$ kg SO_2/t H_2SO_4 *Ans. (e)*

Example 8.2 A fertilizer complex uses naphtha (C/H = 6.0) as a raw material to manufacture ammonia. the naphtha is partially reformed with steam in the primary reformer. The off-gases from the primary reformer are fed into the secondary reformer along with the calculated quantity of air. The composition of off-gases and the air fed to the secondary reformer are given in Table 8.2.

Table 8.2 Compositions of Gases

| Component | Mole % (dry basis) | |
	Off-gases from primary reformer	Air
Methane	8.1	–
Ethane	1.4	–
Carbon monoxide	10.3	–
Carbon dioxide	16.4	–
Hydrogen	62.9	–
Nitrogen	0.9	78.08
Oxygen	–	20.98
Argon	–	0.94

$\dfrac{\text{Steam}}{\text{dry off - gases}} = 1.035$ kmol/kmol

Moisture in air $= 0.0109$ kg/kg dry air

$= 0.0176$ kmol/kmol dry air

The off-gases enter the secondary reformer at 30 bar a and 1089 K (816° C) while the preheated air enters the reformer at 755 K (482°C). The outgoing gases from the secondary reformer have the temperature 1172 K (899°C).

The chief chemical reactions taking place in the reformer are as follow. Combustion reaction: exothermic

$H_2 + 1/2\ O_2 = H_2O$ (A)

Reforming reactions: endothermic

$CH_4 + H_2O = CO + 3 H_2$ (B)

$$CH_4 + 2\ H_2O = CO_2 + 4\ H_2 \tag{C}$$
$$C_2H_6 + 2\ H_2O = 2\ CO + 5\ H_2 \tag{D}$$
$$C_2H_6 + 4\ H_2O = 2\ CO_2 + 7\ H_2 \tag{E}$$

The exact extent of each reaction taking place in the secondary reformer is not known but the chemical equilibrium of the shift reaction at 1172 K (899°C) dictates that

$$\frac{(n_{CO_2})\ (n_{H_2})}{(n_{CO})\ (n_{H_2O})} = 0.642$$

where n_i is the number of moles of the ith component in the outgoing gases.

Assume that 96% methane is consumed. The aim of feeding air to the reformer is to provide sufficient nitrogen so that after shift converters, the ratio of $N_2 : H_2$ (on mole basis) becomes 1 : 3 (stoichiometric ratio for ammonia synthesis).

The oxygen entering with air is completely consumed in the secondary reformer. Based on 1000 kmol/h dry feed gas mixture, find the composition of the outgoing gases from the secondary reformer. Also, establish the heat balance over the reformer.

Solution: Basis: 1000 kmol/h dry incoming gases

The gas mixture contains 14 kmol C_2H_6, 81 kmol CH_4, 103 kmol CO, 164 kmol CO_2, 629 kmol H_2 and 9 kmol N_2 on hourly basis. Steam entering with the mixture is 1035 kmol/h.

Let a be the kmol/h of dry air fed
   b be the kmol/h of CO in the product gas
   c be the kmol/h of CO_2 in the product gas
   d be the kmol/h of H_2 in the product gas
   e be the kmol/h of steam in the product gas

Ethane is completely reformed, but methane is reformed to the extent of 96%.

Leftover methane in the product gas = $81 \times 0.04 = 3.24$ kmol/h

Balance of carbon:

Carbon in the incoming gas mixture = $14 \times 2 + 81 + 103 + 164$
$$= 376\ \text{kmol/h}$$

Carbon in the outgoing gas mixture = $b + c + 3.24$ kmol/h
$$b + c = 3.24 = 376$$
$$b + c = 372.76 \tag{1}$$

Balance of hydrogen:

Hydrogen in the incoming gas mixture = $3 \times 14 + 2 \times 81 + 629 + 1035$
$$= 1868\ \text{kmol/h}$$

Hydrogen in the moisture, entering with air = $0.0176a$ kmol/h

Total hydrogen, entering the reformer = $(1868 + 0.0176a)$ kmol/h

Hydrogen in the outgoing gas mixture = $(d + e + 3.24 \times 2)$ kmol/h
$$d + e + 6.48 = 1868 + 0.0176a$$
$$d + e - 0.0176a = 1861.52 \tag{2}$$

Balance of oxygen:

Oxygen in the incoming gas mixture = $\left(\dfrac{103}{2}\right) + 164 + \left(\dfrac{1035}{2}\right)$
$$= 733\ \text{kmol/h}$$

$$\text{Oxygen entering through air} = 0.2098a + \left(\frac{0.0176}{2}\right)a$$

$$= 0.2186a \text{ kmol/h}$$

$$\text{Oxygen in the outgoing gas mixture} = (b/2) + c + (c/2)$$

$$(b/2) + c + (e/2) = 733 + 0.2186a$$

$$b + 2c + e - 0.4372a = 1466 \tag{3}$$

Ratio of N_2: H_2:

In shift reactors, the reaction taking place is:

$$CO + H_2O = CO_2 + H_2 \tag{F}$$

Thus, in shift reactors, all CO will be consumed. At the outlet of the shift reactor, b kmol/h of H_2 will be added to the gaseous mixture.

Total H_2 in the gas mixture

$$\text{at the outlet of shift reactor} = (b + d) \text{ kmol/h}$$

$$\text{Total } N_2 \text{ in the reformer} = (0.7808a + 9) \text{ kmol/h}$$

$$\frac{\text{No. of moles of } H_2}{\text{No. of moles of } N_2} = 3.0 \text{ (requirement)}$$

$$\frac{b + d}{(0.7808a + 9)} = 3$$

$$b + d = 2.3424a + 27 \tag{4}$$

At the outlet of the secondary reformer, shift conversion will be in accordance with

$$\frac{(n_{CO_2})(n_{H_2})}{(n_{CO})(n_{H_2O})} = 0.642$$

$$\frac{cd}{be} = 0.642 \tag{5}$$

Mathcad solution:

Guess values:

$a := 400 \quad b := 190 \quad c := 175 \quad d := 700 \quad e := 1000$

Given

$b + c = 372.76$

$d + e - 0.0176\,a = 1861.52$

$b + 2\,c + e - 0.4372\,a = 1466$

$b + d = 2.3424a + 27$

$$\frac{c \cdot d}{b \cdot e} = 0.642$$

$vec := \text{Find}(a, b, c, d, e)$

$$vec = \begin{bmatrix} 403.345 \\ 195.7852 \\ 176.9747 \\ 776.0110 \\ 1.09261 \cdot 10^3 \end{bmatrix} \quad \text{all in kmol/h}$$

Argon in the outlet mixture = 403.35×0.0094

$$= 3.79 \text{ kmol/h}$$

Heat balance:

Table 8.3 Enthalpy of Incoming Gas Mixture

Temperature of gas mixture = 1089 K (816° C)

Component	n_i kmol/h,	$(H^\circ - H_0^\circ + \Delta H_f^\circ)_i^*$ kJ/kmol	$n_i \cdot (H^\circ - H_0^\circ + \Delta H_f^\circ)_i$ kW
CH_4	81	– 12 066	– 271.474
C_2H_6	14	+ 18 221	+ 70.861
CO	103	– 80 632	– 2 306.973
CO_2	164	– 345 840	– 15 754.947
H_2	629	+ 31 785	+ 5 553.536
N_2	9	+ 32 993	+ 82.483
H_2O	1035	– 199 564	– 57 374.506
Total	2035		– 70 142.742

* From Table 5.21

Table 8.4 Enthalpy of Supply Air

Temperature of air = 755 K (482°C)

Component	n_i kmol/h	$(H^\circ - H_0^\circ + \Delta H_f^\circ)_i$ kJ/kmol	$n_i \cdot (H^\circ - H_0^\circ + \Delta H_f^\circ)_i$ kW
N_2	314.94	+ 22 253	+ 1 946.733
O_2	84.62	+ 22 921	+ 538.780
Ar	3.79	—	—
H_2O	7.10	– 213 001	– 420.086
Total	410.45		+ 2065.427

Table 8.5 Enthalpy of Product Stream

Temperature of product stream = 1172 K (899°C)

Component	n_i kmol/h	Mole % (dry)	$(H^\circ - H_0^\circ + \Delta H_f^\circ)_i$ kJ/kmol	$n_i \cdot (H^\circ - H_0^\circ + DH_f^\circ)_i$ kW
CH_4	3.24	0.22	– 5 682	– 5.114
CO	195.79	13.23	– 77 823	– 4 232.296
CO_2	176.98	11.96	– 341 171	– 16 722.367
H_2	776.01	52.44	+ 34 335	+ 7 401.123
N_2	323.94	21.89	+ 35 762	+ 3 218.028
Ar	3.79	0.26	—	—
H_2O	1092.60	—	– 196 002	– 59 486.610
Total	2572.30	100.00		– 69827.236

Heat added to argon = $3.79 \times 20.7723 (1172 - 755)$

$$= 32\,829 \text{ kJ/h} \equiv 9.199 \text{ kW}$$

Heat of reaction, $\Delta H_R = -69\,827.236 + 9.119 - (-70\,142.742$

$$+ 2065.427)$$

$$= -1740.802 \text{ kW (exothermic)} \qquad \textit{Ans.}$$

Note: (i) In this example, it is said that 96% of CH_4 entering the reformer is reformed. During actual design calculations, the approach to the equilibrium of methane-steam reforming is also to be considered. This will complicate the problem further.

(ii) For heat balance calculation, absolute enthalpies at 1 bar a are used. However, actual reactions take place at 30 bar a which means ΔH_R will slightly vary at high pressure. In actual practice, ΔH_R is marginally exothermic which indicates heat loss from the system.

Example 8.3 Portland cement (33 grade) is manufactured by the dry process conforming to the following specifications[2].

(i) Lime saturation ratio: $\dfrac{(CaO - 0.7\ SO_3)}{(2.8\ SiO_2 + 1.2\ Al_2O_3 + 0.65\ Fe_2O_3)} = 0.9$

(ii) Iron ratio, $\dfrac{Al_2O_3}{Fe_2O_3} = 2.4$ (0.66 min.)

(iii) Magnesia content and sulphur (as SO_3) should not exceed 1.0% and 2.4% (by mass) respectively.

(iv) Silica content of 23% (by mass) is normally acceptable.

The above cement is manufactured in a rotary kiln by using Milliolite limestone and clay as raw materials. The analysis of the raw materials is given in Table 8.6. Both the raw materials are to be mixed in 72 : 28 proportion by mass.

Table 8.6 Analysis of Raw Materials

Compound	Milliolite limestone (Porbandar, Gujarat), mass %	Clay, mass %
CaO	54.50	7.13
Fe_2O_3	0.42	7.68
Al_2O_3	0.83	17.15
SiO_2	1.72	55.14
MgO	0.85	2.16
Loss on ignition	41.68	10.74

In the kiln, Andrew Yule's coal (West Bengal's colliery) is also added to supply the heat of combustion. Coal contains C: 67.2%, H: 4.0%, S: 1.7%, O: 2.2%, H_2O: 2.6% and ash: 22.3% (by mass). The gross calorific value of the coal is 25 620 kJ/kg on dry ash-free basis. It is burnt with 10% excess air.

The details of fresh air entering the kiln and the Orsat analysis of stack gases are given in Table 8.7.

Table 8.7 Conditions of Fresh Air and Stack Gases

Inlet fresh air:	300 K (27°C) Dry-bulb temperature
	293 K (20°C) Wet-bulb temperature
	100 kPa (750 torr) Barometric pressure
Stack gases:	1073 K (800°C) Dry-bulb temperature
	101.3 kPa (760 torr) Barometric pressure

The CO_2 content of the stack gas mixture needs to be limited to 23.5% by volume. The clinker obtained from the end of the kiln is cooled and gypsum (essentially pure $CaSO_4$), amounting to 3% (by mass) is added to it. The final mixture is the required product, which is crushed to the desired fineness. On the basis of 20 t/day production of portland cement, calculate

  (a) The composition of the final portland cement.
  (b) The hydraulic modulus of the cement, i.e., evaluate the ratio $CaO/(SiO_2 + Al_2O_3 + Fe_2O_3)$.
  (c) The lime-silica ratio CaO/SiO_2,
  (d) The silica modulus $SiO_2/(Al_2O_3 + Fe_2O_3)$.
  (e) The analysis of the clinker, obtained from the kiln.
  (f) It is known that the iron in the clinker is present in the form of tetracalcium aluminoferrite ($4\ CaO.Al_2O_3 . Fe_2O_3$). The remaining alumina combines with burnt lime to form tricalcium aluminate ($3\ CaO . Al_2O_3$). Remaining silica and burnt lime form dicalcium ($2\ CaO . SiO_2$) and tricalcium ($3\ CaO . SiO_2$) silicates. Based on this information, find the chemical constitution of the clinker.
  (g) The analysis of raw mix.
  (h) The Orsat analysis of stack gases.
  (i) The percentage of total sulphur of the coal going into the stack gases.
  (j) The amount of limestone, clay and coal required to be fed to the kiln per hour.
  (k) The volumetric flow rate of the fresh air.
  (l) The volumetric flow rate of dry stack gas and the dew point of stack gases.

The following assumptions can be made in the calculations.

  (i) Complete combustion of the coal takes place.
  (ii) Negligible SO_2 or SO_3 is present in the stack gases. It may be deleted while calculating the analysis of stack gases.
  (iii) No significant calcined products of raw materials are lost in the stack gases (in the form of dust).
  (iv) Sulphur present in the clinker is absorbed in it in the form of SO_3 and forms sulphate.

Solution: Basis: 100 kg portland cement

SO_3 content of the cement = 2.4 kg

Now let a, b and c be the mass (in kg) of CaO, Al_2O_3 and Fe_2O_3 respectively in the cement.

$$a + b + c = 100 - (23.0 + 1.0 + 2.4) = 73.6 \text{ kg} \qquad (1)$$

$$\frac{(CaO - 0.7\ SO_3)}{(2.8\ SiO_3 + 1.2\ Al_2O_3 + 0.65\ Fe_2O_3)} = 0.9$$

$$\frac{(a - 0.7 \times 2.4)}{(2.8 \times 23 + 1.2\ b + 0.65\ c)} = 0.9$$

$$a - 1.08\ b - 0.585\ c = 59.68 \qquad (2)$$

Also,
$$\frac{Al_2O_3}{Fe_2O_3} = 2.4$$

$$\frac{b}{c} = 2.4$$

or, $$b = 2.4\,c \qquad (3)$$

Solving the three equations

$$a = 66.4 \text{ kg CaO}$$
$$b = 5.08 \text{ kg Al}_2O_3$$
$$c = 2.12 \text{ kg Fe}_2O_3$$

Hydraulic modules:

$$\frac{CaO}{(SiO_2 + Al_2O_3 + Fe_3O_3)} = \frac{66.4}{(23.0 + 5.08 + 2.12)} = 2.2 \qquad \textit{Ans. (b)}$$

Lime-silica ratio:

$$\frac{CaO}{SiO_2} = \frac{66.4}{23.0} = 2.887 \qquad \textit{Ans. (c)}$$

Silica modules:

$$\frac{SiO_2}{(Al_2O_3 + Fe_2O_3)} = \frac{23.0}{(5.08 + 2.12)} = 3.19 \qquad \textit{Ans. (d)}$$

Let d be the mass of the clinker.

$$CaSO_4 \text{ added to the clinker} = 0.03\,d \text{ kg}$$
$$\text{Total cement} = 1.03 \times d \text{ kg} = 100 \text{ kg}$$
$$d = 97.1 \text{ kg}$$
$$CaSO_4 \text{ in the clinker} = 100 - 97.1 = 2.9 \text{ kg}$$
$$1 \text{ kmol of } CaSO_4 \equiv 1 \text{ kmol of CaO}$$
$$\equiv 1 \text{ kmol of } SO_3$$
$$2.9 \text{ kg } CaSO_4 \equiv 2.9 \left(\frac{56}{136}\right) \equiv 1.2 \text{ kg CaO}$$
$$2.9 \text{ kg } CaSO_4 \equiv \left(\frac{80}{136}\right) \times 2.9 \equiv 1.7 \text{ kg } SO_3$$

Using the above figures, Table 8.8 is prepared.

Table 8.8 Composition of Clinker and Cement

Compound	Molar mass	Clinker		Cement	
		kg	mass %	kg	mass %
CaO	56	65.20	67.15	66.40	66.40
Al_2O_3	102	5.08	5.23	5.08	5.08
Fe_2O_3	160	2.12	2.18	2.12	2.12
SiO_2	60	23.00	23.69	23.00	23.00
MgO	40.3	1.00	1.03	1.00	1.00
SO_3	80	0.70	0.72	2.40	2.40
Total		97.10	100.00	100.00	100.00

Ans. (a) & (e)

Chemical constitution of the clinker:

Table 8.9 Molar Mass of Clinker Forming Compounds

Compound	Molar Mass
$4\,CaO.Al_2O_3.Fe_2O_3$	486
$3\,CaO.Al_2O_3$	270
$2\,CaO.SiO_2$	172
$3\,CaO.SiO_2$	228

Basis: 97.10 kg clinker
All iron is present in the form of $4\,CaO.Al_2O_3.Fe_2O_3$.
Clinker contains 2.12 kg Fe_2O_3.

$$4\,CaO.Al_2O_3.Fe_2O_3 = \left(\frac{486}{160}\right) \times 2.12 = 6.44 \text{ kg}$$

$$Al_2O_3 \text{ in the above complex} = \left(\frac{102}{160}\right) \times 2.12 = 1.35 \text{ kg}$$

$$CaO \text{ in the above complex} = \frac{(56 \times 4 \times 2.12)}{160} = 2.97 \text{ kg}$$

$$\text{Remainder } Al_2O_3 = 5.08 - 1.35 = 3.73 \text{ kg}$$

This remainder Al_2O_3 forms $3\,CaO.Al_2O_3$.

$$\text{Amount of } 3\,CaO.Al_2O_3 = \left(\frac{270}{102}\right) \times 3.73 = 9.87 \text{ kg}$$

As per IS: 269-1989, tricalcium aluminate is also calculated by

$$\text{Amount of } 3\,CaO.Al_2O_3 = 2.65 \text{ (Amt. of } Al_2O_3) - 1.69 \text{ (Amt. of } Fe_2O_3)$$
$$= 9.88 \text{ kg}$$

This tallies closely with 9.87 kg calculated above. For tricalcium aluminate content of more than 5%, SO_3 content up to 3% is permitted.

$$CaO \text{ in this complex} = 9.87 - 3.73 = 6.14 \text{ kg}$$

$$CaO \text{ remained unaccounted} = 65.20 - (2.97 + 6.14) = 56.09 \text{ kg}$$

The remainder CaO forms dicalcium and tricalcium silicates.
Let e be the weight of $2\,CaO.SiO_2$ and f be the mass of $3\,CaO.SiO_2$.

$$e + f = 56.09 + 23 = 79.09 \qquad (4)$$

Balance of SiO_2:

$$\left(\frac{60}{172}\right)e + \left(\frac{60}{228}\right)f = 23.0$$

$$e + 0.754f = 65.90 \qquad (5)$$

Solving Eqs. (4) and (5),

$$e = 25.47 \text{ kg}$$
$$f = 53.62 \text{ kg}$$

The raw mix is a mixture of milliolite limestone and clay in 72 : 28 proportion.
Basis: 100 kg raw mix

$$CaO \text{ in the raw mix} = 0.545 \times 72 + 0.0713 \times 28 = 41.24 \text{ kg}$$

$$SiO_2 \text{ in the raw mix} = 0.0172 \times 72 + 0.5514 \times 28 = 16.68 \text{ kg}$$

Table 8.10 Chemical Construction of Clinker

Compound	Mass, kg	Mass %
4 CaO.Al$_2$O$_3$.Fe$_2$O$_3$	6.44	6.63
3 CaO.Al$_2$O$_3$	9.87	10.17
2 CaO.SiO$_2$	25.47	26.23
3 CaO.SiO$_2$	53.62	55.22
SO$_3$	0.70	0.72
MgO	1.00	1.03
Total	97.10	100.00

Ans. (f)

$$Fe_2O_3 \text{ in the raw mix} = 0.0042 \times 72 + 0.0768 \times 28 = 2.45 \text{ kg}$$

$$Al_2O_3 \text{ in the raw mix} = 0.0083 \times 72 + 0.1715 \times 28 = 5.40 \text{ kg}$$

$$MgO \text{ in the raw mix} = 0.0085 \times 72 + 0.0216 \times 28 = 1.22 \text{ kg}$$

$$\text{Loss on ignition} = 100 - (41.24 + 16.88 + 2.45 + 5.40 + 1.22)$$

$$= 33.01 \text{ kg (assumed to be } CO_2)$$

The above calculations give mass percentage analysis of raw-mix directly as the basis of calculations in 100 kg. Also, it can be regarded that loss on ignition is due to CO_2 alone. All other volatile matters like moisture will be very little and can be neglected.

Ans. (g)

Basis: 100 kg coal
The oxygen requirement is shown in Table 8.11.

Table 8.11 Oxygen Requirement of Coal

Element	Mass, kg	kmol	O$_2$ requirement, kmol
Carbon	67.2	5.600	5.6
Hydrogen	4.0	2.000	1.0
Sulphur	1.7	0.053	0.053
Total	72.9	7.653	6.653

$$\text{Oxygen present in coal} = 2.2 \text{ kg} = 0.069 \text{ kmol}$$

$$\text{Theoretical oxygen requirement} = 6.653 - 0.069 = 6.584 \text{ kmol}$$

$$\text{Excess } O_2 \text{ supply} = 10\%$$

$$\text{Actual } O_2 \text{ supply} = 1.1 \times 6.584 = 7.242 \text{ kmol}$$

$$N_2 \text{ entering with } O_2 \text{ in air} = \left(\frac{79}{21}\right) \times 7.242 = 27.244 \text{ kmol}$$

$$\text{Fresh dry air supply} = 27.244 + 7.242 = 34.486 \text{ kmol}$$

Assuming complete combustion, O_2 consumption can be calculated. For CO_2 and H_2O formation, O_2 consumption will be the same as listed above in Table 8.11. However, S gets oxidised to SO_3 and not to SO_2.

$$O_2 \text{ consumption for } SO_3 = \left(\frac{3}{2}\right) \times 0.053 = 0.08 \text{ kmol}$$

$$\text{Total } O_2 \text{ consumed} = 5.6 + 1.0 + 0.08 = 6.68 \text{ kmol}$$

$$\text{Oxygen unreacted} = 7.242 + 0.069 - 6.68$$

$$= 0.631 \text{ kmol}$$

This unreacted O_2 will appear in stack gases.

$$\text{Ratio } O_2/N_2 \text{ in stack gases} = \frac{0.631}{27.244} = \frac{1}{43.176}$$

Composition of stack gases:

Basis: 100 kmol stack gases

$$CO_2 \text{ in the stack gases} = 23.5 \text{ kmol}$$

$$(O_2 + N_2) \text{ in the stack gases} = 100 - 23.5 = 76.5 \text{ kmol}$$

Let g be the kmoles of O_2 in stack gases.

$$g + 43.176 \, g = 76.5 \qquad\qquad (6)$$

$$g = 1.732 \text{ kmol } O_2 \qquad\qquad Ans. \text{ (h)}$$

Table 8.12 Analysis of Stack Gases

Component	Mole % (dry basi)
CO_2	23.50
O_2	1.732
N_2	74.768
Total	100.00

In order to evaluate the actual consumptions of limestone, clay and coal, refer to the basis of the 100 kg clinker.

Let h be the mass of the raw mix, i be the mass of coal and j be the kmol of stack gases.

For finding the three unknowns, three simultaneous equations are required.

Now considering the analysis of the raw mix, coal and clinker, it will superficially appear that the S balance is the easiest balance. However, this balance should not be tried as it will lead to a wrong answer because it is assumed that all the S will be absorbed in the clinker in the form of SO_3 to form sulphate. This is not cent per cent true. The distribution of S in the clinker and stack gases is usually unknown.

Balance of non-volatile oxides:

From the analysis of the clinker [Ans. (e)] it is clear that $(100 - 0.72 =) 99.28$ kg is the total amount of non-volatile oxides.

$$\text{Amount of non-volatile oxides from raw mix} = \frac{(100 - 33.01) \, h}{100}$$

$$= 0.6699 \, h$$

Ash present in the coal comprises non-volatile oxides.

$$\text{Amount of ash in coal} = 0.223 \, f \text{ kg}$$

$$0.6699 \, h + 0.223 \, i = 99.28 \qquad\qquad (7)$$

Balance of carbon:

$$\text{Carbon present in the coal} = \left(\frac{67.2}{100}\right) \times i \times \left(\frac{1}{12}\right) = 0.056 \, i \text{ kmol}$$

CO_2 (ignition loss) in the raw mix is the source of carbon in the mix.

$$\text{Carbon from the raw mix} = \left(\frac{33.07}{44}\right)\left(\frac{1}{100}\right)h = 0.0075\,h \text{ kmol}$$

The stack gases have 23.5 mole % CO_2.

$$0.056\,i + 0.0075\,h = 0.235\,j \tag{8}$$

Balance of oxygen:

(O_2 from air) + (O_2 from raw mix)

+ (O_2 from coal) = (O_2 in stack gas) + (O_2 for H in coal)

+ (O_2 for S in coal)

$$\left[\left(\frac{21}{79}\right)\times(0.7477)\right]j + \left[\frac{33.07}{(44\times100)}\right]h$$

$$+ \left[\frac{2.2}{(32\times100)}\right]i = \left(\frac{23.5}{100}\right)j + \left(\frac{1.732}{100}\right)j + \left(\frac{4}{(2\times2\times100)}\right)i$$

$$+ \left[\frac{(3\times1.7)}{(2\times100\times32)}\right]i$$

$$0.75\,h - 0.39\,i = 5.33\,j \tag{9}$$

Solving Eqs. (7), (8) and (9),

$$h = 132.77 \text{ kg raw-mix}$$
$$i = 46.39 \text{ kg coal}$$
$$j = 15.29 \text{ kmol stack gases}$$

(Note that in above calculations, the moisture entering with the air is neglected. However, it does not affect the final results of h, i and j).

Now, the balance of S can be made.

$$\text{S present in coal} = 46.39 \times 0.017 = 0.79 \text{ kg}$$
$$\text{S in the clinker} = \left(\frac{32}{80}\right)\times0.72 = 0.29 \text{ kg}$$
$$\text{Unaccounted S} = 0.79 - 0.29 = 0.5 \text{ kg}$$

This S goes into stack gases.

$$\text{% S going into the stack gases} = \left(\frac{0.5}{0.79}\right)100 = 63.3\% \qquad \textit{Ans. (i)}$$

All the above results can be converted into a basis of 20000 kg/h of portland cement.

Basis: 20000 kg/h portland cement

$$\text{Clinker output of the kiln} = 20000 \times 0.971 = 19420 \text{ kg/h}$$
$$\text{Raw mix required} = \left(\frac{132.77}{100}\right)\times19420 = 25784 \text{ kg/h}$$
$$\text{Limestone required} = 0.72 \times 25784 = 18564 \text{ kg/h}$$
$$\text{Clay required} = 25784 - 18564 = 7220 \text{ kg/h}$$
$$\text{Coal required} = \left(\frac{46.39}{100}\right)\times19420 = 9009 \text{ kg/h}$$

$$\frac{\text{Coal}}{\text{Raw mix ratio}} = \frac{9009}{25\,784} = 0.349 \text{ kg/kg} \qquad Ans. \text{ (j)}$$

Dry-air required, $n_1 = 34.486 \times \left(\frac{9009}{100}\right) = 3106.8 \text{ kmol/h}$

From Fig. 6.11, specific volume of air, $V_H = 25.523 \text{ m}^3 \times 1.813/\text{kg dry air}$

Volumetric flow rate of dry air $= 3106.8 \times 25.523$

$$= 79\,295 \text{ m}^3/\text{h} \qquad Ans. \text{ (k)}$$

Stack gases, $n_2 = 15.29 \times \left(\frac{19\,420}{100}\right) = 2969.3 \text{ kmol/h}$

Volumetric flow rate of stack gases $= n_2 R T_2/p_2$

$$= \frac{(2969.3 \times 8.3145 \times 1073)}{101.325}$$

$$= 261\,441 \text{ m}^3/\text{h} \qquad Ans. \text{ (1-i)}$$

From the psychrometric chart (Fig. 6.11), at 300 K (27°C) *DB* and 293 K (20°C) *WB*,

Absolute humidity $= 0.0118 \text{ kg moisture/kg dry air}$

$$= 0.019 \text{ kmol moisture/kmol dry air}$$

Basis: 100 kg coal

Moisture entering the system through air $= 0.019 \times 34.486 = 0.655 \text{ kmol}$

Free moisture of coal $= 2.8 \text{ kg} = 0.156 \text{ kmol}$

Moisture produced by burning net hydrogen of coal $= \frac{4}{2} = 2 \text{ kmol}$

Total moisture in stack gases $= 0.655 + 0.155 + 2 = 2.811 \text{ kmol}$

$$\text{Stack gas} = \frac{(15.29 \times 100)}{46.39} = 32.96 \text{ kmol}$$

Mole fraction of moisture in stack gases $= \dfrac{2.811}{(32.96 + 2.811)} = 0.0786$

Partial pressure of water in stack gases, $p_w = 101.325 \times 0.0786$

$$= 7.962 \text{ kPa}$$

Dew point $= 314.5 \text{ K}$ (Refer Table 6.8)

$$\equiv 41.5°C \qquad Ans. \text{ (1-ii)}$$

Notes: (i) Various ratios, such as hydraulic modules, silica modules, etc. are calculated as these ratios are very well known in the cement industry. The quality of the cement can be judged if these ratios are known.

(ii) Chemical constitution of the clinker (Ans. (f)) gives an idea about the complexes forming in the cement and the crystallinity of the clinker.

(iii) In the example cited, raw mix is composed of limestone and clay. However, the use of blast furnace slag is also common. Separate specifications are available for the cement manufactured by using blast furnace slag (IS: 455)

(iv) It was assumed that stack gases do not contain carbon monoxide. However, this is rarely true. A small amount of CO is also present in the stack gases.
(v) Before utilizing the waste heat of stack gases, the particulate matter is usually removed by using a cyclone separator and/or an electrostatic precipitator. Later, they are passed through a heat exchanger where the water is heated and steam is generated (in waste heat boiler).
(vi) It is interesting to study the heat balance of the cement manufacture. Lewis et al[3] have worked out the heat balance to which the reference is made.

Example 8.4 A single stage ammonia-water absorption refrigeration plant is employed as shown in Fig. 8.3 for production of aqueous monoethylene glycol (MEG) brine at 268 K(– 5°C).

Liquid ammonia is evaporated in the chiller at 263 K(–10°C). Heat load of the chiller is 200 kW. Assume 2.5% increase in the heat load due to heat gain through insulation of the chiller and heat loss from hot surfaces of the system. Saturated ammonia vapours from the chiller enter the absorber in which they are absorbed at ~ 10 kPa less pressure than that in the chiller in weak aqueous (WA) ammonia solution. Heat of absorption is removed by cooling water.

Strong aqueous (SA) ammonia solution leaves the absorber at saturated conditions at 315 K(42°C), exchanges heat with incoming WA solution in the heat exchanger and enters a packed distillation column at 2.5 K(2.5°C) lower temperature than the saturation temperature of SA solution at the column pressure. Generator (essentially a reboiler) is fed with saturated steam at 3 bar a. From the bottom of the generator, WA solution, having 6.5% (by mass) lower concentration than SA solution (also called *split*), is drawn. Saturated WA solution enters the heat exchanger, exchanges heat with SA solution and enters the absorber.

From the absorber top ammonia vapours are taken to a condenser in which they are condensed with help of cooling water. Liquid ammonia at saturated conditions at 313 K(40°C) from the condenser is divided into two portions. One portion is sent to the chiller for the refrigeration duty while another portion is recycled to the column as reflux at the rate of 0.08 kg/kg ammonia fed to the column. Purity of ammonia (~ 100%) in the chiller is maintained by periodic bleed of a liquid mass from the bottom of the absorber. Thus the refrigeration cycle is completed.

Cooling water is supplied at 2 bar g and 305 K(32°C) in the absorber and the condenser. A rise of 5 K(5°C) is permitted to the cooling water. Use Fig. 5.19 for the enthalpy data.

Table 8.13 Properties of Ammonia[4]

Temperature K(°C)	Saturation pressure, kPa a	Enthalpy, kJ/kg	
		Liquid	Vapour
263(–10)	290.75	301.4	1597.8
313(40)	1555.5	538.5	1637.2

Basis: Specific enthalpy of liquid ammonia at 196 K(– 77°C) = 0 kJ/kg
Make complete material and energy balances of the refrigeration system.

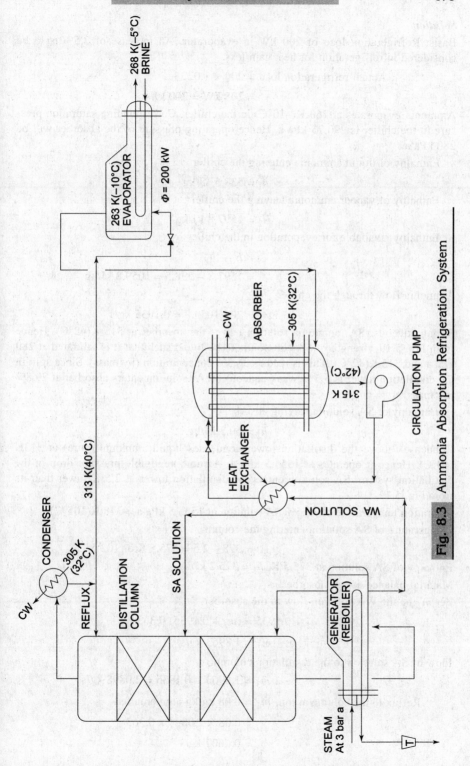

Fig. 8.3 Ammonia Absorption Refrigeration System

Solution

Basis: Refrigeration load of 200 kW in evaporator. An increase of 2.5% is to be considered in refrigeration for heat gain/loss.

$$\text{Actual refrigeration load} = 200 \times 1.025$$
$$= 205 \text{ kW} = 200 \text{ kJ/s}$$

Ammonia evaporates at 263 K($-10°C$) in the chiller. Corresponding saturation pressure in the chiller is 290.75 kPa a. Hence operating pressure of the absorber will be 280 kPa a.

Enthalpy of liquid ammonia entering the chiller

$$h_1 = 538.5 \text{ kJ/kg}$$

Enthalpy of vapour ammonia leaving the chiller

$$H_2 = 1597.8 \text{ kJ/kg}$$

Enthalpy, available for evaporation in the chiller

$$= H_2 - h_1$$
$$= 1597.8 - 538.5 = 1059.8 \text{ kJ/kg}$$

Ammonia flow through the chiller,

$$\dot{m}_1 = 205/1059.8 = 0.1935 \text{ kg/s}$$

Strong aqueous (SA) ammonia solution leaves the absorber at 315 K($42°C$). Hence from Fig. 5.19, strength of SA solution is to be found such that it is saturated at 280 kPa a and 315 K($42°C$). This is read as 36.3% concentration (by mass). Since split in the distillation tower is 6.5%, weak aqueous (WA) solution enters absorber at 29.8% (by mass).

Enthalpy of SA solution leaving absorber

$$h_2 = 60.3 \text{ kJ/kg}$$

Condenser above the distillation tower condenses liquid ammonia (pure) at 313K ($40°C$). Hence it operates at 1555.5 kPa a. Assume negligible pressure drop in the distillation system. SA solution enters the distillation tower at 2.5 K lower than its from Fig. 5.19,

Saturation temperature of 36.5% SA solution at 1555.5 kPa a = 378 K($105°C$)

Temperature of SA solution entering the column

$$= 378 - 2.5 = 375.5 \text{ K or } 102.5°C$$

Enthalpy of SA solution at 375.5 K, $h_3 = 325.2 \text{ kJ/kg}$

Material balance across absorber:

Let $\dot{m}_2$ be the WA solution flow to the absorber.

$$0.298 \ \dot{m}_2 + 0.1935 = (\dot{m}_2 + 0.1935) \ 0.363$$

$$\text{or} \quad \dot{m}_2 = 1.8963 \text{ kg/s}$$

Flow of SA solution to the distillation column

$$\dot{m}_3 = 1.8963 + 0.1935 = 2.0898 \text{ kg/s}$$

Reflux to the column at top, $\dot{m}_4 = 0.08$ kg/kg ammonia fed

$$= 0.08 \times 2.0898 \times 0.363$$
$$= 0.0607 \text{ kg/s}$$

Heat balance across heat exchanger:

Heat gained by SA solution $\phi_1 = (h_3 - h_2) \, 2.0898$

$$= (325.2 - 60.3) \, 2.0898$$

$$= 553.59 \text{ kJ/s or kW}$$

Heat gain by SA solution = Heat loss by WA solution

WA solution leaves the generation under saturated conditions at 1555.5 kPa a. Its temperature and enthalpy are read from Fig. 5.19 as 390 K(117°C) and 412.1 kJ/kg (h_4). Assume heat capacity of WA and SA solutions to be same.

$$1.8963 \, (412.1 - h_5) = 553.59$$

or $\quad h_5 = 120.2$ kJ/kg

For WA solution (of 30% strength), this enthalpy corresponds to a temperature of 327.3 K(54.3°C) in Fig. 5.19.

Heat balance across absorber:

Enthalpy of vapours entering the absorber,

$$\phi_2 = 1597.8 \times 0.1935$$

$$= 309.17 \text{ kJ/s or kW}$$

Enthalpy of WA solution entering the absorber,

$$\phi_3 = 120.2 \times 1.8963$$

$$= 227.94 \text{ kJ/s or kW}$$

Enthalpy of SA solution leaving the absorber

$$\phi_4 = 2.0898 \times 60.3$$

$$= 126.01 \text{ kJ/s or kW}$$

Cooling load of absorber, $\phi_1 = \phi_2 + \phi_3 - \phi_4$

$$= 309.17 + 227.94 - 126.01$$

$$= 411.1 \text{ kJ/s or kW}$$

Heat balance across the distillation column:

Ammonia condensed in the condenser

$$\dot{m}_5 = 0.1935 + 0.0607 = 0.2542 \text{ kg/s}$$

Heat removal in condenser, $\phi_5 = 0.2542 \, (1637.2 - 538.5)$

$$= 279.29 \text{ kJ/s or kW}$$

Enthalpy of vapours at the top,

$$\phi_6 = 1637.2 \times 0.2542$$

$$= 416.18 \text{ kJ/s or kW}$$

Enthalpy of reflux fed back to column,

$$\phi_7 = 0.0607 \times 538.5$$

$$= 32.69 \text{ kJ/s or kW}$$

Enthalpy of SA solution fed to the column,

$$\phi_8 = 325.2 \times 2.0898$$

$$= 679.6 \text{ kJ/s or kW}$$

Enthalpy of WA solution, leaving the generator,

$$\phi_9 = 1.8963 \times 412.1$$

$$= 781.47 \text{ kJ/s or kW}$$

Heat to be supplied in the generator,

$$\phi_{10} = \phi_6 + \phi_9 - \phi_7 - \phi_8$$

$$= 416.18 + 781.47 - 32.69 - 679.6$$

$$= 485.36 \text{ kJ/s or kW}$$

A check can be made of overall heat balance.

Heat input:		**Heat Output:**	
Evaporator	205.00 kW	Condenser	279.29 kW
Generator	485.36 kW	Absorber	411.10 kW
Total	690.36 kW	Total	690.39 kW

Efficiency of refrigeration system or

$$\text{Coefficient of Performance} = \frac{\text{Net refrigeration achieved}}{\text{Heat input to generator}}$$

$$= \frac{200}{485.36}$$

$$= 0.4121 \text{ kJ/kJ}$$

At 3 bar a, saturated steam temperature, $T_s = 406.69$ K(133.54°C) Latent heat of evaporation, $\lambda_v = 2163.2$ kJ/kg (Appendix III.2)

$$\text{Steam consumption in generator} = \frac{485.36}{2163.2}$$

$$= 0.2244 \text{ kg/s}$$

$$\equiv 807.7 \text{ kg/h}$$

$$\text{Total cooling load} = 690.39 \text{ kW}$$

$$\text{Total cooling water flow} = \frac{690.39}{5}$$

$$= 138.08 \text{ kg/s}$$

$$\equiv 497.1 \text{ m}^3/\text{h} \qquad \qquad Ans.$$

On Fig. 5.19, take a point on y-axis at $x = 1.0$ and enthalpy = 1597.8 kJ/kg which represents the incoming ammonia vapours. Take another point, representing WA solution at $x = 0.298$ and temperature of 331 K(58°C). Line joining both the points crosses SA solution strength abscissa; $x = 0.365$ at 363 K(90°C) and has enthalpy $h_6 = 260.1$ kJ/kg solution. However, it shows higher saturation pressure (> 900 kPa a) which does not allow flow of ammonia vapours from the chiller to the absorber. Hence the solution must be cooled to its saturature temperature of 315 K(42°C) at 280 kPa a.

Heat removal rate in absorber = $\dot{m}_3 (h_6 - h_2)$

$$= 2.0898 (260.1 - 60.3)$$

$$= 417.5 \text{ kJ/s or kW}$$

This agrees well with earlier calculated value of 411.1 kJ/s. Flow $\dot{m}_2$ can also be calculated from this line using geometric principles.

Example 8.5 A pilot plant employs aqueous methyl diethanolamine (MDEA) solution for the removal of acid gases from a gas mixture in a coal liquefaction plant. The composition of the saturated gas mixture entering the absorber is as follows (dry volume %):

H_2: 28.4%, CO: 9.1%, CO_2: 38.4%, CH_4: 22.3%, C_2H_6: 0.7%, N_2: 0.4% and H_2S: 0.7%.

The process[5] is depicted in Fig. 3.3. The absorber has 20 trays and operates at 45 bar g while the stripper has 17 trays and operates at 125 kPa a. The feed gas and aqueous solution enter at 314 K (41°C) and 311 K (38°C) respectively. Based on the following data, make a complete material and energy balance of the acid gas removal system.

(i) The flow rate of the incoming dry gas mixture is 8500 Nm³/h from a coal gasification unit employing the Synthane process[6].
(ii) Rich MEDA solution contains 0.6 kmol acid gas per kmol MDEA. With 35% (by mass) concentration of MDEA, 65% CO_2 is absorbed from the gas mixture while H_2S absorption can be assumed complete. In actual practice, H_2S slip will be around 50 ppm (v/v).
(iii) Lean MDEA solution should not contain more than 0.15 kmol acid gas per kmol MDEA of which the H_2S concentration should not exceed 0.002 kmol/kmol MDEA. For achieving this concentration in the lean solution, one kmol of water reflux is required per kmol of MDEA is the stripper.
(iv) Physical properties of MDEA:

Molar mass of MDEA = 119.2

Specific gravity: 1.04 at 293 K (20°C) of 100% solution
1.03 at 303 K (30°C) of 35% solution
1.00 at 373 K (100°C) of 35% solution

Heat capacity: 3.77 kJ/(kg · K) over the temperature range of calculations

Normal boiling point (T_B) at 101.3 kPa = 503.6 K (230.6°C)

Vapour pressure at 293 K (20°C) = 1.33 Pa (0.01 torr)

Latent heat of vaporization, λ_v = 518.7 kJ/kg at T_B

(v) Exothermic heat of reaction at 298.15 K (25°C):

For H_2S absorption = 1047 kJ/kg

For CO_2 absorption = 1342 kJ/kg

(vi) Assume negligible energy consumption in the vaporizer.

Solution: Basis: Feed gas rate = 8500 Nm³/h = 379.23 kmol/h

Ingoing CO_2 = 379.23 × 0.384 = 145.62 kmol/h

Ingoing H_2S = 379.23 × 0.007

= 2.65 kmol/h ≡ 90.31 kg/h

CO_2 absorbed = 145.62 × 0.65

= 94.65 kmol/h ≡ 4165.55 kg/h

Unabsorbed CO_2 in the outgoing

gas mixture = 145.62 − 94.65 = 50.97 kmol/h

Total acid gas removed = 94.65 + 2.65 = 97.30 kmol/h

Absorption of acid gas in the

$$\text{circulating solution} = 0.60 - 0.15 = 0.45 \text{ kmol/kmol MDEA}$$

$$\text{Circulation rate requirement} = \frac{97.30}{0.45} \text{ (100\% MDEA basis)}$$

$$= 216.22 \text{ kmol/h} \cong 25\,767 \text{ kg/h}$$

Ciculation rate of 35% (mass)

$$\text{strength solution} = \frac{25767}{0.35} = 73\,621 \text{ kg/h}$$

$$H_2S \text{ in lean MDEA} = 216.22 \times 0.002 = 0.43 \text{ kmol/h}$$

$$CO_2 \text{ in lean MDEA} = 216.22 \times 0.148 = 32.00 \text{ kmol/h}$$

$$\text{MDEA soln. with acid gases} = 73\,621 + 0.43 \times 34 + 32 \times 44$$

$$= 75\,044 \text{ kg/h}$$

$$\text{Circulation rate of MDEA solution} = \frac{75\,044}{(1.03 \times 1000)} = 72.86 \text{ m}^3/\text{h}$$

Vapour pressure of water:

$$\text{at } 314 \text{ K } (41^\circ\text{C}), \ p_{w1} = 7.777 \text{ kPa} \quad \text{(Refer Table 6.8)}$$

$$\text{at } 311 \text{ K } (38^\circ\text{C}), \ p_{w2} = 6.624 \text{ kPa} \quad \text{(Refer Table 6.8)}$$

Mole fraction of water in 35%

$$\text{MDEA solution} = 0.9144$$

Partial pressure of water at

$$\text{the absorber top} = 6.624 \times 0.9144 = 6.056 \text{ kPa}$$

Total pressure in the absorber, $p_{T_1} = 45$ bar g $= 4601.3$ kPa a
Pressure drop in the absorber is neglected.

$$H_2O \text{ in the outgoing gas mixture} = \left[\frac{6.056}{(4601.3 - 6.056)} \right] (379.23 - 97.30)$$

$$= 0.372 \text{ kmol/h}$$

$$H_2O \text{ in the ingoing gas mixture} = \left[\frac{7.777}{(4601.3 - 7.777)} \right] 379.23$$

$$= 0.642 \text{ kmol/h}$$

$$H_2O \text{ condensed} = 0.642 - 0.372 = 0.27 \text{ kmol/h}$$

$$\cong 4.86 \text{ kg/h}$$

$$H_2S \text{ in rich MDEA solution} = 0.43 + 2.65 = 3.08 \text{ kmol/h}$$

$$CO_2 \text{ in rich MDEA solution} = 32.0 + 94.65 = 126.66 \text{ kmol/h}$$

Heat balance in the absorber:

Base temperature $T_0 = 298.15$ K (25°C)

$$\text{Heat generated due to absorption} = 90.31 \times 1047 + 4165.5 \times 1342$$

$$= 5684\,723 \text{ kJ/h} \cong 1579.09 \text{ kW}$$

Table 8.14 Sour Gas Enthalpy Calculations

| Component | n_i kmol/h | kg | \multicolumn{4}{c}{Heat capacity equation constants} |
			$n_i \cdot a_i$	$n_i \cdot b_i \times 10^3$	$n_i \cdot c_i \times 10^6$	$n_i \cdot d_i \times 10^9$
H_2	107.70	215.40	3081.35	109.79	− 15.90	82.82
CO	34.51	966.28	1001.76	− 97·20	401.82	− 162.41
CO_2	145.62	6407.28	3111.24	9361.05	− 5977.79	1427.06
CH_4	84.57	1353.121	1627.92	4407.24	1012.56	− 957.10
C_2H_6	2.66	79.80	14.40	473.71	− 184.54	23.18
N_2	1.52	42.56	44.98	− 7.81	20.04	− 7.55
H_2S	2.65	90.10	90.65	–	–	–
H_2O	0.642	11.56	20.86	0.05	8.48	− 2.92
Total	379.872	9166.10	8993.16	14 246.83	− 4735.33	403.08

$$\text{Average molar mass of dry sour gas} = \frac{9166.10 - 11.56}{379.872 - 0.642} = 24.14$$

Table 8.15 Treated Gas Enthalpy Calculations

| Component | n_i kmol/h | kg | \multicolumn{4}{c}{Heat capacity equation constants} |
			$n_i \cdot a_i$	$n_i \cdot b_i \times 10^3$	$n_i \cdot c_i \times 10^6$	$n_i \cdot d_i \times 10^9$
H_2	107.70	215.40	3081.35	109.79	− 15.90	82.82
CO	34.51	966.28	1001.76	− 97.20	401.82	− 162.41
CO_2	50.97	2242.68	1089.00	3276.56	− 2092.35	499.50
CH_4	84.57	1353.12	1627.92	4407.24	1012.56	− 957.10
C_2H_6	2.66	79.80	14.40	473.71	− 184.54	23.18
N_2	1.52	42.56	44.98	− 7.81	20.04	− 7.55
H_2S	Nil	–	–	–	–	–
H_2O	0.372	6.70	12.09	0.03	4.91	− 1.69
Total	282.302	4906.54	6871.50	8162.32	− 853.46	− 523.25

$$\text{Average molar mass of dry treated gas} = \frac{4906.54 - 6.70}{282.302 - 0.372} = 17.38$$

Enthalpy of sour gas at 314 K over 298.15 K

$$= \int_{298.15}^{314} (8993.16 + 14\,246.83 \times 10^{-3}T - 4735.33 \times 10^{-6}\,T^2$$

$$+ 403.08 \times 10^{-9}\,T^3)\,dT$$

$$= 206\,732 \text{ kJ/h}$$

$$\equiv 57.42 \text{ kW}$$

Enthalpy of treated gas at 311 K over 298.15 K $= \int_{298.15}^{311} (6871.50 + 8162.32 \times 10^{-3}\,T$

$$- 853.46 \times 10^{-6}\,T^2$$

$$- 523.25 \times 10^{-6}\,T^3)\,dT$$

$$= 120\,420 \text{ kJ/h} \equiv 33.45 \text{ kW}$$

Heat given up in the absorber by the gas mixture = $57.42 - 33.45 = 23.97$ kW

Heat given up by condensation of water = 4.86×2411.7

$$= 11\ 721\ \text{kJ/h} \equiv 3.26\ \text{kW}$$

Heat in the lean MDEA solution = $75\ 044 \times 3.77\ (311 - 298.15)$

$$= 3677\ 906\ \text{kJ/h}$$

$$\equiv 1021.64\ \text{kW}$$

Total heat in the rich MDEA solution = $1021.64 + 23.97$

$$+ 3.26 + 1579.09$$

$$= 2627.96\ \text{kW}$$

$$79\ 302.8 \times 3.77 \times (T_1 - 295) = 2627.96 \times 3600$$

Temperature of the rich MDEA

solution leaving absorber, $T_1 = 329.6$ K (56.6°C)

Material and energy balance across the stripper:

Total acid gas leaving the stripper = 97.30 kmol/h

Reflux water = 97.30 kmol/h

Acid gas mixture leave the accumulator at 333 K (60°C) in saturated condition.

p_{w3} at 333 K (60°C) = 19.92 kPa   (Refer Table 6.8)

$$p_{T_2} = 125\ \text{kPa a}$$

Moisture leaving with acid gas mixture from

$$\text{condensate accumulator} = \frac{(19.92 \times 97.30)}{(125 - 19.92)} = 18.45\ \text{kmol/h}$$

Total water in the acid gas from stripper = $97.30 + 18.45 = 115.75$ kmol/h

$$\text{Specific moisture content} = \frac{115.75}{97.30} = 1.19\ \text{kmol/kmol dry gas}$$

$$p_3 = 40\ \text{kPa g at stripper top}$$

$$= 141.3\ \text{kPa a}$$

$$p_4/(p_3 - p_4) = 1.19$$

$$p_4 = \text{partial pressure of water at the stripper top}$$

$$= 76.79\ \text{kPa a}$$

Vapour pressure of water

at the stripper top, $p_{w4} = \dfrac{76.79}{0.9144} = 83.98$ kPa

Temperature of the gas stream

leaving the stripper = 367.8 K (94.8°C)   (Refer Table 6.8)

Solution interchanger:

In this heat exchanger, lean MDEA solution cools down from 389 K (116°C) to 353 K (80°C).

$$\text{Heat transfer} = 75\,044 \times 3.77\,(389 - 353)$$
$$= 10\,184\,972 \text{ kJ/h} \equiv 2829.16 \text{ kW}$$

Assume 2% radiation loss.

$$\text{Heat picked up by rich MDEA solution} = 2829.16 \times 0.98$$
$$= 2772.58 \text{ kW}$$
$$79\,302.8 \times 3.77\,(T_2 - 329.6) = 2772.58 \times 3600$$
$$T_2 = 363 \text{ K } (90°\text{C}) \text{ (temperature of rich}$$
$$\text{MDEA solution leaving the heat exchanger)}$$

Cooler :

In this heat exchanger, lean MDEA solution is cooled to 311 K (38°C) with the help of cooling water.

$$\text{Heat transfer duty} = 75\,044 \times 3.77\,(353 - 311)$$
$$= 11\,882\,467 \text{ kJ/h} \equiv 3300.69 \text{ kW}$$

Rise in cooling water temperature = 10 K

$$\text{Cooling water flow rate} = \frac{3300.69 \times 3600}{10 \times 4.1868 \times 1000} \equiv 283.7 \text{ m}^3/\text{h}$$

Steam requirement in reboiler:

$$\text{Base temperature, } T_0 = 298.15 \text{ K}$$
$$\text{Enthalpy of rich solution} = 79\,302.8 \times 3.77\,(363 - 298.15)$$
$$= 19\,433\,151 \text{ kJ/h} \equiv 5398.10 \text{ kW}$$
$$\text{Enthalpy of lean solution} = 75\,044 \times 3.77\,(389 - 298.15)$$
$$= 25\,745\,345 \text{ kJ/h} \equiv 7151.48 \text{ kW}$$

Mean heat capacities of CO_2 and H_2S at 367.8 K are 38.67 and 34.42 kJ/(kmol · K), respectively at 367.8 K (94.8°C)

$$\text{Enthalpy of acid gases leaving the stripper} = [94.65 \times 38.67 + 2.65 \times 34.42]\,(367.8$$
$$- 298.15)$$
$$= 261\,843 \text{ kJ/h} \equiv 72.73 \text{ kW}$$
$$\text{Enthalpy of steam at 367 K} = 2667.6 \text{ kJ/kg} \quad \text{(Ref. AIII.2)}$$
$$\text{Enthalpy of water at 298.15 K} = 104.77 \text{ kJ/kg} \quad \text{(Ref. AIII.1)}$$

Enthalpy of water vapour

$$\text{leaving stripper with acid gases} = 115.59 \times 18.0153\,(2667.6 - 104.77)$$
$$= 5\,335\,238 \text{ kJ/h} \equiv 1482.01 \text{ kW}$$

To find the make-up condensate flow rate, material balance across the stripper is required.

Rich MDEA solution + make-up

$$\text{water } (x) + \text{Reflux water} = \text{lean MDEA solution} +$$
$$\text{moist gas at the stripper overhead}$$
$$79\,302.8 + x + 97.3 \times 18.0153 = 75\,044 + 90.3 + 4165.6$$
$$+ 115.59 \times 18.0153$$
$$x = 327.3 \text{ kg/h}$$

Total condensate entering the stripper = $97.3 \times 18.0153 + 327.3$

$$= 2079.6 \text{ kg/h}$$

Enthalpy of condensate = $(251.09 - 104.77)\, 2079.6$

$$= 304\,287 \text{ kJ/h} \equiv 84.52 \text{ kW}$$

Assuming 2% radiation loss,

[Enthalpy of rich solution

+ enthalpy of condensate

+ enthalpy of supplied by steam (ϕ)] 0.98 = enthalpy of moist acid gas at stripper top + enthalpy of lean solution + enthalpies of desorption

$$(5398.10 + 84.52 + \phi)\, 0.98 = 72.73 + 1482.01 + 7151.48 + 1579.09$$

$$\phi = 5012.594 \text{ kW}$$

Latent heat of steam at 4 bar a = 2133.0 kJ/kg

Steam consumption in reboiler = $5012.59 \times \dfrac{3600}{2133}$

$$= 8460 \text{ kg/h}$$

Acid gas cooler:

Acid gas is cooled to 333 K (60°C) in the cooler.

Enthalpy of water vapour at 333 K = 2609.7 kJ/kg   (Ref. A III.2)

Mean heat capacities of CO_2 and H_2S are 38 and 34.3 kJ/(kmol · K) respectively at 333 K (60°C).

Enthalpy of acid gases

leaving the cooler = $[94.65 \times 38 + 2.65 \times 34.3]\,(333 - 298.15)$

$$= 129\,066 \text{ kJ/h} = 35.85 \text{ kW}$$

Enthalpy removed in the cooler = $1482.01 + 72.73 - 35.85 - [18.29 \times 18.0153$

$$(2609.7 - 104.77) + 97.3 \times 18.0153$$

$$\times 4.1868\,(333 - 298.15)]/3600$$

$$= 1218.36 \text{ kW}$$

Cooling water flow = $\dfrac{1218.36 \times 3600}{(10 \times 4.1868 \times 1000)}$

$$\equiv 104.8 \text{ m}^3/\text{h}$$

Ans.

Note: For the heat exchanger in which heat is exchanged between lean and rich MDEA solutions, radiation loss (2%) was assumed but in coolers, radiation loss was not assumed. This is deliberately done to have conservative designs. By assuming radiation loss in the interchanger, the steam requirement in the reboiler will be high. By not assuming radiation loss in coolers, cooling water flows are high. Thus both result in conservative utilities' consumptions.

The complete material and energy balance of the system is given in Table 8.16.

Table 8.16 Material and Energy Balance of Acid Gas Removal System

A. Gas Streams

				Gas component								
		H_2	CO	CO_2	CH_4	C_2H_6	N_2	H_2S	H_2O	Total	Pressure	Temperature K (°C)
Molar mass		2.02	28.01	44.01	16.04	30.07	28.01	34.08	18.01			
1. Sour gas flow, entering absorber,	kmol/h	107.7	34.51	145.62	84.57	2.66	1.52	2.65	0.642	379.872	45 bar g	314 (41)
	kg/h	217.55	966.63	6408.74	1356.50	79.99	42.58	90.31	11.56	9178.86		
	Mole % (dry)	28.4	9.1	38.4	22.3	0.7	0.4	0.7	–	100.00		
2. Treated gas flow, leaving absorber,	kmol/h	107.7	34.51	50.97	84.57	2.66	1.52	Nil	0.372	282.302	45 bar g	311 (38)
	kg/h	217.55	966.63	2243.19	1356.5	79.99	42.58	Nil	6.70	4913.14		
	Mole % (dry)	38.2	12.2	18.1	30.0	0.9	0.6	Nil	—	100.00 (< 50 ppm)		
3. Acid gas flow, leaving condensate accumulator	kmol/h	—	—	94.65	—	—	—	2.65	18.45	115.75	125 kPa a	333 (60)
	kg/h	—	—	4165.55	—	—	—	90.31	332.28	4588.14		
	Mole % (dry)	—	—	97.3	—	—	—	2.7	—	100.00		

(Contd.)

Table 8.16 Contd.

B. Liquid Streams

	Component					Pressure	Temperature, K (°C)
	MDEA	H_2O	H_2S	CO_2	Total		
Molar mass	119.12	18.01	34.08	44.01	—		
1. Lean MDEA solution flow to absorber, kmol/h	216.22	2656	0.43	32.01	2905.00	165 kPa a (at the bottom of the stripper)	389 (116)
kg/h	25767	47 854	14.7	1408.3	75044.0	47 bar g (at the inlet of the absorber)	311 (38)
mass %	34.34	63.76	0.02	1.88	100		
2. Rich MDEA solution flow from absorber, kmol/h	216.22	2656.48	3.08	126.66	3.002.44	45 bar g (at the bottom of the absorber)	329.6 (56.6)
kg/h	25767	47 856.5	105.0	5574.3	79 203.8	150 kPa a (at the inlet of the stripper)	363 (90)
mass %	32.49	60.35	0.13	7.03	100.00		
3. Reflux flow to stripper, kmol/h	—	97.30	—	—	97.30	125 kPa a (at the bottom of the stripper)	333 (60
kg/h	—	1752.30	—	—	1752.30	(at the bottom of the reflux drum)	
mass %	—	100.0	—	—	100.00		
4. Make-up consensate flow, kmol/h	—	18.17	—	—	18.17	140 kPa a	333 (60)
kg/h	—	327.3	—	—	327.3		
mass %	—	100.0	—	—	100.0		

Example 8.6 A caustic soda plant is power intensive. Due to the frequent power interruptions experienced in one plant, it is decided to change the critical drives in the plant by steam-driven turbines and also generate the required power with the help of a steam turbine-alternator set for electrolysis and driving the rest of the rotating machinery with motors.

For a 50 t/d caustic soda plant, the power requirement is nearly 3200 kW for electrolysis. In addition, power is also required for refrigerant and chlorine compressors, cooling water pump and other rotating machinery. The total power requirement at the power turbine shaft is estimated at 6832 kW, thus making available 6500 kW at the alternator shaft, i.e. ~ 95% efficiency.

A four-level cascade steam system is proposed. High pressure (HP) steam is generated at 115 bar a and 713 K (440°C) in the boiler. It is proposed to pass nearly the entire quantity of the HP steam through the power turbine. From this turbine, a definite quantity of medium pressure (MP) steam at 39 bar a and 593 K (320°C) is extracted. The balance of HP and MP steam is further utilised in the power turbine and the final exhaust at 323 K (50°C) and 12 kPa a (95% dry) is taken to a surface condenser (SC). The cascade steam system is shown in Fig. 8.4

MP steam is utilised in four equipments. Saturated steam @ 3 t/h at 15 bar a is required in the second-stage evaporator. This is obtained by letting down MP steam and desuperheating it.

The boiler has a balanced draft furnace. Based on start-up considerations, it is decided to have a forced-draft (FD) fan with a steam turbine driver and the induced-draft fan with a motor. Normal running boiler feed water (BFW) pump is a steam turbine driven while a motor driven BFW pump is a standby and is useful for start-up purpose. This arrangement also satisfies Indian Boiler Regulations requirements. Both, FD fan and BFW pump turbines, are back-pressure type. MP steam is introduced in these turbines while the exhaust steam at 4.4 bar a and 443 K (170°C) join the low-pressure (LP) steam header.

Large cooling water (CW) circulation will be required in the plant. One motor driven CW pump will be used during the start-up and not in normal run. The circulation rate will be stepped up to full requirements when a turbine driven CW pump is also put in operation. This turbine is proposed to be a condensing type and it utilises MP steam.

LP superheated steam is desuperheated and is used in the first stage evaporator (@ 9 t/h), ejectors for SC (@ 0.5 t/h), vacuum ejectors for evaporators (@ 2 t/h) and coil-type brine heater (@ 2 t/h).

Ejector steam from SC is condensed in inter/after condesners and the condensate is recycled with the condensate from the SC, evaporators and brine heater. The make-up boiler feed water @ 2 t/h is fed to the deaerator, the function of which is to remove oxygen from the water. This is done by boiling and stripping with saturated LP steam. BFW at 378 K (105°C) is pumped at 123.5 bar g and is fed to the boiler. A small amount of BFW is used for desuperheating. Based on these details, establish a steam balance in which HP steam generation is minimum.

Data:

Deaerator steam requirement = 0.11 kg/kg condensate

FD fan power requirement = 2.47 kW/t steam generated per hour

Energy conversion in turbine = 97% (including gland losses)

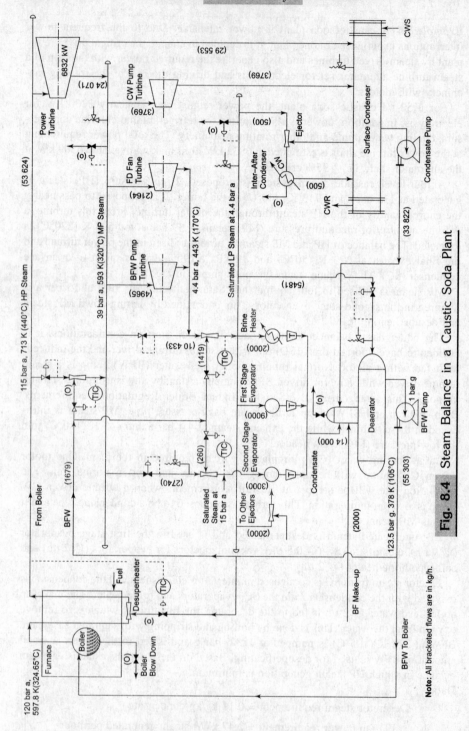

Fig. 8.4 Steam Balance in a Caustic Soda Plant

Note: All bracketed flows are in kg/h.

Specific volume of compressed water

at 123.5 bar g and 378 K(105° C) = 0.955 m^3/kg

Efficiency of BFW pump = 65%

Miscellaneous CW requirement excluding that in SC = 600 m^3/h

Permitted rise in CW temperature in SC = 10 K (10°C)

Discharge pressure of CW pump = 5 bar g

Efficiency of CW pump = 60%

Neglect losses between the machine and the driver, excluding that specified for the power turbine.

Solution:

Let a = Saturated LP steam input to deaerator, t/h

b = MP steam input to CW pump turbine, t/h

c = MP steam input to BFW pump turbine, t/h

d = MP steam input to FD fan turbine, t/h

e = Exhaust (under vacuum) from power turbine, t/h

g = Letdown from MP steam to LP steam, t/h

h = Letdown from HP steam to MP steam, t/h

Before making the balance of steam at each pressure level, it is necessary to find the specific steam consumptions in different turbines and also, BFW requirement in different desuperheaters.

Table 8.17 Specific Steam Requirements of Turbines

Initial steam conditions	Final steam conditions	Enthalpy available for energy conversion, kJ/kg	Actual energy conversion (97%), kJ/kg	Specific steam consumption in turbine, kg/kWh
115bar a 713 K (440°C) 3190.7 kJ/kg	39 bar a 593 K (320°C) 3020.4 kJ/kg	170.3	165.2	21.79
39 bar a 593 K (320°C) 3020.4 kJ/kg	4.4 bar a 443 K (170°C) 2793.3 kJ/kg	227.1	220.3	16.34
115 bar a 713 K (440°C) 3190.7 kJ/kg	12 kPa a 323 K (50°C) 2472.0 kJ/kg 95% dry	718.7	697.1	5.16
39 bar a 593 K (320°C) 3020.4 kJ/kg	12 kPa a 323 K (50°C) 2472.0 kJ/kg 95% dry	548.4	532.0	6.77

Table 8.18 BFW Requirements for Desuperheating
Enthalpy of BFW at 378 K (105°C) = 440.17 kJ/kg

Initial steam conditions			Final steam conditions			BFW Requirement kg/kg initial steam
Pressure bar a	Temp., K (°C)	Enthalpy, kJ/kg	Pressure bar a	Temp., K (°C)	Enthalpy, kJ/kg	
115	713 (440)	3190.7	39	593 (320)	3020.4	0.066
39	593 (320)	3020.4	15	Satd.	2789.9	0.095
39	593 (320)	3020.4	4.4	Satd.	2741.9	0.095
4.4	443 (170)	2793.3	4.4	Satd.	2741.9	0.022

Saturated 15 bar a steam

requirement in the second-stage evaporator = 3 t/h

$$\text{Equivalent MP steam} = \frac{3}{(1 + 0.095)} = 2.74 \text{ t/h}$$

Saturated LP steam header:

$$\text{Requirement} = 9 + 2 + 0.5 + 2 + a = 13.5 + a$$

Production of superheated LP steam = $c + d$

Equivalent saturated LP steam production = $(1 + 0.022)(c + d) + 1.121 g$

$$1.022 (c + d) + 1.121 g = 13.5 + a \tag{1}$$

Deaerator:

Condensate from LP steam consumers = $9 + 2 = 11$ t/h

Condensate from the second-stage evaporator = 3 t/h

at 123.5 bar g and 378 K (105°C) = 0.955 m³/kg

Boiler feed make-up water = 2 t/h

Condensate from SC = $b + e + 0.5$ t/h

$$a = 0.11 (b + e + 16.5)$$

$$a - 0.11 b - 0.11 e = 1.815 \tag{2}$$

Power turbine:
This turbine is a special turbine in which steam is partly extracted at a back pressure and also a part is exhausted under vacuum with 5% wetness.
If this turbine is totally a back pressure one,

$$\text{HP steam requirement} = 6832 \times 21.79 = 148\,869.3 \text{ kg/h}$$

$$\equiv 148.87 \text{ t/h}$$

If this turbine is totally a condensing type,

$$\text{HP steam requirement} = 6832 \times 5.16 = 35\,253.1 \text{ kg/h}$$

$$\equiv 35.25 \text{ t/h}$$

Both the above cases are extreme cases and the optimum consumption of HP steam will be between 35.25 and 148.87 t/h.

$$\text{MP steam consumption} =$$

$$b + c + d + g + 2.74$$

MP steam produced by direct letdown = $1.066 h$

HP steam through power turbine,
produced as MP steam = $b + c + d + g + 2.74 - 1.066 h$

$$\frac{(b+c+d+g+2.74-1.066h)\,1000}{21.79} + \frac{1000\,e}{5.16} = 6832$$

$$5.16\,b + 5.16\,c + 5.16\,d + 21.79\,e + 5.16\,g - 5.50\,h = 754.03 \qquad (3)$$

FD fan:

$$\text{Total HP steam produced} = b + c + d + g + 2.74 - 1.066\,h + h + e$$

$$= b + c + d + g + 2.74 - 0.066\,h + e \text{ t/h}$$

$$\text{FD fan power requirement} = 2.47\,(b + c + d + e + g - 0.066\,h + 2.74) \text{ kW}$$

FD fan turbine steam consumption $= d$

$$= \frac{2.47(b + c + d + e + g - 0.066h + 2.74)\,16.34}{1000}$$

or, $b + c - 23.78\,d + e + g - 0.066\,h = -2.74 \qquad (4)$

BFW pump:

$$\text{Total BFW} = a + b + e + 16.5 \text{ t/h}$$

$$\text{Head developed} = 123.5 \text{ bar}$$

$$\equiv 1310.7 \text{ m } H_2O \text{ at } 378 \text{ K } (105°C)$$

$$\text{Power requirement of the pump} = \frac{(a + b + e + 16.5)\,1310.7 \times 0.7355 \times 1000}{3600 \times 75 \times 0.65}$$

$$= 5.493\,(a + b + e + 16.5) \text{ kW}$$

BFW pump turbine steam requirement $= c$

$$= 5.493\,(a + b + e + 16.5)\,\frac{16.34}{1000}$$

$$a + b + e - 11.14\,c = -16.5 \qquad (5)$$

CW pumps:

$$\text{Enthalpy is given up in SC} = 2472.0 - 209.2 = 2262.8 \text{ kJ/kg}$$

$$\text{CW requirement in SC} = (b + e)\,\frac{2262.8}{(10 \times 4.1868)}$$

$$= 54.05\,b + 54.05\,e \text{ m}^3/\text{h}$$

$$\text{Total CW requirement} = 54.05\,b + 54.05\,e + 600 \text{ m}^3/\text{h}$$

$$\text{Head developed} = 5 \text{ bar g} = 51 \text{ m } H_2O \text{ at } 323 \text{ K}$$

Power requirement

$$\text{of CW pump} = \frac{(54.05\,b + 54.05\,e + 600)\,51 \times 0.7355 \times 1000}{3600 \times 75 \times 0.60}$$

$$= 0.2315\,(54.05\,b + 54.05\,e + 600) \text{ kW}$$

Steam consumption

$$\text{in CW pump turbine} = b$$

$$= \frac{0.2315\,(54.05\,b + 54.05\,e + 600)\,6.77}{1000}$$

$$584.01\,b - 54.05\,e = 600 \qquad (6)$$

Thus, six equations are available with seven unknowns. This is an optimization problem in which the aim is to minimize the production of HP steam, i.e. the boiler capacity. Since all the unknowns are positive (value ≥ 0) and all the equations are linear in nature, linear programming can be applied.

The objective function to be minimised is

$$Z = b + c + d + e + g - 0.066\,h + 2.74$$

subject to constraint equations developed earlier.

The Simplex method in linear algebra states that whenever there exists an optimum-feasible solution, it coincides with one of the basis feasible solutions. To determine the basis solution, the Gauss-Jordan reduction method can be adopted. The coefficient matrix of the constraint equation is

Table 8.19 Coefficients of Simultaneous Equations

Eq. No.	a	b	c	d	g	h	e	Constant
2	1	− 0.11	0	0	0	0	− 0.11	1.815
6	0	9.109	0	0	0	0	− 0.843	9.358
5	8.977	8.977	−100	0	0	0	8.977	− 148.115
4	0	− 4.037	− 4.037	96	− 4.037	0.266	− 4.037	11.061
3	0	5.16	5.16	5.16	5.16	− 5.50	21.79	754.03
1	− 1	0		1.022	1.022	1.121	0	0	13.5

The rows of the matrix are arranged to preserve the zeros.

Choosing e as a non-basic variable, the matrix can be converted to canonical form, which is given as follows.

Table 8.20 Coefficients of Simultaneous Equations in Canonical Form

Eq. No.	a	b	c	d	g	h	e	Constant
2	1	0	0	0	0	0	− 0.1202	1.9282
6	0	1	0	0	0	0	− 0.0927	1.0291
5	0	0	1	0	0	0	− 0.1089	1.7466
4	0	0	0	1	0	0	− 0.049	0.7163
3	0	0	0	0	1	0	0.0367	11.5172
1	0	0	0	0	0	1	− 3.9821	−117.683

From the above matrix, the solutions are:

$$a = 1.9282 + 0.1202\,e$$

$$b = 1.0291 + 0.0927\,e$$

$$c = 1.7466 + 0.1089\,e$$

$$d = 0.7163 + 0.049\,e$$

$$g = 11.5172 - 0.0367\,e$$

$$h = -117.683 + 3.9821\,e$$

Substituting the above value in the objective function,

$$Z = 25.5163 + 0.9511\,e$$

If e is taken as zero, h is negative which is not feasible. Further, h cannot assume a negative value and e should have a minimum value. Therefore h should be zero.

When $h = 0$,

$$e = 29.553 \text{ t/h}$$
$$a = 5.481 \text{ t/h}$$
$$b = 3.769 \text{ t/h}$$
$$c = 4.965 \text{ t/h}$$
$$d = 2.164 \text{ t/h}$$
$$g = 10.433 \text{ t/h}$$

and $Z_{min} = 53.624$ t/h

Mathcad solution:

Using 6 equations, following two matrices are defined.

$$M := \begin{bmatrix} 1 & 0 & -1.022 & -1.022 & 0 & -1.121 \\ 1 & -0.11 & 0 & 0 & -0.11 & 0 \\ 0 & 5.16 & 5.16 & 5.16 & 21.79 & 5.16 \\ 0 & 1 & 1 & -23.78 & 1 & 1 \\ 1 & 1 & -11.14 & 0 & 1 & 0 \\ 0 & 584.01 & 0 & 0 & -54.05 & 0 \end{bmatrix} \qquad v := \begin{bmatrix} -13.5 \\ 1.815 \\ 754.03 \\ -2.74 \\ -16.5 \\ 600 \end{bmatrix}$$

$$\text{soln} := \text{lsolve}(M, v)$$

$$\text{soln} = \begin{bmatrix} 5.48 \\ 3.763 \\ 4.964 \\ 2.164 \\ 29.555 \\ 10.433 \end{bmatrix}$$

$a := \text{soln}_0 \quad b := \text{soln}_1 \quad c := \text{soln}_2 \quad d := \text{soln}_3 \quad e := \text{soln}_4 \quad g := \text{soln}_5$

$a = 5.48 \quad b = 3.763 \quad c = 4.964 \quad d = 2.164 \quad e = 29.555 \quad g = 10.433$ all in t/h

$Z := b + c + d + e + g + 2.74$

$Z = 53.618$ t/h

All these steam consumptions are given in Fig. 8.4.

Note: In this example, it was proved that $h = 0$ only yields an optimal solution. However, a case can arise in which more then one variable can become negative when the solution is expressed in terms of a basic variable (such as e in this example). In such a case, the Simplex criterion can help in arriving at the optimal solution.

Example 8.7 In an effort to conserve energy, it is decided to incorporate two boiler feed water (BFW) heaters in the cascade steam system of Example 8.6. BFW from the discharge of the pump enters BFW Heater I where it will be heated from 378 K

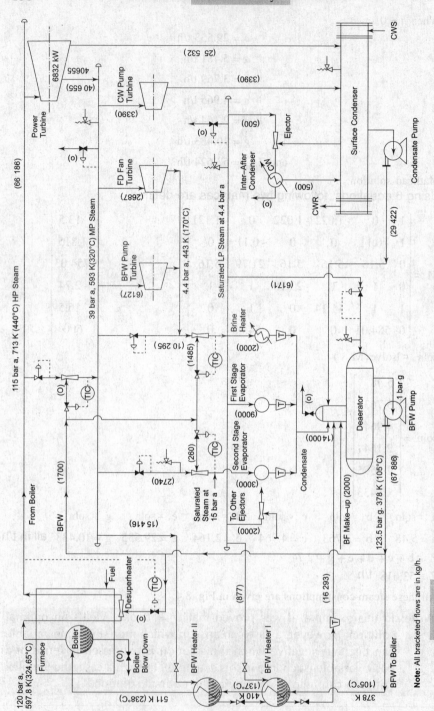

Fig. 8.5 Steam balance in a Caustic Soda plant with BFW Heaters.

Note: All bracketed flows are in kg/h.

(105°C) to 410 K (137°C) with the help of saturated LP steam. Further BFW will be heated to 511 K (238°C) with the help of superheated MP steam in BFW Heater II. Both the BFW Heaters are operated at header pressures with negligible pressure drops. Deaerator steam requirement will be reduced to 0.10 kg/kg condensate as a result of receipt of hot condensates from BFW heaters. Revised steam system is shown in Fig. 8.5.

Considering all other parameters unchanged, establish the steam balance.

Solution: Basis: 100 kg BFW, entering BFW Heaters I and II Heat balance across BFW Heater II:

Enthalpy of superheated steam at 39 bar a and 593 K (320°C) = 3020.4 kJ/kg

From A III.2, at 39 bar a, T_s = 521.99 K (248.84°C),

h = 1080.13 kJ/kg and λ_v = 1720.6 kJ/kg

Heat transferred to BFW = 3020.4 – 1080.1

= 1940.3 kJ/kg steam

Enthalpy of condensate at 410 K (137°C) and 511 K (238°C) are read as 576.2 and 1028.1 kJ/kg, respectively from A III.2.

Heat picked up by BFW in Heater II = 1028.1 – 576.2

= 451.9 kJ/kg

Superheated MP steam input = $\dfrac{451.9 \times 100}{1940.3}$

= 23.29 kg

Further, steam condensate at 521.99 K (248.84°C) will enter BFW Heater I.

Heat balance across BFW Heater I:

Steam condensate at 521.84 K (248.84°C) enters BFW Heater I and flashes at 4.4 bar a.

From A III.2, at 4.4 bar a, T_s = 420.24 K(147.09°C),

h = 619.6 kJ/kg and λ_v = 2122.3 kJ/kg

Heat available from MP steam condensate

= 1080.1 – 619.6 = 460.5 kJ/kg condensate

Total heat available = 460.5 × 23.29

= 10 725kJ

Now BFW is heated from 378 K(105°C) to 410 K(137°C), increasing its enthalpy from 440.2 to 576.2 kJ/kg.

Heat picked up by BFW in Heater I = 100 (576.2 – 440.2)

= 13 600 kJ

Heat required from saturated LP steam

= 13600 – 10 725 = 2875 kJ

LP steam condensed = 2875/2122.3

= 1.325 kg

Total condensate from BFW Heaters, entering deaerator

= 23.29 + 1.325

= 24.615 kg

Thus MP steam and LP steam consumptions are 0.2329 kg and 0.013 25 kg per kg condensate passed through the BFW Heater II and BFW Heater I respectively.

Condensate enters deaerator at 420.24 K(147.09°C) and flashes at 1 bar g. Availability of flash steam will result in less LP saturated steam requirement in deaerator which is estimated at 0.01 kg/kg total condensate, entering deaerator.

New basis: 6832 kW at power turbine shaft

Let j = Total BFW pumped by BFW pump, t/h and

   m = BFW used for quenching in desuperheaters, t/h

Assume $h = 0$.

Total BFW, $j = a + b + e + 16.5 + 0.246\,15\,(j - m)$

and $m = 0.121\,g + 0.260 + 0.022\,(c + d)$

Saturated LP Steam Header:

$$\text{Requirement} = 9 + 2 + 0.5 + 2 + a + 0.013\,25\,(j - m)$$

Production of saturated LP steam = $1.022\,(c + d) + 1.121\,g$

Equating the requirement and production, substituting values of j and m and simplifying,

$$1.022\,(c + d) + 1.121\,g - 13.5 + a + 0.013\,25\,(j - m) \tag{1}$$

Deaerator:

$$\begin{aligned}\text{Total condensate} = &\text{ condensate from SC} + 16.0\text{ t/h from}\\ &\text{ejectors and BF make-up} + \text{condensate}\\ &\text{from BFW Heaters}\end{aligned}$$

$$= b + e + 0.5 + 16.0 + 0.246\,15\,(j - m)$$

$$a = 0.1\,[b + e + 0.5 + 16.0 + 0.246\,15\,(j - m)] \tag{2}$$

Power Turbine:

Total MP superheated steam consumption,

$$x = b + c + d + g + 2.74 + 0.2329\,j$$

$$\frac{x \times 1000}{21.79} + \frac{1000\,e}{5.16} = 6832 \tag{3}$$

FD Fan:

Total HP steam produced = $x + e$

$$d = \frac{2.47 \times 16.34\,(x + e)}{1000} \tag{4}$$

BFW Pump:

$$c = \frac{5.493 \times 16.34\,j}{1000} \tag{5}$$

CW Pump:

Balance remains unchanged.

$$584.01\,b - 54.05\,e = 600 \tag{6}$$

Mathcad solution:
Guess values:

a := 5.5   c := 5   g := 10.5   m := 1.5   x := 40

b := 3.8   d := 2.2   e := 3.3   j := 16   Z := 66

Given

$j = a + b + e + 16.5 + 0.24615(j - m)$

$m = 0.121 \cdot g + 0.26 + 0.022(c + d)$

$1.022(c + d) + 1.121 \cdot g = 13.5 + a + 0.01325(j - m)$

$a = 0.1 \cdot (b + e + 16.5 + 0.24615(j - m))$

$x = b + c + d + g + 2.74 + 0.2329j$

$\dfrac{x \cdot 1000}{21.79} + \dfrac{1000 \cdot e}{5.16} = 6832$

$d = \dfrac{2.47 \cdot 16.34 (x + e)}{1000}$

$c = \dfrac{5.493 \cdot 16.43j}{1000}$

$584.01 \cdot b - 54.05 \cdot e = 600$

$Z = b + c + d + e + g + 2.74 + 0.2329(j - m)$

vec := Find(a, b, c, d, e, g, j, m, x, Z)

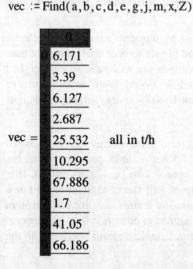

vec =   all in t/h

6.171
3.39
6.127
2.687
25.532
10.295
67.886
1.7
41.05
66.186

All the steam flows are given in Fig. 8.5.

It may be noted that boiler will generate 66.186 t/h HP superheated steam as compared to 53.624 t/h, calculated in Example 8.6. Apparently it looks like spending more energy than the original case. A closer look reveals actual energy savings.

For the original case (Example 8.6),

Heat pick-up in the boiler = 3190.7 − 440.2

= 2750.2 kJ/kg steam

Total heat absorption, $\phi_1 = 53\,624 \times 2750.2$

$$= 147\,476\,725 \text{ kJ/h}$$

$$\equiv 40\,965.8 \text{ kW}$$

In the steam system with BFW heaters,

Heat pick-up in the boiler $= 3190.7 - 1028.1$

$$= 2162.6 \text{ kJ/kg steam}$$

Total heat absorption, $\phi_2 = 66\,186 \times 2162.6$

$$= 143\,133\,844 \text{ kJ/h}$$

$$\equiv 39\,759.4 \text{ kW}$$

Assume boiler efficiency of 75% with NCV of fuel as 40 000 kJ/kg.

$$\text{Energy saving} = \frac{(147\,476\,725 - 143\,133\,844)\,100}{147\,476\,725}$$

$$= 2.95\%$$

$$\text{Fuel saving} = \frac{(147\,476\,725 - 143\,133\,844)}{0.75 \times 40\,000}$$

$$= 144.8 \text{ kg/h}$$

There is also a substantial reduction in cooling load of the surface condenser. Steam condensation requirement in the surface condenser will reduce from 33 822 to 29 422 kg/h, representing a reduction of 13.0%.

It is now clear that there are all-around benefits by introduction of BFW Heaters. Howevers, cost of BFW Heaters, bigger boiler and bigger turbine will be higher than those for the original case. Additional cost of equipments will have to be weighed against savings in fuel consumption and reduction in cooling tower load. Return of investment will determine the selection of system. Usually energy saving outweighs the investment in such a case.

Example 8.8 In another energy conservation exercise to the steam system described in Example 8.7, it is decided to draw steam at 7.5 bar a (back pressure) from the turbine as shown in Fig. 8.7. Its temperature is expected to be 473 K(200°C). It is compressed in a thermocompressor with the help of MP steam to achieve 15 bar a steam which will then be desuperheated to its saturation temperature for utilization in second stage evaporator. Thermocompressor is designed to compress 0.45 kg steam at 7.5 bar a and 473 K(200°C) with 1 kg of MP steam. Establish steam balance with the thermocompressor and BFW Heaters.

Solution:

Basis: 45 kg steam at 7.5 bar a and 473 K(200°C)

Enthalpy of steam at 7.5 bar a and 473 K = 2841.4 kJ/kg   (Ref. A III.3)

Total enthalpy of compressed steam at 15 bar a

$$= 45 \times 2841.4 + 100 \times 3020.4$$

$$= 429\,903 \text{ kJ/145 kg steam}$$

$$\equiv 2964.85 \text{ kJ/kg steam}$$

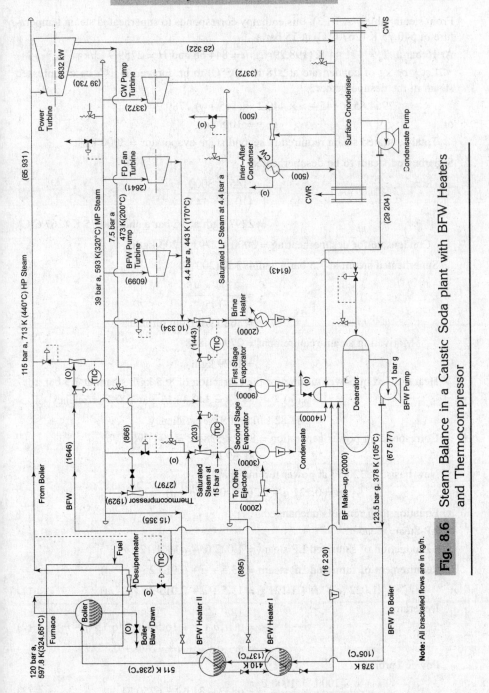

Fig. 8.6 Steam Balance in a Caustic Soda plant with BFW Heaters and Thermocompressor

Note: All bracketed flows are in kg/h.

From steam tables (A III.3), this enthalpy corresponds to superheated steam temperature of 540.75 K (267.6°C) at 15 bar a.

At 15 bar a, $T_s = 471.44$ K (198.29°C), $h = 844.66$ and $H = 2789.9$ kJ/kg

Let y be kg of condensate at 378 K (105°C) to be sprayed in 145 kg compressed steam in the desuperheater.

$$2964.85 \times 145 + y \times 440.2 = (145 + y)\, 2789.9$$

or $\qquad\qquad y = 10.8$ kg

Total saturated steam required in second stage evaporator = 3000 kg/h

Superheated steam to be desuperheated

$$= \frac{145 \times 3000}{(10.5 + 145)}$$

$$= 2797 \text{ kg/h at 15 bar a and 540.75 K (267.6°C)}$$

Condensate for desuperheating = 3000 − 2797 = 203 kg/h

Superheated steam at 7.5 bar a and 473 K (200°C)

$$= \frac{2797 \times 45}{145}$$

$$= 868 \text{ kg/h from turbine}$$

Motivating steam requirement = 2797 − 868

$$= 1929 \text{ kg/h}$$

Heat utilised in power turbine for the extraction of 868 kg/h steam at 7.5 bar a

$$= 3190.7 - 2841.4 = 349.3 \text{ kJ/kg at 100\% efficiency}$$

$$\equiv 338.82 \text{ kJ/kg at 97\% efficiency}$$

Corresponding power generation = 868 × 338.82 = 294 096 kJ/h

$$\equiv 81.69 \text{ kW}$$

New basis: 6832 kW at power turbine shaft

$$m = 0.121\, g + 0.203 + 0.22\, (c + d)$$

Equation for j remains unchanged.

LP Steam Header:

Production of saturated LP steam = $1.022\, (c + d) + 1.121\, g$

Requirement of saturated LP steam = $13.5 + a + 0.013\,25\, (j - m)$

$$1.022\, (c + d) + 1.121\, g = 13.5 + a + 0.013\,25\, (j - m) \qquad (1)$$

Deaerator:

$$a = 0.1\,[b + e + 16.5 + 0.246\,15\,(j - m) \qquad (2)$$

$$x = b + c + d + g + 1.929 + 0.2329\, j$$

Power Turbine:

$$\frac{x \times 1000}{21.79} \times \frac{1000\, e}{5.16} = 6832 - 81.69 = 6750.31 \qquad (3)$$

Equations for FD Fan, BFW Pump and CW Punp turbines remain uncharged

Mathcad solution:

Guess values:

$a := 5.5$ $c := 5$ $g := 10.5$ $m := 1.5$ $x := 40$

$b := 3.8$ $d := 2.2$ $e := 3.3$ $j := 16$ $Z := 66$

Given

$j = a + b + e + 16.5 + 0.24615(j - m)$

$m = 0.121 \cdot g + 0.203 + 0.022(c + d)$

$1.022(c + d) + 1.121 \cdot g = 13.5 + a + 0.01325(j - m)$

$a = 0.1 \cdot (b + e + 16.5 + 0.24615(j - m))$

$x = b + c + d + g + 1.929 + 0.2329j$

$\dfrac{x \cdot 1000}{21.79} + \dfrac{1000e}{5.16} = 6750.3$

$d = \dfrac{2.47 \cdot 16.34 (x + e)}{1000}$

$c = \dfrac{5.493 \cdot 16.43j}{1000}$

$584.01 \cdot b - 54.05e = 600$

$Z = b + c + d + e + g + 2.797 + 0.2329(j - m)$

$vec := Find(a, b, c, d, e, g, j, m, x, Z)$

vec =	0	
	0	6.143
	1	3.372
	2	6.099
	3	2.641
	4	25.332	all in t/h
	5	10.334
	6	67.577
	7	1.646
	8	40.114
	9	65.931

All the steam flows are given in Fig. 8.6

> *Note:* This indicates a marginal reduction in HP steam production (255 kg/h) and may not prove economically attractive as the cost of the power turbine may offset the savings. However, the example indicates yet another possibility of energy saving.

Multistage efficient turbines with multiple extraction facilities have resulted in economizing the steam consumptions. The trend is to select an efficient turbine. When all these conditions are taken into account, the most optimal steam balance is obtained.

Steam balance has assumed considerable importance in the process industry. Apart from the increased reliability, it has been proved to be an excellent working tool and an energy-saving measure. Frequent checks of the actual steam balance in the plant enables visualization of the plant's overall steam, condensate and BFW demands, as well as quick identification of upset conditions and their effects[7].

Steam balance making is an art. Brinkso[8] and Matas-Valiente[8] have given a step-by-step procedure for making a steam balance. Useful guidelines can be derived from these articles for making a steam balance for any plant. Using these guidelines, various steam balances are developed in this book. To start with, a steam balance is made with theoretical considerations as is the case with Example 8.6. A number of overriding parameters, based on process conditions, are to be kept in mind before selecting a type of turbine for a particular machine. Start-up requirements, power failure, boiler trip, etc. are some of these process conditions. Subsequently, exact consumptions, specified by selected turbine vendors (inclusive of gland losses), are inserted in the balance and thereby the actual working steam balance is obtained.

Example 8.9 Methyl tertialy butyl ether (MTBE) is produced by reaction between methanol and i-butene. This is a well-known oxygenating product for improvement of octane number of gasolines. This is a catalytic reaction and in a typical process, sulphuric acid is used as a catalyst[10].

The feed to the plant is a C_4-cut stream of a steam cracker which contains 45% i-butent and 55% other C_4-hydrocarbons by mass (having average molar mass = 56). It is mixed with methanol such that mole ratio of methanol to i-butene at the reactor inlet (mixed feed) is 1.1. Sulphuric acid in the mixed feed is 5% (by mass). Two reactors are used in series. In the first reactor, 90% conversion of i-butene is achieved while total conversion of 98% of i-butent is achieved at the outlet of the second reactor. While fresh methanol is of 100% strength, recycle methanol stream contains 2% water, 2% MTBE and 6% C_4-hydrocarbons (on mole basis). Water, recycled with methanol, reacts with i-butene to form tertiary butyl alcohol (TBA). Also nearly 0.35% i-butene is converted to Di-iso-butene (DIB). Reactions taking place in the reactors are given as follows.

$$CH_3-CH_2-CH{=}CH_2 + CH_3OH = H_3C-\underset{\underset{CH_3}{|}}{\overset{\overset{CH_3}{|}}{C}}-O-CH_3 \qquad (A)$$

i-Butene \qquad MeOH \qquad MTBE

$$CH_3-CH_2-CH{=}CH_2 + H_2O = H_3C-\underset{\underset{CH_3}{|}}{\overset{\overset{CH_3}{|}}{C}}-OH \qquad (B)$$

i-Butene \qquad\qquad Water \qquad TBA

$$2C_4H_8 \qquad = \qquad (C_4H_8)_2 \qquad (C)$$

i-Butene \qquad\qquad DIB

In the first reactor (R1), reaction mixture enters at 20 bar a and 343 K (70°C). Reaction temperature is controlled below 393 K (120°C) in the reactor. Product mixture is cooled to 313 K (40°C) and sent to second reactor (R2), operating at 16.2 bar a. Exit temperature from R2 is controlled to 322 K (49°C) by cooling within the reactor.

Product mixture from R2 is cooled to 313 K (40°C) and allowed to separate into two phases; an organic phase and an acid phase in Settler (S). 90% acid is recovered from the settler in T1 with negligible organic impurities. Recovered acid alongwith fresh acid (of 100% strength) is fed to the mixed feed.

Organic phase from S is sent to Water Washing Column (C1) which is a rotating disc conactor. It operates at 10 bar a. Caustic soda solution of 46% (by mass) strength is used as make-up. Diluted solution is introduced to C1 is stoichiometric quantity.

The extract phase is fed to a packed column (C2) which operates at 1.5 bar a. Live steam at 15 bar a is used for stripping off methanol alongwith organic impurities at the rate of 4.2 kmol steam per kmol methanol. Overhead vapours are recycled to the reactor at 345 K (72°C). Bottom product from C2 leaves at 384 K (111°C) and sent to Water Purge Tank (T2) in which Na_2SO_4 concentration is maintained at 10% (by mass). Methanol in the bottom product from C2 is approximately 0.5% (by mass).

In column C3, overhead product is C_4-hydrocarbons which contains unconverted i-butent and a small amount of MTBE. Loss of MTBE in the overhead is 1.3% of the total production. Bottom product from C3 contains 99 mole % MTBE, balance being TBA and DIB. C_4-hydrocarbons in the bottom product is approximately 0.5 mole %. This column operates at nearly 10 bar a. Steam 15 at bar a is supplied to the reboiler. Both the products from the column are cooled and sent to storage. The process flow diagram is given in Fig. 8.7.

For a production rate of 15 t/h of MTBE (100%), establish the material balance of each process stream.

Solution: Basis: 15 000 kg/h MTBE (100%)

Overall material balance:

$$\text{Desired MTBE production rate} = \frac{15\,000}{88} = 170.45 \text{ kmol/h}$$

$$\text{Bottom product from C3} = \frac{170.45}{0.99} = 172.18 \text{ kmol/h}$$

Loss of MTBE in the overhead

$$\text{stream from C3} = 170.45 \times \frac{1.3}{98.7}$$

$$= 2.25 \text{ kmol/h}$$

$$\text{Total MTBE production} = 170.45 + 2.25 = 172.70 \text{ kmol/h}$$

Let fresh feed be F_1 kmol/h (of i-butene + C_4s)

$$i\text{-butene feed rate} = 0.55\ F_1 \text{ kmol/h}$$

Note that i-butene and C_4s have the same molar mass and hence mass % equals mole %.

$$\text{Conversion of } i\text{-butene} = 0.98 \times 0.55\ F_1 \text{ (overall)}$$

$$= 0.539\ F_1 \text{ kmol/h}$$

$$i\text{-butene converted to DIB} = 0.0035 \times 0.55\ F_1 = 0.002\ F_1 \text{ kmol/h}$$

Let fresh methanol feed be F_2 kmol/h and recycle stream be R kmol/h of methanol recycle.

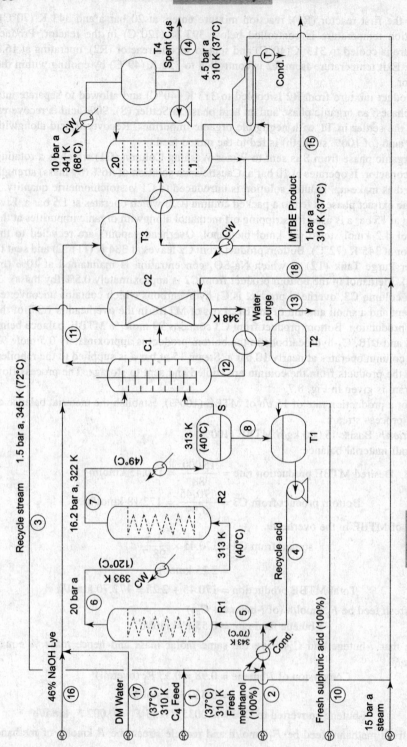

Fig. 8.7 Manufacture of MTBE Using Sulphuric Acid as Catalyst

Methanol content of recycle stream = $0.9\,R$ kmol/h

Total methanol charged = $(F_2 + 0.9\,R)$ kmol/h

$$\frac{\text{Methanol}}{i - \text{butane}} = 1.1$$

$$\frac{F_2 + 0.9\,R}{0.55\,F_1} = 1.1 \text{ or}$$

$$F_2 + 0.9\,R = 0.605\,F_1 \tag{1}$$

Water content of recycle stream = $0.02\,R$ kmol/h

i-butene consumed for TBA production = $0.02\,R$ kmol/h

$$
\begin{aligned}
\text{i-butene consumed to MTBE} &= 0.539\,F_1 - 0.02\,R - 0.002\,F_1 \\
&= 0.537\,F_1 - 0.02\,R \text{ kmol/h}
\end{aligned}
$$

Methanol consumed = $0.537\,F_1 - 0.02\,R$ kmol/h

$$
\begin{aligned}
\text{Unconverted methanol} &= F_2 + 0.9\,R - 0.537\,F_1 + 0.02\,R \\
&= F_2 - 0.537\,F_1 + 0.92\,R \text{ kmol/h}
\end{aligned}
$$

Acid content of mixture = 5% by mass

Table 8.21 Composition of Mixed Feed (without Acid)

Component	kmol/h	Molar mass	kg/h
i-butene	$0.55\,F_1$	56	$30.8\,F_1$
C_4s	$0.45\,F_1 + 0.06\,R$	56	$25.2\,F_1 + 3.36\ R$
Water	$0.02\,R$	18	$0.36\,R$
MTBE	$0.02\,R$	88	$1.76\,P$
CH_3OH	$F_2 + 0.9\,R$	32	$32\,F_2 + 28.8\,R$
Total	$F_1 + F_2 + R$		$56\,F_1 + 32\,F_2 + 34.28\,R$

$$
\begin{aligned}
\text{Acid content of mixed feed} &= \frac{(56\,F_1 + 32\,F_2 + 34.28\,R)0.05}{0.95} \\
&= 2.947\,F_1 + 1.684\,F_2 + 1.804\,R \text{ kg/h}
\end{aligned}
$$

$$
\begin{aligned}
\text{Acid in the feed to C1} &= 0.1\,(2.947\,F_1 + 1.684\,F_2 + 1.804\,R) \\
&= 0.2947\,F_1 + 0.1684\,F_2 + 0.1804\,R \text{ kg/h}
\end{aligned}
$$

$$2\,NaOH + H_2SO_4 = Na_2SO_4 + 2\,H_2O \tag{D}$$

$$2 \times 40 \qquad 98 \qquad 142 \qquad 2 \times 18$$

$$
\begin{aligned}
Na_2SO_4 \text{ produced} &= (0.2947\,F_1 + 0.1684\,F_2 + 0.1804\,R)\frac{142}{98} \\
&= 0.427\,F_1 + 0.244\,F_2 + 0.2613\,R \text{ kg/h}
\end{aligned}
$$

Water purge contains 10% Na_2SO_4.

$$
\begin{aligned}
\text{Water purge flow rate (stream 13)} &= \frac{0.427\,F_1 + 0.244\,F_2 + 0.2613\,R}{0.1} \\
&= 4.27\,F_1 + 2.44\,F_2 + 2.613\,R \text{ kg/h}
\end{aligned}
$$

Methanol in water purge (i.e., loss in stream 13)

$$
\begin{aligned}
&= \text{Water purge flow} \times 0.005 \\
&= 0.02135\,F_1 + 0.0122\,F_2 + 0.0131\,R \text{ kg/h} \\
&\equiv 0.00067\,F_1 + 0.00038\,F_2 + 0.00041\,R \text{ kmol/h}
\end{aligned}
$$

Methanol recycled = methanol unconverted − methanol lost in water purge

$$= F_2 - 0.537\ F_1 + 0.92\ R - 0.000\ 67\ F_1$$
$$- 0.000\ 38\ F_2 - 0.000\ 41\ R$$
$$= 0.999\ 62\ F_2 - 0.537\ 67\ F_1 + 0.919\ 59\ R \text{ kmol/h}$$
$$= 0.9\ R \quad \text{(given)}$$
$$0.999\ 62\ F_2 - 0.537\ 67\ F_1 = -0.019\ 59\ R$$

or
$$F_2 - 0.537\ 87\ F_1 = -0.0196\ R \tag{2}$$
$$\text{MTBE produced} = 0.537\ F_1 - 0.02\ R = 172.7 \tag{3}$$

Solving the three equations:
$$F_1 = 322.511 \text{ kmol/h}$$
$$F_2 = 172.987 \text{ kmol/h}$$
$$R = 24.592 \text{ kmol/h}$$
$$\text{Total methanol fed} = 172.987 + 22.133 = 195.120 \text{ kmol/h}$$

$$\text{Mole ratio of } \frac{\text{methanol}}{i-\text{butane}} = \frac{195.120}{177.381} = 1.1 \text{ (Check !)}$$

Acid content of mixed feed (Stream 5) $= 2.947 \times 322.511 + 1.684$
$$\times\ 172.987 + 1.804 \times 24.592]$$
$$= 950.44 + 291.31 + 44.36$$
$$= 1286.11 \text{ kg/h} \equiv 13.123 \text{ kmol/h}$$

$$\text{Recycle acid} = 1286.11 \text{ kg/h} \qquad \text{(Stream 4)}$$
$$\text{Make-up acid} = 1286.11 \times 0.1 = 128.61 \text{ kg/h} \quad \text{(Stream 10)}$$

Material balance across Reactor R1:

Conversion of i-butene in R1 = 90%   (given)

Assume conversion of water to TBA = 100% in R1

Conversion of i-butene $= 177.381 \times 0.9 = 159.643$ kmol/h

TBA formed = water consumed
$$\doteq 0.492 \text{ kmol/h} = i\text{-butene consumed}$$

i-butene consumed to MTBE $= 159.643 - 0.492 = 159.151$ kmol/h
$$= CH_3OH \text{ consumed} = \text{MTBE produced}$$

Material balance across rector R2:

Total i-butene conversion = 98%

Additional i-butene conversion in R2 $= 98 - 90 = 8\%$

i-butene consumed $= 177.381 \times 0.08 = 14.191$ kmol/h

i-butene converted to DIB $= 177.381 \times 0.0035 = 0.621$ kmol/h

$$\text{DIB formed} = \frac{0.621}{2} = 0.3105 \text{ kmol/h}$$

i-butene converted to MTBE $= 14.191 - 0.621 = 13.57$ kmol/h
$$= CH_3OH \text{ consumed} = \text{MTBE produced}$$

Material balance across Column C2:

Steam input $= 4.2 \times$ moles of CH_3OH in extract phase
$$= 4.2 \times 22.399 = 94.076 \text{ kmol/h}$$
$$\equiv 1701.37 \text{ kg/h} \qquad \text{(Stream-18)}$$

$$Na_2SO_4 \text{ produced} = 0.427 \, F_1 + 0.244 \, F_2 + 0.2613 \, R$$
$$= 137.71 + 42.21 + 6.43 = 186.35 \text{ kg/h}$$

Acid neutralized = 128.61 kg/h

Na_2SO_4 production, based on

$$\text{acid consumption} = \frac{142 \times 128.61}{98} = 186.35 \text{ kg/h} \qquad \text{(Check !)}$$

$$H_2O \text{ produced} = \frac{36 \times 128.61}{98} = 47.24 \text{ kg/h}$$

NaOH required for neturalization = 186.35 + 47.24 − 128.61
$$= 104.98 \text{ kg/h}$$

$$\text{Bottom product from C2} = \frac{186.35}{0.09} = 2070.55 \text{ kg/h}$$

Recycle stream R = 24.592 kmol/h = 843.02 kg/h

Extract phase from C1 = 843.02 + 2070.55 − 1710.37
$$= 1203.20 \text{ kg/h}$$

Methanol loss in bottom

$$\text{Product from C2} = 0.021 \, 35 \, F_1 + 0.0122 \, F_2 + 0.0131 \, R$$
$$= 6.89 + 2.11 + 0.32 = 9.32 \text{ kg/h}$$

Total methanol consumption = 159.151 + 13.57 = 172.721 kmol/h

This figure matches well with Stream 2.

Water entering in extract phase of C1 = 174.28 kg/h

$$\text{NaOH strength required} = \frac{104.98 \times 100}{(104.98 + 174.28)} = 37.6\%$$

NaOH strength of lye = 46.0%

$$\text{Lye supply} = \frac{104.98}{0.46} = 228.22 \text{ kg/h} \qquad \text{(Stream 16)}$$

Fresh water added = 279.26 − 228.22 = 51.04 kg/h   (Stream 17)

$$\text{Loss of MTBE} = \frac{199.44 \times 100}{15199.44} = 1.31\% \qquad \qquad Ans.$$

Material balance results are summarised in Table 8.22.

EXERCISES

8.1 A packed column is packed with carbon Raschig rings[11]. It is used to absorb CO_2 in the solution containing $KHCO_3$. The solution is 3 N, based on potassium content. At the inlet, 30% of K in the solution is found to be in the form of bicarbonates. In the exit solution, bicarbonate amounts to 68% of the total K. The entering gas contains 18% CO_2 while the CO_2 content of the leaving gas is 6.9%, both on dry volume % basis. The solution flow rate is 1.65 L/s. Calculate

    (a) the analysis of entering and leaving solution in g/L,

    (b) the absorption rate of CO_2 in kg/h,

Table 8.22 Material Balance of MTBE Production Plant

Component	Stream 1				Stream 2				Stream 3			
	kg/h	mass%	kmol/h	mole%	kg/h	mass%	kmol/h	mole %	kg/h	mass%	kmol/h	mole %
i-butene	9 939.34	55.0	177.391	55.0					82.60	9.80	1.475	6.0
C_4s	8 127.28	45.0	145.130	45.0					708.26	84.01	22.133	90.0
MeOH					5535.58	100.0	172.987	100.0	43.30	5.14	0.492	2.0
MTBE									43.30	5.14	0.492	2.0
H_2O									8.86	1.05	0.492	2.0
Total	18066.62	100.0	322.521	100.0	5535.58	100.0	172.987	100.0	843.02	100.0	24.592	100.0

Component	Stream 4				Stream 5				Stream 6			
	kg/h	mass%	kmol/h	mole%	kg/h	mass%	kmol/h	mole %	kg/h	mass%	kmol/h	mole %
i-butene	9933.34	38.61	177.381	33.27	993.33	3.86	17.738	4.75	196.63	0.77	3.547	0.99
C_4s	8209.88	31.91	146.605	27.50	8209.88	31.91	146.605	39.24	8209.88	31.91	146.605	40.76
MeOH	6243.84	24.27	195.12	36.59	1151.01	4.45	35.969	9.63	716.77	2.79	22.399	6.21
MTBE	43.30	0.17	0.492	0.09	14048.58	54.61	159.643	42.74	15242.74	59.25	173.213	48.16
H_2O	8.86	0.04	0.492	0.09	Nil	Nil	Nil	Nil	Nil	Nil	Nil	Nil
H_2SO_4	1286.11	5.00	13.123	2.46	1 286.11	5.00	13.123	3.51	1286.11	5.00	13.123	3.65
TBA					36.41	0.14	0.492	0.13	36.41	0.14	0.492	0.14
DIB									34.76	0.14	0.310	0.09
Total	25 725.33	100.00	533.213	100.00	25725.32	100.00	373.570	100.00	25725.32	100.00	359.689	100.00

(Contd.)

Table 8.22 (Contd.)

Component	Stream 11				Stream 12				Stream 13			
	kg/h	mass%	kmol/h	mole%	kg/h	mass%	kmol/h	mole%	kg/h	mass%	kmol/h	mole%
i-butene	198.63	0.84	3.547	1.10	—	—	—	—	—	—	—	—
C$_4$s	8127.28	34.44	145.130	45.04	82.60	6.87	1.475	4.24	—	—	—	—
MeOH	—	—	—	—	716.77	59.57	22.399	64.35	8.51	0.41	0.266	0.25
MTBE	15197.44	64.41	172.721	53.61	43.30	3.6	0.492	1.41	—	—	—	—
H$_2$O	—	—	—	—	174.28	14.48	9.682	27.81	1875.69	90.59	104.205	99.02
TBA	36.41	0.16	0.492	0.15	—	—	—	—	—	—	—	—
DIB	34.76	0.15	0.310	0.10	186.35	15.48	0.762	2.19	186.35	9.00	0.762	0.73
Na$_2$SO$_4$	—	—	—	—	—	—	—	—	—	—	—	—
Total	23596.52	100.00	322.200	100.00	1203.20	100.00	34.810	100.00	2070.55	100.00	105.233	100.00

Component	Stream 14				Stream 15			
	kg/h	mass%	kmol/h	mole%	kg/h	mass%	kmol/h	mole%
i-butene	198.63	2.35	3.547	2.36	51.97	0.34	0.928	0.54
C$_4$s	8075.31	95.30	144.202	96.13	15000.00	99.19	170.455	99.00
MTBE	199.44	2.35	2.266	1.51	—	—	—	—
TBA	—	—	—	—	36.41	0.24	0.492	0.28
DIB	—	—	—	—	34.76	0.23	0.310	0.18
Total	8473.38	100.00	150.015	100.00	15123.14	100.0	172.185	100.00

(c) the % recovery of CO_2 from the incoming gas and

(d) the molar flow rate of inlet gas.

> [*Ans*. (a) K_2CO_3: 66.24 g/L, $KHCO_3$: 204 g/L in outgoing solution
> K_2CO_3: 144.9 g/L and $KHCO_3$: 90 g/L in incoming solution
> (b) CO_2 absorption rate = 149 kg/h
> (c) Per cent recovery = 66
> (d) Molar flow rate of inlet gas = 28.4 kmol/h]

8.2 Regenerative (Ljungstrom) type combustion air preheater (RAH) has heat transfer elements, packed in a cylindrical housing in compartments as shown in Fig. 8.8. This rotor is rotated at a constant slow speed (~ 5 rpm) by an electric motor and thereby elements come in contact alternately with flue gas and combustion air streams. In this process, some air (being at a higher pressure) mixes with the flue gas, necessitating higher capacities of combustion air fan and induced draft (ID) fan. Variety of elements are available in different materials of construction. Effective cleaning of the heat transfer elements by soot blowing is provided. While low pressure drop and less space requirement for RAH are claimed to have been major advantages over recuperative tubular type air heater, mixing of air in flue gas is a major disadvantage. RAH is particularly economical for high capacity boilers. In an oil fired boiler of 100 t/h steam generation at 62 bar g and 673 K(400°C), flue gas is found to contain 14.0% CO_2, 3%, O_2 and 83.0% N_2 on dry basis at the outlet of boiler furnace. Its dew point is measured to be 319.3 K(46.3°C) at 100 kPa a. Based on combustion stoichiometry, 1.045 kmol wet flue gas are produced per kmol wet combustion air, entering the furnace. Flue gas, passed through RAH, is cooled from 523 K(250°C) to 433 K(160°C). Flue gas at outlet of the RAH is analyzed to contain 12.5% CO_2 on dry basis due to air mixing with flue gas. Combustion air enters RAH at 313 K(40°C) *DB* and 295 K(22°C) *WB*.

Calculate

(a) kmol of dry air mixed with kmol of dry flue gas,

(b) heat transferred in RAH in kJ/kmol,

(c) temperature of combustion air, leaving RAH, and

(d) increase in volumetric capacity of combustion air fan.

> [*Ans*. (a) 0.12 kmol/kmol dry flue gas, entering RAH,
> (b) 2773.5 kJ/kmol dry flue gas, entering RAH,
> (c) 396.95 K(123.8°C) and
> (d) 12.82%]

Note: If a tubular heater is used in place of RAH, heat transfer duty and air temperature at the outlet of the heater are calculated to be 3206.7 kJ/kmol and 412.25 K(139.1°C), respectively.

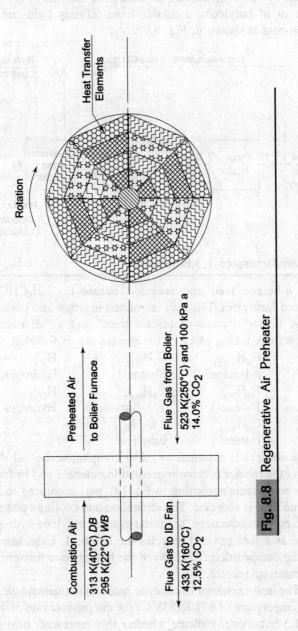

Fig. 8.8 Regenerative Air Preheater

Heat Transfer Elements

Rotation

Preheated Air to Boiler Furnace

Flue Gas from Boiler
523 K(250°C) and 100 kPa a
14.0% CO₂

Combustion Air
313 K(40°C) *DB*
295 K(22°C) *WB*

Flue Gas to ID Fan
433 K(160°C)
12.5% CO₂

8.3 1, 3-Butadiene (CH_2: CH—CH: CH_2) of rubber grade purity is manufactured by several methods, including the dehydrogenation of normal
butane or of butylenes, available from refinery light-end fractions[12].
The process is shown in Fig. 8.9.

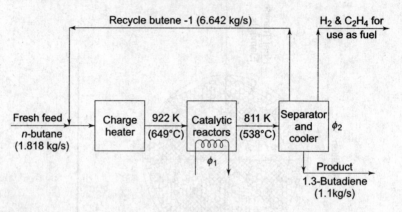

Fig. 8.9 Manufacture of 1,3-Butadiene

Fresh *n*-butane feed and recycled butene-1 ($C_2H_5CHCH_2$) at the
indicated flow rates (Fig. 8.9) are mixed together and passed through a
"charge heater", "catalytic reactor train" and a "separation system".
The reactions taking place in the reactor are as follows:

$$C_4H_{10(g)} \quad = \quad C_4H_{8(g)} \quad + \quad H_{2(g)} \tag{1}$$
$$\text{n-Butane} \qquad \text{Butene-1} \qquad \text{Hydrogen}$$

$$C_4H_{8(g)} \quad = \quad C_4H_{6(g)} \quad + \quad H_{2(g)} \tag{2}$$
$$\text{Butene-1} \qquad \text{1, 3-Butadiene} \qquad \text{Hydrogen}$$

$$C_4H_{8(g)} \quad = \quad 2\,C_2H_{4(g)} \tag{3}$$
$$\text{Butene-1} \qquad \text{Ethylene}$$

Reaction (1) is assumed to go to completion, i.e. all the *n*-butane
entering the reactor is dehydrogenated to butene-1 and hydrogen. A part
of butene-1 reacts according to Eq. (2), part according to Eq. (3) and
the remainder is recycled. The separation and cooling system condenses
out the product butadiene, sends the gaseous ethylene-hydrogen mixture
for use as a fuel gas and recycles the butene-1. Calculate

(a) the composition (mole %) of the hot gaseous mixture leaving the
catalytic reactor.

(b) The heat exchange in catalytic reactors to maintain the desired exit
temperature of 811 K(538°C) for the product rate of 4000 kg/h of
1,3-butadiene. Indicate whether this represents heat added to or
heat removed from the reactor. Use absolute enthalpies given in
Table 5.21.

(c) The vapour pressure to which the butadiene will have to be
flashed to cool down to 273.15 K(0°C) for condensation. Use may
be made of the Antoine equation (Table 5.4).

(d) The butadiene is to be cooled from the gaseous state at 811 K (538°C) to the liquid state of 273.15 K(0°C). Calculate the heat that will have to be removed from the product butadiene to accomplished this cooling and condensation. Assume condensation of all butadiene.

[*Ans.* (a) Butene-1: 55.77%, 1, 3-butadiene: 9.68%, hydrogen: 24.42% and ethylene: 10.13% (on mole basis)

(b) ϕ_1 = 4528.84 kW (endothermic)

(c) p = 120.2 kPa

(d) ϕ_2 = 1797 kW]

8.4 A demineralizing plant, using ion-exchange technology, produces boiler feed quality water. It employs a strong cation exchanger, a weak anion exchanger and mixed bed units.

The cation exchanger is regenerated with hydrochloric acid solution of about 4% (by mass) strength. At first, acidic solution is introduced in a countercurrent manner. At the end of acid introduction, slow rinse is carried out with the help of pure water. Samples were taken periodically of the effluents during both the regeneration steps and were analysed for total chlorides (as Cl) and free mineral acidity (FMA) as HCl.

The analytical data are presented as shown[13] in Table 8.23.

Table 8.23 Analyses of Effluent Samples Collected During Regeneration

Regeneration step	Time from start, min.	Flow rate of effluent, m³/h	Total chlorides as Cl, mg/L	FMA as HCl, mg/L
Acid introduction	0 (start)	—	—	—
	10	63	1 500	—
	15	63	9 000	—
	27	63	50 000	65.8
	44	63	56 000	28 636
	52	63	55 000	46 447
Slow rinse	0 (start)	—	—	—
	15	54	42 000	39 133
	30	54	6 000	2 560
	45	54	2 000	1 097

The chlorides content of the effluents above 600 ppm is objectionable as per IS: 2490 (Part - I) which prescribes limits for effluents to be discharged on land for irrigation purpose. For this reason, it was considered to segregate the effluents into two streams, concentrated and dilute, such that nearly 85% of total chlorides eluated are to be segregated in the concentrated stream.

(a) Suggest the duration in which the effluents are to be segregated as concentrated effluents.

(b) Calculate the quantities of concentrated and weak effluents.

(c) Calculate the average concentrations of chlorides and FMA of the concentrated stream.

(d) Calculate the consumption of 31.5% (by mass) HCl for regeneration.

(e) Calculate, the excess acid, fed over stoichiometric requirements assuming that the resins are completely regenerated.

[Ans. (a) Period: 50 min, starting from 20 min from start of acid introduction step.

(b) Volume of concentrated effluents = 49.8 m^3

Volume of dilute effl   ats = 45.3 m^3

(c) Chlorides in concentrated effluents = 49 203 mg/L

FMA in concentrated effluent = 24 982 mg/L

(d) 9.27 t,

(e) 43.5% excess acid]

8.5 In a chemical plant, a bullet (high pressure storage tank) is used for storing liquefied petroleum gas (LPG). Over a period of its utilization, it required repairs, involving hotwork (cutting/welding). Its geometric volume is 22 m^3. For issuance of safety work permit, preparations are to be made.

At first, the bullet is emptied out of LPG such that its pressure is reduced to 0.25 bar g (in gaseous form) and 308 K(35°C). Composition of LPG may be taken as: C_2H_6: 1.2%, C_3H_8: 25.2%, i-C_4H_{10}: 23.9% and n-C_4H_{10}: 49.7% (by volume). It is pressure purged with pure dry nitrogen (having less than 0.1% O_2 by volume). Pressure purging is carried out by pressurising the bullet with nitrogen upto 2.5 bar g and depressursing it to 0.25 bar g during each cycle. Bullet is considered safe for hotwork if the concentration of each hydrocarbon is brought down below its lower flammability limit. Finally bullet is depressurized to atmospheric pressure for hotwork.

Table 8.24 Data on Flammability Limits[14]

Gas	Flammability limits in air at 101.325 kPa a and 298.15 K (25°C)	
	Higher limit	Lower limit
Ethane	12.5	3.0
Propane	9.5	2.3
Butane (any isomer)	8.5	1.9

(a) Calculate the number of cycles of pressure purging for safe hotwork permit issuance.

(b) Calculate final concentration of each hydrocarbon.

(c) Calculate nitrogen requirement for all cycles of purging.

[Ans. (a) 4 cycles, (b) ethane: 0.02%,

propane: 0.42% and butane: 1.23% (by vol.)

(c) 173.2 Nm^3 nitrogen]

8.6 The LPG bullet, described in Exercise 8.5, is to be prepared for man-entry for thorough inspection. This requires that oxygen content of LPG tank environment should be 18% by volume (min.). For this purpose, compressed dry air at 6 bar g and 308 K(35°C) is used for pressurisation after nitrogen purging. Bullet at atmospheric pressure is pressurized with air to 4 bar g and depressurised to atmospheric pressure during each cycle. Calculate the number of cycles of pressurisation required to attain oxygen level of 18% by volume and also compressed air requirement. Assume ideal gas law.

[*Ans.* 2 cycles, air requirement = 154 Nm^3]

8.7 A three-stage calcination process is used for the solidification of Purex waste[15]. First, an aqueous solution containing 31.55% solids (by mass) is fed to a bent-tube evaporator where it is concentrated to a 60% solution by condensing saturated steam at 185 kPa g pressure. Partially concentrated solution (60%) is sent to a wiped-film evaporator where it is further concentrated to 90% solids by condensing saturated steam at 12 bar g pressure. A slurry containing 90% is fed to an Auger-agitated calciner where the leftover water is removed by electric heating. The system is shown in Fig. 8.10. The operating details of the plant have been given in Table 8.25.

At 60% solids concentration, the solids remain dissolved in the solution. At 90% concentration, 50% of Na_2CO_3 and Na_2SO_4 (each) precipitate out and a slurry is thus obtained. In the calciner Na_2NO_3 and $NaOH$ are in liquid state at 623 K(350°C) while the rest are in solid state. In the Auger-agitated calciner, the vapours are at 473 K (200°C) although the product solid mixture is at 623 K(350°C). In the other two evaporators; the boiling point elevations in the bent-tube evaporator and wiped-film evaporator are 10 K and 23 K respectively.

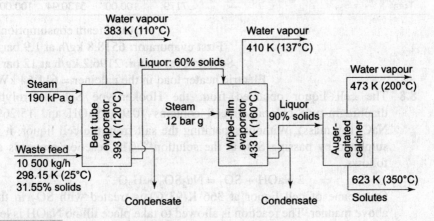

Fig. 8.10 Three-stage Calcination Process

Table 8.25 Operating Details of the Calcination Plant

	Temperature, K (°C)	Enthalpy, kJ/kg solution
Feed	298.15 (25)	0 (Basis)
Bent-tube evaporator	393 (120)	225.7
Wiped-film evaporator	433 (160)	202.2
Auger-agitated calciner	623 (350)	581.5 (of final solid mixture)

Table 8.26 Composition of Feed

Component	mass %
$NaNO_3$	23.12
Na_2CO_3	2.96
Na_2SO_4	0.91
$NaAlO_2$	3.60
NaOH	0.96
H_2O	68.45
Total	100.00

Establish the material and energy balances of the plant.

Table 8.27 Summary of Results

Stage	Type of concentrator	Feed, kg/h	Water evaporated		Heat load	
			kg/h	mass %	kW	%
1st	Bent-tube evaporator	10 500	4979	69.36	3923.24	68.46
2nd	Wiped-film evaporator	5 522	1832	25.52	1196.06	20.87
3rd	Auger-agitated calciner	3 681	368	5.12	611.64	10.67
Total		—	7179	100.00	5730.94	100.00

[*Ans.* Steam consumptions:
First evaporator: 6518.8 kg/h at 1.9 bar g
Second evaporator: 2196.2 kg/h at 12 bar g
Electric heater load in the calciner = 611.64 kW]

8.8 The cell liquor obtained from the Hooker-type S-1 electrolytic diaphragm-type chloralkali cell contains 10.9% NaOH and 15.26% NaCl (by mass). Without separating the salt from the cell liquor, it is sulphited by passing SO_2 in the solution[16]. The reaction proceeds as follows.

$$2\,NaOH + SO_2 = Na_2SO_3 + H_2O$$

One tonne of cell liquor at 366 K(93°C) is treated with SO_2 in the above manner. The reaction is allowed to take place till no NaOH is left over in the solution. The reaction is quite exothermic and hence the evaporation amounting to 71 kg water takes place. The final temperature of the sulphited liquor is kept at 373 K(100°C).

Use Fig. 8.11 and make the following calculations. (a) Find the yield of Na_2SO_3 at 373 K(100°C). (b) The above mass is concentrated by evaporating the water at 373 K(100°C). The evaporation is carried out till the invariant composition is reached. Find the yield of Na_2SO_3 at the end of evaporation process and also the amount of evaporation taken place. (c) Instead of evaporation as suggested in (b), salt is added to the solution to the extent that the composition of the solution reaches that of invariant point at 373 K(100°C). Find the quantity of salt to be added to the solution and also the yield of Na_2SO_3. (d) As an alternative to (b), the cooling of sulphited liquor is carried out to 273.15 K(0°C). It is known that below 305.5 K(32.5°C), the crystals are hepta-hydrated. Find the yield of crystals.

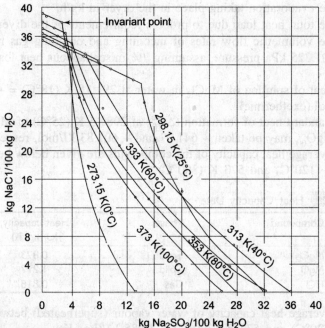

Fig. 8.11 NaCl-Na$_2$SO$_3$-H$_2$O System from 273.15 K(0°C) to 373.15 K (100°C)

(Reproduced with the permission of the American Chemical Society, USA)

[*Ans.* (a) 118.1 kg or 68.8% yield
(b) 159.7 kg or 93.0% yield
(c) 150.9 kg or 87.9% yield
(d) 148.5 kg as Na_2SO_3 or 297 kg $Na_2SO_3.7H_2O$; 86.5% yield]

8.9 A spray drier is used to produce crystals of magnesium chloride from its aqueous solution. The object of the operation is to dry $MgCl_2$ to the lowest possible level. However, during the operation, $MgCl_2$ is also subjected to hydrolysis, leading to oxide formation. The reaction is

$$MgCl_2 \quad + \quad H_2O \quad = \quad MgO \quad + \quad 2\,HCl$$

Typical operating conditions of the dryer are given below.

Feed: Aqueous solution containing 48% $MgCl_2$ by mass

Feed temperature: 393 K (120°C) (boiling point of the solution at 101.325 kPa)

Product rate: 5000 kg/h $MgCl_2$

Analysis of the final product: 90% $MgCl_2$, 5% MgO and balance water (by mass)

Hot flue gas inlet temperature: 798 K (525°C)

Hot flue gas outlet temperature: 573 K (300°C)

Inlet hot flue gases contain 0.03 kg moisture per kg dry flue gas and has an average molar mass equal to 29. Calculate,

(a) the evaporation taking place in the dryer in kg/h,
(b) the total heat load due to process requirements of the dryer and
(c) the volumetric flow rates of incoming and outgoing gas mixtures at 101.325 kPa pressure, assuming 7% miscellaneous heat loss.

Data:

(i) Heat of solution of $MgCl_2$ in water at 291.15 K (18°C) = + 153.2 kJ/mol (exothermic)

(ii) Standard heat of formation (ΔH_f°) at 298.15 K (25°C) of $MgCl_{2(s)}$ and $MgO_{(s)}$ may be taken – 641.07 and – 601.83 kJ/mol, respectively.

(iii) Average heat capacity of the compounds are given below between 393 K (120°C) and 573 K (300°C):

Table 8.28 Heat Capacity Data

Compound	Phase	Heat capacity, kJ/(kg · K)
$MgCl_2$	Solid	0.873
MgO	Solid	1.277
HCl	Gas	0.816

(iv) Average heat capacity of water vapour (superheated) between 393 K (120°C) and 573 K (300°C) = 1.985 kJ/(kg · K)

Assume that the product discharge temperature is equal to the outlet flue gas temperature.

[*Ans.* (a) 5726.4 kg/h (b) 7815.11 kW (c) (i) Incoming flue gases = 276 921 m³/h (ii) Outgoing flue gases = 214 124 m³/h]

8.10 In the steel industry, semifinished steel is treated with dilute sulphuric acid to remove iron oxide scale from the surface. Waste pickle liquor is obtained after the treatment. This liquor will pose an effluent problem and will also result in the loss of valuable acid. Electrolysis can be of use in recovering the acid.

A batch-type electrolytic cell is used to treat the waste sulphate pickle liquor as shown in Fig. 8.12[17]. It consists of an anion exchange membrane, a stainless steel cathode and an antimonial lead anode. The membrane is prepared by embedding anion exchange resin in the normal osmotic membrane matrix such as that of cellulose acetate or polyamide. Such a membrane allows only anions to migrate through it.

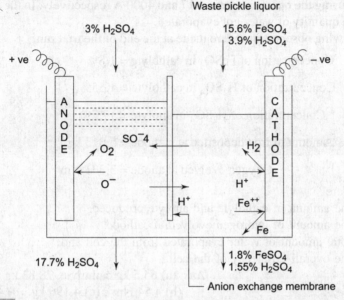

Fig. 8.12 Treatment of Waste Sulphate Pickle Liquor in an Electrolytic Cell

In the cathode compartment, $FeSO_4$ and H_2SO_4 of the waste liquor get electrolysed. Sulphate ions migrate to the anode compartment. Hydrogen ions and iron ions loose the charge to the cathode. As a result, hydrogen gas is evolved and iron is deposited at the cathode. In the anode compartment, water is electrolysed into H^+ and O^- ions. Sulphate ions combine with protons to form H_2SO_4, thereby increasing the strength of the electrolyte. Some protons migrate to the cathode compartment due to high mobility although such migration is deliberately slowed down by anion exchange membrane. The reactions are summarised as follows.

Cathode reactions:

$$FeSO_4 = Fe^{++} + SO_4--$$
$$H_2SO_4 = 2\ H^+ + SO_4--$$
$$Fe^{++} + 2\ e = Fe$$
$$2\ H^+ + 2e = H_2$$

Anode reactions:

$$2\ H_2O = 4\ H^+ + 2\ O--$$
$$4\ H^+ + 2\ SO_4^{--} = 2\ H_2SO_4$$
$$2\ O^{--} = O_2 + 2\ e$$

A trial run of the cell was taken. The catholyte charge amounted to 100 kg, yielding an analysis of 15.6% $FeSO_4$ and 3.9% H_2SO_4 (by mass). The anode compartment was filled with 59 kg of 3% H_2SO_4 (by mass) solution so as to make the solution conductive. As electrolysis progresses, the concentration of H_2SO_4 in the catholyte reduces thereby requiring higher voltage. Beyond 1.8%

$FeSO_4$ (mass %) concentration in the catholyte, the voltage rise is steep and therefore the operation had to be stopped after 186 min. The average voltage and current during the operation were 4.17 and 4000 A respectively. In the process, a definite quantity of water got evaporated.

The following observations were made at the end of the trial run.

Concentration of $FeSO_4$ in catholyte = 1.8%

Concentration of H_2SO_4 in catholyte = 1.55%

Concentration of H_2SO_4 in anolyte = 17.7%

Amount of iron deposited at cathode = 5.313 kg

Oxygen evolved at anode = 3.331 Nm^3

Calculate
(a) the amount of catholyte and anolyte produced,
(b) the amount of hydrogen evolved at cathode,
(c) total amount of water evaporated from the cell and
(d) the overall efficiency of the cell.

[*Ans.* (a) 65.5 kg catholyte, 78.83 kg anolyte,
(b) 4.54 Nm^3, (c) 4.196 kg, (d) 41.05%]

8.11 Synthesis gas for ammonia production can be obtained in a number of ways. One such method is partial oxidation of hydrocarbons. In a typical plant, natural gas is used with the following composition[18].
CH_4: 93.25%, N_2: 1.95%, Ar: 0.4%, C_2H_6: 3.32%, C_3H_8: 0.88% and n-C_4H_{10}: 0.2% (by volume)
Oxygen with 98% purity (rest argon) is fed to the unit. The chemistry of partial oxidation of methane can be represented by the following equations:

$$CH_4 + 2\,O_2 = CO_2 + 2\,H_2O$$

$$CH_4 + CO_2 = 2\,CO + 2\,H_2$$

$$CH_4 + H_2O = CO + 3\,H_2$$

$$CO + H_2O = CO_2 + H_2 \quad \text{shift reaction}$$

Similar reactions can be written for other hydrocarbons also.
Natural gas and oxygen enter the reactor at 422 K(149°C) and 400 K (127°C) respectively. The reactor is to be designed in such a way that the gas mixture leaves the reactor at 1395 K(1122°C) and the methane slip (on wet basis) is 0.35% (v/v). The reactor is designed to operate at 20 bar a. The design approach to equilibrium of steam-methane reforming reaction is 30 K and that of shift reaction is 0 K. Equilibrium constants[19] for the reforming and shift reactions are given below:

$$K_{p1} = \frac{p_{CH_4} \times p_{O_2}}{p_{CO} \times p_{H_2}^3} = 2.5207 \times 10^{-5} \text{ at 1365 K(1092°C)}$$

$$K_{p2} = \frac{p_{H_2} \times p_{CO}}{p_{CO} \times p_{H_2O}} = 0.4465 \text{ at } 1395 \text{ K}(1122°C)$$

Where p_i = partial pressure of ith component, kPa.

Calculate

(a) the oxygen stream supply in kmol/kmol natural gas,

(b) dry analysis of exit gas mixture,

(c) steam to dry exit gas mole ratio and

(d) net heat transfer in the reactor per kmol feed gas using absolute enthalpies, listed in Table 5.21.

[*Ans.* (a) 0.7644 kmol O_2/kmol feed gas
(b) Composition of dry mixture, leaving the reactor:
H_2: 60.03%, CO: 34.50%, CO_2: 3.62%
CH_4: 0.40%, N_2: 0.73%, and Ar: 0.72%
(c) Steam/dry gas ratio = 0.141 kmol/kmol
(d) Net heat transfer = 5776 kJ/kmol feed gas (exothermic)]

8.12 Sulphuric acid is one of the most widely-used basic chemicals. The major part of sulphuric acid consumption, however, is not bound in a marketable end product but generally ends up as spent acid, creating a waste disposal problem. In the organic chemical industry such as plastics, synthetic fibres including caprolactum, methylacrylate and others, the spent acid with organic impurities, metal sulphates and ammonium hydrogen sulphate is found to be the waste. In the phosphoric acid plant and nitrogenous fertilizer plant, the waste consists of spent acid, containing metal sulphates and ammonium sulphate. In some textile mills, acid waste contains fibrous organic impurities.

To solve the waste problem, recycling the sulphur within the process can become useful. Dilute spent acids can be reconcentrated, but in most cases, the remaining impurities in the reconcentrated acid do not permit the reuse of reconcentrated acid in the original process.

Regeneration of sulphuric acid can be attained by thermal degradation to SO_2 at high temperatures[20] where all organic compounds are completely burnt. SO_2 thus obtained is reprocessed by the constant process to produce concentrated acid or oleum.

An acid regeneration plant, equipped with two parallel spent acid decomposition units, is designed for processing 860 t/d spent acid that has ammonia content. The average chemical composition of spent acid is H_2SO_4: 20%, NH_4HSO_4: 45%, H_2O: 30% and organics: 5% (by mass). For calculation purposes, C:H ratio (mass) and NCV of the organic compounds can be taken as 5.1 and 41 870 kJ/kg, respectively. This spent acid is decomposed by firing with fuel oil [C : H ratio = 6.2 : 1 (by mass) and NCV = 43 000 kJ/kg]. In the decomposition furnace hot air at 723 K(450°C) is introduced. Gas mixture leaves the furnace at 106.7 kPa (800 torr) and at about 1275 K(1002°C), the SO_2 content of the exit gas mixture should be less than 6% (v/v). Oxygen requirement in the exit gas mixture is 1.2 kmol per kmol SO_2 for further conversion to SO_3.

In the heat recovery section, the exit gas mixture from the furnace exchanges heat with air and cools down to 623 K(350°C). Subsequently, the gas mixture is cooled and used for acid production. Ambient air at 308 K(35°C) *DB* and 296 K(23°C) *WB* is first heated in a steam heater above the dew point of the gas mixture from the furnace and then further heated to 723 K(450°C) in the gas/air heat exchanger. Hot air from the exchanger is divided into two parts. One part is used as combustion air in the furnace, while the rest of the quantity is taken to a waste heat boiler, generating saturated steam at 11 bar a. Figure 8.13 schematically represents the process.

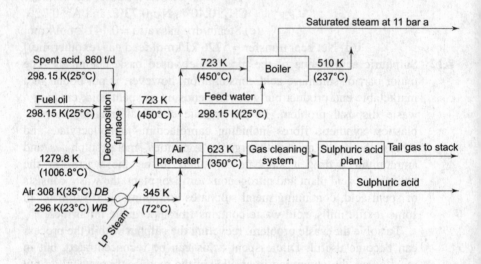

Fig. 8.13 Regeneration of Spent Sulphuric Acid

Make a complete material and energy balance of the plant up to the heat recovery system. The heat of solution of NH_4HSO_4 is + 2.34 kJ/mol (exothermic).

[*Ans.* (i) Composition and temperature of exit gas mixture, SO_2: 5.51%, CO_2: 9.13%, O_2: 6.61% and balance N_2 (v/v), 1279.8 K (1006.8°C)
(ii) Water dew point of exit gas mixture = 341.6 K (68.6°C)
(iii) Fuel oil required = 8.9 kg/100 kg spent acid = 76.54 t/d
(iv) Steam generation at 11 bar a = 14.81 t/h]

8.13 Benzene can be produced from toluene economically. Thermal dealkylation[21] with hydrogen results in benzene and methane at 34.5 bar a and 923 K(650°C).

Side reaction results in the undesired product diphenyl which is controlled by excess hydrogen.

Based on experience, it was decided to use excess hydrogen in such a way that the moles of H_2 in the gross feed should be five times that of 'oil' in the gross feed. Here 'oil' denotes the mixture of benzene, toluene and diphenyl. The process is shown in Fig. 3.4. The gross feed enters the plug flow reactor and the product stream goes to the phase separator. Based on thermodynamic considerations in the separator, the mole ratio of each component in the gas phase and liquid phase is given as, H_2: ∞, CH_4: ∞, C_6H_6: 0.005, C_7H_8: 0.001 and diphenyl: 0. A part of the flash gas mixture is recycled after compression and joins the make-up hydrogen stream, containing 95% H_2 and 5% CH_4 (v/v). Recycle gas stream contains 50% H_2 (v/v).

To avoid accumulation of inerts (CH_4) in the loop, a fixed amount of the flash gas mixture is purged from the separator. The liquid stream leaving the phase separator is treated in successive distillation columns to separate benzene, toluene and diphenyl. The recovered toluene with small amounts of benzene and diphenyl is recycled to feed the toluene header. The benzene column is designed to separate 95% of the benzene and the toluene column can separate 75% of the diphenyl. Based on an experimental study, following data were found.

Table 8.29 Dealkylation of Toluene[21]

Conversion, %	50	66	70	75	85
Yield, %	99	98.5	97.7	97	93

As the conversion increases, the recycle stream will reduce and the compression cost as well as equipment cost will reduce. But as the conversion increases, formation of undesirable products will also increase which in turn will increase the operational cost as well as call for larger separation towers. To find the optimum conversion, a cost study was performed. Such a study revealed that the profit increases directly with the square root of the conversion and with the cube of the yield. Make the material balance of the plant for producing 1000 kg/h or benzene.

[*Ans.* See Table 8.30]

8.14 Refer Fig. 8.14. Calculate the requirement of the HP steam and boiler feed water (BFW) based on following assumptions:
(a) Consider 95% energy conversion in each turbine.
(b) Consider 5% loss of energy in the condensate from the condensate system to the deaerator.

[*Ans.* HP steam flow = 75 254 kg/h
BFW flow = 78 645 kg/h]

Table 8.30 Material Balance for Dealkylation of Toluene to Benzene

Basis: Benzene product rate = 1000 kg/h

Component/ Conditions	Toluene	Hydrogen	Methane	Diphenyl	Benzene	Total	Pressure, bar a	Temperature, K (°C)
Molar mass	92	2	16	154	78			
Fresh toluene feed								
kmol/h	13.24	—	—	—	—	13.24	41.6	308 (35)
kg/h	1218.2	—	—	—	—	1218.2		
Fresh hydrogen feed								
kmol/h	—	27.74	1.46	—	—	29.2	33	288 (15)
kg/h	—	55.48	23.38	—	—	78.86		
Mole %	—	95.0	5.0	—	—	—		
Recycle gas stream								
kmol/h	0.009	63.41	63.35	—	0.055	126.824	32	311 (38)
kg/h	0.9	126.82	1013.6	—	4.29	1145.61		
Mole %	0.007	50.0	49.95	—	0.043	—		
Toluene recycled								
kmol/h	4.17	—	—	0.07	0.66	4.9	41.7	394 (121)
kg/h	383.64	—	—	10.78	52.22	446.64		
Mass %	85.90	—	—	2.41	11.69	100.0		
Reactor inlet								
kmol/h	17.419	91.15	64.81	0.07	0.715	174.164	36.5	923 (650)
kg/h	1602.74	182.3	1036.98	10.78	56.51	2889.31		

(Contd.)

Table 8.30 (Contd.)

Component/Conditions	Toluene	Hydrogen	Methane	Diphenyl	Benzene	Total	Pressure bar a	Temperature K(°C)
Reactor outlet								
kmol/h	4.18	78.12	78.05	0.28	13.56	174.19	34.5	977 (704)
kg/h	384.63	156.24	1248.76	42.78	1057.89	2890.3		
Vapour stream from phase separator								
kmol/h	0.01	78.54	78.46	—	0.069	157.079	32	311 (38)
kg/h	1.01	157.08	1255.36	—	5.38	1418.83		
Mole %	0.007	50.0	49.95		0.043	100.00		
Purge stream (total)								
kmol/h	0.002	14.71	14.70	—	0.013	29.425	3.4	293 (20)
kg/h	0.2	29.42	235.2		1.0	265.82		
Mole %	0.007	50.00	49.95		0.043	100.00		
Liquid stream from phase separator								
kmol/h	4.17	—	—	0.28	13.49	17.94	11.8	311 (38)
kg/h	383.64	—	—	42.12	1052.22	1477.98		
Mass %	25.96	—	—	2.85	71.19	100.00		
Benzene product from benzene column								
kmol/h	—	—	—	—	12.83	12.83	1.7	371 (98)
kg/h	—	—	—	—	1000.0	1000.0		
Diphenyl from toluene column								
kmol/h	—	—	—	0.22	—	0.22	1.4	477 (204)
kg/h	—	—	—	32.34	—	32.34		

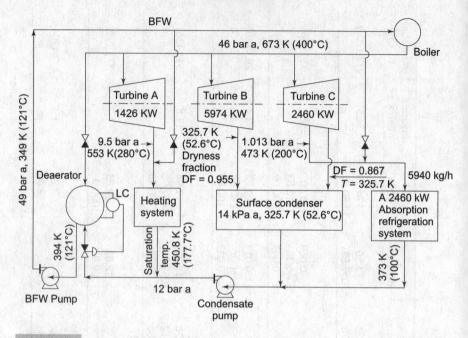

BFW

46 bar a, 673 K (400°C)

Boiler

49 bar a, 349 K (121°C)

Turbine A	Turbine B	Turbine C
1426 KW	5974 KW	2460 KW

9.5 bar a →
553 K(280°C)

325.7 K
(52.6°C)
Dryness
fraction
DF = 0.955

1.013 bar a →
473 K (200°C)

DF = 0.867
T = 325.7 K

5940 kg/h

Deaerator

LC

Heating
system

Surface condenser
14 kPa a, 325.7 K (52.6°C)

A 2460 kW
Absorption
refrigeration
system

394 K
(121°C)

Saturation
temp.
450.8 K
(177.7°C)

373 K
(100°C)

BFW Pump

12 bar a

Condensate
pump

Fig. 8.14 Steam Balance in a Chemical Plant

8.15 Refer Example 8.6. LP steam header pressure is proposed to be reduced to 4 bar a. As a result

(i) Temperature of LP steam from BFW pump and FD fan turbines will be reduced to 438 K(165°C),

(ii) Consumption in ejectors operating with LP steam as motivating fluid will increase by 10% and

(iii) Consumption of LP steam in heaters will reduce by 1.75% due to increase in latent heat of LP steam. Establish the steam balance.

[*Ans*. Refer Fig. 8.15]

Note: It can be seen that HP steam generation will be lower by 529 kg/h, representing nearly 1% reduction. Thus, operation of a given cascade steam balance can be optimized by selecting right operation parameters (without any modifications).

Cooling tower load will increase marginally (~ 0.6%).

8.16 In Example 8.6, letdown of MP steam is substantial which can be reduced gainfully by converting the CW pump turbine from a condensing one to the back-pressure type. Establish the revised steam balance in which the HP steam generation is again minimum.

[*Ans*. Refer Fig. 8.16]

Note: It may be noted that HP steam generation is lower (by 4.8%) as there is a reduction in letdown from MP steam to LP steam. There is also a reduction of heat load (by 8.8%) on the surface condenser.

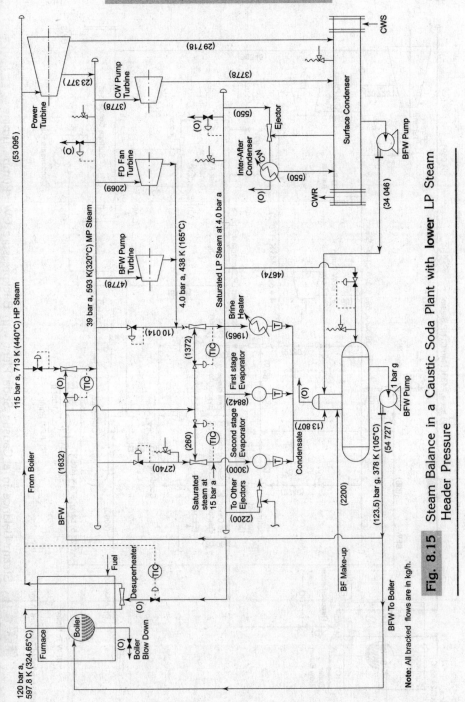

Fig. 8.15 Steam Balance in a Caustic Soda Plant with **lower LP Steam** Header Pressure

Note: All bracketed flows are in kg/h.

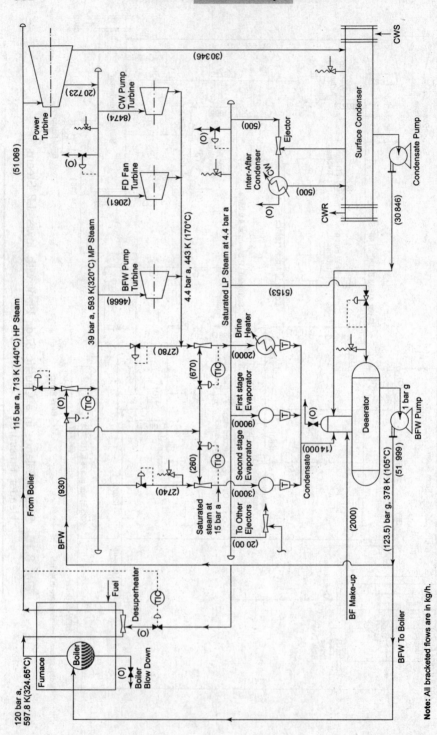

Fig. 8.16 Steam Balance in a Caustic Soda Plant with Backpressure CW Pump Turbine

Note: All bracketed flows are in kg/h.

8.17 In Example 8.6, MP steam is available at 39 bar a and 593 K(320°C). A part of MP steam is reheated in the boiler furnace to 673 K(400°C) as shown in Fig. 8.17. Reheated MP steam is fed to FD Fan, BFW Pump and CW Pump turbines. Total pressure drop in the reheating coils and desuperheater is calculated to be 3 bar. LP steam from these turbines is obtained at 4.4 bar a and 458 K(185°C). Establish steam balance with revised conditions.

[*Ans*. Refer Fig. 8.17]

Note: Conversion of condensing turbine to a back pressure one (Exercise 8.16), incorporation of BFW Heaters (Example 8.7), reheating of intermediate pressure steam (Exercise 8.17), adoption of thermocompressor (Example 8.8), lowering header pressure (Exercise 8.15), etc. could prove useful in minimizing HP steam generation (thereby reduction in fuel consumption) and in heat load of cooling tower. Careful design of a cascade steam system at the project stage can pay rich dividends.

8.18 Polypropylene (PP) drying (i.e. *n*-hexane removal) can be performed in different types of dryers. One such dryer is a flash dryer (convective drying) in which the feed cake is dispersed in a venturi throat with hot recycle gas (nitrogen). Such a dryer requires gas circulation rate of about 1 kg dry nitrogen per kg PP which acts as a heat carrier for drying. In another spiral dryer [22], indirect heating and convective drying are performed thereby nitrogen circulation is significantly reduced. In this type of dryer, heat is transmitted to the thin fast moving product film rising in a spiral path along the inner wall surface. Conveying medium is nitrogen. For PP, the nitrogen circulation requirement is only 0.18 kg dry nitrogen per kg PP. Spiral dryer is also claimed to prevent corrosion due to the avoidance of hexane condensation.

In both the cases, nitrogen at 403 K(130°C) enters the dryer having a *n*-hexane dew point of 307 K(34°C). Nitrogen leaves the dryer at 363 K (90°C) in either case. PP enters the dryer with 35% *n*-hexane on a wet basis at 338 K(65°C). Product PP leaves flash dryter at 328 K (55°C) with *n*-hexane content of 0.05 kg per kg dry PP while the product leaves spiral dryer at 353 K(80°C) with *n*-hexane content of 0.02 kg per kg dry PP. Steam is used in the jacket of the spiral dryer at 4 bar a to maintain the heat transfer surface temperature of 383 K (110°C). The process of spiral drying is shown in Fig. 8.18.

Nitrogen rich in *n*-hexane leaves the dryer at 363 K(90°C) and is sent to a direct contact scrubber to separate *n*-hexane from nitrogen. An external water cooler cools recycled *n*-hexane used for scrubbing. Cooled liquid *n*-hexane, equivalent to the amount evaporated in the dryer, is bled out from the circulating solution. Nitrogen at 307 K (34°C), saturated with *n*-hexane, is recycled back to the dryer via a

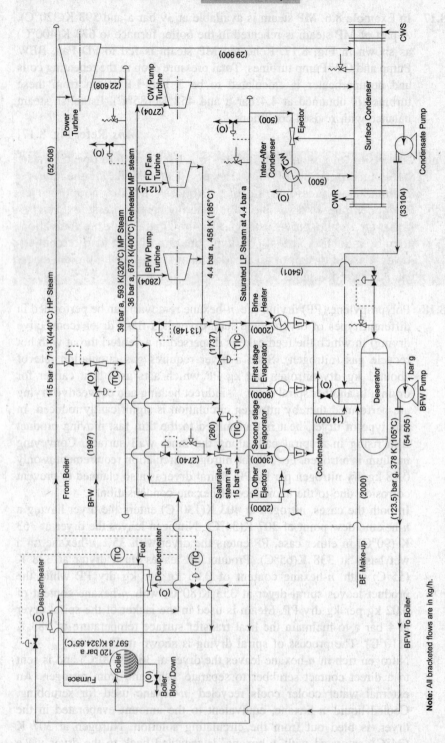

Note: All bracketed flows are in kg/h.

Fig. 8.17 Steam Balance in a Caustic Soda Plant with Reheat of MP Steam

blower through an indirect steam-gas heater. Suction pressure of blower is 102 kPa (765 torr). Average heat capacity of solid PP and liquid n-hexane may be taken as 1.926 and 2.512 kJ/(kg · K) respectively. For a drying plant having a capacity of 10 000 kg/h dry PP rate, calculate the followings.

(a) Steam requirement in nitrogen heater for spiral dryer,
(b) Steam requirement in the jacket of the spiral dryer and
(c) Temperature of gas mixture, leaving the interchanger.

[*Ans.* (a) 181.2 kg/h
(b) 950.0 kg/h
(c) 348.5 K (75.5°C)]

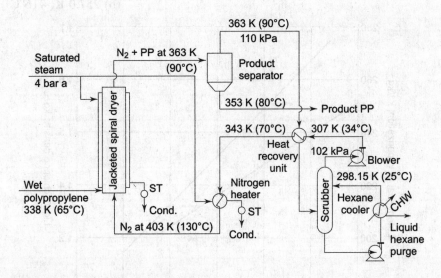

Fig. 8.18 Drying of Polypropylene

8.19 A chlorine ton container is utilised for chlorinating cooling water. Outside diameter and effective length of the container are 760 mm and 1800 mm respectively. It is a known fact that when the halogen is consumed from the container, the temperature of the liquid halogen (and so of the container) will drop due to flashing of the halogen from the liquid surface.

(a) When the container is full, it contains 900 kg liquid chlorine. Chlorination of cooling water is desired at 5.56 g/s (≈ 20 kg/h) at an uniform rate. For steady-state conditions, the rate at which heat is transmitted by ambient air into the container must equal the rate at which chlorine is vaporized, thereby no change in temperature of liquid chlorine will take place. For a fresh full container, calculate the steady-state temperature of liquid chlorine assuming the ambient temperature to be 303 K(30°C).

(b) Assume that the container has 100 kg liquid chlorine at ambient temperature after certain use. Calculate the temperature of liquid chlorine with the same drawl rate after 3600 s (1 h) taking five iterations of 720 s (0.2 h) each.

For the above calculations, assume an overall heat transfer coefficient[23] of 11.4 W/(m^2·K) based on the effective area of the container which is defined as the area in contact with liquid chlorine. Properties of chlorine can be read from Fig. 8.19.

Hint: Neglect sensible heat in the metal and mass of gaseous chlorine in the empty space of the container.

[*Ans.* (a) 261.3 K(– 11.7°C)
(b) 257.0 K(– 16°C)]

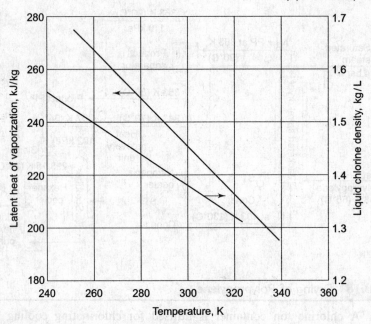

Fig. 8.19 Properties of Chlorine[24]

8.20 A distillation tower is designed for aromatics separation. Design conditions of the column are as follows[25]:

Table 8.31 Composition of Distillation Column Streams

Component	Composition, mole %		
	Feed	Distillate	Bottoms
Benzene	2.2	22.8	0
Toluene	7.4	72.2	0.5
Ethyl benzene	43.4	5.0	47.5
Styrene	47.0	0	52.0

Based on various considerations, a reflux ratio of 6.0 is selected for design. Design pressure of the column is fixed at 21.3 kPa a (160 torr). All the streams may be taken as saturated liquids. Also assume that the mixtures are ideal mixtures.

For a design feed rate of 100 kmol/h, calculate,

(a)   the flow rates of distillate and bottom products,
(b)   bubble point and dew point of distillate products,
(c)   the heat removal in the overhead condenser assuming that condensation takes place at an average temperature of the dew point and bubble point of the distillate product and
(d)   the heat duty and saturated steam consumption at 2 bar a of the reboiler.

[*Ans.* (a) D = 9.63 kmol/h, B = 90.37 kmol/h

(b) T_{DP} = 334.7 K (61.7°C) and T_{BB} = 328.3 K (55.3°C)

(c) Heat load of condenser = 662.26 kW

(d) Heat load of reboiler = 593.88 kW

Steam consumption = 971 kg/h]

8.21   A carbon black plant generates 40 000 Nm³/h off gas mixture having following composition by volume on dry basis.

H_2: 15.3%, N_2: 61.9%, Ar: 0.9%, CH_4: 0.4%, CO: 17.2%, CO_2: 3.9% and C_2H_2: 0.4%

Moisture content: 0.15 kmol/kmol dry gas mixture. Off gas mixture (free from any solid) is available at 0.25 bar g and 523 K(250°C). Following alternatives are considered for its utilization.

(a)   Case-I: Offgas mixture is fired in a boiler to generate steam at 43 bar a and 698.15 K (425°C). Calculate steam generation rate of the boiler.

(b)   Case-II: Offgas mixture is treated in a CO_2-removal plant in which 1% loss of gas mixture is envisaged. CO_2 recovery is considered 97% from the mixture of which 95% product can be made available either in liquid or solid (dry ice) form for sale. Gas mixture from CO_2-absorber is available at 0.10 bar g and 328 K(55°C), saturated with water vapours. This gas mixture is utilized for steam generation at 43 bar a and 698.15 K(425°C). Calculate CO_2 production and steam generation rate.

(C)   Case-III: Gas mixture from CO_2-absorber (of Case-II) is compressed, dried and passed through a cold box for cryogenic recovery of H_2 and CO for methanol production by the reaction: CO + 2 H_2 = CH_3OH. Hydrogen availability being limiting, equivalent CO is utilized and balance is mixed with reject stream of the cold box. Assume 1% loss of gas-mixture from second CO_2 absorber before cryogenic processing. Neglect CO_2 so recovered from second absorber. Reject stream from cold box at 1 bar g and 298.15 K(25°C) (including excess CO), having practically no moisture, is utilized in boiler to generate steam at 43 bar a and

698 K(425°C). In the cold box, hydrogen recovery is 90% and overall methanol conversion (inducing recovery) from the recovered hydrogen is 90%.

Calculate methanol production and steam generation rate.

Following general assumptions can be made for stoichiometric calculations.

(i) Boiler is supplied feed water at 303 K(30°C).

(ii) Gas mixture is fired with 10% excess air in the boiler. Ambient air at 313 K(40°C) has humidity of 0.017 kmol/kmol dry air.

(iii) Flue gases leave boiler furnace at 745 torr and 448 K(175°C).

(iv) Unaccounted heat loss in the boiler is 1.5% of total heat input to it.

[*Ans.* Case-I: Steam generation = 30.82 t/h

Case-II: Steam generation = 27.3 t/h

CO_2 production = 58.9 t/d

Case-III: Steam generation = 8.76 t/h

CO_2 production = 58.9 t/d

Methanol production = 72.5 t/d]

Note: It can be seen in this example that offgas mixture is a valuable input for various products. Cost of the plant and revenue generation from the products will have to be techno-commercially evaluated for deciding over the best alternative to be adopted.

8.22 Offgases from an adipic acid plant have following composition:

N_2O: 30%, CO_2: 3%, O_2: 8% and balance nitrogen (on volume basis) It is saturated with water at 2 bar g and 313 K(40°C).

Nitrous oxide (N_2O), being a greenhouse gas having many-fold potential than that of CO_2 is required to be dissociated to nitrogen and oxygen before the gases are letout to atmosphere.

Reaction: $N_2O = N_2 + 1/2\ O_2$

In a newly developed process[26, 27] nitrous oxide is dissociated over mixed transition metal oxides (as catalyst) in a series of beds. The process is shown in enclosed Fig. 8.20.

In this process a portion of offgas mixture is diluted with a definite quantity of treated gas mixture, being letout to atmosphere such that the temperature of the treated gas mixture from the 1st bed is limited to 973 K(700°C). Reaction initiation temperature is 723 K(450°C) and hence the mixed gas is heated in E2 to 723 K(450°C) before being introduced to the 1st bed.

Gas mixture, leaving the 1st bed, is quenched with definite (bypass) quantity of offgas mixture such that the gas mixture, entering the 2nd bed, is at 723 K(450°C). In a similar manner, the gas mixture from the 2nd bed is quenched with definite quantity of offgas mixture. Treated gas mixture from the 3rd bed is found to contain 200 ppm (v/v) N_2O

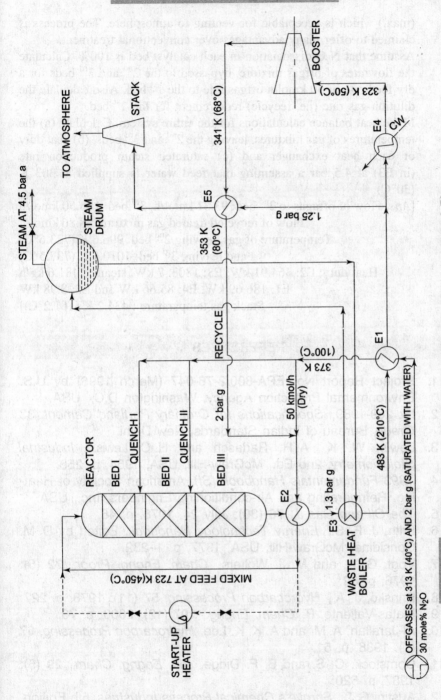

Fig. 8.20 Nitrous Oxide Removal from Offgases of Adipic Acid Plant

(max.) which is acceptable for venting to atmosphere. The process is claimed to offer many advantages over conventional treatment.

Assume that N_2O dissociation in each catalyst bed is 100%. Calculate the flowrates of offgas mixture, bypassed to the 2nd and 3rd beds for a dry feed rate of 50 kmol/h offgas rate to the 1st bed. Also calculate the dilution gas rate (i.e. recycle) requirement for the 1st bed.

Make heat balance calculations for the entire system. Calculate (a) the temperatures of gas mixtures, leaving the 2nd and 3rd beds, (b) heat duty of each heat exchanger and (c) saturated steam production rate (in E3) at 4.5 bar a assuming that feed water is supplied at 303 K (30°C).

[*Ans.* Flow of offagas to 2nd bed: 93.31 kmol/h, 3rd bed: 185.50 kmol/h
Flow of recycled treated gas mixture: 88.86 kmol/h
Temperature of gas, leaving 2nd bed: 996.6 K (723.6°C)
and leaving 3rd bed: 1010.5 K (737.5°C)
Heat duty: E2: 464.91 kW, E3: 1803. 7 kW, steam: 2481.6 kg/h
E1: 186.69 kW, E4: 85.66 kW and E5: 8.98 kW
Stack gas temparature : 434.2 K (161.2°C)]

REFERENCES

1. Project Report No. EPA-600/2-76-047 (March 1996) by U.S. Environmental Protection Agency, Washington D.C., USA.
2. IS: 269-1989, *Specifications for Ordinary Portland Cement*, 33 *Grade*, Bureau of Indian Standards, New Delhi.
3. Lewis, W. K., A. H. Radasch and H. C. Lewis. *Industrial Stoichiometry*, 2nd Ed., McGraw-Hill, USA, 1954, p. 258.
4. *1993 Fundamentals Handbook (SI)*, American Society of Heating, Refrigerating and Air-conditioning Engineers, Inc., USA.
5. *The Oil and Gas J.*, **76** (30): July 24, 1978. p. 46.
6. Frith, J. F. S., *Energy Technology Handbook*, Edited by D. M. Considine, McGraw-Hill, USA, 1977, p. 1–232.
7. Vogt, G. A. and M. J. Wolters, *Chem. Engng. Progr.*, **72** (5): 1976, p. 62.
8. Brinsko, J. A., *Hydrocarbon Processing*, **57** (11): 1978, p. 227.
9. Matas-Valiente, P. *Chem. Engng.*, **107** (12), 2000, p. 70.
10. Al-Jarallah, A. M. and A. K. K. Lee, *Hydrocarbon Processing*, **67** (7): 1988, p. 51.
11. Comstock, C. S. and B. F. Didge, *Ind. Engng. Chem.*, **29** (5): 1937, p. 520.
12. Austin, G.T., *Shreve's Chemical Process Industries*, 5th Edition, McGraw-Hill, USA, 1984, p. 696.
13. Sabadra, P. N. and K. K. Therat, *Treatment and Optimization of Process Waters*— A paper presented at the Seminar on Water

Management in Process Industries, organized by the Indian Institute of Chemical Engineers, New Delhi, 1977.

14. Dean, J. A., *Lange's Handbook of Chemistry*, 14th Ed., McGraw-Hill, USA, 1992, pp. 5.135 – 5.141.

15. Cordiner, J. B. and H. L. Bull, *Low Temperature Waste Solidification in Environmental Engineering*, Edited by G. Lindner and K. Nyberg, D. Reidel Publishing Co., Holland, 1973, p. 413.

16. Kobe, K. A. and K. C. Hellwig, *Ind. Engng. Chem.*, **47** (6): 1955, p. 1120.

17. Horner, C., A. G. Winger, G. W. Bodamer and R. K. Kunin, *Ind. Engng. Chem.*, **46** (6): 1955, p. 1121.

18. Strelzoff, S., and L. C. Pan, *Synthetic Ammonia*, Chemical Construction Corporation, USA, p. 9.

19. *Catalyst Handbook*, Springer-Verlag, New York, USA, 1970.

20. Sander, U. and G. Daradimos, *Chem. Engng. Progress*, **74** (9): 1978. p. 57.

21. *AIChE Student Contest Problem 1967*.

22. Hess, D. and R. A. Rossi, *Chem. Engng. Progress*, **79** (14), 1983 p. 43.

23. Horwitz, B. A., *Chem. Engng.*, **90** (13), June 27. 1983, p. 68.

24. White, G. C., *Handbook of Chlorination*, Van Nostrand Reinhold Co., USA, 1972.

25. Venkateswara, K. and A. Raviprasad, *Chem, Engng.*, **94** (14), Oct. 12. 1987, p. 137.

26. *Chemical Engineering*, **110** (2), p. 15.

27. Private communication with Radici Chimica S. P. A., Italy.

Chapter 9

Stoichiometry and Digital Computation

9.1 INTRODUCTION

In the rapidly-growing technology of this modern world, computers play a key role in analyzing complex problems using sophisticated mathematics. The use of various size computers for research and problem-solving, both in industry and education, has increased dramatically in the last two and half decades. In addition, the accelerating growth of personal computers (PCs) has further increased the role of digital computation in routine process engineering work. This chapter briefly introduces the applications of computers in stoichiometry. This is illustrated by using some selected examples from previous chapters.

9.2 APPLICATION/JUSTIFICATION

Process engineers use computers in routine and special jobs for a variety of reasons:

(a) To minimize time for performing repetitive calculations and time-consuming data analyses, e.g. (i) performing battery limit material and energy balances to determine yields and to identify losses, (ii) computing detailed balances for equipment characterization and to identify instrument malfunction by comparing the computer results with plant measurements and laboratory analysis.

(b) To increase the accuracy and reliability of engineering calculations with improved handling of the complex process flow system, e.g., (i) solving atmospheric dispersion models to analyze the effect of a particulate stack emission(s) on the plant surroundings, (ii) establishing a control philosophy for a multi-feed/product distillation columns, reactors, etc.

(c) To provide a valuable predictive tool (model) for process evaluation, e.g. (i) optimizing the process design by simulation or defining optimum operating conditions to attain maximum benefit of multi process variable systems, (ii) computing vapour-liquid equilibria for mixtures to predict and simulate separation/distillation column behaviour, (iii) evaluating process equipment, such as reboilers, condensers, etc., and (iv) modeling and designing CSTR, batch, and other reactors.

In using computers, a deep understanding of the theories and principles are needed to solve the (complex) problems. One also must be able to state the problem correctly and estimate the expected answers to confirm the validity of the algorithm. Although, the knowledge of programming languages is valuable, a number of software packages are available which are user friendly and require a little skill to use them for various tasks of process engineering.

9.3 ANALOG COMPUTATION vs DIGITAL COMPUTATION

This chapter mainly deals with digital computation of stoichiometric problems. However, a comparison between analog and digital computers seems very appropriate. An analog computer uses a continuous variable of electricity, namely, a dc "voltage" to represent continuous variables, such as fluid flow, temperatures, compositions, velocities, volumes, pressures, etc. The main advantages of the analog system include: (a) it is a continuous system and it simulates parameters by actual measurement, (b) it can perform integration and differentiation in addition to the four basic arithmetic functions of addition, subtraction, multiplication and division, and (c) it can handle parallel modes of operation and can therefore be operated on a real-time basis. The use of the analog machine requires lengthly set-up time due to voltage and time scaling and patching of wires. The probability of errors in patching and component malfunctions is significant. Also, the accuracy of results is limited.

All these problems are practically eliminated in a digital computer which is a discrete machine, simulating continuous parameters with frequent sampling/counting. All integrations and differentiations must be done numerically which involve approximating continuous differential equations with a discrete finite-difference equation. The selection of the algorithm is a key in solving/simulating the problem. Despite these minor problems, the digital computer is more powerful because of its capability in logical functionality and memory. The digital computers are also superior with regard to flexibility of operation and precision of calculations. Some of the functions cannot conveniently be accomplished with analog computers but they can be performed using the digital machines. Particularly in process control, these unique functions include feed forward and cascade controls, non-interacting multi-variables, compensation of process variables, online and automatic tuning, automatic start-up and shutdown, and optimal control.

When a digital computer is used, it is unusual to obtain the correct solution to an engineering problem in the first trial. At the same time a variety of *canned* (library) computer programmers are widely available for solving specific problems and they simplify the use of computers.

9.4 USE OF PROGRAMMABLE CALCULATORS

Since 1859, the slide rule has been a handy calculating tool for scientists and engineers. But it had been replaced by an electronic marvel—the calculator which incorporates a solid circuit. The emergence of hand-held programmable calculators permitted the engineer to solve effortlessly all his complex problems elegantly at his desk that were formerly relegated to full scale computer solution.

In a keystroke programmable calculator, the program is introduced with the help of keystrokes. Having programmed, data can be fed in with the help of keys and the calculator runs the entire computations at a single keystroke. In a fully programmable calculator, complex problems are permanently stored on small magnetic cards or magnetic taps and used in the calculator over and over again.

Rapier[1] has given an excellent introduction to calculators. Benenati[2,3] has given examples to demonstrate the capabilities of programmable calculators in solving complex chemical engineering problems.

Certain limitations of the programmable calculators may be worth mentioning here. The memory storage is usually limited in such a calculator. However, such a limitation can be overcome to a certain extent by connecting an additional memory pack to the calculator. Also, the calculator gives only the final answer. If this answer is incorrect, it is difficult to find the step where calculations went wrong. If a printer is attached with the calculator and if certain intermediate answers are also printed on it, it may become possible to check the wrong step. Properties of chemical compounds can be fed in the form of an empirical equation in the calculator. Data in the tabular form occupy a large memory storage and hence when tabular data are to be used for substitution, a computer may be needed. Nevertheless the emergence of programmable calculators increased the ability of an engineer to a great extent.

9.5 PROGRAMMING LANGUAGES

Programming is the set of instructions and logic used by a computer to perform a specific task correctly. Therefore, programming language is the method of communication between man and machine. There are many languages in use and each of them has its own operational limitations. Among engineers, originally developed in the 1950s for technical applications, FORTRAN (FORmula TRANslator) was the universal language being used for problem-solving and process simulation. Of its versions, the FORTRAN IV was the most versatile language through mid 70s.

American National Standards Institution (ANSI) had published an improved set of standards in 1977 FORTRAN X 3.9-1978 or FORTRAN 77. Etter[4] has summarized a variety of real world applications using these revised standards, which include new features and structures to write more versatile and powerful programmes. Another improved version, FORTRAN 90, (ANSI X3.198-1991, identical to International FORTRAN Standards, ISO/IEC 1539:1991) has been established making the language stronger ever for its use in the technical applications.

FORTRAN 90 includes several significant additions to its special character sets that can be used for special purposes and also include symbols for mathematics, chemistry, etc.

9.6 GENERAL PROCEDURE

A proper approach must be followed for an effective and efficient use of computers. A general procedure described below may be used as a guideline.

1. Define the problem clearly with the input (available) and output (desired to be calculated) data
2. Develop the algorithm (logic) considering all principles and details.
3. Draw a flow chart, a pictorial step-by-step description of the input data, algorithm, and the output data.
4. Write the computer programme or select an appropriate canned programme (software).
5. Debug and confirm the validity of the programme.
6. Use the programme for solving the defined problem.

In the following presentation, some of the important and useful numerical methods[5-10] are introduced in order of increasing complexity. For simulating more complicated and highly complex systems, reader should refer to advanced books and literature references in related fields.

Combination of FORTRAN 77 and IV standards, spreadsheet software (Microsoft Excel©) and Mathcad software are used throughout this text.

9.7 APPLICATIONS OF FORTRAN

9.7.1 Roots of Equations

One common problem in digital computation is the solution of algebraic and transcendental equations. When these equations are complex or nonlinear, analytical solutions are not practical and then an iterative trial-and-error method is used. An initial value is assumed and used as a trial solution. If the first trial is not sufficiently accurate, a second is generated and the whole process is repeated until the iteration converges within some desired tolerance limit.

A variety of techniques can be used for the initial guess and subsequent new guesses to rapidly arrive at the correct answer. The selection of the technique depends upon the nature of the equations. Sometimes, numerical instability is experienced such that the solution diverges or oscillates around the correct solution.

The computer solution to an algebraic equation can best be illustrated by using some stoichiometric examples. As discussed in chapter 2, van der Waals equation accounts for non-ideal behaviour of gases. This equation [Eq. (2.25)], which is of third order cannot be easily solved. Two different computation techniques for solving this equation are introduced in the following illustration.

Example 9.1 Generate a computer solution to Example 2.20(b) by (a) trial-and-error and (b) Newton-Raphson methods.

Solution In this example it is proposed to calculate the specific volume of super-heated steam at 10MPa a (100 bar a) and 623 K (350°C) using the van der Waals equations of state.

$$(p + a / V^2) (V - b) = RT \tag{2.25}$$

where,

$$a = 27R^2T_c^2/64p_c \ (m^3)^2 MPa \ /(kmol)^2 \tag{2.26}$$

$$b = RT_c / 8p_c \ m^3/kmol \tag{2.27}$$

(a) Trial-and-Error Method

Rearranging Eq. (2.25):

$$F(V) = V - \frac{RT}{\left(p + \dfrac{a}{V^2}\right)} - b = 0 \tag{9.1}$$

Calculate V such that $F(V) = 0$. the constants and conditions are known. At random, the initial value of V is selected as 0.1; it is also the initial increment to be added or subtracted from V for successive guesses. The increment ΔV is reduced depending upon the value of the function $F(V)$. the iterations are continued until $F(V)$ is within some desired tolerance. Also, calculations are discontinued if they exceed some pre-set number of iterations; this is done to check for and avoid diverging or oscillating instability. In such a case, this successive guess technique will be unsuccessful and must be changed.

The flow chart for this example is shown in Fig. 9.1 and the FORTRAN names of the variables are given in Table 9.1.

A digital computer program and the solution are shown in Figs. 9.2 and 9.3, respectively.

(b) Newton-Raphson Method

Rearranging the equation in polynomial form,

$$F(V) = pV^3 - (bp + RT)V^2 + aV - ab$$

As discussed earlier in Chapter 2, this method requires the evaluation of first derivative.

$$F'(V) = 3pV^2 - 2(bp + RT)V + a$$

Subsequent guesses are based on the slope of this function which can be illustrated as

$$V_{n+1} = V_n - F(V_n) / F'(V_n) \tag{2.41}$$

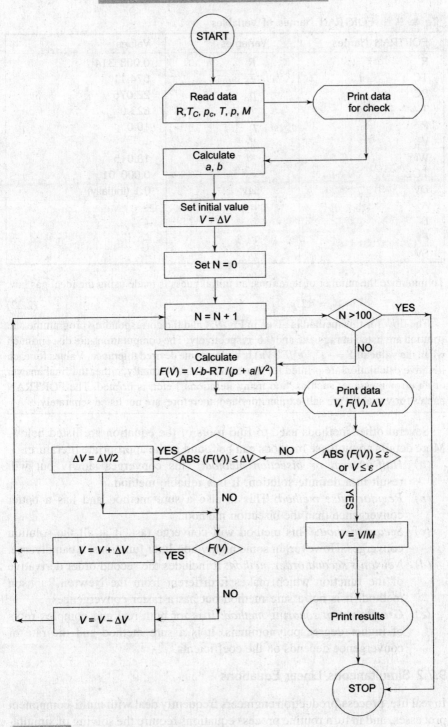

Fig. 9.1 Flow Chart of Example 9.1(a)

Table 9.1 FORTRAN Names of Variables

FORTRAN Names	Variables	Values
R	R	0.008 314
TC	T_c	674.11
PC	p_c	22.076
T	T	623.0
P	p	10.0
V	V	–
WM	M	18.015
TOL	e	0.000 01
DV	ΔV	0.1 (initially)
A	a	–
B	b	–
FV	$F(V)$	–
SV	v	–

To minimize the number of iterations, an initial guess is made using the ideal gas law,

$$V_0 = RT/p \tag{2.22}$$

The flow for this method is given in Fig. 9.4 and the corresponding programme and solution are listed in Figs. 9.5 and 9.6, respectively. The computations are discontinued when the value of $Y = -F(Vn)/F'(Vn)$ is within some desired tolerance. Values for each iterative calculation are printed for illustration only. Normally, either the final answer or an error message, such as "too many iterations," etc., is printed. The FORTRAN names for variables are self-explanatory and, therefore, are not listed separately.

Several other methods used to find roots of the equation are listed below. More details about these methods can be found in the appropriate literature.

(a) *Half-interval or bisection method*: This converges slowly but will result in a definite solution. It is a reliable method.

(b) *Regular false method*: This is also a sure method and has a better convergence than the bisection method.

(c) *Secant method*: This method will converge fast, if at all the solution converges. However, in some highly non-liner functions, it can diverge.

(d) *Newton's second order method*: It includes the second order derivative of the function which makes it different from the Newton-Raphson method. It is not a sure method but has a faster convergence.

(e) *Graeffe's root squaring method*: It is for both real and complex roots of higher degree polynominals. It is a sure method and the rate of convergence depends on the coefficients.

9.7.2 Simultaneous Linear Equations

In real life, process/production engineers frequently deal with multi-component processes, and in turn routine process equations require the solving of simultaneous linear algebraic equations. Such evaluations include (a) determining the

```
C       EXAMPLE  9.1 (A)
C
C       THIS PROGRAMME SOLVES VAN DER WAAL'S EQUATION
C
C       READ CONSTANTS

        READ(5,*)R,TC,PC,T,P,WM,TOL,DV
        WRITE(6,12)R,TC,PC,T,P,WM,TOL,DV
12      FORMAT(9X,'DATA INPUT' /9X, 'R = ', F10.4, 5X, 'TC = ',F10.4,5X,'PC='
     1  10.4/9X,'T=',F10.4,5X,'P=',F10.4,5X'WM=',F10.4/9X,'TOL=',
     2  F10.5,5X,'DV=',F10.4////14X,'SOLUTION BY TRIAL AND ERROR......'/
     3  17X,'V',13X,'FV',13X,'DV')
        WRITE(*,*) "PRESS ANY KEY TO CONTINUE"
        A=(27. * (R*TC)**2.)/(64. * PC)
        B=R*TC/(8. * PC)
        V=DV
        N=0
5       N=N+1
        IF (N .GT. 100) STOP
        FV=V-R*T/(P+A/(V**2.))-B
        WRITE(6,13) V,FV,DV
13      FORMAT(5X,3(5X,F10.5))
        IF(ABS(FV) .LE. TOL .OR. DV .LE. TOL) GOTO 6
        IF(ABS(FV) .LE. DV) DV=DV/2
        IF(FV .LT. 0.) V= V+DV
        IF(FV .GT. 0.) V= V-DV
        GOTO 5
6       SV=V/WM
C
C       PRINT RESULTS
C
        WRITE(6,14)SV
14      FORMAT(//10X, 'SPECIFIC VOLUME = ',F10.5,2X,'M3/KG')
        END
```

Fig. 9.2 Computer Program for Trial and Error Solution of van der Waals Equation

```
DATA INPUT
R   =        .0083    TC  =   647.1100   PC  =    22.0760
T   =     623.0000    P   =    10.0000   WM  =    18.0150
TOL=        .00001    DV  =      .1000
```

```
          SOLUTION BY TRIAL AND ERROR......
              V             FV            DV
           .10000        -.00977        .10000
           .17500        -.04004        .02500
           .20000        -.04783        .02500
           .22500        -.05298        .02500
           .25000        -.05524        .02500
           .27500        -.05462        .02500
           .30000        -.05126        .02500
           .32500        -.04540        .02500
           .35000        -.03730        .02500
           .37500        -.02720        .02500
           .40000        -.01536        .02500
           .41250        -.00885        .01250
           .41875        -.00547        .00625
           .42188        -.00374        .00313
           .42500        -.00199        .00313
           .42656        -.00111        .00156
           .42734        -.00067        .00078
           .42773        -.00045        .00039
           .42813        -.00022        .00039
           .42832        -.00011        .00020
           .42842        -.00006        .00010
           .42847        -.00003        .00005
           .42849        -.00002        .00002
           .42850        -.00001        .00001
```

```
SPECIFIC VOLUME =      .02379   M3/KG
```

Fig. 9.3 Computer Output for Example 9.1(a)

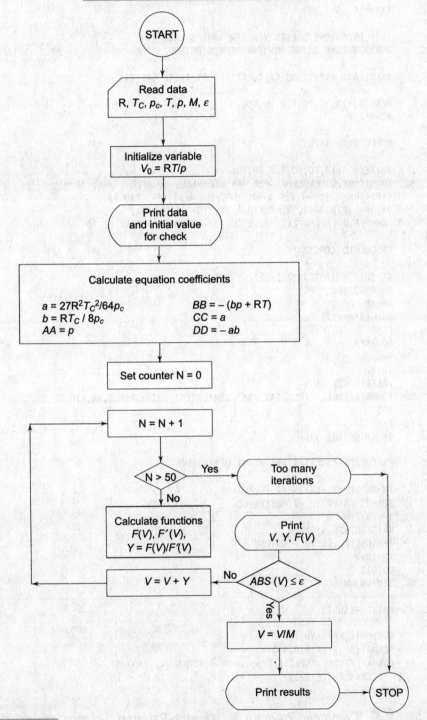

Fig. 9.4 Flow Chart of Example 9.1(b)

```
C       EXAMPLE  9.1 (B)
C
C       THIS PROGRAMME SOLVES VAN DER WAAL'S EQUATION
C       FOR V-VOLUME USING NEWTON-RAPHSON METHOD
C
C       READ DATA INPUT AND CALCULATE VO BY IDEAL GAS LAW

        READ(5,*)R,TC,PC,T,P,WM,TOL
        VO=R*T/P
C
C       CHECK DATA INPUT
C
        WRITE(6,51)R,TC,PC,T,P,VO,TOL,WM
   51   FORMAT(9X,'DATA INPUT FOR VAN DER WAALS EQUATION' /9X, 'R =',
       1 F10.4/9X, 'TC =',F10.4/9X, 'PC='10.4/9X,'T=',F10.4/,
       2 9X,'P=',F10.4/9X,'VO=',F10.4/9X,'TO=',F10.6/9X,
       3 'WM=',F10.4///// 2X, 'SOLUTION BY NEWTON-RAPHSON.... ')
C
C       CALCULATE CONSTANTS
C
        A =(27. * (R*TC)**2.)/(64. * PC)
        B =R*TC/(8. * PC)
        AA =P
        BB=-(B*P+R*T)
        CC=A
        DD=-A*B
        Y=0.
        VN=VO
        WRITE(6,52) VN,Y
   52   FORMAT(//16X, 'VN' ,14X, 'Y' ,14X, 'FN' //10X,F10.5,5X,F10.5)
        N=0
   12   N=N+1
        IF (N.GE.50) STOP
C
C       CALCULATE FUNCTION AND FIRST DERIVATIVE
C
        FN=AA*VN**3.+BB*VN**2.+CC*VN+DD
        FDN=3.*AA*VN**2.+2.*BB*VN+CC
        Y=-FN/FDN
        WRITE(6,53) VN,Y,FN
        IF(ABS(Y) .LE.TOL) GOTO50
        VN=VN+Y
        GOTO12
   50   SVN=VN/WM
C
C       PRINT RESULTS
C
        WRITE (6,54) SVN,Y
   53   FORMAT(5X,3(5X,F10.5))
   54   FORMAT(//10X, 'SPECIFIC VOLUME =',F10.5,2X, 'M3/KG',5X,
       1 'TOLERANCE=',E12.5)
        END
```

Fig. 9.5 Computer Program for Newton-Raphson Solution of van der Waals Equation

DATA INPUT FOR VAN DER WAALS EQUATION

R	=	.0083
TC	=	647.1100
PC	=	22.0760
T	=	623.0000
P	=	10.0000
VO	=	.5180
TO	=	.000010
WM	=	18.0150

SOLUTION BY NEWTON-RAPHSON....

VN	Y	FN
.51796	.00000	
.51796	-.06435	.18793
.45361	-.02226	.03897
.43135	-.00279	.00392
.42856	-.00004	.00006
.42852	.00000	.00000

SPECIFIC VOLUME   = .02379 M3/KG TOLERANCE = -.12037E-06

Fig. 9.6 Computer Output of Example 9.1 (b)

performance of distillation column, (b) calculating the battery limit material and energy balances, (c) rating heat exchangers, etc.

The number of equations must be equal to the number of unknowns. All of these equations need to be independent for obtaining unique solutions. In general,

$$a_{11} X_1 + a_{12} X_2 + \ldots + a_{1n} X_n = C_1$$
$$a_{21} X_1 + a_{22} X_2 + \ldots + a_{2n} X_n = C_2$$
$$\vdots \qquad \vdots \qquad \vdots \qquad \vdots \qquad \vdots$$
$$a_{n1} X_1 + a_{n2} X_2 + \ldots + a_{nn} X_n = C_n \qquad (9.2)$$

If all Cs are zero, the set is considered homogeneous; otherwise, the set is non-homogeneous.

Example 9.2 Solve Example 8.6 with the help of the FORTRAN using Gauss-Jordan elimination method.

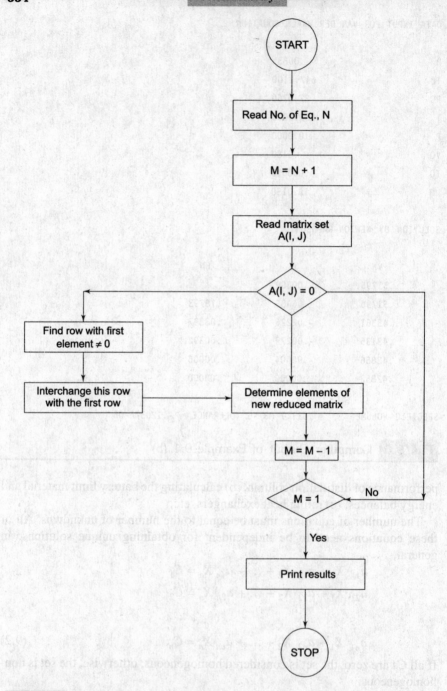

Fig. 9.7 Flow Chart of Example 9.2

```
C       EXAMPLE 9.2
C
C       THIS PROGRAMME SOLVES SIMULTANEOUS EQUATIONS
C       BY GAUSS-JORDAN ELIMINATION METHOS
C       ALLOCATE MATRIX
C
        DIMENSION A(10,11) B(10,10)
C
C       READ NO. OF EQUATIONS AND THEN MATRIX ELEMENTS BY ROW. .
C
        READ(5,*) N
        M=N+1
        DO 10 I=1,N
   10   READ(5,*)(A(I,J),J=1,M)
C       DATA CHECK
C
        WRITE(6,103)N,M
  103   FORMAT(////5X,'INPUT DATA.....'//11X,'NO. OF EQUATIONS =',I3,5X,   1'M
       ='I3///)
        DO 20 I=1,N
   20   WRITE(6,104)  (A(I,J),J=1,M)
  104   FORMAT(5X,8E12.4)
C       CHECK FOR FIRST ZERO ELEMENT
C
        EPS=.0000001
    9   AA=ABS(A(1,1)
        IF(AA .GT. EPS)GOTO 51
        MM=M-1
        DC 30 I=2,MM
        AB=ABS(A(I,1))
        IF(AB .LE. EPS)GOTO 30
        DO 40 J=1,M
        TEMP=A(I,J)
        A(I,J)=A(1,J)
   40   A(1,J)=TEMP
        GOTO51
   30   CONTINUE
        WRITE(6,105)
  105   FORMAT(//'.....ERROR..... -NO UNIQUE SOLUTION')
        STOP
C
   51   DO 50 J=2,M
        DO 50 I=2,N
   50   B(I-1,J-1)=A(I,J)-A(1,J)*A(I,1)/A(1,1)
        DO 60 J=2,M
   60   B(N,J-1)=A(I,J)/A(1,1)
        M=M-1
        DO 70 J=1,M
        DO 70 I=1,N
        IF (ABS(B(I,J)) .LE. 0.0001) B(I,J)=0
   70   A(I,J)=B(I,J)
        IF((M-1) .NE. 0) GOTO 9
        WRITE(6,106)
```

```
106   FORMAT(///15X,'SOLUTION FOR SIMULTANEOUS EQUATIONS.....'/)
      DO 80 I=1,N
80    WRITE(6,107)I,(A(I,1))
107   FORMAT(15X,'X(',I2,') =',E12.4/)
      END
```

Fig. 9.8   Computer Program for solving Simultaneous Equations using Gauss-Jordan Elimination Method

Solution   There are six simultaneous equations and six unknowns. These equations can be solved by using flowchart, given in Fig. 9.7, and programme, given in Fig. 9.8. Computer output is given in Fig. 9.9.

```
INPUT DATA......

NO. OF EQUATIONS  =  6 M = 7

-.1000E+01  .0000E+00  .1022E+01  .1022E+01  .1211E+01  .0000E+00  .1350E+02
 .1000E+01 -.1100E+00  .0000E+00  .0000E+00  .0000E+00  .1100E+00 -.1815E+01
 .0000E+00  .5160E+01  .5160E+01  .5160E+01  .5160E+01  .2179E+02  .7540E+03
 .0000E+00 -.4037E+01 -.4037E+01  .9600E+02 -.4037E+01 -.4037E+01  .1106E+02
 .8977E+01  .8977E+01 -.1000E+03  .0000E+00  .0000E+00  .8977E+01 -.1481E+03
 .0000E+00  .9109E+01  .0000E+00  .0000E+00  .0000E+00 -.8403E+00  .9358E+01


SOLUTION FOR SIMULTANEOUS EQUATIONS ....

    X( 1)  =  .5480E+01
    X( 2)  =  .3762E+01
    X( 3)  =  .4964E+01
    X( 4)  =  .2164E+01
    X( 5)  =  .1043E+02
    X( 6)  =  .2955E+02
```

Fig. 9.9   Computer Output for Example 9.2

Ans.

$a = 5.480$ t/h	$b = 3.762$ t/h
$c = 4.964$ t/h	$d = 2.164$ t/h
$e = 29.55$ t/h	$g = 10.43$ t/h

Other methods used to solve simultaneous linear algebraic equations are listed below and related literature should be referred to for detailed explanation and applications [5, 6, 7, 11].

1. Matrix-inversion method
2. Gaussian elimination method
3. Jacobi-iteration method
4. Gauss-Seidel iteration method

9.7.3 Numerical Integration and Differentiation

Process engineers are often required to solve problems which are best described with integration or differentiating functions. Various numerical methods can be used to obtain a higher degree of accuracy. One of these is introduced in Example 9.3 with stoichiometric application.

Example 9.3 Pure ethylene is heated from 303 to 523 K (30 to 250°C) at a constant pressure. Generate a computer solution to calculate the heat added per kmol of ethylene using the following two equations.

(a) $C^o_{mp} = 11.8486 + 119.7 \times 10^{-3}\, T - 365 \times 10^{-7}\, T^2$

(b) $C^o_{mp} = 51.012 + 16.24 \times 10^{-3}\, T - (10.806 \times 10^5)/T^2$

where C^o_{mp} is in kJ /(kmol · K) and T is in K.

Solution:

$$Q = \int_{T_1}^{T_2} C^o_{mp}\, dT$$

$$= \frac{\Delta T}{3}\left(C^o_{mp1} + C^o_{mpn+1}\; 4\sum_{j=2,4,6}^{n} C^o_{mpj} + 2\sum_{j=3,5,7}^{n-1} C^o_{mpj} \right)$$

where
$$C^o_{mp1} = C^o_{mp} \text{ at } T_1$$
$$C^o_{mpn+1} = C^o_{mp} \text{ at } T_2$$
$$\Delta T = (T_2 - T_1)/n$$
$$n = \text{even number of intervals}$$
$$C^o_{mpj} = C^o_{mp} \text{ at } T_j$$
$$T_j = T_1 + (j-1)\,\Delta T$$

A flow chart to solve this equation is given in Fig. 9.10. The program and the results are shown in Figs. 9.11 and 9.12 (a) and (b), respectively.

Ans. (a) Q = 12 083 kJ/kmol ethylene

(b) Q = 11 299 kJ/kmol ethylene

The above problem can be conveniently solved by analytical integration but one may often face the situation in which tabulated data (such as steam tables) are to be utilized for integration. In such a situation, numerical integration with the help of a computer is valuable.

Other methods of numerical integration include:

1. Trapezoid rule
2. Romberg method (extension of trapezoid rule)
3. Gauss quadrature (uses unequally spaced intervals)

   For details of these methods the reference is made to related literature in this field.[7-9]

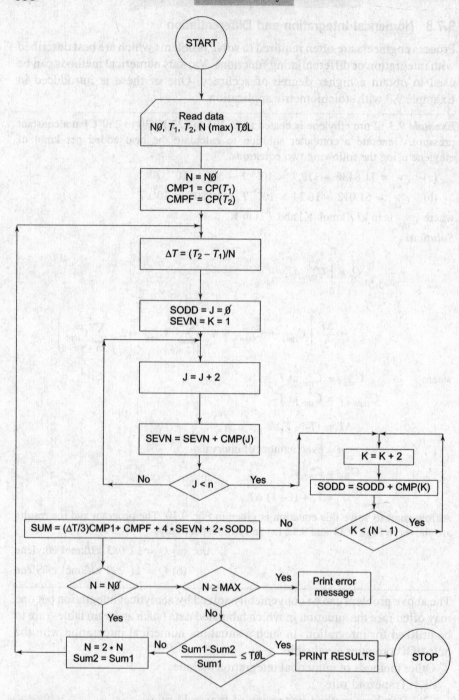

Fig. 9.10 Flow Chart of Example 9.3

```
C
C      EXAMPLE 9.5
C
C      PROGRAM SIMPSON'S RULE FOR INTEGRATION.....
C
C      READ CONSTANTS AND LIMITS
C
       READ (5,*)NO,NMAX,T1,T2,TOL,A,B,C,M
       WRITE(6,12) NO,NMAX,T1,T2,TOL,A,B,C,M
   12  FORMAT(///15X,'DATA INPUT :'//15X, 'NO=I4,11X,'NMAX =',I5/15X,'T1
      1 =',E12.5,3X,'T2 =',E12.5,3X,'TOL =',E12.5///15X,'EQUATION... '/15X,
      2 'COP=',E12.5, ' + ',E12.5,'* T + ',E12.5,'* T **',I4//15X,
      3 'SOLUTION..... '//20X, 'NN'M 7X, 'N',9X,ÉRROR',10X, 'SUM1
         ',11X, 'SUM2')
       CPI=A+B*T1+C*T1**M
       CPF=A+B*T2+C*T2**M
       N=NO
   5   DT=(T2-T1)/N
       NN=NN+1
       SODD=0
       SEVN=0
       J=0
       K=1
       KF=N-1
   6   J=J+2
       TJ=T1+J*DT
       CPJ=A+B*TJ+C*TJ**M
       SEVN=SEVN+CPJ
       IF(J.LT.N) GOTO6
   7   K=K+2
       TK=T1+K*DT
       CPK=A+B*TK+C*TK**M
       SODD=SODD+CPK
       IF(K.LT.KF)GOTO7
       SUM1=(DT/3.)*(CPI+CPF+4.*SEVN+2.*SODD)
       IF(N.W.NO)GOTO8
       IF(NNN.GE.20) GOTO9
       EROR=ABS((SUM1-SUM2)/SUM1)
       IF(EROR.LE.TOL) GOTO99
   8   WRITE(6,15) NN,N,EROR,SUM1,SUM2
   15  FORMAT(15X,I7,3X,I7,3X,E12.5,3X,E12.5,3X,E12.5)
       N=2*N
       SUM2=SUM1
       GOTO5
   9   WRITE(6,13)
   13  FORMAT(15X, '...TOO MANY INTERVALS .... '/5X, '..CHECK DATA.. '///)
  99WR ITE(6,15)NN,N,EROR,SUM1,SUM2
       WRITE(6,14)N,DT,CPI,CPF,EROR,SUM2
   14  FORMAT(///15X, 'INTERVALS',5X, '=',I5,10X, 'DT',10X, '=',E12.5/
      11.5X, 'INITIAL VALUE =',E12.5,3X, 'FINAL VALUE ='E12.5/15X,
      2'ERROR= ',E12.5//15X, 'Q =',E12.5,2X, 'KCAL/KG MOL')
       END
```

Fig. 9.11 Computer Program for Integration of Polynomial Equation with the help of Simpson's Rule

```
DATA INPUT
          NO = 4                  NAMX = 10000
          T1 = .30300E+03          T2 = .52300E+03      TOL =.10000E-03

EQUATION...
CPO = .11849E+02  +  .114970E+00  * T  +  -.36500E-04 * T ** 2

SOLUTION.....

       NN            N            ERROR              SUM1                SUM2
        1            4         .00000E+00         .12963E+05          .00000E+00
        2            8         .31154E-01         .12572E+05          .12963E+05
        3           16         .18877E-01         .12339E+05          .12572E+05
        4           32         .10309E-01         .12213E+05          .12339E+05
        5           64         .53780E-02         .12148E+05          .12213E+05
        6          128         .27457E-02         .12114E+05          .12148E+05
        7          256         .13871E-02         .12097E+05          .12114E+05
        8          512         .69746E-03         .12089E+05          .12097E+05
        9         1024         .34901E-03         .12085E+05          .12089E+05
       10         2048         .17498E-03         .12083E+05          .12085E+05
       11         4096         .87863E-04         .12082E+05          .12083E+05

          INTERVALS = 4096                       DT = .53711E-01
    INITIAL VALUE = .4476E+02          FINAL VALUE = .64468E+02
          ERROR = .87863E-04
              Q = .12083E+05 KJ/KMOL
```

Fig. 9.12 (a) Computer Output for Example 9.3(a)

```
DATA INPUT
          NO = 4                  NAMX = 10000
          T1 = .30300E+03          T2 = .52300E+03      TOL = .10000E-03

EQUATION...
CPO = .51012E+02  +  .162400E-01  * T  +  -.10086E+07 * T ** -2

SOLUTION.....

       NN            N            ERROR              SUM1                SUM2
        1            4         .00000E+00         .11720E+05          .00000E+00
        2            8         .14785E-01         .11549E+05          .11720E+05
        3           16         .99945E-02         .11435E+05          .11549E+05
        4           32         .57595E-02         .11370E+05          .11435E+05
        5           64         .30873E-02         .11335E+05          .11370E+05
        6          128         .15979E-02         .11316E+05          .12148E+05
        7          256         .81296E-03         .11307E+05          .11335E+05
        8          512         .40971E-03         .11303E+05          .11316E+05
        9         1024         .20620E-03         .11300E+05          .11303E+05
       10         2048         .10268E-03         .11299E+05          .11300E+05
       11         4096         .51600E-04         .11299E+05          .11299E+05

          INTERVALS = 4096                       DT = .53711E-01
    INITIAL VALUE = .44947E+02         FINAL VALUE = .55818E+02
          ERROR = .51600E-04
              Q = .11299E+05        KJ/KMOL
```

Fig. 9.12 (b) Computer Output for Example 9.3(b)

9.7.4 Ordinary Differential Equations

A number of chemical engineering problems are described by a set of differential equations of order one or higher. Normally equations describing a dynamic or transient process become highly non-linear when combined with chemical reaction(s). To solve such equations, a suitable numerical integration technique must be used for which an approximate solution of predetermined accuracy can be obtained. In the following example, initial value ordinary differential equations are solved by using a Runge-Kutta numerical technique. This method is one of the most popular methods and its derivation can be easily found in the literature.

Example 9.4 Consider a single continuous stirred tank reactor with a second-order irreversible exothermic reaction

$$2A \rightarrow B + C$$

The heat generated by the reaction is removed with cooling water being circulated in a jacket (ref. Fig. 9.13).

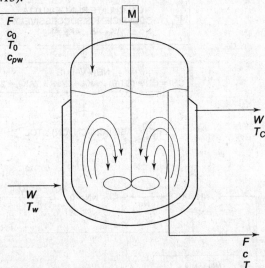

Fig. 9.13 Continuous Stirred Tank Reactor

All related process conditions and parameter values are given below. Generate a computer solution for transient concentration of the reactant A when the feed is entering at the steady-state reaction temperature 360 K (87°C).

V = reactor volume, 700 L

c_0 = concentration of reactant A in feed, 140 g/L

c = concentration of reactant A in product stream, g/L

r = reaction rate

    = $-k c^2$, g/(L·s)

k = reaction rate constant, $1.488 \times 10^{-3} \exp(-1421/T)$, L/(g·s)

T = product stream temperature, K

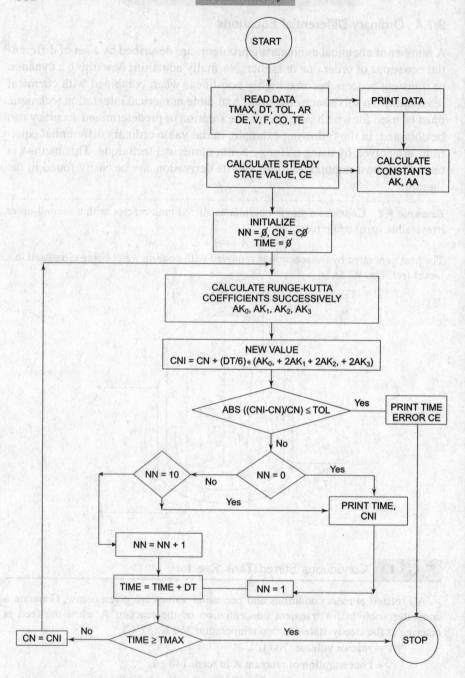

Fig. 9.14   Flow Chart of Example 9.4

T_∞ = steady–state reaction temperature, 360 K(87°C)

T_0 = feed temperature, 360 K(87°C)

T_w = cooling water supply temperature, 300 K(27°C)

T_c = cooling water return temperature, K

T'_c = average cooling water temperature $(T_w + T_c)/2$, K

θ = time, s

F = feed rate = 7.5 L/s

W = cooling water rate, g/s

ΔH = heat of reaction = 2100 J/g

ρ = reactant/product density at reaction temperature = 960 g/L

Cps = heat capacity of solution = 3.77 kJ(kg·K)

Cpw = heat capacity of cooling water = 4.1868 kJ/ (kg·K)

UA = heat transfer rate = 18 850 W/K

$$\left(\begin{array}{c}\text{Flow of}\\\text{reactant in}\end{array}\right) - \left(\begin{array}{c}\text{Flow of}\\\text{reactant out}\end{array}\right) - \left(\begin{array}{c}\text{Reactant}\\\text{disappearance}\\\text{by reaction}\end{array}\right) - \left(\begin{array}{c}\text{Material}\\\text{accumulation}\end{array}\right)$$

$$Fc_0 = Fc - (kc^2)\,V = d(Vc)d\theta \qquad (9.3)$$

where
$$k = 1.488 \times 10^{-3} \exp (-1421/T)$$

Rearranging the above equation,

$$dc/d\theta = (F/V)(c_0 - c) - kc^2$$

Assuming $T = 360$ K the above equation is solved for concentration c as function of time θ using the fourth order Runge-Kutta method. The flow chart is given in Fig. 9.14. the computer programme and the solution are given in Figs. 9.15 and 9.16 respectively. The transient behaviour is plotted in Fig. 9.17.

```
C

C       EXAMPLE 9.4

C

C       PROGRAM RUNGE-KUTTA : 4TH- ORDER

C

C       READ DATA

C

        READ (5,*)TMAX,DT,TOL,AR,DE,V,F,CO,TE
        WRITE(6,12)TMAX,DT,TOL,AR,DE,V,F,CO,TE
    12 FORMAT(///15X,'DATA INPUT:'//15X,'TMAX =',E12.5,3X,'DT =',F10.2,
      1 5X,'TOL =',E12.5,/15X,'AR =',E12.5,3X,'DE =',E12.5/15X,'VOL =',
      2 E12.5,3X,'FEED =',E12.5/15X, 'CO =',E12.5,3X,'TE =',E12.5)

    14 FORMAT(///15X,'SOLUTION BY RUNGE-KUTTA .......'//16X,'T,SEC',9X,'CON
      1 CN'/)
        RK=AR*EXP(DE/TE)
```

```
      AA=F/V
      CE=(AA/(2. *RK)) * (-1. * (1. *4. *RK*CO/AA) ** 0.5)
      NN=0
      TIME=0
      CN=CO
      WRITE(6,101) TIME,CN
   10 CONTINUE
      AKO=AA * (CO-CN) -RK *CN**2
      AK1=AA * (CO-(CN+AKO/2.)) -RK*(CN+AKO/2.)**2.
      AK2=AA * (CO-(CN+AK1/2.)) -RK*(CN+AK1/2.)**2.
      AK3=AA * (CO-(CN+AK2)) -RK*(CN+AK2/2.)**2.
      CN1=CN+(DT/6.)*(AKO+2.*AK1+2.*AK2+AK3)
      EROR=ABS((CN1-CN)/CN)
      IF(EROR .LE. TOL) GOTO 99
      IF(NN .EQ. 10) GOTO 51
      NN=NN+1
      GOTO 52
   51 WRITE(6,101)TIME,CN1
  101 FORMAT(15X,F8.1,5X,E12.5)
      NN=1
   52 TIME=TIME+DT
      IF(TIME .GE. TMAX) STOP
      CN=CN1
      GOTO 10
   99 WRITE(6,101) TIME,CN1
      WRITE(6,102)EROR,CE,CN1
  102 FORMAT(//15X,'ERROR =',E12.5,5X,' EQUI. CONC. = ', E12.5/39X, 'CONV.
     1CONCN.  =',E12.5)
      END
```

Fig. 9.15 Computer Program for Evaluation of Transient Behaviour of CSTR

DATA INPUT :

TMAX	=	.10000E+06	DT	=	10.00	TOL	=	.10000E-04
AR	=	.14880E-02	DE	=	-.14210E+04		
VOL	=	.70000E+04	FEED	=	.75000E+01		
CO	=	.14000E+03	TE	=	.36000E+03		

SOLTUION BY RUNGA-KUTTA.....

T, SEC	CONCN
.0	.14000E+03
100.0	.98288E+02
200.0	.80695E+02
300.0	.71016E+02
400.0	.65340E+02
500.0	.61886E+02
600.0	.59738E+02
700.0	.58383E+02
800.0	.57522E+02
900.0	.56971E+02
1000.0	.56617E+02
1100.0	.56390E+02
1200.0	.56243E+02
1300.0	.56149E+02
1400.0	.56088E+02
1500.0	.56048E+02
1600.0	.56023E+02
1700.0	.56007E+02
1800.0	.55996E+02
1900.0	.55989E+02

ERROR = .99473E-05 EQUI. CONCN = .55977E+02

CONV. CONCN = .55989E+02

Fig. 9.16 Computer Output of Example 9.4

Fig. 9.16 Computer Output of Example 9.4

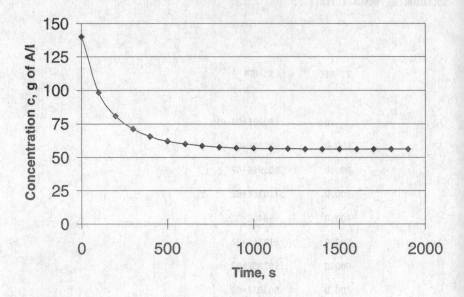

Transient Solution of Example 9.4

Other methods used for solving initial value differential equation are listed below. Derivations and details of using these methods can be found in the literature.

1. Euler's method
2. Predictor-corrector method (Euler's modified, self-starting)
3. Runge-Kutta methods of different orders (first, second, third, sixth...) for solving single and simultaneous equations.
4. Milne's method.
5. Hamming's method

The numerical solution of boundary-value problems is somewhat difficult. Mainly, shooting method[9], instead of the previously used trial-and-error method, is used to solve such problems. No further details are given in this book and the reader is advised to refer to the appropriate literature. Similarly, quite a few chemical engineering problems are described by partial differential equations[10]. These problems include calculation of partial molar enthalpies, and so on. Details about various numerical methods used for solving partial differential equations is beyond the scope of this book.

In Example 9.4, a simple case of CSTR is described. However, a complex problem will result when kinetics and thermodynamics are coupled with stoichiometry. Kunzru et al[12] have demonstrated the capability of a computer in simulating a catalytic reformer unit. In this application, calculations are made for a plant in which naphtha is reformed in the presence of hydrogen-rich gas to yield high octane gasoline. Such a programme can be used in a wide variety of applications such as selection of (a) operating conditions; (b) number of reactors, (c) catalyst bed depth, etc.

9.8 APPLICATIONS OF SPREADSHEET SOFTWARE IN STOICHIOMETRY

Spreadsheet softwares for personal computers were initially introduced as accounting tools. However, these softwares find applications in chemical engineering and other disciplines. Two most widely used spreadsheet softwares are Microsoft Excel© and LOTUS 1–2–3©. Several spreadsheet applications involving process flowsheeting and mass balances have appeared in literature. These softwares are well known for simplicity in use and also for sensitivity analysis that can be performed with case.

In the preceding sections, use of FORTRAN-77 was made to write specific programs. While developing these programs, knowledge of numerical methods and development of a flowchart were necessary. Programming based on the flow chart is a task by itself and usually debugging of the program is necessary before the final program can be put into use.

Real advantage of a spreadsheet software over conventional computer methods, for instance use of FORTRAN, lies in the simplicity of the numerical formulation. Shorter programming and less debugging time are other benefits. Spreadsheet programs suit the occasional user who does not have the time and resources of a programming facility to help formulate and debug the source code. A few hours of learning a spreadsheet package will enable one to start, using software immediately and produce valuable results. Formulas can be entered easily.

Spreadsheets can be easily manipulated for process calculations and optimization. Input variables and parameters can be varied both manually and automatically. A macro can be built in the spreadsheet to optimize a process design automatically thereby one can appreciate the ability of the spreadsheet to iterate to converge. Spreadsheets also contain readymade programs that will allow one to conduct standard calculations, such as regration analysis for solving simultaneous equations, once data are entered in an appropriate format. In the following examples, the use of a spreadsheet software (Excel© of Microsoft Corporation, USA) is demonstrated in a variety of stoichiometric problems.

Example 9.5 Solve Example 9.1 using a spreadsheet program.
Solution
a. by Trial and Error method

Rearranging the equation, $F(V) = V - R*T / (p + a/V^2) - b$

Input Data:

Pressure, p	10	MPa
Temperature, T	623.00	K
Critical Presure, p_c	22.1	MPa

Critical Temperature, T_c 647.11 K
Gas Constant, R   0.008314 $m^3 \times MPa/(kmol \times K)$
Molar Mass, M_m 18.015
Tolerance, e   0.00001
Initial delta V, dV   0.10

Calculation:

$a = 27*R^2*T_c^2/(64*p_c)$ a = 552545.2 $(m^3)^2 \times MPa/(kmol)^2$
$b = R*T_c/(8*p_c)$ b = 0.030430 $m^3/kmol$

Trial	V	F(V)	dV	New dV	test	Sp. Vol
0	0.1	-0.00981	0.10000	0.05000	FALSE	#N/A
1	0.15000	-0.03031	0.05000	0.02500	FALSE	#N/A
2	0.17500	-0.04014	0.02500	0.02500	FALSE	#N/A
3	0.20000	-0.04794	0.02500	0.02500	FALSE	#N/A
4	0.22500	-0.05309	0.02500	0.02500	FALSE	#N/A
5	0.25000	-0.05535	0.02500	0.02500	FALSE	#N/A
6	0.27500	-0.05472	0.02500	0.02500	FALSE	#N/A
7	0.30000	-0.05136	0.02500	0.02500	FALSE	#N/A
8	0.32500	-0.04550	0.02500	0.02500	FALSE	#N/A
9	0.35000	-0.03739	0.02500	0.02500	FALSE	#N/A
10	0.37500	-0.02728	0.02500	0.02500	FALSE	#N/A
11	0.40000	-0.01543	0.02500	0.01250	FALSE	#N/A
12	0.41250	-0.00893	0.01250	0.00625	FALSE	#N/A
13	0.41875	-0.00554	0.00625	0.00313	FALSE	#N/A
14	0.42188	-0.00381	0.00313	0.00313	FALSE	#N/A
15	0.42500	-0.00206	0.00313	0.00156	FALSE	#N/A
16	0.42656	-0.00118	0.00156	0.00078	FALSE	#N/A
17	0.42734	-0.00074	0.00078	0.00039	FALSE	#N/A
18	0.42773	-0.00051	0.00039	0.00039	FALSE	#N/A
19	0.42813	-0.00029	0.00039	0.00020	FALSE	#N/A
20	0.42832	-0.00018	0.00020	0.00010	FALSE	#N/A
21	0.42842	-0.00012	0.00010	0.00010	FALSE	#N/A
22	0.42852	-0.00007	0.00010	0.00005	FALSE	#N/A
23	0.42856	-0.00004	0.00005	0.00002	FALSE	#N/A
24	0.42859	-0.00003	0.00002	0.00002	FALSE	#N/A
25	0.42861	-0.00001	0.00002	0.00001	FALSE	#N/A
26	0.42863	-0.00001	0.00001	0.00001	TRUE	0.023792 m^3/kg

b. by Newton – Raphson method:

Rearranging the equation: $F(V) = p*V^3 - (b*p + R*T)*V^2 + a*V - a*b$
Derivative w.r.t V $F'(V) = 3*p*V^2 - 2*(b*p + R*T)*V + a$
$$V_{n+1} = V_n - F(V) / F'(V)$$

Trial	V_n	$F(V_n)$	$F'(V_n)$	$F(V_n)/ F'(V_n)$	test	Sp. Vol.
0	0.517962	187743.5	2920158.9	0.064292252	FALSE	#N/A
1	0.453669	38904.51	1751254.1	0.022215234	FALSE	#N/A
2	0.431454	3900.765	1405009.9	0.002776326	FALSE	#N/A
3	0.428678	57.28540	1363819.9	4.20036E-05	FALSE	#N/A
4	0.428636	0.013013	1363200.3	9.54631E-09	FALSE	#N/A
5	0.428636	7.38510E	1363200.1	5.41747E-16	TRUE	0.023793 m^3/kg

Fig. 9.18 Spreadsheet Outputs of Example 9.1

> **Note:** Advantage of using of numerical method (i.e. Newton-Raphson method) is evident as less number of trials are required for getting the solution.

Example 9.6 In Example 8.6 steam balance of a caustic soda plant is given. Its flowchart and solution using FORTRAN are given in Example 9.2. Solve the example using a spreadsheet.

Solution Refer Fig. 9.19 for the computer output using spreadsheet program.

OPTIMIZATION OF STEAM BALANCE

Notations: a = Saturated Low Pressure Steam Input to Deaerator, t/h
b = Medium Pressure Steam Input to CW Pump Turbine, t/h
c = Medium Pressure Steam Input to BFW Pump Turbine, t/h
d = Medium Pressure Steam Input to FD Fan Turbine, t/h
e = Exhaust (under vacuum) from Power Turbine, t/h
g = Letdown from Medium Pressure to Low Pressure Header, t/h
h = Letdown from High Pressure to Medium Pressure Header, t/h
Z = Total high Pressure Steam Produced, t/h

a	b	c	d	E	g	H	k
-1	0	1.022	1.022	0	1.121	0	13.5
1	-0.11	0	0	-0.11	0	0	1.815
0	5.16	5.16	5.16	21.79	5.16	-5.5	754.03
0	-4.037	-4.037	96	-4.037	-4.037	0.266	11.061
8.977	8.977	-100	0	8.977	0	0	-148.115
0	9.109	0	0	-0.843	0	0	9.358

Z_{min} = b + c + d + e + g + 2.745, for h=0

Solution
Regression Statistics
Multiple R	1
R Square	1
Adjusted R Square	0
Standard Error	0
Observations	6

Analysis of variance
	df	Sum of Squares	Mean Square	F	Significance F
Regression	6	522275.8497	87045.97495	0	#N/A
Residual	0	5.42036E-24	0		
total	6	522275.8497			

	Coefficients	Standard error	Statistics	P – value	Lower 95%	Upper 95%
Intercept	0	#N/A	#N/A	#N/A	#N/A	#N/A
a	5.47992043	0	0	0	#N/A	#N/A
b	3.76252185	0	0	0	#N/A	#N/A
c	4.9639907	0	0	0	#N/A	#N/A
d	2.1637615	0	0	0	#N/A	#N/A
e	29.5549366	0	0	0	#N/A	#N/A
g	10.4329685	0	0	0	#N/A	#N/A

Z_{min} = 53.6231791, for h = 0

Fig. 9.19 Spreadsheet Output for Example 9.6

Example 9.7 In Example 4.15, material balance of a typical ammonia synthesis loop is given in which the inerts content of the mixed feed stream is restricted to 10 mole %. It is desired to carry out the sensitivity analysis of the synloop by changing the inerts content in the mixed feed stream from 10 mole % to 15 mole % in the steps of 0.5 mole %. Using a spreadsheet program, calculate the flow rates of mixed feed, recycle stream and product ammonia stream for a fresh feed rate of 100 kmol/s.

Solution Simulation of Ammonia Synthesis Loop

```
Notations:   a = Nitrogen in mixed feed, kmol/s
             I = Inerts in mixed feed, mole fraction
             M = Mixed feed, kmol/s
             P = Purge rate, kmol/s
             R = Recycle flow, kmol/s
             N = Ammonia production rate, kg/s

Equations:   a = 24.75*I*M/(0.75+0.25*I*M)
             (M-100)/(I*M-1) = (0.35*M+065*I*M+1.775*a)/(I*M)
             P = (M-100)/(I*M-1)
             R = M-100,  R >= 100
             N = 0.65*(M*(I-1)-3.5*A)*17.031

Solution:    M^2+B*M+C = 0, where
             B = (3.5385 − 426.1926*I)/(I*(1-I)) and
             C = (1.6154 − 188.192*I)/(I^2 − I^3)
```

I	B	C	M	a	P	R	N
0.100	-434.2307	-1911.5333	438.5890	92.6618	7.9001	338.5890	779.4908
0.105	-438.5392	-1838.8639	442.6930	92.9979	7.5346	342.6930	782.8542
0.110	-442.7241	-1772.2834	446.6916	93.3034	7.2023	346.6916	785.9117
0.115	-446.8057	-1711.0788	450.6030	93.5822	6.8990	350.6030	788.7032
0.120	-450.8013	-1654.6433	454.4423	93.8378	6.6210	354.4423	791.2620
0.125	-454.7253	-1602.4576	458.2224	94.0728	6.3653	358.2224	793.6161
0.130	-458.5901	-1554.0747	461.9542	94.2898	6.1292	361.9542	795.7890
0.135	-462.4063	-1509.1079	465.6472	94.4906	5.9107	365.6472	797.8009
0.140	-466.1833	-1467.2212	469.3096	94.6771	5.7077	369.3096	799.6691
0.145	-469.9288	-1428.1211	472.9484	94.8507	5.5188	372.9484	801.4084
0.150	-473.6501	-1391.5503	476.5700	95.0126	5.3425	376.5700	803.0317

Fig. 9.20 Spreadsheet Output for Example 9.7

Example 9.6 is a steam balance which can be performed for variety of conditions as discussed in Chapter 8. In Example 9.7, simulation is carried out for different inerts in the mixed feed. Such iterative calculations enable a designer to select optimum design based on cost of equipment, type of equipment and other considerations. Simulation can also be used for plant troubleshooting, controllability and maintenance[13]. A detailed plant simulation enables one to understand interdependency of performance of one equipment on another and helps in their quantitative evaluation. Plant simulation can also help in achieving better quality in terms of product specifications. Sowa[14] has demonstrated the use of process plant simulation in minimizing the waste generation and also in increasing the plant safety.

9.9 APPLICATIONS OF MATHEMATICAL SOFTWARE IN STOICHIOMETRY

In Sec. 9.8, use of spreadsheet program was demonstrated in solving stoichiometric problems. However, use of a spreadsheet required the knowledge of algorithm to perform iterations and to specify the condition(s) to terminate the iteration.

Limitation of a spreadsheet can be overcome by use of a mathematical software, which is a versatile, highly functional tool that can solve symbolic and numerical mathematical problems on a personal computer. Phillips[15] et al reviewed five well known software packages; Mathcad, Maple, Matlab, Mathematica and TK Solver. All these packages run on Windows operating system.

In this book, Mathcad is selected for solving variety of stoichiometric problems. It is developed by Mathsoft, Inc., USA. It is easy and ideal for repetitive engineering calculations where the objective is to determine the effects of change of a variable on calculated parameters thereby finding an optimum value. Data can be entered in vectors or metrices or can be imported from a spreadsheet. The software has also an ability to do unit conversions.

User interface with Mathcad is done by selecting an icon from a toolbar that represents the desired calculation. For example, choosing the icon for an integral from calculus toolbar generates an integral sign with place holders for the integrand and limits of integration. By filling the placeholders, numerical subroutine is performed by Mathcad and calculates the value of the integral. Similar toolbars exist for arithmetics, calculus, matrix, symbolic keywords, graph, etc.

Iteration is an integral part of the software. Algorithms are built-in for solving the equations. Starting value (called 'Guess') is required and it must be appropriate to the particular root of equation.

In Chapters 2 to 8, use of Mathcad was demonstrated as a tool in solving polynomial and simultaneous equations. These are relatively simple applications of Mathcad. In this chapter, small programmes are developed to perform repetitive calculations by varying a parameter. Some are general (e.g. equations of state) while some are specific (e.g. ammonia synthesis loop).

User friendly Mathcad can boost efficiency of an engineer and save his considerable time. Reader is advised to refer the website for knowing more capabilities of Mathcad.

Example 9.8 Write a generalized program in Mathcad to solve van der Waals equation [Eq. (2.25)] of state. Solve Example 2.20(b) using the program.

Solution

$$a\left(R, T_c, p_c\right) := 27 \cdot R^2 \cdot \frac{\left(T_c\right)^2}{64 \cdot p_c}$$

$$b\left(R, T_c, p_c\right) := R \cdot \frac{T_c}{8 \cdot p_c}$$

$$f\left(V, p, R, T, T_c, p_c\right) := \left[\left(p + \frac{a\left(R, T_c, p_c\right)}{V^2}\right) \cdot \left(V - b\left(R, T_c, p_c\right)\right)\right] - (R \cdot T)$$

Guess value of V may be taken from the Ideal Gas Law.

$$V := 0.518$$

$$\text{soln} := \text{root}\left(f\left(V, p, R, T, T_c, p_c\right), V\right)$$

Solution of Example 2.20 (b)

$$V := 0.518$$

$$V := \text{root}(f(V, 10, 0.008314623, 647.11, 22.076), V)$$

$$V = 0.4285 \quad \text{m}^3/\text{kmol}$$

$$\text{spvol} := \frac{V}{18.0115}$$

$$\text{spvol} = 0.02379 \quad \text{m}^3/\text{kg}$$

Fig. 9.21 Mathcad Program for van der Waals Equation

In Chapter 2, use of Mathcad was demonstrated to solve the equation with a single unknown (i.e. V). However, before solving the equation with a built-in root function, basic equation was simplified. By writing a specific program for the basic equation in Mathcad, it can be seen in Fig. 9.21 that substitution of parameters is the only requirement.

Example 9.9 Solve Example 2.21 using the program, developed in Example 9.9, and calculating pseudo-critical properties by inserting a table.

Solution

ttable :=

	0	1	2
0	0.352	32.200	1.297
1	0.148	190.500	4.604
2	0.128	282.340	5.039
3	0.339	132.850	3.494
4	0.015	304.120	7.374
5	0.018	126.090	3.394

$$T_c := \sum_{i=0}^{5} \text{table}_{i,0} \cdot \text{table}_{i,1} \qquad p_c := \sum_{i=0}^{5} \text{table}_{i,0} \cdot \text{table}_{i,2}$$

$T_c = 127.535$ K $\qquad\qquad\qquad p_c = 3.139$ MPa

$$a(R) := \frac{27 \cdot R^2 \cdot T_c^2}{64 \cdot p_c} \qquad\qquad b(R) := \frac{R \cdot T_c}{8 \cdot p_c}$$

$$f(V, p, R, T) := \left[\left(p + \frac{a(R)}{V^2} \right) \cdot (V - b(R)) \right] - (R \cdot T)$$

Guess value of V may be taken from the Ideal Gas Law.

$V := 16$

$\text{soln}(V, p, R, T) := \text{root}(f(V, p, R, T), V)$

$\text{soln}(V, 0.4, 0.008314773) = 16.086$ L/mol

Fig. 9.22 Mathcad Solution for Example 2.21

Example 9.10 Write a generalized program in mathcad to solve Beattie-Bridgeman equation of state. Solve Exercise 2.32 using the program.

$$A(a_0, a, V) := a_0 \cdot \left(1 - \frac{a}{V} \right) \qquad B(b_0, b, V) := b_0 \cdot \left(1 - \frac{b}{V} \right) \qquad \varepsilon(c, T, V) := \frac{c}{V \cdot T^3}$$

$$f(a_0, b_0, a, b, c, T, R, p, V) := p - \left[\frac{R \cdot T \cdot (1 - \varepsilon(c, T, V))}{V^2} \cdot (V + B(b_0, b, V)) \right] + \frac{A(a_0, a, V)}{V^2}$$

Guess value of V may be taken from the Ideal Gas Law.

$V := \blacksquare$

$\text{soln} := \text{root}\left(f(a_0, b_0, a, b, c, T, R, p, V), V \right)$

$\text{soln} =$
Solution of Exercise 2.32

$V := 0.482$

$V := \text{root}\left(f(0.588, 0.094, 0.05861, 0.01915, 90 \cdot 10^4, 423, 0.008314, 7.3, V), V \right)$

$V = 0.4002$ m³/kmol

Fig. 9.23 Mathcad Program for Solving Beattie-Bridgeman Equation of State

---

Example 9.11 Write a generalized program in Mathcad for recycle loop of ammonia synthesis. Solve Example 4.15 using the program.
Solution

$N_{2m}(a) := a$ $\qquad\qquad\qquad\qquad$ N₂ in Mixed feed

$H_{2m}(a) := 3 \cdot a$ $\qquad\qquad\qquad\qquad$ H₂ in Mixed feed

$I_m(M,y) := y \cdot M$ — Inerts in Mixed Feed

$NH_{3m}(M,a,y) := M - a - H_{2m}(a) - I_m(M,y)$ — NH$_3$ in Mixed Feed

N$_2$ Reacted : $\qquad N_{2r}(a,x) := x \cdot a$

H$_2$ Reacted : $\qquad H_{2r}(a,x) := 3 \cdot x \cdot a$

NH$_3$ Produced : $\qquad NH_{3p}(a,x) := 2 \cdot x \cdot a$

N$_2$ Unreacted : $\qquad N_{2ur}(a,x) := (1-x) \cdot a$

H$_2$ Unreacted: $\qquad H_{2ur}(a,x) := (1-x) \cdot 3 \cdot a$

Total NH$_3$ in Outlet gas after converter

$NH_{3c}(M,a,x,y) := NH_{3p}(a,x) + NH_{3m}(M,a,y)$

NH$_3$ Separated in the Separator

$NH_{3s}(M,a,x,y,z) := NH_{3c}(M,a,x,y) \cdot z$

NH$_3$ uncondensed

$NH_{3un}(M,a,x,y,z) := (1-z) \cdot NH_{3c}(M,a,x,y)$

Total Gas mixture after separator :

$G_s(M,a,x,y,z) := N_{2ur}(a,x) + H_{2ur}(a,x) + NH_{3un}(M,a,x,y,z) + I_m(M,y)$

Recycle stream

$R(M,a,x,y,z,P) := G_s(M,a,x,y,z) - P$

N$_2$ lost in Purge

$$N_{2p}(M,a,x,y,z,P) := N_{2ur}(a,x) \cdot \frac{P}{G_s(M,a,x,y,z)}$$

N$_2$ in Recycle

$N_{2rec}(M,a,x,y,z,P) := N_{2ur}(a,x) - N_{2p}(M,a,x,y,z,P)$

Guess Value for M, P, a. Use guess value of M more than F.

$M := 200 \qquad P := 1 \qquad a := 1$

Given

$$I_m(M,y) \cdot \frac{P}{G_s(M,a,x,y,z)} = y_f F$$

$F + R(M,a,x,y,z,P) = M$

$N_{2rec}(M,a,x,y,z,P) + a_f = a$

$vec(F, a_f, y_f, x, y, z) := Find(M, P, a)$

Solution of Example of 4.15 :

$$vec(100, 24.75, 0.01, 0.25, 0.1, 0.65) = \begin{bmatrix} 438.589 \\ 7.9 \\ 92.662 \end{bmatrix}$$

$M := vec(100, 24.75, 0.01, 0.25, 0.1, 0.65)_0$

$P := vec(100, 24.75, 0.01, 0.25, 0.1, 0.65)_1$

$a := vec(100, 24.75, 0.01, 0.25, 0.1, 0.65)_2$

$M = 438.589$ $P = 7.9$ $a = 92.662$ all in kmol/s

$R(F, M) := M - F$

$R(100, M) = 338.589$ kmol/s

$rr(F, M) := \dfrac{R(F, M)}{F}$

$rr(100, M) = 3.386$

$NH_{3s}(M, a, 0.25, 0.1, 0.65) = 45.769$ kmol/s

Fig. 9.24 Mathcad Program for Ammonia Synthesis Loop

Note: It can be seen in Fig. 9.24 that all parameters can be varied at will. Exercise 4.30 (ref. Exercise 9.3) can be easily solved by the above program.

Example 9.12 In Example 4.15, fresh feed composition shows that N_2: H_2 ratio is 1:3 on volume basis. Vary this ratio from 1:2.8 to 1:3.2 in increments of 0.05, keeping inerts in feed and purge at 1% and 10% mole%, respectively. Assume 25% conversion per pass and 65% separation of ammonia in the separator. It is desired that N_2:H_2 ratio be 1:3 on molar basis in the mixed feed. Evaluate the material balance of the synthesis loop.

Solution With feed gas containing 99% N_2 + H_2 and a molar ratio of 1:2.8 of N_2 : H_2, nitrogen content of feed gas works out to 26.053 mole%. Substitution of these parameters in the programme does not yield the results and computer shows an error in calculations. This is because dynamic conditions of the loop do not permit achievement of exact 1:3 molar ratio in the mixed feed. In such cases, Mathcad provides a solution with minimum error which is difficult to achieve by manual calculations.

Approximate results are tabulated in Table 9.2 which are derived using Mathcad program, given in Fig. 9.24 with minimum errors, except for N_2:H_2 ratio of 1:3 in mixed feed.

Table 9.2 Effect of Varying Feed Composition of Ammonia Synthesis Loop

Basis : 100 kmol/s fresh feed

Molar ratio of N_2:H_2 in fresh feed	N_2 content in Fresh Feed, mole %	Mixed Feed, M kmol/s	Purge Rate, P kmol/s	Ammonia Production Rate, kmol/s
2.80	26.053	453.9078	7.9726	43.1518
2.85	25.714	449.9192	7.9542	43.8326
2.90	25.385	446.0503	7.9360	44.4934
2.95	25.063	442.2658	7.9179	45.1402
3.00	24.750	438.5891	7.9001	45.7690 (Exact)
3.05	24.444	434.9967	7.8823	46.3838
3.10	24.146	431.5000	7.8648	46.9825
3.15	23.855	428.0874	7.8473	47.5672
3.20	23.571	424.7587	7.8301	48.1378

Ans.

Note: It is interesting to analyse the data of Table 9.2. It can be seen that purge rate P does not vary so significantly as seen in the table. This leads to valuable information concerning control philosophy of the loop. When inerts in the fresh feed does not vary significantly, minor variations in purge rate is able to control the N_2:H_2 in the mixed feed effectively. Thus in this case, purge gas flow needs to be controlled in a very narrow range. However, when there is a significant variation in inerts in fresh feed, purge gas flow needs to be varied significantly which is obvious because inerts, entering the system, must be purged out in the concentrated form.

Example 9.13 Write a generalized program in Method for solving steam balance (Example 8.6).

It is decided to carryout simulation of the steam balance by varying temperature of superheated HP steam from 713 K (440°C) to 793 K (520°C). Anticipated operating conditions of the cascade steam system are given in Table 9.3.

Solution HP steam enthalpy = H_1 kJ/kg
MP superheated steam enthalpy = H_2 kJ/kg
LP superheated steam enthalpy = H_3 kJ/kg
LP saturated steam enthalpy = H_4 kJ/kg
15 bar saturated steam enthalpy = H_5 kJ/kg
Surface condenser steam enthalpy = H_6 kJ/kg
BFW enthalpy = H_7 kJ/kg
Surface condenser steam enthalpy = H_8 kJ/kg
Let x_1 kg BFW required to quench 1kg of 39 bar MP superheated steam to 15 bar saturated steam

$$x_1(H_2, H_5, H_7) := \frac{H_2 - H_5}{H_5 - H_7}$$

$$Q_1(H_2, H_5, H_7) := \frac{3}{1 + x_1(H_2, H_5, H_7)} \text{ t MP steam required/h}$$

Let x2 kg BFW required to quench 1kg of 39 bar MP superheated steam to 4.4 bar saturated steam

$$x_2(H_2, H_4, H_7) := \frac{H_2 - H_4}{H_4 - H_7}$$

Let x3 kg BFW required to quench 1kg of 4.4 bar superheated steam to 4.4 bar saturated steam

$$x_3(H_3, H_4, H_7) := \frac{H_3 - H_4}{H_4 - H_7}$$

Power Turbine:
Specific steam consumption in Power Turbine from HP to MP steam:

$$S_1(H_1, H_2) := \frac{3600}{(H_1 - H_2) \cdot 0.97}$$

Specific steam consumption in Steam turbine from MP to LP:

$$S_2(H_2, H_3) := \frac{3600}{(H_2 - H_3) \cdot 0.97}$$

Table 9.3 Anticipated Operating Conditions of a Cascade Steam System (Base Case: Example 8.6)

Units	Case – I Initial	Case – I Final	Case – II Initial	Case – II Final	Case – III Initial	Case – III Final	Case – IV Initial	Case – IV Final	Case – V Initial	Case – V Final
(a) Power turbine – (i) Extraction										
MPa a	11.5	3.9	11.5	3.9	11.5	3.9	11.5	3.9	11.5	3.9
K (°C)	713 (440)	593 (320)	733 (460)	612 (339)	753 (489)	631 (358)	773 (500)	650 (377)	793 (520)	669 (396)
kJ/kg	3190.7	3020.4	3247.8	3069.7	3320.7	3117.1	3356.0	3163.0	3408.1	3207.9
(a) Power turbine – (ii) Condensing										
MPa a	11.5	0.012	11.5	0.012	11.5	0.012	11.5	0.012	11.5	0.012
K (°C)	713 (440)	323 (50)	733 (460)	323 (50)	753 (480)	323 (50)	773 (500)	323 (50)	793 (520)	332 (58)
		95% dryness		96.5% dryness		98% dryness		99.5% dryness		
kJ/kg	3190.7	2472.0	3247.8	2507.7	3320.7	2543.5	3356.0	2578.7	3408.1	2607.4
(b) Medium pressure turbine – (ii) Extraction										
MPa a	3.9	0.44	3.9	0.44	3.9	0.44	3.9	0.44	3.9	0.44
K (°C)	593 (320)	443 (170)	612 (339)	462 (189)	631(358)	480.6 (207.6)	650 (337)	499 (226)	669 (396)	516 (243)
kJ/kg	3020.4	2793.3	3069.7	2834.9	3117.1	2874.4	3163.0	2913.1	3207.9	2948.6
(b) Medium pressure turbine – (ii) Condensing										
MPa a	3.9	0.012	3.9	0.012	3.9	0.012	3.9	0.012	3.9	0.012
K (°C)	593 (320)	323 (50)	612 (339)	323 (50)	961 (358)	323 (50)	650 (377)	323 (50)	669 (396)	332 (58)
		95% dryness		96.5% dryness		98% dryness		99.5% dryness		
kJ/kg	3020.4	2472.0	3069.7	2507.7	3117.1	2543.5	3163.0	2578.7	3207.9	2607.4
(c) Cooling water requirement										
m³/h	600		635		670		710		740	

Note: Anticipated operating conditions are calculated by assuming constant thermodynamic efficiency of different turbines.

Specific steam consumption in Power turbine from HP to SC steam:

$$S_3(H_1, H_6) := \frac{3600}{(H_1 - H_6) \cdot 0.97}$$

Specific steam consumption in Steam turbine from MP to surface condenser:

$$S_4(H_2, H_6) := \frac{3600}{(H_2 - H_6) \cdot 0.97}$$

Cooling water requirement in surface condenser:

$$Q_{cw}(H_6, H_8) := \frac{H_6 - H_8}{10 \cdot 4.1868}$$

Guess

$$a := 1 \qquad b := 1 \qquad c := 1 \qquad d := 1 \qquad e := 1 \qquad g := 1$$

Given

$$13.5 + a = (1 + x_3(H_3, H_4, H_7)) \cdot (c + d) + (1 + x_2(H_2, H_4, H_7)) \cdot g$$

$$a = 0.11 \cdot (b + e + 16.5)$$

$$\frac{(b + c + d + g + Q_1(H_2, H_5, H_7))}{S_1(H_1, H_2)} + \frac{e}{S_3(H_1, H_6)} = \frac{6832}{1000}$$

$$2.47 \cdot (b + c + d + e + g + Q_1(H_2, H_5, H_7)) \cdot S_2(H_2, H_3) = 1000d$$

$$5.493(a + b + e + 16.5) \cdot S_2(H_2, H_3) = 1000c$$

$$0.2315 \left[Q_{cw}(H_6, H_8) \cdot (b + e) + 600 \right] \cdot S_4(H_2, H_6) = 1000 \cdot b$$

$$vec(H_1, H_2, H_3, H_4, H_5, H_6, H_7, H_8) := find(a, b, c, d, e, g)$$

$$vec(3190.7, 3020.4, 2793.3, 2741.9, 2800.8, 2472.0, 440.17, 209.2) = \begin{bmatrix} 5.482 \\ 3.763 \\ 4.966 \\ 2.165 \\ 29.577 \\ 10.43 \end{bmatrix}$$

$$H_1 := 3190.7 \qquad H_2 := 3020.4 \qquad H_3 := 2793.3 \qquad H_4 := 2741.9$$

$$H_5 := 2800.8 \qquad H_6 := 2472.0 \qquad H_7 := 440.17 \qquad H_8 := 209.2 \qquad \text{all in kJ/kg}$$

$$a := vec(H_1, H_2, H_3, H_4, H_5, H_6, H_7, H_8)_0$$

$$b := vec(H_1, H_2, H_3, H_4, H_5, H_6, H_7, H_8)_1$$

$$c := vec(H_1, H_2, H_3, H_4, H_5, H_6, H_7, H_8)_2$$

$$d := vec(H_1, H_2, H_3, H_4, H_5, H_6, H_7, H_8)_3$$

$$e := vec(H_1, H_2, H_3, H_4, H_5, H_6, H_7, H_8)_4$$

$$a = 5.482 \text{ t/h} \qquad b = 3.763 \text{ t/h} \qquad c = 4.966 \text{ t/h}$$

$$d = 2.165 \text{ t/h} \qquad e = 29.577 \text{ t/h} \qquad g = 10.430 \text{ t/h}$$

$$Z := b + c + d + e + g + Q_1\left(H_2, H_5, H_7\right)$$
$$Z = 53.646 \ \text{t/h}$$

Fig. 9.25 Mathcad Solution for Cascade Steam Balance

Using the above program, steam flows for all five cases are calculated and tabulated in Table 9.4.

Table 9.4 Evaluation of Cascade Steam Balance for Different Operating Conditions

Case	Steam flow, t/h						
	a	b	c	d	e	g	Z
I	5.482	3.763	4.966	2.165	29.577	10.430	53.646
II	5.367	3.681	4.702	2.034	28.607	10.380	52.097
III	5.136	3.525	4.353	1.867	26.663	10.368	49.421
IV	5.183	3.592	4.266	1.818	27.023	10.267	49.567
V	5.076	3.448	4.027	1.704	26.158	10.255	48.191

Note: From the above table, it can be seen that steam balance with 753 K (480°C) (Case-iII) is probably the best. It is important to note that downstream conditions of various turbines matter significantly in optimization.

Example 9.14 Refer Exercise 8.11. Write a Mathcad Program to solve the problem. Using the program, calculate (a) oxygen requirement in kmol/kmol NG and (b) steam to dry exit gas mole ratio for operating pressures 1.8, 1.9, 2.0, 2.1 and 2.2 MPa a for each of the temperatures; 1340, 1395 and 1450 K (1067, 1122 and 1177 °C). Assume design approach to equilibrium of steam-reforming reaction as 30 K (30°C). Equilibrium constants for the steam reforming and shift reaction are given in Table 9.5.

Table 9.5 Values of Equilibrium Constants[16]

Temperature of reforming reaction	K_{P1}	Temperature of shift reaction	K_{P2}
K(°C)		K(°C)	
1310 (1037)	5.8789×10^{-5}	1340 (1067)	0.4993
1365 (1092)	2.5207×10^{-5}	1395 (1122)	0.4465
1420 (1147)	1.1542×10^{-5}	1450 (1177)	0.4038

Solution Reforming reactions :

$$CH_4 + H_2O = CO + 3 H_2 \tag{A}$$
$$C_2H_6 + 2 H_2O = 2 CO + 5 H_2 \tag{B}$$

$$C_3H_8 + 3\,H_2O = 3\,CO + 7\,H_2 \tag{C}$$

$$C_4H_{10} + 4\,H_2O = 4\,CO + 9\,H_2 \tag{D}$$

Shift reaction :

$$CO + H_2O = CO_2 + H_2O \tag{E}$$

Reactions (B), (C) and (D) go to 100% completion while reactions (A) and (E) go to completion as per the equilibrium.

Reaction (A) is endothermic and hence the methane slip will be determined by the chemical equilibrium at $1395 - 30 = 1365$ K.

Reaction (E) is exothermic and the operating temperature is quite high. Hence its chemical equilibrium at 1395 K will have to be taken for calculations.

Based on above understandings, Mathcad program and computer output for $p = 2.0$ MPa a and $T = 1395$ K (1122°C) are given below in Fig. 9.26.

Solution

$$n_i(F, f_i) := \frac{F \cdot f_i}{100}$$

$$p_1(p) := p \cdot 9.86923$$

$$n(n_{H2}, n_{CO}, n_{CO2}, n_{H2O}, n_{CH4}, f_{O2}, y, f_i, F) := n_{H2} + n_{CO} + n_{CO2} + n_{H2O} \cdots$$
$$+ n_i(F, f_i) + n_{CH4} + (1 - y) f_{O2}$$

Guess the values:

$n_{H2} := 150$ $\quad n_{CO} := 200$ $\quad n_{CO2} := 10$

$n_{H2O} := 40$ $\quad n_{CH4} := 1$ $\quad f_{O2} := 10$

Given
CH$_4$ Balance:

$$n(n_{H2}, n_{CO}, n_{CO2}, n_{H2O}, n_{CH4}, f_{O2}, y, f_i, F) = \frac{n_{CH4}}{s_{CH4}} \cdot 100$$

H$_2$ Balance:

$$n_{H2} + n_{H2O} + 2 \cdot n_{CH4} = F \cdot \frac{(2 \cdot f_m + 3 \cdot f_e + 4 \cdot f_p + 5 \cdot f_{nb} + 5 \cdot f_{ib})}{100}$$

Carbon Balance:

$$n_{CO} + n_{CO2} + n_{CH4} = \frac{F \cdot (f_m + 2 \cdot f_e + 3 \cdot f_p + 4 \cdot f_{nb} + 4 \cdot f_{ib})}{100}$$

O$_2$ Balance:

$$0.5 \cdot n_{CO} + n_{CO2} + 0.5 \cdot n_{H2O} = y \cdot f_{O2}$$

$$K_{p1} = \frac{n_{CH4} \cdot n_{H2O} \cdot n(n_{H2}, n_{CO}, n_{CO2}, n_{H2O}, n_{CH4}, f_{O2}, y, f_i, F)^2}{n_{H2}^3 \cdot n_{CO} \cdot p_1(p)^2}$$

$$K_{p2} = \frac{n_{H2} \cdot n_{CO2}}{n_{CO} \cdot n_{H2O}}$$

$$vec\left(F, f_m, f_e, f_p, f_{nb}, f_{ib}, f_i, y, p, K_{p1}, K_{p2}, s_{CH4}\right):$$
$$= find\left(n_{H2}, n_{CO}, n_{CO2}, n_{H2O}, n_{CH4}, f_{O2}\right)$$

$$vec\left(100, 93.25, 3.32, 0.88, 0.2, 0, 2.35, 0.98, 2.0, 2.5207 10^{-5}, 0.4465, 0.35\right) = \begin{bmatrix} 161.0174 \\ 92.5524 \\ 9.7065 \\ 37.8203 \\ 1.0712 \\ 76.4212 \end{bmatrix}$$

$$n_{H2} := vec\left(100, 93.25, 3.32, 0.88, 0.2, 0, 2.35, 0.98, 2.0, 2.5207 10^{-5}, 0.4465, 0.35\right)_0$$

$$n_{CO} := vec\left(100, 93.25, 3.32, 0.88, 0.2, 0, 2.35, 0.98, 2.0, 2.5207 \cdot 10^{-5}, 0.4465, 0.35\right)_1$$

$$n_{CO2} := vec\left(100, 93.25, 3.32, 0.88, 0.2, 0, 2.35, 0.98, 2.0, 2.5207 \cdot 10^{-5}, 0.4465, 0.35\right)_2$$

$$n_{H2O} := vec\left(100, 93.25, 3.32, 0.88, 0.2, 0, 2.35, 0.98, 2.0, 2.5207 \cdot 10^{-5}, 0.4465, 0.35\right)_3$$

$$n_{CH4} := vec\left(100, 93.25, 3.32, 0.88, 0.2, 0, 2.35, 0.98, 2.0, 2.5207 \cdot 10^{-5}, 0.4465, 0.35\right)_4$$

$$f_{O2} := vec\left(100, 93.25, 3.32, 0.88, 0.2, 0, 2.35, 0.98, 2.0, 2.5207 \cdot 10^{-5}, 0.4465, 0.35\right)_5$$

$$f_{O2} = 76.421 \quad \text{kmol oxygen}$$

$$r_1(F) := \frac{f_{O2}}{F}$$

$$r_1(100) = 0.764 \quad \text{kmol / kmol Feed}$$

Total outgoing gas mixture (wet)

$$n\left(n_{H2}, n_{CO}, n_{CO2}, n_{H2O}, n_{CH4}, f_{O2}, 0.98, 2.35, 100\right) = 306.046$$

Total outgoing dry gas mixture

$$d_g\left(y, f_i, F\right) := n\left(n_{H2}, n_{CO}, n_{CO2}, n_{H2O}, n_{CH4}, f_{O2}, y, f_i, F\right) - n_{H2O}$$

$$d_g(0.98, 2.35, 100) = 268.226 \quad \text{kmol}$$

$$r_2\left(y, f_i, F\right) := \frac{n_{H2O}}{d_g\left(y, f_i, F\right)}$$

$$r_2(0.98, 2.35, 100) = 0.141 \quad \text{kmol steam / kmol dry gas}$$

Fig. 9.26 Mathcad Program for Solving Exercise 8.9

Substitution of values of p, T, K_{p1} and K_{p2} in the program permit calculations of material balances. Table 9.6 is the summary of results.

Table 9.6 Oxygen Requirement and Steam in Exit Gas Stream

Exist gas temperature K(°C)	Operating pressure MPa a	Oxygen requirement, kmol/kmol NG	Steam/dry exit gas mole ratio
1340 (1067)	1.8	0.8617	0.2019
	1.9	0.8787	0.2137
	2.0	0.8950	0.2252
	2.1	0.9107	0.2365
	2.2	0.9272	0.2484
1395 (1122)	1.8	0.7364	0.1232
	1.9	0.7505	0.1322
	2.0	0.7642	0.1410
	2.1	0.7775	0.1497
	2.2	0.7921	0.1592
1450 (1177)	1.8	0.6480	0.0710
	1.9	0.6582	0.0771
	2.0	0.6683	0.0832
	2.1	0.6785	0.0894
	2.2	0.6885	0.0955

9.10 OPTIMIZATION

Optimization is a very important tool in every aspect of chemical engineering. Starting from project scheduling, equipment design, construction, operational analysis of existing processes and improving them, all of these are ultimately required to minimize cost and maximize profit. The capability of the digital computer for performing complex computations can be best used in determining the optimal criteria of all activities. Various optimization techniques are available and their applicability depends upon the nature of the problem to be optimized. If the process can be described by a set of linear equations, linear programming can be used as the most powerful technique for optimization. Typically, this has been widely used to maximize the profit of a petroleum refinery operation by adjusting product cuts based on their demands, prices, and production costs. Optimization of a steam balance is another classical example of linear programming. If the activity or a process is described in stages with branches and loops, dynamic programming is a more suitable technique. Determining the optimum number of effects in case of a multiple effect evaporator system[17] is a typical application of dynamic programming. In general, any decision analysis can use this technique to determine the optimum criteria. The EVolutionary OPeration (EVOP) technique can also be used for optimization. The design of multiple effect evaporator system can also be optimized with the help of EVOP[18]. Geometric programming can conveniently be used in the case of linear problems.

For a highly complex system, numerical search techniques are used. In one dimensional search techniques, Sequential, Golden-search, Lattice, Fibonacci, and Dichotomous are a few of the widely used methods. Some of the multi-dimensional search techniques include Successive Quadratic Programming (SQP), steep ascent, steep ascent pattern and gradient search methods. No one method can be said as being better than another because there is no criterion for defining the effectiveness of a particular numerical optimization technique. The effectiveness depends upon the problem model to be optimized. Optimization can be of the entire system or of a subsystem. A detailed discussion of optimization techniques is beyond the scope of this book.

9.11 CONTROL OF PLANT OPERATION WITH THE HELP OF A COMPUTER

With growing energy crisis and emphasis on quality control, trimming of plant operation has assumed great importance for maximum productivity and efficiency. Computers are increasingly used in the heavy chemical industry for the purpose. A classical example is ammonia synthesis. A computer-controlled quench bed reactor can result in the optimum ammonia production with the minimum energy input in the compression equipment. Similarly, a computer check on the cascade steam balance can result in a significant fuel saving. The computer analyses the plant operating data using stoichiometric principles and prints out the important parameters for a quick check by a production manager. Operators can then be advised suitably for adjusting the operating parameters.

EXERCISES

9.1 A process vent gas the following composition by volume :
H_2 : 81%, C_2H_6 : 2%, C_2H_4 : 4%, C_3H_8 : 1%, C_3H_6 : 2%, N_2 : 8 % and NH_3 : 2%
Calculate the molar volume of the gas mixture at 2.0 MPa a and 333 K (60°C) using van der Waals equation by (a) spreadsheet (by trial and error method) and (b) Mathcad program.

[*Ans.* 0.19345 m^3/kg]

9.2 Calculate the temperature at which ethane gas will have density of 50 kg/m^3 at a pressure of 4.2 MPa a. Assume Beatti-Bridgeman equation of state (ref. Exercise 2.32). Use the Mathcad program for calculations.

[*Ans.* 835.18 K(562°C)]

9.3 Refer Exercise 4.30. Calculate recycle ratio and purge rate for both the cases using Mathcad program.

Ans. (a) Recycle ratio = 3.553, P = 7.971 kmol/s
(b) Recycle ratio = 3.328, P = 7.871 kmol/s

9.4 Refer Exercise 8.16. Establish the steam balance in Mathcad and calculate the high pressure steam generation for all the five cases, tabulated in Table 9.3.

[Ans. Table 9.7]

Table 9.7 Evaluation of Cascade Steam Balance for Different Operation Conditions

Case	Steam flow, t/h						
	a	b	c	d	e	g	Z
I	5.156	8.480	4.670	2.063	30.369	2.769	51.095
II	5.048	8.228	4.423	1.937	29.392	2.950	49.675
III	4.837	7.795	4.100	1.780	24.476	3.332	47.228
IV	4.874	7.852	4.012	1.731	27.808	3.185	47.333
V	4.777	7.562	3.079	1.623	26.923	3.441	46.083

9.5 Refer Exercise 4.35. Write a Mathcad program for establishing material balance of the synloop. Using the programme, calculate various parameters for mixed feed containing inerts from 0.09 to 0.13 (mole fraction) in increments of 0.05 for the ethylene oxide production rate of 3500 kg/h. Assume other parameters to be constant.

[Ans. Table 9.8]

Table 9.8 Effects of Inerts in Mixed Feed on Ethylene Oxide Manufacture

Inerts in mixed feed mole fraction	Fresh feed F kmol/h	Recycle R_2 kmol/h	Purge P kmol/h	Recycle ratio = R_2/F	Ethylene feed rate kg/h
0.090	262.20	2007.8	44.07	7.6575	3252.5
0.095	262.07	2007.9	41.70	7.6617	3248.9
0.100	261.95	2008.0	39.58	7.6656	3245.6
0.105	261.85	2008.1	37.66	7.6690	3242.7
0.110	261.76	2008.2	35.92	7.6722	3240.0
0.115	261.67	2008.3	34.33	7.6750	3237.6
0.120	261.60	2008.4	32.88	7.6777	3235.4
0.125	261.52	2008.5	31.55	7.6801	3233.3
0.130	261.45	2008.5	30.32	7.6823	3231.4

9.6 Purge stream from the ammonia synthesis loop (ref. Example 4.15) contains nearly 60 mole % H_2. This stream is normally burnt as a fuel in reformer furnace. As an energy conservation measure, a cryogenic separation plant (similar to Exercise 4.34), also known as Purge Gas Recovery (PGR) Plant, is installed to recover hydrogen. Figure 9.27 gives the flow scheme.

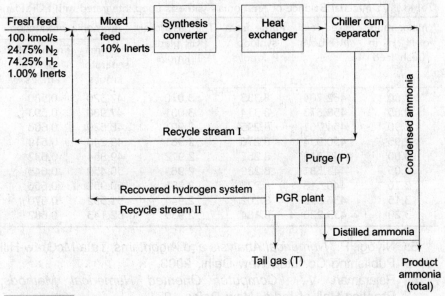

Fig. 9.27 Recycle Loop of Ammonia Synthesis with PGR Plant

In the PGR plant, at first ammonia is scrubbed out in aqueous solution form and concentrated to pure (100%) ammonia by distillation. Ammonia-free dry purge gas is passed through a single stage cold box (similar to the one, described in Example 5.22) in which hydrogen rich stream is separated at about 86 K(–187°C) and 45 bar g which contains 90% H_2, 10% N_2 and 5% inerts, contained in the purge gas (P). Rest gas mixture leaves the cold box as a tail gas stream for use as a fuel in the reformer furnace.

For the ammonia synthesis loop with PGR plant, vary $N_2:H_2$ molar ratio of fresh feed from 1:2.8 to 1:3.2 in increments of 0.05, keeping inerts in the fresh feed and mixed feed streams at 1% and 10% by mole respectively. Assume 25% conversion per pass and 65% separation of ammonia in chillers. Further it is desired that $N_2 : H_2$ molar ratio in the mixed feed be 1:3. Write a Mathcad program for the synthesis loop integrated with the PGR plant and evaluate the material balance of the system.

[*Ans.* Table 9.9]

REFERENCES

1. Rapier, P.M., *Chem. Engg.* **80** (19), Aug. 20, 1973, p. 114.
2. Benenati, R.F., *Chem. Engg.* **84**(5), Feb. 28, 1977, p. 201.
3. _____, **84** (6), March 14, 1977, p. 129.
4. Etter, D.M., *Structured FORTRAN 77 for Engineers and Scientists,* 4th Ed., The Benjamin/Cummings Publishing Co. Inc., Redwood City, USA, 1993.

Table 9.9   Material Balance of Ammonia Synthesis Loop integrated with PGR Plant

Molar ratio of $N_2:H_2$ in fresh feed	Mixed feed, M kmol/s	Purge from synloop, P kmol/s	Tail gas from PGR plant, T kmol/s	Ammonia production	
				From separator kmol/s	From PGR plant kmol/s
2.80	462.704	8.333	3.010	47.320	0.580
2.85	458.673	8.314	3.001	47.980	0.593
2.90	454.761	8.295	2.991	48.620	0.606
2.95	450.934	8.276	2.981	49.246	0.619
3.00	447.216	8.257	2.972	49.854	0.632
3.05	443.581	8.239	2.963	50.459	0.645
3.10	440.518	8.223	2.955	50.950	0.656
3.15	436.590	8.202	2.944	51.592	0.670
3.20	433.220	8.184	2.935	52.143	0.682

5. Niyogi, P., *Numerical Analysis and Algorithms,* Tata McGraw-Hill Publishing Co. Ltd., New Delhi, 2003.

6. Rajaraman, V., *Computer Oriented Numerical Methods,* Prentice-Hall of India, New Delhi, 1971.

7. Forsythe, G. E., M. A. Malcolm and C. B. Moler, *Computer Methods for Mathematical Computations,* Prentice-Hall, Englewood Cliff, NJ, USA, 1977.

8. Johnston, R. L., *Numerical Methods — A Software Approach,* John Wiley & Sons, New York, NY, USA, 1982.

9. Davis, M. E., *Numerical Methods and Modeling for Chemical Engineers,* John Wiley & Sons, New York, NY, USA, 1984.

10. Finlayson, B. A., *Nonlinear Analysis in Chemical Engineering,* McGraw-Hill, New York, NY, 1980.

11. Lapidus, L., *Digital Computation for Chemical Engineers,* McGraw-Hill, New York, USA, 1972.

12. Kunzru, D. and V. Kumar, *Indian Chem. Engg., Transactions,* Vol. XXII, No. 1, p. 35.

13. Dimian, A., *Chem. Engg. Progress,* **90** (9), 1994, p. 58.

14. Sowa, C. J., *Chem. Engg. Progress,* **90** (11), 1994, p. 40.

15. Phillips, J. E. and J. D. DeCicco, *Chem. Engg. Progress,* **95** (7), 1999, p. 69.

16. *Catalyst Handbook,* Springer-Verlag, New York, USA, 1970.

17. Itahara, S. and L. L. Stiel, *Ind. Engng. Chem. Proc. Des. and Develop.,* **5**; 1966, p. 309.

18. Bhatt, B. I., S. P. Deshpande and K. Subrahmanyam, *Chemical Age of India,* **20** (12): 1970, p. 1135.

Conversion Tables

Table AI.1 Length Units

	Metres (m)	Centimetres (cm)	Inches (in)	Feet (ft)	Yards (yd)
m	1	100	39.37008	3.28084	1.093613
cm	0.01	1	0.393701	3.28084×10^{-2}	1.093613×10^{-2}
inch	0.0254	2.54	1	8.333333×10^{-2}	2.777778×10^{-2}
ft	0.3048	30.48	12	1	0.333333
yd	0.9144	91.44	36	3	1

Table AI.2 Area Units

	Square Metres (m^2)	Square Centimetres (cm^2)	Square Inches (in^2)	Square Feet (ft^2)	Square Yards (yd^2)
m^2	1	10^4	1550.003	10.76391	1.19599
cm^2	10^{-4}	1	0.155	1.076391×10^{-3}	1.19599×10^{-4}
in^2	6.4516×10^{-4}	6.4516	1	6.944444×10^{-3}	7.716049×10^{-4}
ft^2	0.092903	929.0304	144	1	0.111111
yd^2	0.836127	8361.273	1296	9	1

Table AI.3 Volume and Capacity Units

	Cubic Metres (m³)	Cubic Centimetres (cm³)	Cubic Inches (inch³)	Cubic Feet (ft³)	UK (Imperial) gallons (UK gal)	US gallons (US gal)
m³	1	10^6	6.102374×10^4	$35.314\,67$	$219.96\,25$	264.172
cm³	10^{-6}	1	6.102374×10^{-2}	$3.531\,467 \times 10^{-5}$	$2.199\,69 \times 10^{-4}$	$2.641\,722 \times 10^{-4}$
in³	$1.638\,706 \times 10^{-5}$	$16.387\,06$	1	$5.787\,037 \times 10^{-4}$	$3.604\,651 \times 10^{-3}$	$4.329\,007 \times 10^{-3}$
ft³	$2.831\,685 \times 10^{-2}$	$28.316\,85 \times 10^3$	1728	1	$6.228\,9$	$7.480\,52$
UK gal	$4.546\,095 \times 10^{-3}$	$4.546\,095 \times 10^3$	$2.774\,194 \times 10^2$	$0.160\,54$	1	$1.200\,95$
US gal	$3.785\,412 \times 10^{-3}$	$37.854\,12 \times 10^2$	2.31×10^2	$0.133\,681$	$0.832\,674$	1

Table AI.4 Mass Units

	Kilograms (kg)	Grams (g)	Tonnes (t)	Pounds (av.) (lb)	Tons (T)	Tons (short) (Ts)
kg	1	1000	10^{-3}	2.204623	9.8421×10^{-4}	1.102312×10^{-3}
g	10^{-3}	1	10^{-6}	2.204623×10^{-3}	9.8421×10^{-7}	1.102312×10^{-6}
t	1000	10^6	1	2204.623	0.98421	1.102312
lb	$453.592\,37 \times 10^{-3}$	$453.592\,37$	$4.535\,924 \times 10^{-4}$	1	$4.464\,3 \times 10^{-4}$	5×10^{-4}
T	1016.047	$1.016\,271 \times 10^6$	$1.016\,271$	2240	1	1.12
Ts	907.185	$9.071\,847 \times 10^5$	$0.907\,185$	2000	0.89286	1

Table AI.5 Density and Concentration Units

	Kilograms per cubic metre (kg/m³)	Grams per cubic centimetre (g/cm³)*	Pound per cubic foot (lb/ft³)	Pound per UK gallon (lb/UK gal)	Pound per US gallon (lb/US gal)
kg/m³	1	10^{-3}	$6.242\,795 \times 10^{-2}$	1.0022×10^{-2}	$8.345\,402 \times 10^{-3}$
g/cm²	1000	1	62.427 95	10.0224	8.345 402
lb/ft³	16.018 462	$1.601\,846 \times 10^{-2}$	1	0.160 54	0.133 681
lb/UKgal	99.776 5	9.978×10^{-2}	6.228 842	1	0.832 675
lb/USgal	119.8264	0.119 826	7.480 518	1.20095	1

* 1 g/cm³ = 1 t/m³ = 1.000 028 g/mL = 1.000 028 kg/L

Table AI.6 Force Units

	Newtons (N)	Kilograms force (kgf)	Dynes (dyn)	Pounds force (lbf)	Poundals (pdl)
N	1	0.101972	10^{5}	0.224809	7.223
kgf	9.806 65	1	$9.806\,65 \times 10^{5}$	2.20462	70.932
dyn	10^{-5}	1.01972×10^{-6}	1	2.2×10^{-6}	7.233×10^{-5}
lbf	4.448 22	0.453592	4.44822×10^{5}	1	32.174
pdl	0.138 256	1.4098×10^{-2}	1.38225×10^{4}	3.1081×10^{-2}	1

Table AI.7.1   Pressure Units

	Newtons per Square Metre (N/m² (Pa))	Bars (bar)	Standard Atmospheres (atm)	Kilograms-force per Square Centimetre (kgf/cm²)	Dynes per Square Centimetre (dyn/cm²)
N/m² (Pa)	1	10^{-5}	9.869223×10^{-6}	1.019716×10^{-5}	10
bar	10^{5}	1	0.986923	1.019 716	10^{6}
atm	101.325×10^{3}	1.013 25	1	1.033 227	101.325×10^{4}
kgf/cm²	908.665×10^{2}	0.980 665	0.967 841	1	$9.806\ 65 \times 10^{5}$
dyn/cm²	0.1	10^{-6}	$9.869\ 233 \times 10^{-7}$	$1.019\ 716 \times 10^{-6}$	1
torr	133.3224	$1.333\ 224 \times 10^{-3}$	$1.315\ 79 \times 10^{-3}$	$1.359\ 51 \times 10^{-3}$	1 333.224
in Hg	3 386.388	$3.386\ 395 \times 10^{-2}$	$3.342\ 105 \times 10^{-2}$	$3.453\ 155 \times 10^{-2}$	$33.863\ 886 \times 10^{3}$
m H₂O	9 806.65	9.8067×10^{-2}	$9.678\ 4 \times 10^{-2}$	0.1	$9.806\ 65 \times 10^{4}$
ft H₂O	2 989.063	2.989×10^{-2}	$2.949\ 89 \times 10^{-2}$	3.048×10^{-2}	$2.989\ 067 \times 10^{4}$
lbf/in²	6 894.757	$6.894\ 757 \times 10^{-2}$	$6.804\ 596 \times 10^{-2}$	$7.030\ 696 \times 10^{-2}$	$6.894\ 757 \times 10^{4}$

Table AI.7.2   Pressure Units (Contd.)

	Torr or Barometric millimetres of mercury (torr)	Barometric inches of mercury (in Hg)	Head of water m H₂O	Head of water ft H₂O	Pounds-force per square inch (lbf/in²)
N/m² (Pa)	7.500616×10^{-3}	2.952999×10^{-4}	1.01972×10^{-4}	$3.345\ 53 \times 10^{-4}$	1.450377×10^{-4}
bar	750.0616	29.52999	10.1972	33.4554	14.50377
atm	760	29.92126	10.33227	33.8985	14.69595
kgf/cm²	735.559 2	28.959 03	10	32.8084	14.223 34
dyn/cm²	$7.500\ 617 \times 10^{-4}$	2.952999×10^{-5}	1.01972×10^{-5}	$3.345\ 53 \times 10^{-5}$	$1.450\ 377 \times 10^{-5}$
torr	1	$3.937\ 008 \times 10^{-2}$	$1.359\ 15 \times 10^{-2}$	$4.460\ 351 \times 10^{-2}$	$1.933\ 678 \times 10^{-2}$
in Hg	25.4	1	0.345 316	1.13292	0.491154
m H₂O	73.555 6	2.895 9	1	3.280 84	1.422 334
ft H₂O	22.419 8	0.882 67	0.304 8	1	0.433 526
lbf/in²	51.714 93	2.036 021	0.703072	2.306 67	1

Table AI.8.1 Energy and Heat Units

	Joules (J)	Kilowatt hours (kWh)	Kilocalories (kcal$_{IT}$)	Kilogram-force metres (kgf·m)
J	1	2.777778×10^{-7}	2.388459×10^{-4}	0.101972
kWh	3.6×10^{6}	1	859.8452	3.67098×10^{5}
kcal$_{IT}$	4186.8	1.163×10^{-3}	1	426.935
kgf.m	9.80665	2.72407×10^{-6}	2.3423×10^{-3}	1
L.atm	101.325	2.814583×10^{-5}	2.420107×10^{-2}	10.33231
Btu$_{IT}$	1055.056	2.930711×10^{-4}	0.251996	107.586
lbf·ft	1.355818	3.766161×10^{-7}	3.238315×10^{-4}	0.138255

Table AI.8.2 Energy and Heat Units (Contd.)

	Litre atmospheres (L·atm)	British thermal units (Btu$_{IT}$)	Pound-force feet (lbf·ft)
J	9.869233×10^{-3}	9.478172×10^{-4}	0.737562
kWh	3.552924×10^{4}	3.412142×10^{3}	2.655224×10^{6}
kcal$_{IT}$	41.3205	3.968321	3088.96
kgf.m	9.67838×10^{-2}	9.29488×10^{-3}	7.233
L.atm	1	9.603759×10^{-2}	74.73351
Btu$_{IT}$	10.41259	1	778.1693
lbf·ft	1.338088×10^{-2}	1.285067×10^{-3}	1

Table AI.9 Specific Energy Units

	Joules per kilogram (J/kg)	Kilocalories per kilogram (kcal$_{IT}$/kg)	British thermal unit per pound (Btu$_{IT}$/lb)
J/kg	1	2.388459×10^{-4}	4.299226×10^{-4}
kcal$_{IT}$/kg	4186.8	1	1.8
Btu$_{IT}$/lb	2326	0.555556	1

Table AI.10 Power Units

	Kilowatts (kW)	Kilogram force metre per second (kgf·m/s)	Metric horse-powers (mhp)	Pound-force feet per second (lbf·ft/s)	Horsepowers (hp)
kW	1	101.97144	1.35962	737.5622	1.341022
kgf·m/s	9.8066×10^{-3}	1	1.3333×10^{-2}	7.233	1.3151×10^{-2}
mhp	0.7355	75	1	542.4764	0.98632
lbf·ft/s	1.35582×10^{-3}	0.13825	1.8434×10^{-3}	1	1.8182×10^{-3}
hp	0.7457	75.0395	1.01387	550	1

Table AI.11   Temperature Units

	Degrees Kelvin (K)	Degrees Celcius (°C)	Degrees Fahrenheit (°F)	Degrees Rankine (°R)
K	T	$t + 273.15$	$5/9\ (t' + 459.67)$	$5/9\ T'$
°C	$T - 273.15$	t	$5/9\ (t' - 32)$	$5/9\ (T' - 459.67)$
°F	$9/5\ T - 459.67$	$9/5\ t + 32$	t'	$T' - 459.67$
°R	$9/5\ T$	$9/5\ t + 459.67$	$t' + 459.67$	T'

Reproduced with the permissions of

(i) *Thermodynamics Research Centre (TRC)*, USA from its Publication: Reprint of the Introduction to the TRC Thermodynamic Tables: Non-Hydrocarbons, December 31, 1991 and

(ii) *International Union of Pure and Applied Chemistry (IUPAC)*, UK from its Publication: Quantities, Units and Symbols in Physical Chemistry, Edited by I. Mills, T. Cvitas, K. Homann, N. Kallay and K. Kuchitsu, 2nd Ed., 1993.

List of Elements

Table AII	List of Elements in Alphabetical Order Based on $^{12}C = 12$		
Element	Symbol	Atomic Number	Atomic Mass (Atomic Weight)
Actinium	Ac	89	227.027 750*
Aluminium (Aluminum)	Al	13	26.981 538
Americium	Am	95	243.061 375*
Antimony (Stibium)	Sb	51	121.760
Argon	Ar	18	39.948
Arsenic	As	33	74.921 60
Astatine	At	85	209.987 126*
Barium	Ba	56	137.327
Berkelium	Bk	97	247.070 300*
Beryllium	Be	4	9.012 182
Bismuth	Bi	83	208.980 38
Bohrium	Bh	107	264.12
Boron	B	5	10.811
Bromine	Br	35	79.904
Cadmium	Cd	48	112.411
Caesium (Cesium)	Cs	55	132.905 45
Calcium	Ca	20	40.078
Californium	Cf	98	
Carbon	C	6	12.010 7
Cerium	Ce	58	140.116
Chlorine	Cl	17	35.453
Chromium	Cr	24	51.996 1
Cobalt	Co	27	58.933 200
Copper (Cuprum)	Cu	29	63.546

(Contd.)

Table AII (Contd.)

Element	Symbol	Atomic Number	Atomic Mass (Atomic Weight)
Curium	Cm	96	247.070 347*
Dubnium	Db	105	262.1141*
Dysprosium	Dy	66	162.500^2
Einsteinium	Es	99	252.082 944*
Erbium	Er	68	167.259
Europium	Eu	63	151.964
Fermium	Fm	100	257.095 099*
Fluorine	F	9	18.998 403 2
Francium	Fr	87	223.019 733*
Gadolinium	Gd	64	157.25
Gallium	Ga	31	69.723
Germanium	Ge	32	72.64
Gold (Aurum)	Au	79	196.966 55
Hafnium	Hf	72	178.49
Hassium	Hs	108	
Helium	He	2	4.002 602
Holmium	Ho	67	164.930 32
Hydrogen (Protium)	^{1}H	1	1.007 94
Hydrogen (Deuterium)	^{2}H (also D)	1	2.014 102
Hydrogen (Tritium)	^{3}H (also T)	1	3.016 049
Indium	In	49	114.818
Iodine	I	53	126.904 47
Iridium	Ir	77	192.217
Iron (Ferrum)	Fe	26	55.845
Krypton	Kr	36	83.798^2
Lanthanum	La	57	138.905 5
Lawrencium	Lr	103	260.105 320*
Lead (Plumbum)	Pb	82	207.2
Lithium	Li	3	6.941
Lutetium	Lu	71	174.967
Magnesium	Mg	12	24.305 0
Manganese	Mn	25	54.938 049
Meitnerium	Mt	109	268.138 8*
Mendelevium	Md	101	258.098 57*
Mercury (Hydragyrum)	Hg	80	200.59
Molybdenum	Mo	42	95.94^2
Neodymium	Nd	60	144.24
Neon	Ne	10	20.179 7
Neptunium	Np	93	237.048 167 8*
Nickel	Ni	28	58.693 4
Niobium	Nb	41	92.906 38
Nitrogen	N	7	14.006 7
Nobelium	No	102	259.100 931*
Osmium	Os	76	190.23
Oxygen	O	8	15.999 4
Palladium	Pd	46	106.42
Phosphorus	P	15	30.973 761
Platinum	Pt	78	195.078

(Contd.)

Table AII (Contd.)

Element	Symbol	Atomic Number	Atomic Mass (Atomic Weight)
Plutonium	Pu	94	244.064 199*
Polonium	Po	84	208.982 404*
Potassium (Kalium)	K	19	39.098 3
Praseodymium	Pr	59	140.907 65
Promethium	Pm	61	144.912 743*
Protactinium	Pa	91	231.035 88
Radium	Ra	88	226.025 403*
Radon	Rn	86	222.017 571*
Rhenium	Re	75	186.207
Rhodium	Rh	45	102.905 50
Rubidium	Rb	37	85.467 8
Ruthenium	Ru	44	101.07
Rutherfordium	Rf	104	261.108 8*
Samarium	Sm	62	150.36
Scandium	Sc	21	44.955 910
Seaborgium	Sg	106	266.1219*
Selenium	Se	34	78.96
Silicon	Si	14	28.085 5
Silver (Argentum)	Ag	47	107.868 2
Sodium (Natrium)	Na	11	22.989 770
Strontium	Sr	38	87.62
Sulphur	S	16	32.065
Tantalum	Ta	73	180.9479
Technetium	Tc	43	97.907215*
Tellurium	Te	52	127.60
Terbium	Tb	65	158.925 34
Thallium	Tl	81	204.383 3
Thorium	Th	90	232.038 1
Thulium	Tm	69	168.934 21
Tin (Stannum)	Sn	50	118.710
Titanium	Ti	22	47.867
Tungsten (Wolfram)	W	74	183.84
Ununbium	Uub	112	
Ununhexium	Uuh	116	
Ununnilium	Uun	110	
Ununoctium	Uuo	118	
Ununquadium	Uuq	114	
Unununium	Uuu	111	272.1535
Uranium	U	92	238.02891*
Vanadium	V	23	50.9415
Xenon	Xe	54	131.293
Ytterbium	Yb	70	173.04
Yttrium	Y	39	88.905 85
Zinc	Zn	30	65.409^2
Zirconium	Zr	40	91.224

* The value represent atomic mass (weight) of the isotope having the longest half-time.

(Contd.)

Reprinted with permission of **International Union of Pure and Applied Chemistry (IUPAC)** from

1. Coplen, T. B., *Pure Appl. Chem.*, Vol. 73, No. 4, (2001), pp 667–683, © 2001.
2. Private Communication with Dr. T. B. Coplen based on **IUPAC** General Assembly in Brisbane, July 2001.
3. Quantities, Units and Symbols in Physical Chemistry by Mills, I., T. Cvitas, K. Homann, N. Kallay, and K. Kuchitsu, Blackwell Science Ltd., UK, 2nd Edition, 1993 (1998 Reprint).

Notes: 1. **IUPAC** do not recommend change of the term "atomic weight" to "atomic mass" because the former is clearly understood and widely accepted by chemists without ambiguity.
2. Names of elements with atomic numbers 110 to 118 are provisonal.

Steam Tables

NOTATION

p = Absolute pressure in torr, kPa or MPa

t = Saturation temperature in °C

T = Saturation temperature in K

v = Specific volume of superheated steam in m^3/kg

v' = Specific volume of saturated or compressed water in m^3/kg

v'' = Specific volume of saturated steam in m^3/kg

h = Specific enthalpy of saturated or compressed water in kJ/kg

H = Specific enthalpy of saturated steam in kJ/kg

i = Specific enthalpy of superheated steam in kJ/kg

λ_v = Latent heat of vaporization of saturated water in kJ/kg

s = Specific entropy of superheated steam in kJ/(kg · K)

s' = Specific entropy of saturated or compressed water in kJ/(kg · K)

s'' = Specific entropy of saturated steam in kJ/(kg · K)

Table AIII.1 Properties of Saturated Water and Saturated Steam Up to 1 Atmospheric Pressure

Pressure, p		Temperature		Specific volume, m³/kg		Specific Enthalpy, kJ/kg			Specific Entropy, kJ/(kg·K)		Pressure, p
kPa	torr or mm Hg	t °C	T K	v'	v''	h	H	λ_v	s'	s''	kPa
0.6108	4.6	0	273.15	0.00100022	206.305	– 0.042	2501.6	2501.6	– 0.000 15	9.15773	0.6108
0.6112	**4.6**	**0.01**	**273.16***	**0.00100022**	**206.163**	**0**	**2501.6**	**2501.6**	**0**	**9.15746**	**0.6112**
1.0	7.5	6.983	280.133	0.00100007	129.209	29.335	2514.4	2485.0	0.106 04	8.97667	1
1.5	11.3	13.036	286.186	0.00100057	87.9821	54.715	2525.5	2470.7	0.195 67	8.82883	1.5
2.0	15.0	17.513	290.663	0.00100124	67.0061	73.457	2533.6	2460.2	0.260 65	8.72456	2
2.5	18.8	21.096	294.246	0.00100196	54.2562	88.446	2540.2	2451.7	0.311 91	8.64403	2.5
3.0	22.5	24.100	297.250	0.00100266	45.6673	101.003	2545.6	2444.6	0.354 36	8.57848	3.0
3.166	**23.7**	**25.000**	**298.150**	**0.00100289**	**43.4017**	**104.767**	**2547.3**	**2442.5**	**0.367 01**	**8.55916**	**3.166**
3.5	26.3	26.694	299.844	0.00100334	39.4787	111.845	2550.4	2438.5	0.390 68	8.52322	3.5
4.0	30.0	28.983	302.133	0.00100400	34.8022	121.412	2554.5	2433.1	0.422 46	8.47548	4.0
4.5	33.8	31.03	304.18	0.00100463	31.1408	129.988	2558.2	2428.2	0.450 75	8.43347	4.5
5.0	37.5	32.90	306.05	0.00100523	28.1944	137.772	2561.6	2423.8	0.476 26	8.39596	5.0
5.5	41.3	34.61	307.76	0.00100582	25.7707	144.908	2564.7	2419.8	0.499 51	8.36210	5.5
6.0	45.0	36.18	309.33	0.00100637	23.7410	151.502	2567.5	2416.0	0.520 88	8.33124	6.0
6.5	48.8	37.65	310.80	0.00100691	22.0159	157.636	2570.2	2412.5	0.540 66	8.30289	6.5
7.0	52.5	39.02	312.17	0.00100743	20.5310	163.376	2572.6	2409.2	0.559 09	8.27669	7.0
7.5	56.3	40.32	313.47	0.00100793	19.2391	168.771	2574.9	2406.2	0.576 33	8.25233	7.5
8.0	60.0	41.53	314.68	0.00100842	18.1046	173.865	2577.1	2403.2	0.592 55	8.22956	8.0
8.5	63.8	42.69	315.84	0.00100889	17.1001	178.691	2579.2	2400.5	0.607 86	8.20821	8.5
9.0	67.5	43.79	316.94	0.00100935	16.2043	183.279	2581.1	2397.9	0.622 35	8.18810	9.0

* reference state

(Contd.)

Table AIII.1 (Contd.)

Pressure, p	Pressure, p	Temperature	Temperature	Specific volume, m³/kg	Specific volume, m³/kg	Specific Enthalpy, kJ/kg	Specific Enthalpy, kJ/kg	Specific Enthalpy, kJ/kg	Specific Entropy, kJ/(kg·K)	Specific Entropy, kJ/(kg·K)	Pressure, p
kPa	torr or mm Hg	t °C	T K	v'	v''	h	H	λ_v	s'	s''	kPa
9.5	71.3	44.83	317.98	0.00100980	15.4003	187.652	2383.0	2595.3	0.636 13	8.169 09	9.5
10	75.0	45.83	318.98	0.00101023	14.6746	191.832	2584.8	2392.9	0.649 25	8.151 08	10
11	82.5	47.71	320.86	0.00101106	13.4161	199.680	2588.1	2388.4	0.673 78	8.117 66	
12	90.0	49.45	322.60	0.00101186	12.3619	206.938	2591.2	2384.3	0.696 34	8.087 21	12
13	97.5	51.06	324.21	0.00101262	11.4657	213.695	2594.0	2380.3	0.717 23	8.059 24	13
14	105.0	52.57	325.72	0.001013 34	10.694 2	220.022	2596.7	2376.7	0.736 69	8.033 38	14
15	112.5	54.00	327.15	0.001014 04	10.022 8	225.973	2599.2	2373.2	0.754 92	8.009 33	15
16	120.0	55.34	328.49	0.001014 71	9.433 14	231.595	2601.6	2370.0	0.772 07	7.986 87	16
17	127.5	56.61	329.76	0.001015 36	8.910 95	236.925	2603.8	2366.9	0.788 26	7.965 80	17
18	135.0	57.83	330.98	0.001015 99	8.445 21	241.994	2605.9	2363.9	0.803 60	7.945 95	18
19	142.5	58.98	332.13	0.001016 60	8.027 16	246.829	2607.9	2361.1	0.818 18	7.927 20	19
20	150.0	60.09	333.24	0.001017 19	7.649 77	251.453	2609.9	2358.4	0.832 07	7.909 43	20
21	157.5	61.14	334.29	0.001017 76	7.307 32	255.884	2611.7	2355.8	0.845 35	7.892 54	21
22	165.0	62.16	335.31	0.001018 32	6.995 14	260.139	2613.5	2353.3	0.858 05	7.876 45	22
23	172.5	63.14	336.29	0.001018 86	6.709 34	264.234	2615.2	2350.9	0.870 24	7.861 08	23
24	180.0	64.08	337.23	0.001019 39	6.446 69	268.180	2616.8	2348.6	0.881 96	7.846 39	24
25	187.5	64.99	338.14	0.001019 91	6.204 47	271.990	2618.3	2346.4	0.893 24	7.832 30	25
26	195.0	65.87	339.02	0.001020 41	5.980 34	275.673	2619.9	2344.2	0.904 11	7.818 78	26
27	202.5	66.72	339.87	0.001020 91	5.772 35	279.238	2621.3	2342.1	0.914 61	7.805 78	27
28	210.0	67.55	340.70	0.001021 39	5.578 79	282.693	2622.7	2340.0	0.924 76	7.793 26	28
29	217.5	68.35	341.50	0.001021 86	5.398 20	286.045	2624.1	2338.1	0.934 59	7.781 18	29
30	225.0	69.12	342.27	0.001022 32	5.229 30	289.302	2625.4	2336.1	0.944 11	7.769 53	30

(Contd.)

Table AIII.1 (Contd.)

Pressure, p		Temperature		Specific volume, m³/kg		Specific Enthalpy, kJ/kg			Specific Entropy, kJ/(kg·K)		Pressure, p
kPa	torr or mm Hg	t °C	T K	v'	v''	h	H	λ_v	s'	s''	kPa
31	232.5	69.88	343.03	0.001 022 78	5.070 98	292.468	2626.7	2334.3	0.953 35	7.758 26	31
32	240.0	70.61	343.76	0.001 023 22	4.922 27	295.549	2628.0	2332.4	0.962 32	7.747 36	32
33	247.5	71.33	344.48	0.001 023 66	4.782 32	298.550	2629.2	2330.6	0.971 03	7.736 79	33
34	255.0	72.03	345.18	0.001 024 08	4.650 36	301.476	2630.4	2328.9	0.979 52	7.726 55	34
35	262.5	72.71	345.86	0.001 024 51	4.525 71	304.330	2631.5	2327.2	0.987 77	7.716 61	35
36	270.0	73.37	346.52	0.001 024 92	4.407 79	307.116	2632.6	2325.5	0.995 82	7.706 96	36
37	277.5	74.02	347.17	0.001 025 33	4.296 05	309.838	2633.7	2323.9	1.003 66	7.697 57	37
38	285.0	74.66	347.81	0.001 025 73	4.190 03	312.500	2634.8	2322.3	1.011 32	7.688 44	38
39	292.5	75.28	348.43	0.001 026 12	4.089 28	315.103	2635.9	2320.8	1.018 79	7.679 55	39
40	300.0	75.89	349.04	0.001 026 51	3.993 42	317.650	2636.9	2319.2	1.026 10	7.670 89	40
41	307.5	76.48	349.63	0.001 026 89	3.902 10	320.145	2637.9	2317.7	1.033 23	7.662 45	41
42	315.0	77.06	350.21	0.001 027 26	3.815 00	322.589	2638.9	2316.3	1.040 22	7.654 21	42
43	322.5	77.63	350.78	0.001 027 64	3.731 83	324.985	2639.8	2314.8	1.047 05	7.646 18	43
44	330.0	78.19	351.34	0.001 028 00	3.652 32	327.335	2640.7	2313.4	1.053 74	7.638 32	44
45	337.5	78.74	351.89	0.001 028 36	3.576 25	329.640	2641.7	2312.0	1.060 29	7.630 65	45
46	345.0	79.28	352.43	0.001 028 72	3.503 38	331.904	2642.6	2310.7	1.066 72	7.623 15	46
47	352.5	79.81	352.96	0.001 029 07	3.433 52	334.126	2643.4	2309.3	1.073 02	7.615 82	47
48	360.0	80.33	353.48	0.001 029 41	3.366 49	336.309	2644.3	2308.0	1.079 19	7.608 64	48
49	367.5	80.84	353.99	0.001 029 76	3.302 10	338.455	2645.2	2306.7	1.085 26	7.601 61	49
50	375.0	81.35	354.50	0.001 030 09	3.240 22	340.564	2646.0	2305.4	1.091 21	7.594 72	50
52	390.0	82.33	355.48	0.001 030 76	3.123 38	344.679	2647.6	2302.9	1.102 79	7.581 37	52
54	405.0	83.27	356.42	0.001 031 40	3.014 94	348.665	2649.2	2300.5	1.113 99	7.568 52	54

(Contd.)

Table AIII.1 (Contd.)

Pressure, p kPa	Pressure, p torr or mm Hg	Temperature t °C	Temperature T K	Specific volume, m³/kg v'	Specific volume, m³/kg v''	Specific Enthalpy, kJ/kg h	Specific Enthalpy, kJ/kg H	Specific Enthalpy, kJ/kg λ_v	Specific Entropy, kJ/(kg·K) s'	Specific Entropy, kJ/(kg·K) s''	Pressure, p kPa
56	420.0	84.19	357.34	0.001032 04	2.914 01	352.529	2650.7	2298.2	1.124 81	7.556 15	56
58	435.0	85.09	358.24	0.001032 66	2.819 84	356.280	2652.1	2295.9	1.135 29	7.544 22	58
60	450.0	85.95	359.10	0.001033 26	2.731 75	359.925	2653.6	2293.6	1.145 44	7.532 70	60
62	465.0	86.80	359.95	0.001033 86	2.649 18	363.471	2654.9	2291.5	1.155 30	7.521 56	62
64	480.0	87.62	360.77	0.001034 44	2.571 62	366.923	2656.3	2289.4	1.164 87	7.510 79	64
66	495.0	88.42	361.57	0.001035 01	2.498 61	370.286	2657.6	2287.3	1.174 18	7.500 35	66
68	510.0	89.20	362.35	0.001035 57	2.429 76	373.566	2658.8	2285.3	1.183 24	7.490 22	68
70	525.0	89.96	363.11	0.001036 12	2.364 73	376.768	2660.1	2283.3	1.192 05	7.480 40	70
72	540.0	90.70	363.85	0.001036 66	2.303 20	379.894	2661.3	2281.4	1.200 65	7.470 85	72
74	555.0	91.43	364.58	0.001037 19	2.244 90	382.949	2662.4	2279.5	1.209 03	7.461 57	74
76	570.0	92.14	365.29	0.001037 71	2.189 57	385.937	2663.6	2277.6	1.217 21	7.452 54	76
78	585.0	92.83	365.98	0.001038 23	2.136 99	388.860	2664.7	2275.8	1.225 20	7.443 75	78
80	600.0	93.51	366.66	0.001038 74	2.086 96	391.722	2665.8	2274.0	1.233 01	7.435 19	80
82	615.0	94.18	367.33	0.001039 23	2.039 30	394.526	2666.8	2272.3	1.240 65	7.426 84	82
84	630.1	94.83	367.98	0.001039 73	1.993 83	397.274	2667.9	2270.6	1.248 12	7.418 69	84
86	645.1	95.47	368.62	0.001040 21	1.950 41	399.969	2668.9	2268.9	1.255 43	7.410 74	86
88	660.1	96.10	369.25	0.001040 69	1.908 91	402.613	2669.9	2267.3	1.262 59	7.402 97	88
90	675.1	96.71	369.86	0.001041 16	1.869 60	405.207	2670.9	2265.6	1.269 60	7.395 38	90
92	690.1	97.32	370.47	0.001041 62	1.831 15	407.755	2671.8	2264.0	1.276 48	7.387 96	92
94	705.1	97.91	371.06	0.001042 08	1.794 67	410.257	2672.7	2262.5	1.283 22	7.380 70	94
96	720.1	98.49	371.64	0.001042 53	1.759 67	412.716	2673.7	2260.9	1.289 84	7.373 59	96
98	735.1	99.07	372.22	0.001042 98	1.726 05	415.133	2674.6	2259.4	1.296 33	7.366 63	98
100	750.1	99.63	372.79	0.001043 42	1.693 73	417.510	2675.4	2257.9	1.302 71	7.359 82	100
101.325	760.0	100.00	373.15	0.001043 71	1.673 00	419.064	2676.0	2256.9	1.306 87	7.355 38	101.325

Table AIII.2 Properties of Saturated Water and Saturated Steam from 1 to 150 bar

Pressure, p bar	Temperature t °C	Temperature T K	Specific volume, m³/kg v'	Specific volume, m³/kg v''	Specific Enthalpy, kJ/kg h	Specific Enthalpy, kJ/kg H	Specific Enthalpy, kJ/kg λ_v	Specific Entropy kJ/(kg·K) s'	Specific Entropy kJ/(kg·K) s''	Pressure, p bar
1.0	99.63	372.78	0.00104342	1.69373	417.510	2675.4	2257.9	1.302 71	7.359 82	1.0
1.1	102.32	375.47	0.00104554	1.549 24	428.843	2679.6	2250.8	1.332 97	7.327 69	1.1
1.2	104.81	377.96	0.00104755	1.428 13	439.362	2683.4	2244.1	1.360 87	7.298 39	1.2
1.3	107.13	380.28	0.00104947	1.325 09	449.188	2687.0	2237.8	1.386 76	7.271 46	1.3
1.4	109.32	382.47	0.00105129	1.236 33	458.417	2690.3	2231.9	1.410 93	7.246 55	1.4
1.5	111.37	384.52	0.00105303	1.159 04	467.125	2693.4	2226.2	1.433 61	7.223 37	1.5
1.6	113.32	386.47	0.00105471	1.091 11	475.375	2696.2	2220.9	1.454 98	7.201 69	1.6
1.7	115.17	388.32	0.00105632	1.030 93	483.217	2699.0	2215.7	1.475 20	7.181 34	1.7
1.8	116.93	390.08	0.00105788	0.977 227	490.696	2701.5	2210.8	1.494 39	7.162 17	1.8
1.9	118.62	391.77	0.00105938	0.928 999	497.846	2704.0	2206.1	1.512 65	7.144 03	1.9
2.0	120.23	393.38	0.00106084	0.885 441	504.700	2706.3	2201.6	1.530 08	7.126 83	2.0
2.1	121.78	394.93	0.00106226	0.845 900	511.284	2708.5	2197.2	1.546 76	7.110 47	2.1
2.2	123.27	396.42	0.00106363	0.809 839	517.622	2710.6	2193.0	1.562 75	7.094 87	2.2
2.3	124.71	397.86	0.00106497	0.776 813	523.732	2712.6	2188.9	1.578 11	7.079 97	2.3
2.4	126.09	399.24	0.00106628	0.746 451	529.634	2714.5	2184.9	1.592 89	7.065 71	2.4
2.5	127.43	400.58	0.00106755	0.718 439	535.343	2716.4	2181.0	1.607 14	7.052 02	2.5
2.6	128.73	401.88	0.00106879	0.692 512	540.873	2718.2	2177.3	1.620 89	7.038 88	2.6
2.7	129.98	403.13	0.00107001	0.668 443	546.235	2719.7	2173.6	1.634 19	7.026 22	2.7
2.8	131.20	404.35	0.00107119	0.646 037	551.443	2721.5	2170.1	1.647 06	7.014 03	2.8
2.9	132.39	405.54	0.00107236	0.625 125	556.504	2723.1	2166.1	1.659 53	7.002 27	2.9

(Contd.)

Table AIII.2 (Contd.)

Pressure, p bar	Temperature t °C	Temperature T K	Specific volume, m³/kg v'	Specific volume, m³/kg v''	Specific Enthalpy, kJ/kg h	Specific Enthalpy, kJ/kg H	Specific Enthalpy, kJ/kg λ_v	Specific Entropy kJ/(kg·K) s'	Specific Entropy kJ/(kg·K) s''	Pressure, p bar
3.0	133.54	406.69	0.001073 50	0.605 562	561.429	2724.7	2163.2	1.671 64	6.990 90	3.0
3.1	134.66	407.81	0.001074 62	0.587 219	566.226	2726.1	2159.9	1.683 39	6.979 90	3.1
3.2	135.75	408.90	0.001075 72	0.569 985	570.902	2727.6	2156.7	1.694 81	6.969 25	3.2
3.3	136.82	409.97	0.001076 79	0.553 761	575.464	2729.0	2153.5	1.705 93	6.958 93	3.3
3.4	137.86	411.01	0.001077 85	0.538 459	579.918	2730.3	2150.4	1.716 75	6.948 91	3.4
3.5	138.87	412.02	0.001078 90	0.524 003	584.270	2731.6	2147.4	1.727 30	6.939 18	3.5
3.6	139.86	413.01	0.001079 92	0.510 323	588.525	2732.9	2144.4	1.737 59	6.929 72	3.6
3.7	140.83	413.98	0.001080 93	0.497 357	592.688	2734.1	2141.4	1.747 63	6.920 52	3.7
3.8	141.78	414.93	0.001081 92	0.485 051	596.764	2735.3	2138.6	1.757 44	6.911 56	3.8
3.9	142.71	415.86	0.001082 90	0.473 355	600.757	2736.5	2135.7	1.767 03	6.902 83	3.9
4.0	143.62	416.77	0.001083 87	0.462 224	604.670	2737.6	2133.0	1.776 40	6.894 33	4.0
4.1	144.52	417.67	0.001084 82	0.451 618	608.507	2738.7	2130.2	1.785 57	6.886 02	4.1
4.2	145.39	418.54	0.001085 75	0.441 500	612.272	2739.8	2127.5	1.794 55	6.877 92	4.2
4.3	146.25	419.40	0.001086 68	0.431 836	615.967	2740.9	2124.9	1.803 34	6.870 00	4.3
4.4	147.09	420.24	0.001087 59	0.422 597	619.596	2741.9	2122.3	1.811 96	6.862 26	4.4
4.5	147.92	421.07	0.001088 49	0.413 754	623.161	2742.9	2119.7	1.820 41	6.854 70	4.5
4.6	148.73	421.88	0.001089 38	0.405 283	626.665	2743.9	2117.2	1.828 70	6.847 30	4.6
4.7	149.53	422.68	0.001090 26	0.397 160	630.111	2744.8	2114.7	1.836 83	6.840 05	4.7
4.8	150.31	423.46	0.001091 13	0.389 364	633.499	2745.7	2112.2	1.844 82	6.832 95	4.8
4.9	151.08	424.23	0.001091 99	0.381 875	636.833	2746.6	2109.8	1.852 66	6.826 00	4.9

(Contd.)

Table AIII.2 (Contd.)

Pressure, p bar	Temperature t °C	T K	Specific volume, m³/kg v'	v''	Specific Enthalpy, kJ/kg h	H	λ_v	Specific Entropy kJ/(kg·K) s'	s''	Pressure, p bar
5.0	151.84	424.99	0.00109284	0.374 676	640.115	2747.5	2107.4	1.860 36	6.819 19	5.0
5.2	153.33	426.48	0.00109451	0.361 080	646.530	2749.3	2102.7	1.875 37	6.805 95	5.2
5.4	154.76	427.91	0.00109614	0.348 457	652.755	2750.9	2098.1	1.889 90	6.793 20	5.4
5.6	156.16	429.31	0.00109775	0.336 705	658.805	2752.5	2093.7	1.903 96	6.780 90	5.6
5.8	157.52	430.67	0.00109932	0.325 736	664.691	2754.0	2089.3	1.917 60	6.769 03	5.8
6.0	158.84	431.99	0.00110086	0.315 474	670.422	2755.5	2085.0	1.930 83	6.757 54	6.0
6.2	160.12	433.27	0.00110238	0.305 851	676.009	2756.9	2080.9	1.943 70	6.746 43	6.2
6.4	161.38	434.53	0.00110386	0.296 809	681.458	2758.2	2076.8	1.956 21	6.735 65	6.4
6.6	162.60	435.75	0.00110533	0.288 296	686.779	2759.5	2072.7	1.968 38	6.725 20	6.6
6.8	163.79	436.94	0.00110677	0.280 267	691.978	2760.8	2068.8	1.980 25	6.715 05	6.8
7.0	164.96	438.11	0.00110819	0.272 681	697.061	2762.0	2064.9	1.991 81	6.705 70	7.0
7.2	166.10	439.25	0.00110959	0.265 502	702.034	2763.1	2061.1	2.003 10	6.695 58	7.2
7.4	167.21	440.36	0.00111096	0.258 697	706.903	2764.3	2057.4	2.014 12	6.686 24	7.4
7.6	168.30	441.45	0.00111232	0.252 239	711.674	2765.4	2053.7	2.024 89	6.677 14	7.6
7.8	169.37	442.52	0.00111366	0.246 100	716.349	2766.4	2050.1	2.035 42	6.668 26	7.8
8.0	170.41	443.56	0.00111498	0.240 257	720.935	2767.5	2046.5	2.045 72	6.659 60	8.0
8.2	171.44	444.59	0.00111629	0.234 690	725.434	2768.5	2043.0	2.055 80	6.651 14	8.2
8.4	172.45	445.60	0.00111757	0.229 378	729.852	2769.4	2039.6	2.065 67	6.642 88	8.4
8.6	173.44	446.59	0.00111885	0.224 305	734.190	2770.4	2036.2	2.075 35	6.634 80	8.6
8.8	174.41	447.56	0.00112010	0.219 454	738.453	2771.3	2032.8	2.084 83	6.626 90	8.8

(Contd.)

Table AIII.2 (Contd.)

Pressure, p bar	Temperature t °C	Temperature T K	Specific volume, m³/kg v'	Specific volume, m³/kg v''	Specific Enthalpy, kJ/kg h	Specific Enthalpy, kJ/kg H	Specific Enthalpy, kJ/kg λ_v	Specific Entropy kJ/(kg·K) s'	Specific Entropy kJ/(kg·K) s''	Pressure, p bar
9.0	175.36	448.51	0.00112135	0.214812	742.644	2772.1	2029.5	2.09414	6.61917	9.0
9.2	176.29	449.44	0.00112258	0.210364	746.764	2773.0	2026.2	2.10327	6.61160	9.2
9.4	177.21	450.36	0.00112379	0.206099	750.819	2773.8	2023.0	2.11223	6.60419	9.4
9.6	178.12	451.27	0.00112500	0.202006	754.809	2774.6	2019.8	2.12103	6.59692	9.6
9.8	179.01	452.16	0.00112619	0.198073	758.737	2775.4	2016.7	2.12967	6.58980	9.8
10.0	179.88	453.03	0.00112737	0.194293	762.605	2776.2	2013.6	2.13817	6.58281	10.0
10.5	182.02	455.17	0.00113026	0.185450	772.029	2778.0	2006.0	2.15880	6.56590	10.5
11.0	184.07	457.22	0.00113309	0.177384	781.124	2779.7	1998.5	2.17861	6.54973	11.0
11.5	186.05	459.20	0.00113586	0.169995	789.917	2781.3	1991.3	2.19768	6.53424	11.5
12.0	187.96	461.11	0.00113858	0.163200	798.430	2782.7	1984.3	2.21606	6.51936	12.0
12.5	189.81	462.96	0.00114124	0.156931	806.685	2784.1	1977.4	2.23380	6.50505	12.5
13.0	191.61	464.76	0.00114385	0.151127	814.700	2785.4	1970.7	2.25095	6.49126	13.0
13.5	193.35	466.50	0.00114641	0.145738	822.491	2786.6	1964.1	2.26756	6.47795	13.5
14.0	195.04	468.19	0.00114893	0.140721	830.073	2787.8	1957.7	2.28366	6.46509	14.0
14.5	196.69	469.84	0.00115141	0.136038	837.460	2788.9	1951.4	2.29929	6.45265	14.5
15.0	198.29	471.44	0.00115386	0.131656	844.663	2789.5	1945.2	2.31447	6.44059	15.0
15.5	199.85	473.00	0.00115626	0.127547	851.693	2790.8	1939.2	2.32924	6.42889	15.5
16.0	201.37	474.52	0.00115864	0.123686	858.561	2791.7	1933.2	2.34361	6.41753	16.0
16.5	202.86	476.01	0.00116098	0.120051	865.275	2792.6	1927.3	2.35762	6.40648	16.5
17.0	204.31	477.46	0.00116329	0.116623	871.843	2793.4	1921.5	2.37125	6.39574	17.0

(Contd.)

Table AIII.2 (Contd.)

Pressure, p bar	Temperature t °C	Temperature T K	Specific volume, m³/kg v'	Specific volume, m³/kg v''	Specific Enthalpy, kJ/kg h	Specific Enthalpy, kJ/kg H	Specific Enthalpy, kJ/kg λ_v	Specific Entropy kJ/(kg·K) s'	Specific Entropy kJ/(kg·K) s''	Pressure, p bar
17.5	205.72	478.87	0.001 165 57	0.113 383	878.274	2794.1	1915.9	2.384 27	6.385 27	17.5
18.0	207.11	480.26	0.001 167 83	0.110 317	884.573	2794.8	1910.3	2.397 62	6.375 07	18.0
18.5	208.47	481.62	0.001 170 06	0.107 411	890.749	2795.5	1904.7	2.410 33	6.365 12	18.5
19.0	209.80	482.95	0.001 172 26	0.104 653	896.806	2796.1	1899.3	2.422 77	6.355 41	19.0
19.5	211.10	484.25	0.001 174 45	0.102 031	902.751	2796.7	1893.9	2.434 94	6.345 92	19.5
20.0	212.37	485.52	0.001 176 61	0.099 5361	908.588	2797.2	1888.6	2.446 86	6.336 65	20.0
21.0	214.85	488.00	0.001 180 86	0.094 8898	919.959	2798.2	1878.2	2.469 98	6.318 70	21.0
22.0	217.24	490.39	0.001 185 04	0.090 6516	930.953	2799.1	1868.1	2.492 21	6.301 48	22.0
23.0	219.55	492.70	0.001 189 15	0.086 7692	941.601	2799.8	1858.2	2.513 63	6.284 93	23.0
24.0	221.78	494.93	0.001 193 20	0.083 1994	951.929	2800.4	1848.5	2.534 30	6.268 99	24.0
25.0	223.94	497.09	0.001 197 18	0.079 9053	961.961	2800.9	1839.0	2.554 29	6.253 61	25.0
26.0	226.04	499.19	0.001 201 11	0.076 8560	971.719	2801.4	1829.6	2.573 64	6.238 74	26.0
27.0	228.07	501.22	0.001 204 98	0.074 0247	981.221	2801.7	1820.5	2.592 39	6.224 36	27.0
28.0	230.05	503.20	0.001 208 81	0.071 3887	990.494	2802.0	1811.5	2.610 60	6.210 41	28.0
29.0	231.97	505.12	0.001 212 60	0.068 9282	999.524	2802.2	1802.6	2.628 29	6.196 87	29.0
30.0	233.84	506.99	0.001 216 34	0.066 6261	1008.35	2802.3	1793.9	2.645 50	6.183 72	30.0
31.0	235.67	508.82	0.001 220 05	0.064 4674	1016.99	2802.3	1785.4	2.662 25	6.170 92	31.0
32.0	237.45	510.60	0.001 223 72	0.062 4389	1025.43	2802.3	1776.9	2.678 58	6.158 45	32.0
33.0	239.18	512.33	0.001 227 35	0.060 5290	1033.70	2802.3	1768.6	2.694 51	6.146 30	33.0
34.0	240.88	514.03	0.001 230 96	0.058 7276	1041.81	2802.1	1760.3	2.710 07	6.134 44	34.0

(Contd.)

Table AIII.2 (Contd.)

Pressure, p bar	Temperature t °C	Temperature T K	Specific volume, m^3/kg v'	Specific volume, m^3/kg v''	Specific Enthalpy, kJ/kg h	Specific Enthalpy, kJ/kg H	Specific Enthalpy, kJ/kg λ_v	Specific Entropy kJ/(kg·K) s'	Specific Entropy kJ/(kg·K) s''	Pressure, p bar
35.0	242.54	515.69	0.001 234 54	0.057 0255	1049.76	2802.0	1752.2	2.725 27	6.122 85	35.0
36.0	244.16	517.31	0.001 238 09	0.055 4146	1057.55	2801.7	1744.2	2.740 13	6.111 52	36.0
37.0	245.75	518.90	0.001 241 62	0.053 8877	1065.21	2801.4	1736.2	2.754 67	6.100 43	37.0
38.0	247.31	520.46	0.001 245 12	0.052 4383	1072.73	2801.1	1728.4	2.768 90	6.089 58	38.0
39.0	248.84	521.99	0.001 248 60	0.051 0606	1080.13	2800.8	1720.6	2.782 85	6.078 94	39.0
40.0	250.33	523.48	0.001 252 06	0.049 7493	1087.40	2800.3	1712.9	2.796 52	6.068 51	40.0
42.0	253.24	526.39	0.001 258 93	0.047 3073	1101.60	2799.4	1697.8	2.823 10	6.048 22	42.0
44.0	256.05	529.20	0.001 265 73	0.045 0795	1115.38	2798.3	1682.9	2.848 71	6.028 64	44.0
46.0	258.75	531.90	0.001 272 47	0.043 0383	1128.76	2797.0	1668.3	2.873 46	6.009 69	46.0
48.0	261.37	534.52	0.001 279 17	0.041 1611	1141.78	2795.7	1653.9	2.897 40	5.991 33	48.0
50.0	263.91	537.06	0.001 285 82	0.039 4285	1154.47	2794.2	1639.7	2.920 60	5.973 49	50.0
52.0	266.37	539.52	0.001 292 44	0.037 8242	1166.85	2792.6	1625.7	2.943 12	5.956 14	52.0
54.0	268.76	541.91	0.001 299 03	0.036 3342	1178.94	2790.8	1611.9	2.965 01	5.939 23	54.0
56.0	271.09	544.24	0.001 305 59	0.034 9465	1190.77	2789.0	1598.2	2.986 31	5.922 72	56.0
58.0	273.35	546.50	0.001 312 14	0.033 6506	1202.35	2787.0	1584.7	3.007 06	5.906 58	58.0
60.0	275.55	548.70	0.001 318 68	0.032 4378	1213.69	2785.0	1571.3	3.027 30	5.890 79	60.0
65.0	280.82	553.97	0.001 334 99	0.029 7192	1241.14	2779.5	1538.4	3.075 87	5.852 65	65.0
70.0	285.79	558.94	0.001 351 32	0.027 3733	1267.41	2773.5	1506.0	3.121 89	5.816 16	70.0
75.0	290.50	563.65	0.001 367 72	0.025 3270	1292.69	2766.9	1474.2	3.165 71	5.781 05	75.0
80.0	294.97	568.12	0.001 384 24	0.023 5253	1317.10	2759.9	1442.8	3.207 62	5.747 10	80.0

(Contd.)

Table AIII.2 (Contd.)

Pressure, p bar	Temperature		Specific volume, m³/kg		Specific Enthalpy, kJ/kg			Specific Entropy kJ/(kg·K)		Pressure, p bar
	t °C	T K	v'	v''	h	H	λ_v	s'	s''	
85.0	299.23	572.38	0.001 400 94	0.021 9258	1340.74	2752.5	1411.7	3.247 87	5.714 13	85.0
90.0	303.31	576.46	0.001 417 86	0.020 4953	1363.73	2744.6	1380.9	3.286 66	5.682 01	90.0
95.0	307.21	580.36	0.001 435 05	0.019 2076	1386.14	2736.4	1350.2	3.324 17	5.650 60	95.0
100.0	310.96	584.11	0.001 452 56	0.018 0413	1408.04	2727.7	1319.7	3.360 55	5.619 80	100.0
105.0	314.57	587.72	0.001 470 43	0.016 9790	1429.50	2718.7	1289.2	3.395 92	5.589 48	105.0
110.0	318.05	591.20	0.001 488 72	0.016 0062	1450.57	2709.3	1258.7	3.430 42	5.559 53	110.0
115.0	321.40	594.55	0.001 507 48	0.015 1109	1471.31	2699.5	1228.2	3.464 14	5.529 82	115.0
120.0	324.65	597.80	0.001 526 76	0.014 2830	1491.77	2689.77	1197.4	3.497 18	5.500 22	120.0
125.0	327.78	600.93	0.001 546 64	0.013 5141	1511.99	2678.3	1166.3	3.529 62	5.470 59	125.0
130.0	330.83	603.98	0.001 567 19	0.012 7970	1532.01	2667.0	1135.0	3.561 57	5.440 80	130.0
135.0	333.78	606.93	0.001 588 49	0.012 1256	1551.88	2655.0	1103.1	3.593 08	5.410 73	135.0
140.0	336.64	609.79	0.001 610 63	0.011 4950	1571.64	2642.4	1070.7	3.624 24	5.380 26	140.0
145.0	339.42	612.57	0.001 633 72	0.010 9010	1591.33	2629.0	1037.7	3.655 14	5.349 31	145.0
150.0	342.13	615.28	0.001 657 91	0.010 3402	1611.01	2615.0	1004.0	3.685 85	5.317 82	150.0

Table AIII.3 Properties of Superheated Steam

Pres., kPa (torr) Sat. temp. °C Sat. temp. K	Para- meter	Superheated steam temperature, °C (K)										
		100 (373.15)	120 (393.15)	140 (413.15)	160 (433.15)	180 (453.15)	200 (473.15)	220 (493.15)	240 (513.15)	260 (533.15)	280 (553.15)	300 (573.15)
10(75.0) 45.83 318.98	v	17.195	18.123	19.050	19.975	20.900	21.825	22.750	23.674	24.598	25.521	26.445
	i	2687.5	2725.6	2763.9	2802.3	2840.9	2879.6	2918.6	2957.8	2997.2	3036.8	3076.6
	s	8.4486	8.5481	8.6430	8.7337	8.8208	8.9045	8.9852	9.0630	9.1383	9.2113	9.2820
20(150.0) 60.09 333.24	v	8.585	9.051	9.516	9.980	10.444	10.907	11.370	11.832	12.295	12.757	13.219
	i	2686.3	2724.6	2763.1	2801.6	2840.3	2879.2	2918.2	2957.4	2996.9	3036.5	3076.4
	s	8.1261	8.2262	8.3215	8.4127	8.5000	8.5839	8.6647	8.7426	8.8180	8.8910	8.9618
30(225.0) 69.12 342.27	v	5.714	6.027	6.338	6.648	6.958	7.268	7.577	7.885	8.194	8.502	8.811
	i	2685.1	2723.6	2762.3	2801.0	2839.8	2878.7	2917.8	2957.1	2996.6	3036.2	3076.1
	s	7.9363	8.0370	8.1329	8.2243	8.3119	8.3960	8.4769	8.5550	8.6305	8.7035	8.7744
40((300.0) 75.89 349.04	v	4.279	4.515	4.749	4.982	5.215	5.448	5.680	5.912	6.144	6.375	6.606
	i	2683.8	2722.6	2761.4	2800.3	2839.2	2878.2	2917.4	2956.7	2996.3	3036.0	3075.9
	s	7.8009	7.9023	7.9985	8.0903	8.1782	8.2624	8.3435	8.4217	8.4973	8.5704	8.6413
50((375.0) 81.35 354.5	v	3.418	3.607	3.796	3.983	4.170	4.356	4.542	4.728	4.913	5.099	5.284
	i	2682.6	2721.6	2760.6	2799.6	2838.6	2877.7	2917.0	2956.4	2995.9	3035.7	3075.7
	s	7.6953	7.7972	7.8940	7.9861	8.0742	8.1587	8.2399	8.3182	8.3939	8.4671	8.5380
60(450.0) 85.95 359.1	v	2.844	3.002	3.160	3.317	3.473	3.628	3.783	3.938	4.093	4.248	4.402
	i	2681.3	2720.6	2759.8	2798.9	2838.1	2877.3	2916.6	2956.0	2995.6	3035.4	3075.4
	s	7.6085	7.7111	7.8083	7.9008	7.9891	8.0738	8.1552	8.2336	8.3093	8.3826	8.4536
70((525) 89.96 363.11	v	2.434	2.570	2.706	2.841	2.975	3.108	3.241	3.374	3.507	3.640	3.772
	i	2680.0	2719.6	2759.0	2798.2	2837.5	2876.8	2916.2	2955.7	2995.3	3035.2	3075.2
	s	7.5346	7.6379	7.7355	7.8284	7.9170	8.0019	8.0834	8.1619	8.2377	8.3111	8.3822

(Contd.)

Table AIII.3 (Contd.)

Pres., kPa (torr) / Sat. temp. °C / Sat. temp. K	Para-meter	Superheated steam temperature, °C (K)										
		100 (373.15)	120 (393.15)	140 (413.15)	160 (433.15)	180 (453.15)	200 (473.15)	220 (493.15)	240 (513.15)	260 (533.15)	280 (553.15)	300 (573.15)
80(600) 93.51 366.66	v	2.126	2.246	2.365	2.484	2.601	2.718	2.835	2.952	3.068	3.184	3.300
	i	2678.8	2718.6	2758.1	2797.5	2836.9	2876.3	2915.8	2955.3	2995.0	3034.9	3075.0
	s	7.4703	7.5742	7.6723	7.7655	7.8544	7.9395	8.0212	8.0998	8.1757	8.2491	8.3202
90(675.1) 96.71 369.86	v	1.887	1.994	2.101	2.206	2.311	2.415	2.519	2.623	2.726	2.829	2.933
	i	2677.5	2717.5	2757.3	2796.9	2836.4	2875.8	2915.4	2955.0	2994.7	3034.6	3074.7
	s	7.4132	7.5177	7.6164	7.7099	7.7991	7.8843	7.9662	8.0449	8.1209	8.1944	8.2656
100((750.1) 99.63 372.78	v	1.696	1.793	1.889	1.984	2.078	2.172	2.266	2.359	2.453	2.546	2.639
	i	2676.2	2716.5	2756.4	2796.2	2835.8	2875.4	2915.0	2954.6	2994.4	3034.4	3074.5
	s	7.3618	7.4670	7.5662	7.6601	7.7495	7.8349	7.9169	7.9958	8.0719	8.1454	8.2166
150(1125.1) 111.37 384.52	v		1.188	1.253	1.317	1.381	1.444	1.507	1.570	1.633	1.695	1.757
	i		2711.2	2752.2	2792.7	2832.9	2872.9	2912.9	2952.9	2992.9	3033.0	3073.3
	s		7.2693	7.3709	7.4667	7.5574	7.6439	7.7266	7.8061	7.8826	7.9565	8.0280
200(150.1) 120.23 400.58	v			0.9349	0.9840	1.032	1.080	1.128	1.175	1.222	1.269	1.316
	i			2747.8	2789.1	2830.0	2870.5	2910.8	2951.1	2991.4	3031.7	3072.1
	s			7.2298	7.3275	7.4196	7.5072	7.5907	7.6707	7.7477	7.8219	7.8937
250(1875.1) 127.43 400.58	v			0.7440	0.7840	0.8232	0.8620	0.9004	0.9385	0.9763	1.014	1.052
	i			2743.3	2785.5	2827.0	2868.0	2908.7	2949.3	2989.8	3030.3	3070.9
	s			7.1183	7.2179	7.3115	7.4001	7.4845	7.5651	7.6425	7.7171	7.7891
300(2250.2) 133.54 406.69	v			0.6167	0.6506	0.6837	0.7164	0.7486	0.7805	0.8123	0.8438	0.8753
	i			2738.8	2781.8	2824.0	2865.6	2906.6	2947.5	2988.2	3028.9	3069.7
	s			7.0254	7.1271	7.2222	7.3119	7.3971	7.4783	7.5562	7.6311	7.7034

(Contd.)

Table AIII.3 (Contd.)

Pres., bar / Sat. temp. °C / Sat. temp. K	Parameter	Superheated steam temperature, °C (K)										
		160 (433.15)	180 (453.15)	200 (473.15)	220 (493.15)	240 (513.15)	260 (533.15)	280 (553.15)	300 (573.15)	320 (593.15)	340 (613.15)	360 (633.15)
4 / 143.62 / 416.77	v	0.4837	0.5093	0.5343	0.5589	0.5831	0.6072	0.6311	0.6549	0.6785	0.7021	0.7256
	i	2774.2	2817.8	2860.4	2902.3	2943.9	2985.1	3026.2	3067.2	3108.3	3149.4	3190.6
	s	6.9805	7.0788	7.1708	7.2576	7.3402	7.4190	7.4947	7.5675	7.6379	7.7061	7.7723
4.5 / 147.92 / 421.07	v	0.4283	0.4514	0.4738	0.4958	0.5176	0.5391	0.5605	0.5817	0.6028	0.6238	0.6448
	i	2770.3	2814.6	2857.8	2900.2	2942.0	2983.5	3024.8	3066.0	3107.2	3148.4	3189.8
	s	6.9191	7.0191	7.1123	7.2000	7.2832	7.3625	7.4386	7.5117	7.5824	7.6507	7.7171
5 / 151.84 / 424.99	v	0.3835	0.4045	0.4250	0.4450	0.4647	0.4841	0.5034	0.5226	0.5416	0.5606	0.5795
	i	2766.4	2811.4	2855.1	2898.0	2940.1	2981.9	3023.4	3064.8	3106.1	3147.4	3188.8
	s	6.8631	9.9647	7.0592	7.1478	7.2317	7.3115	7.3879	7.4614	7.5322	7.6008	7.6673
5.5 / 155.47 / 428.62	v	0.3470	0.3664	0.3852	0.4036	0.4216	0.4394	0.4570	0.4745	0.4918	0.5091	0.5264
	i	2762.3	2808.1	2852.5	2895.7	2938.3	2980.3	3022.0	3063.5	3105.0	3146.4	3187.9
	s	6.8117	6.9151	7.0108	7.1004	7.1849	7.2653	7.3421	7.4158	4.4869	7.5556	7.6222
6 / 158.84 / 431.99	v	0.3165	0.3346	0.3520	0.3690	0.3857	0.4021	0.4183	0.4344	0.4504	0.4663	0.4821
	i	2758.2	2804.8	2849.7	2893.5	2936.4	2978.8	3020.6	3062.3	3103.9	3145.4	3187.0
	s	6.7640	6.8691	6.9662	7.0567	7.1419	7.2228	7.3000	7.3740	7.4454	7.5143	7.5810
6.5 / 161.99 / 435.14	v		0.3077	0.3240	0.3398	0.3553	0.3705	0.3856	0.4005	0.4153	0.4300	0.4446
	i		2801.5	2847.0	2891.2	2934.4	2977.0	3019.2	3061.0	3102.7	3144.4	3186.1
	s		6.8263	6.9247	7.0162	7.1021	7.1835	7.2611	7.3355	7.4070	7.4761	7.5431
7 / 164.96 / 438.11	v		0.2846	0.2999	0.3147	0.3292	0.3435	0.3575	0.3714	0.3852	0.3989	0.4125
	i		2798.0	2844.2	2888.9	2932.5	2975.4	3017.7	3059.8	3101.6	3143.4	3185.2
	s		6.7861	6.8859	6.9784	7.0651	7.1470	7.2250	7.2997	7.3715	7.4407	7.5078

(Contd.)

Table AIII.3 (Contd.)

Pres., bar / Sat. temp. °C / Sat. temp. K	Parameter	Superheated steam temperature, °C (K)										
		180 (453.15)	200 (473.15)	220 (493.15)	240 (513.15)	260 (533.15)	280 (553.15)	300 (573.15)	320 (593.15)	340 (613.15)	360 (633.15)	380 (653.15)
7.5 167.76 440.91	v	0.2646	0.2791	0.2930	0.3066	0.3200	0.3332	0.3462	0.3591	0.3719	0.3847	0.3974
	i	2794.6	2841.4	2886.6	2930.6	2973.7	3016.3	3058.5	3100.5	3142.4	3184.3	3226.2
	s	6.7482	6.8493	6.9429	7.0303	7.1128	7.1912	7.2662	7.3382	7.4077	7.4749	7.5401
8 170.41 443.56	v	0.2471	0.2608	0.2740	0.2869	0.2995	0.3119	0.3241	0.3363	0.3483	0.3603	0.3723
	i	2791.1	2838.6	2884.2	2928.6	2972.0	3014.9	3057.3	3099.4	3141.4	3183.4	3225.4
	s	6.7122	6.8148	6.9094	6.9976	7.0806	7.1595	7.2348	7.3070	7.3767	7.4441	7.5094
8.5 172.94 446.09	v	0.2316	0.2447	0.2572	0.2694	0.2814	0.2931	0.3047	0.3162	0.3275	0.3388	0.3501
	i	2787.5	2835.7	2881.9	2926.6	2970.4	3013.4	3056.0	3098.3	3140.4	3182.5	3224.6
	s	6.6780	6.7820	6.8777	6.9666	7.0503	7.1295	7.2051	7.2777	7.3475	7.4150	7.4805
9 175.36 448.51	v	0.2178	0.2303	0.2423	0.2539	0.2653	0.2764	0.2874	0.2983	0.3090	0.3197	0.3304
	i	2783.9	2832.7	2879.5	2924.6	2968.7	3012.0	3054.7	3097.1	3139.4	3181.5	3223.7
	s	6.6452	6.7508	6.8475	6.9373	7.0215	7.1012	7.1771	7.2499	7.3199	7.3876	7.4532
9.5 177.67 450.82	v	0.2055	0.2175	0.2290	0.2400	0.2509	0.2615	0.2719	0.2822	0.2925	0.3027	0.3128
	i	2780.2	2829.8	2877.0	2922.6	2967.0	3010.5	3053.4	3096.0	3138.4	3180.6	3222.9
	s	6.6137	6.7209	6.8187	6.9093	6.9941	7.0742	7.1505	7.2235	7.2938	7.3616	7.4273
10 179.88 453.03	v	0.1944	0.2059	0.2169	0.2276	0.2379	0.2480	0.2580	0.2678	0.2776	0.2873	0.2969
	i	2776.5	2826.8	2874.6	2920.6	2965.2	3009.0	3052.1	3094.9	3137.3	3179.7	3222.0
	s	6.5835	6.6922	6.7911	6.8825	6.9680	7.0485	7.1251	7.1984	7.2689	7.3368	7.4027
11 184.07 457.22	v		0.1859	0.1961	0.2060	0.2155	0.2248	0.2339	0.2429	0.2518	0.2607	0.2695
	i		2820.7	2869.6	2916.4	2961.8	3006.0	3049.5	3092.6	3135.3	3177.9	3220.3
	s		6.6379	6.7392	6.8323	6.9190	7.0005	7.0778	7.1516	7.2224	7.2907	7.3568

(Contd.)

Table AIII.3 (Contd.)

Pres., bar / Sat. temp. °C / Sat. temp. K	Parameter	200 (473.15)	220 (493.15)	240 (513.15)	260 (533.15)	280 (553.15)	300 (573.15)	320 (593.15)	340 (613.15)	360 (633.15)	380 (653.15)	400 (673.15)
12 / 187.96 / 461.11	v	0.1692	0.1788	0.1879	0.1968	0.2054	0.2139	0.2222	0.2304	0.2386	0.2467	0.2547
	i	2814.4	2864.5	2912.2	2958.2	3003.0	3046.9	3090.3	3133.2	3176.0	3218.7	3261.3
	s	6.5872	6.6909	6.7858	6.8738	6.9562	7.0342	7.1085	7.1798	7.2484	7.3147	7.3790
13 / 191.61 / 464.76	v	0.1551	0.1641	0.1727	0.1810	0.1890	0.1969	0.2046	0.2123	0.2198	0.2273	0.2348
	i	2808.0	2859.3	2908.0	2954.7	3000.0	3044.3	3088.0	3131.2	3174.1	3217.0	3259.7
	s	6.5394	6.6457	6.7424	6.8316	6.9151	6.9938	7.0687	7.1404	7.2093	7.2759	7.3404
14 / 195.04 / 468.19	v	0.1429	0.1515	0.1596	0.1674	0.1749	0.1823	0.1896	0.1967	0.2038	0.2108	0.2177
	i	2801.4	2854.0	2903.6	2951.0	2996.9	3041.6	3085.6	3129.1	3172.3	3215.3	3258.2
	s	6.4941	6.6030	6.7016	6.7922	6.8766	6.9561	7.0315	7.1036	7.1729	7.2398	7.3045
15 / 198.29 / 471.44	v	0.1324	0.1406	0.1483	0.1556	0.1628	0.1697	0.1765	0.1832	0.1898	0.1964	0.2029
	i	2794.7	2848.6	2899.2	2947.3	2993.7	3038.9	3083.3	3127.0	3170.4	3213.5	3256.6
	s	6.4508	6.5624	6.6629	6.7550	6.8405	6.9207	6.9967	7.0693	7.1389	7.2060	7.2709
16 / 201.37 / 474.52	v		0.1310	0.1383	0.1453	0.1521	0.1587	0.1651	0.1714	0.1777	0.1838	0.1900
	i		2843.1	2894.7	2943.6	2990.6	3036.2	3080.9	3124.9	3168.5	3211.8	3255.0
	s		6.5237	6.6263	6.7198	6.8063	6.8873	6.9639	7.0369	7.1069	7.1743	7.2394
17 / 204.31 / 477.46	v		0.1225	0.1296	0.1362	0.1427	0.1489	0.1550	0.1610	0.1669	0.1728	0.1785
	i		2837.5	2890.1	2939.8	2987.4	3033.5	3078.5	3122.8	3166.6	3210.1	3253.5
	s		6.4866	6.5912	6.6863	6.7739	6.8557	6.9329	7.0064	7.0767	7.1444	7.2098
18 / 207.11 / 480.26	v		0.1150	0.1217	0.1282	0.1343	0.1402	0.1460	0.1517	0.1573	0.1629	0.1684
	i		2831.7	2885.4	2935.9	2984.1	3030.7	3076.1	3120.6	3164.7	3208.4	3251.9
	s		6.4509	6.5577	6.6543	6.7430	6.8257	6.9035	6.9774	7.0481	7.1160	7.1816

(Contd.)

Table AIII.3 (Contd.)

Pres., bar / Sat. temp. °C / Sat. temp. K	Parameter	\multicolumn{10}{c}{Superheated steam temperature, °C (K)}									
		240 (513.15)	260 (533.15)	280 (533.15)	300 (373.15)	320 (393.15)	340 (613.15)	360 (633.15)	380 (653.15)	400 (673.15)	440 (713.15)
19 / 209.8 / 482.95	v	0.1147	0.1209	0.1268	0.1325	0.1380	0.1435	0.1488	0.1541	0.1593	0.1696
	i	2880.7	2932.0	2980.9	3027.9	3073.6	3118.5	3162.7	3206.6	3250.3	3337.4
	s	6.5254	6.6236	6.7135	6.7970	6.8755	6.9498	7.0209	7.0891	7.1550	7.2806
20 / 212.37 / 485.52	v	0.1084	0.1144	0.1200	0.1255	0.1308	0.1360	0.1411	0.1461	0.1511	0.1610
	i	2875.9	2928.1	2977.5	3025.0	3071.2	3116.3	3160.9	3204.9	3248.7	3336.0
	s	6.4943	6.5941	6.6852	6.7696	6.8487	6.9235	6.9950	7.0635	7.1295	7.2555
22 / 217.24 / 490.39	v	0.097 52	0.1031	0.1084	0.1134	0.1183	0.1231	0.1278	0.1324	0.1370	0.1460
	i	2866.0	2920.0	2970.8	3019.3	3066.2	3111.9	3156.9	3201.4	3245.5	3333.3
	s	6.4349	6.5328	6.6317	6.7179	6.7983	6.8742	6.9464	7.0155	7.0821	7.2088
24 / 221.78 / 494.93	v	0.088 39	0.093 67	0.098 63	0.1034	0.1079	0.1124	0.1167	0.1210	0.1252	0.1335
	i	2855.7	2911.6	2963.8	3013.4	3061.1	3107.5	3153.0	3197.8	3242.3	3330.6
	s	6.3788	6.4857	6.5818	6.6699	6.7517	6.8286	6.9016	6.9714	7.0384	7.1658
26 / 226.04 / 499.19	v	0.080 64	0.085 67	0.090 37	0.094 83	0.099 12	0.1033	0.1073	0.1113	0.1153	0.1230
	i	2845.2	2903.0	2956.7	3007.4	3056.0	3103.0	3149.0	3194.3	3239.0	3327.8
	s	6.3253	6.4360	6.5348	6.6249	6.7082	6.7862	6.8600	6.9304	6.9979	7.1260
28 / 230.05 / 503.2	v	0.073 97	0.788 80	0.083 28	0.087 51	0.091 56	0.095 48	0.099 29	0.1030	0.1067	0.1139
	i	2834.2	2894.2	2949.5	3001.3	3050.8	3098.5	3145.0	3190.7	3235.8	3325.11
	s	6.2738	6.3886	6.4903	6.5824	6.6672	6.7464	6.8210	6.8921	6.9601	7.0890
30 / 233.84 / 506.99	v	0.068 16	0.072 83	0.077 12	0.08116	0.085 00	0.08871	0.092 32	0.095 84	0.099 31	0.1061
	i	2822.9	2885.1	2942.0	2995.1	3045.4	3093.9	3140.9	3187.0	3232.5	3322.3
	s	6.2241	6.3432	6.4479	6.5422	6.6285	7.7088	6.7844	6.8561	6.9246	7.0543

(Contd.)

Table AIII.3 (Contd.)

Pres., bar / Sat. temp. °C / Sat. temp. K	Parameter	Superheated steam temperature, °C (K)									
		280 (553.15)	300 (573.15)	320 (593.15)	340 (613.15)	360 (633.15)	380 (653.15)	400 (673.15)	440 (713.15)	480 (753.15)	520 (793.15)
32 237.45 510.6	v	0.071 73	0.075 59	0.079 26	0.082 79	0.086 21	0.089 55	0.092 83	0.099 25	0.1055	0.1117
	i	2934.4	2988.7	3040.0	3089.2	3136.8	3183.4	3229.2	3319.5	3409.2	3498.8
	s	6.4072	6.5037	6.5917	6.6733	6.7497	6.8221	6.8912	7.0216	7.1439	7.2598
34 240.88 514.03	v	0.066 95	0.070 68	0.074 19	0.077 56	0.080 82	0.084 00	0.087 11	0.093 19	0.099 15	0.1050
	i	2926.2	2982.2	3034.5	3084.4	3132.7	3179.7	3225.9	3316.8	3406.8	3496.7
	s	6.3681	6.4669	6.5566	6.6394	6.7168	6.7833	6.8595	6.9907	7.1135	7.2299
36 244.16 517.31	v	0.062 70	0.066 30	0.069 68	0.072 91	0.076 03	0.079 06	0.082 02	0.087 81	0.093 47	0.099 03
	i	2918.6	2975.6	3028.9	3079.6	3128.4	3175.9	3222.5	3314.0	3404.4	3494.6
	s	6.3302	6.4315	6.5230	6.6070	6.6854	6.7592	6.8294	6.9614	7.0848	7.2015
38 247.31 520.46	v	0.058 88	0.062 37	0.065 64	0.068 75	0.071 74	0.074 64	0.077 47	0.083 00	0.088 38	0.093 67
	i	2910.4	2968.9	3023.3	3074.8	3124.2	3172.2	3219.1	3311.2	3402.0	3492.5
	s	6.2935	6.3973	6.4906	6.5760	6.6553	6.7299	6.8007	6.9336	7.0575	7.1746
40 250.33 523.48	v	0.055 44	0.058 83	0.062 00	0.06499	0.067 87	0.070 66	0.073 38	0.078 66	0.083 81	0.088 86
	i	2902.0	2962.0	3017.5	3069.8	3119.9	3168.4	3215.7	3308.3	3399.6	3490.4
	s	6.2576	6.3642	6.4593	6.5461	6.6265	6.7019	6.7733	6.9069	7.0314	7.1489
42 253.24 526.39	v	0.052 31	0.055 62	0.058 70	0.06160	0.064 37	0.067 06	0.069 67	0.074 74	0.079 67	0.084 50
	i	2893.5	2955.0	3011.6	3064.8	3115.5	3164.5	3212.3	3305.5	3397.1	3488.3
	s	6.2227	6.3320	6.4291	6.5173	6.5987	6.6749	6.7469	6.8815	7.0065	7.1244
44 256.05 529.2	v	0.049 46	0.052 70	0.055 69	0.058 50	0.061 19	0.063 78	0.066 29	0.071 17	0.075 90	0.080 54
	i	2884.7	2947.8	3005.7	3059.7	3111.1	3160.6	3208.8	3302.6	3394.7	3486.2
	s	6.1884	6.3006	6.3998	6.4894	6.5719	6.6489	6.7216	6.8570	6.9826	7.1010

(Contd.)

Table AIII.3 (Contd.)

Pres., bar / Sat. temp. °C / Sat. temp. K	Para-meter	Superheated steam temperature, °C (K)									
		300 (573.15)	320 (593.15)	340 (613.15)	360 (633.15)	380 (653.15)	400 (673.15)	440 (713.15)	480 (753.15)	520 (793.15)	560 (833.15)
46 / 258.75 / 531.9	v	0.050 03	0.052 94	0.055 68	0.058 28	0.060 79	0.063 21	0.067 091	0.072 47	0.076 92	0.08130
	i	2940.5	2999.6	3054.6	3106.7	3156.7	3205.3	3299.8	3392.3	3484.1	3575.8
	s	6.2700	6.3712	6.4624	6.5460	6.6239	6.6972	6.8335	6.9597	7.0784	7.1913
48 / 261.37 / 534.52	v	0.047 57	0.050 42	0.053 09	0.055 61	0.058 04	0.060 39	0.064 93	0.069 31	0.073 60	0.077 82
	i	2933.1	2993.4	3049.3	3102.2	3152.8	3201.8	3296.9	3389.8	3481.9	3573.9
	s	6.2399	6.3434	6.4362	6.5209	6.5996	6.6736	6.8108	6.9376	7.0568	7.1699
50 / 263.91 / 537.06	v	0.045 30	0.048 10	0.050 70	0.053 16	0.055 51	0.057 79	0.062 18	0.0066 42	0.070 55	0.07461
	i	2925.5	2987.2	3044.1	3097.6	3148.8	3198.3	3294.0	3387.4	3479.8	3572.0
	s	6.2105	6.3163	6.4106	6.4966	6.5762	6.6508	6.7890	6.9164	7.0360	7.1494
54 / 268.76 / 541.91	v	0.041 25	0.043 95	0.046 44	0.048 78	0.05102	0.053 17	0.057 29	0.06126	0.065 13	0.068 91
	i	2909.8	2974.3	3033.3	3088.3	3140.7	3191.1	3244.2	3382.5	3475.6	3568.3
	s	6.1530	6.2636	6.3614	6.4498	6.5312	6.6072	6.7473	6.8760	6.9964	7.1105
58 / 273.35 / 546.5	v	0.037 74	0.040 36	0.04276	0.045 01	0.047 13	0.049 18	0.053 08	0.056 82	0.060 45	0.064 00
	i	2893.5	2961.0	3022.2	3078.9	3132.4	3183.8	3282.3	3377.5	3471.3	3564.6
	s	6.0969	6.2128	6.3142	6.4052	6.4885	6.5660	6.7081	6.8381	6.9594	7.0741
62 / 277.7 / 550.85	v	0.034 65	0.037 22	0.039 55	0.04171	0.043 75	0.045 70	0.049 41	0.052 95	0.056 37	0.059 73
	i	2876.3	2947.3	3010.8	3069.2	3124.0	3176.4	3276.3	3372.5	3467.0	3560.8
	s	6.0418	6.1635	6.2688	6.3625	6.4478	6.5268	6.6710	6.8023	6.9245	7.0399
66 / 281.84 / 554.99	v	0.031 91	0.034 45	0.036 72	0.038 81	0.040 77	0.042 64	0.046 18	0.049 54	0.05279	0.055 97
	i	2858.3	2933.1	2999.0	3059.2	3115.5	3168.9	3270.3	3367.5	3462.7	3557.0
	s	5.9872	6.1154	6.2248	6.3214	6.4089	6.4894	6.6358	6.7684	6.8916	7.0076

(Contd.)

Table AIII.3 (Contd.)

Pres., bar / Sat. temp. °C / Sat. temp. K	Para-meter	320 (593.15)	340 (613.15)	360 (633.15)	380 (653.15)	400 (673.15)	440 (713.15)	480 (753.15)	520 (793.15)	560 (833.15)	600 (873.15)	640 (913.15)
70 / 285.79 / 558.94	v	0.031 98	0.03420	0.036 23	0.038 12	0.039 92	0.043 31	0.046 53	0.049 52	0.05264	0.055 59	0.05850
	i	2918.3	2987.0	3049.1	3106.7	3161.2	3264.2	3362.4	3458.3	3553.2	3647.9	3742.6
	s	6.0681	6.1820	6.2817	6.3714	6.4536	6.6022	6.7362	6.8603	6.9771	7.0880	7.1941
74 / 289.57 / 562.72	v	0.029 76	0.031 94	0.033 92	0.035 76	0.037 50	0.040 76	0.043 84	0.046 79	0.049 67	0.052 48	0.055 24
	i	2903.0	2974.6	3038.7	3097.8	3153.5	3258.0	3357.3	3454.0	3549.5	3644.5	3739.7
	s	6.0214	6.1402	6.2432	6.3351	6.4190	6.5700	6.7054	6.8305	6.9480	7.0594	7.1660
78 / 293.21 / 566.36	v	0.027 75	0.029 91	0.03185	0.033 64	0.035 32	0.038 47	0.04142	0.04425	0.047 00	0.049 69	0.052 32
	i	2887.0	2961.8	3028.1	3088.8	3145.6	3251.8	3352.2	3449.6	3545.7	3641.2	3736.7
	s	5.9751	6.0992	6.2056	6.3000	6.3857	6.5390	6.6760	6.8021	6.9202	7.0322	7.1392
82 / 296.7 / 569.85	v	0.025 92	0.028 06	0.029 97	0.031 71	0.033 35	0.036 39	0.039 24	0.04196	0.04459	0.047 17	0.049 69
	i	2870.2	2948.6	3017.2	3079.5	3137.6	3245.5	3347.0	3445.2	3541.8	3637.9	3733.7
	s	5.9288	6.0588	6.1689	6.2659	6.3534	6.5092	6.6477	6.7748	6.8937	7.0062	7.1136
86 / 303.31 / 573.21	v	0.024 24	0.026 38	0.028 26	0.29 97	0.03156	0.03451	0.037 26	0.039 88	0.042 41	0.04488	0.047 30
	i	2852.7	2935.0	3006.1	3070.1	3129.4	3239.1	3341.8	3440.8	3538.0	3634.5	3730.8
	s	5.8823	6.0189	6.1330	6.2326	6.3220	6.4804	6.6205	6.7486	6.8682	6.9813	7.0891
90 / 303.13 / 576.46	v	0.022 69	0.024 84	0.026 69	0.028 37	0.029 93	0.032 80	0.035 46	0.037 99	0.040 42	0.042 80	0.045 12
	i	2834.3	2920.9	2994.7	3060.5	3121.2	3232.7	3336.5	3436.3	3534.2	3631.1	3727.8
	s	5.8355	5.9792	6.0976	6.2000	6.2915	6.4525	6.5942	6.7233	6.8437	6.9574	7.0656
94 / 306.44 / 579.59	v	0.021 24	0.023 41	0.025 26	0.026 91	0.028 43	0.03123	0.033 81	0.036 25	0.03861	0.040 89	0.043 13
	i	2814.8	2906.3	2983.0	3050.7	3112.8	3226.2	3331.2	3431.9	3530.3	3627.8	3724.8
	s	5.7879	5.9397	6.0627	6.1631	6.2617	6.4254	6.5688	6.6990	6.8201	6.9343	7.0430

(Contd.)

Table AIII.3 (Contd.)

Pres., bar / Sat. temp. °C / Sat. temp. K	Para-meter	340 (613.15)	360 (633.15)	380 (653.15)	400 (673.15)	440 (713.15)	480 (753.15)	520 (793.15)	560 (833.15)	600 (873.15)	640 (913.15)	680 (953.15)
					Superheated steam temperature, °C (K)							
98 / 309.48 / 582.63	v	0.022 09	0.023 93	0.025 56	0.027 06	0.029 79	0.032 29	0.034 66	0.036 93	0.039 14	0.041 30	0.04342
	i	2891.2	2970.9	3040.8	3104.2	3219.6	3325.9	3427.4	3526.5	3624.4	3721.8	3819.2
	s	5.9001	6.0282	6.1368	6.2325	6.3990	6.5441	6.6755	6.7974	6.9121	7.0213	7.1257
100 / 310.96 / 584.11	v	0.02147	0.023 31	0.024 93	0.026 41	0.029 11	0.031 58	0.033 91	0.036 15	0.038 32	0.040 44	0.042 52
	i	2883.4	2964.8	3035.7	3099.9	3216.2	3323.2	3425.1	3524.3	3622.7	3720.4	3817.9
	s	5.8803	6.0110	6.1213	6.2182	6.3861	6.5321	6.6640	6.7863	6.9013	7.0107	7.1153
105 / 314.57 / 587.72	v	0.020 00	0.021 84	0.023 44	0.024 89	0.027 52	0.029 92	0.032 16	0.03432	0.036 40	0.03843	0.04043
	i	2863.1	2949.1	3022.8	3089.0	3207.9	3316.4	3419.5	3519.7	3618.5	3716.6	3814.6
	s	5.8303	5.9684	6.0831	6.1829	6.3545	6.5027	6.6360	6.7593	6.8751	6.9850	7.0901
110 / 318.05 / 591.2	v	0.018 64	0.020 49	0.022 08	0.023 51	0.026 08	0.028 40	0.030 58	0.032 65	0.034 66	0.036 61	0.038 52
	i	2841.7	2932.8	3009.6	3077.8	3199.4	3309.6	3413.8	3514.8	3614.2	3712.9	3811.3
	s	5.7797	5.9259	6.0454	6.1483	6.3238	6.4742	6.6091	6.7334	6.8499	6.9604	7.0659
115 / 321.40 / 594.55	v	0.017 38	0.019 26	0.020 84	0.022 25	0.024 76	0.027 02	0.029 12	0.031 13	0.033 06	0.034 94	0.036 78
	i	2819.0	2915.8	2996.0	3066.4	3190.7	3302.7	3408.1	3509.9	3609.9	3709.1	3808.0
	s	5.7279	5.8835	6.0082	6.1144	6.2939	6.4467	6.5830	6.7083	6.8256	6.9367	7.0427
120 / 324.65 / 597.8	v	0.016 19	0.018 11	0.019 69	0.021 08	0.023 55	0.025 75	0.027 79	0.029 73	0.031 60	0.033 42	0.035 19
	i	2794.7	2898.1	2982.0	3054.8	3182.0	3295.7	3402.3	3505.0	3605.7	3705.4	3804.7
	s	5.6747	5.8408	5.9712	6.0810	6.2647	6.4199	6.5578	6.6842	6.8022	6.9139	7.0203
125 / 327.78 / 600.93	v	0.015 08	0.017 04	0.018 63	0.020 01	0.022 43	0.024 58	0.026 57	0.028 45	0.030 26	0.032 01	0.03373
	i	2768.7	2879.6	2967.6	3042.9	3173.1	3288.7	3396.5	3500.0	3601.4	3701.6	3801.3
	s	5.6195	5.7976	5.9345	6.0481	6.2362	6.3939	6.5334	6.6608	6.7796	6.8919	6.9987

(Contd.)

Table AIII.3 (Contd.)

Pres., bar Sat. temp. °C Sat. temp. K	Parameter	Superheated steam temperature, °C (K)										
		340 (613.15)	360 (633.15)	380 (653.15)	400 (673.15)	440 (713.15)	480 (753.15)	520 (793.15)	560 (833.15)	600 (873.15)	640 (913.15)	680 (953.15)
130 330.83 603.98	v	0.014 01	0.016 04	0.017 64	0.019 02	0.021 40	0.023 50	0.025 44	0.027 27	0.029 02	0.030 72	0.032 37
	i	2740.6	2860.2	2952.7	3030.7	3164.1	3281.6	3390.6	3495.1	3597.1	3697.8	3798.0
	s	5.5618	5.7539	5.8979	6.0155	6.2082	6.3685	6.5096	6.6381	6.7577	6.8706	6.9779
135 333.78 606.93	v	0.012 99	0.015 10	0.016 72	0.018 09	0.020 44	0.022 50	0.024 39	0.026 17	0.027 87	0.029 52	0.031 12
	i	2709.9	2839.7	2937.3	3018.3	3155.0	3274.4	3384.7	3490.1	3592.8	3694.1	3794.7
	s	5.5007	5.7093	5.8612	5.9833	6.1808	6.3437	6.4865	6.6161	6.7365	6.8499	6.9578
140 336.64 609.79	v	0.0120 00	0.014 21	0.015 86	0.017 23	0.019 55	0.021 57	0.023 42	0.025 15	0.026 80	0.028 40	0.029 96
	i	2675.7	2818.1	2921.4	3005.6	3145.0	3267.1	3378.8	3485.1	3588.5	3690.3	3791.3
	s	5.4348	5.6636	5.8243	5.9513	6.1538	6.3194	6.4639	6.5947	6.7159	6.8299	6.9382
145 339.42 612.57	v	0.011 00	0.013 37	0.015 05	0.016 42	0.018 72	0.020 70	0.022 51	0.024 20	0.025 81	0.027 37	0.028 88
	i	2635.8	2795.2	2904.9	2992.5	3136.4	3259.8	3372.8	3480.0	3584.1	3686.5	3788.0
	s	5.3603	5.6165	5.7872	5.9194	6.1272	6.2957	6.4419	6.5738	6.6959	6.8105	6.9193
150 342.13 615.28	v		0.012 56	0.014 28	0.015 66	0.017 94	0.019 89	0.021 66	0.023 31	0.024 88	0.026 40	0.027 87
	i		2770.8	2887.7	2979.1	3126.9	3252.4	3366.8	3475.0	3579.8	3682.7	3784.7
	s		5.5677	5.7497	5.8876	6.1010	6.2724	6.4204	6.5535	6.6764	6.7917	6.9009

(Reproduced with the permission of *The Japan Society of Mechanical Engineers, Japan* from *1980 JSME Steam Tables in SI*.)

Heats of Formation of Inorganic Compounds and of Formation and Combustion of Organic Compounds

Table AIV.1 Heats of Formation of Inorganic Compounds

Substance	Formula	Molar mass kg/kmol	ΔH_f^0, kJ/mol at 298.15 K (25°C) and 1 bar		
			Gas	Liquid	Solid
Oxygen	O_2	31.9988	0.0		
Ozone	O_3	47.9982	142.70		
Hydrogen	H_2	2.0159	0.0		
Water	H_2O	18.0153	−241.82	−285.83	
Hydrogen peroxide	H_2O_2	34.0147	−136.30	−187.80	
Fluorine	F_2	37.9968	0.0		
Hydrogen fluoride	HF	20.0063	−273.30	−299.78	
in H_2O	HF, aq.			−332.63	
Chlorine	Cl_2	70.906	0.0		
Hydrogen chloride	HCl	36.4609	−92.31		
in H_2O	HCl, aq.			−167.169	
Hypochlorous acid	HClO	52.4603	−78.70		
Chlorine dioxide	ClO_2	67.4518	102.50		
Perchloric acid	$HClO_4$	100.4585		−40.58	
in H_2O	$HClO_4$, aq.			−129.33	
Bromine	Br_2	159.808	30.91		0.0
Hydrogen bromide	HBr	80.9119	−28.56		
in H_2O	BHr, aq.			−121.55	
Bromine dioxide	BrO_2	111.9028			48.53
Iodine	I_2	253.8089	62.421		0.0

(Contd.)

Table AIV.1 (Contd.)

Substance	Formula	Molar mass kg/kmol	ΔH_f^o, kJ/mol at 298.15 K (25°C) and 1 bar		
			Gas	Liquid	Solid
Hydrogen iodide	HI	127.9124	26.50		
in H_2O	HI, aq.			– 55.19	
Iodic acid	HIO_3	175.9106			– 230.12
Sulphur	S	32.065	276.98		
rhombic	S	32.065			0.0
monoclinic	S	32.065			0.33
Sulphur, diatomic	S_2	64.13	128.49		
Sulphur dioxide	SO_2	64.0638	– 296.81	– 320.49	
Sulphur trioxide	SO_3	80.0632	– 395.72	– 441.04	– 454.51
Sulphuric acid	H_2SO_4	98.0785		– 813.99	
in H_2O	H_2SO_4, aq.			– 909.27	
Hydrogen sulphide	H_2S	34.0809	– 20.63		
Thionyl chloride	$SOCl_2$	118.9704	– 212.55	– 245.6	
Nitrogen	N_2	28.0134	0.0		
Nitrogen oxide	NO	30.0061	90.25		
Nitrogen dioxide	NO_2	46.0055	33.18		
Nitrogen trioxide	NO_3	62.0049	71.00		
Nitrous oxide	N_2O	44.0128	82.05		
(Di)nitrogen dioxide	N_2O_2	60.0123	168.60		
(Di)nitrogen pentoxide	N_2O_5	108.0104	11.30		– 43.1
(Di)nitrogen tetroxide	N_2O_4	92.011	9.16	– 19.50	
(Di)nitrogen trioxide	N_2O_3	76.0116	84.61		
Ammonia	NH_3	17.0305	– 45.94		
Hydrazine	N_2H_4	32.0452	95.4 50.63		
Nitrous acid (cis)	HNO_2	47.0134	– 77.99		
Nitric Acid	HNO_3	63.0128	– 135.06	– 174.10	
in H_2O	HNO_3, aq.			– 207.36	
Ammonium hydroxide	NH_4OH	35.0458		– 361.20	
in H_2O	NH_4OH, aq.			– 362.50	
Ammonium nitrate	NH_4NO_3	80.0434			– 365.56
in H_2O	NH_4NO_3, aq.			– 339.87	
Nitrosyl chloride	NOCl	65.4591	51.71		
Ammonium chloride	NH_4Cl	53.4915			– 314.43
in H_2O	NH_4Cl, aq			– 299.66	
Ammonium bromide	NH_4Br	97.9425			– 270.83
in H_2O	NH_4Br, aq.			– 254.05	
Ammonium iodide	NH_4I	144.9429			– 201.42
in H_2O	NH_4I, aq			– 187.69	
Sulphamic acid	H_2NSO_3H	97.0937			– 674.9
Ammonium hydrogen sulphate	NH_4HSO_4	115.109			– 1026.96
Ammonium sulphate	$(NH_4)_2SO_4$	132.1395			– 1180.85
in H_2O	$(NH_4)_2SO_4$, aq.			– 1174.28	

(Contd.)

622 — Stoichiometry

Table AIV.1 (Contd.)

Substance	Formula	Molar mass kg/kmol	ΔH_f^0, kJ/mol at 298.15 K (25°C) and 1 bar Gas	Liquid	Solid
Phosphorus	P	30.9738	314.64		
α, white	P	30.9738			0.0
triclinic red	P	30.9738			− 17.6
black	P	30.9738			− 39.3
amorphous red	P	30.9738			− 7.5
Phosphorous pentoxide					
hexagonal crystals	P_4O_{10}	283.8890			− 2984.0
amorphous	P_4O_{10}	283.8890			− 3042.0
Phosphoric acid (ortho)	H_3PO_4	97.9952		− 1266.9	− 1279.0
Phosphine	PH_3	33.9976	5.4		
Metaphosphoric acid	HPO_3	79.9799			− 948.5
Pyrophosphoric acid	$H_4P_2O_7$	177.9592		− 2231.7	− 2241.0
Ammonium dihydrogen phosphate	$NH_4H_2PO_4$	115.0257			− 1445.07
Ammonium hydrogen phosphate	$(NH_4)_2HPO_4$	132.0562			− 1566.91
Ammonium phosphate					
α, crystal	$(NH_4)_3PO_4$	149.0867			− 1671.9
amorphous	$(NH_4)_3PO_4$	149.0867			− 1254.53
Boron	B	10.811			0.0
Diborane	B_2H_6	27.6696	35.6		
Boric oxide	B_2O_3	69.6202	− 843.79		− 1272.77
Boric acid	H_3BO_3	61.8330	− 994.1	− 1094.33	
Silicon	Si	28.0855			0.0
Silicon dioxide	SiO_2	60.0843	− 322.0		
quartz	SiO_2	60.0843			− 910.94
amorphous	SiO_2	60.0843			− 903.94
Silane	SiH_4	32.1773	34.3		
Disilane	Si_2H_6	62.2186	80.3		
Silicon tetrachloride	$SiCl_4$	169.8975	− 657.01	− 687.0	
Sodium	Na	22.9898	107.32		0.0
Sodium oxide	Na_2O	61.9789	− 35.6	− 414.22	
Sodium hydroxide	NaOH	39.9971	− 207.1	− 425.609	
in H_2O	NaOH, aq.			− 470.11	
Sodium, fluoride	NaF	41.9882	− 291.2	− 573.647	
in H_2O	NaF, aq.			− 572.75	
Sodium chloride	NaCl	58.4428	− 176.65		− 411.153
in H_2O	NaCl, aq.			− 407.27	
Sodium bicarbonate	$NaHCO_3$	84.0066			− 950.81
Sodium carbonate	Na_2CO_3	105.9884			− 1130.68
Sodium formate	$NaCHO_2$	68.0072			− 666.5
Sodium acetate	$NaC_2H_3O_2$	82.0338			− 708.81
in H_2O	$NaC_2H_3O_2$, aq.			− 726.13	
Potassium	K	39.0983	89.24		0.0
Potassium oxide	K_2O	94.196	− 63.0	− 361.5	

(Contd.)

Table AIV.1 (Contd.)

Substance	Formula	Molar mass kg/kmol	ΔH_f^o, kJ/mol at 298.15 K (25°C) and 1 bar		
			Gas	Liquid	Solid
Potassium hydroxide	KOH	56.1056	– 23.10		– 424.764
in H_2O	KOH, aq.			– 482.37	
Potassium fluoride	KF	58.0967	– 325.43		– 567.27
in H_2O	KF, aq.			– 585.01	
Potassium chloride	KCl	74.5513	– 214.14		– 436.747
in H_2O	KCl, aq.			– 419.53	
Potassium chloride	KCl	74.5513	– 214.14		– 296.25
in H_2O	KCl, aq.				
Potassium chlorate	$KClO_3$	122.5495		– 356.35	
in H_2O	$KClO_3$, aq.				
Carbon, graphite	C	12.0107	716.67		0.0
Carbon monoxide	CO	28.0101	– 110.53		
Carbon dioxide	CO_2	44.0095	– 393.51		

Table AIV.2 Heats of Formation and Heats of Combustion of Organic Compounds

Substance	Formula and state	Molar mass kg/kmol	kJ/mol at 298.15 K (25°C) and 1 bar		
			ΔH_f^o	$-\Delta H_c^o$	
				Gross	Net
Methane	CH_4,g[a]	16.0425	– 74.52	890.65	802.62
Ethane	C_2H_6,g	30.069	– 83.82	1560.69	1428.64
	C_2H_6,l*		– 93.46	1551.05	1419.00
Propane	C_3H_8,g	44.0956	– 104.68	2219.17	2043.11
	C_3H_8,l*		– 121.08	2202.77	2026.71
n-Butane	C_4H_{10},g	58.1222	– 125.79	2877.40	2657.32
	C_4H_{10},l*		– 147.53	2855.66	2635.58
2-Methyl propane	C_4H_{10},g	58.1222	– 134.99	2868.20	2648.12
(iso-butane)	C_4H_{10},l*		– 155.22	2847.97	2627.89
n-Pentane	C_5H_{12},g	72.1488	– 146.76	3535.77	3271.67
	C_5H_{12},l		– 173.49	3509.04	3244.94
2-Methylbutane	C_5H_{12},g	72.1488	– 153.70	3528.83	3264.73
(iso-pentane)	C_5H_{12},l[a]		– 178.89	3503.64	3239.54
2,2-Dimethyl propane	C_5H_{12},g	72.1488	– 167.92	3514.61	3250.51
(neo-pentane)	C_5H_{12},l		– 190.31	3492.22	3228.12
n-Hexane	C_6H_{14},g	86.1754	– 166.92	4194.95	3886.84
	C_6H_{14},l		– 198.66	4163.21	3855.10
n-Heptane	C_7H_{16},g	100.2019	– 187.78	4853.43	4501.30
	C_7H_{16},l		– 224.35	4816.86	4464.73
n-Octane	C_8H_{18},g	114.2285	– 208.75	5511.80	5115.66
	C_8H_{18},l		– 250.26	5470.29	5074.15

(Contd.)

Table AIV.2 (Contd.)

Substance	Formula and state	Molar mass kg/kmol	ΔH_f^o	$-\Delta H_c^o$ Gross	$-\Delta H_c^o$ Net
n-Nonane	C_9H_{20},g	128.2551	− 228.74	6171.15	5730.99
	C_9H_{20},l		− 275.18	6124.71	5684.55
n-Decane	$C_{10}H_{22}$,g	142.2817	− 249.46	6829.77	6345.59
	$C_{10}H_{22}$,l		− 300.83	6778.40	6294.22
Cyclopropane	C_3H_6,g	42.0797	53.3	2091.3	1959.3
	C_3H_6,l*		35.2	2073.2	1941.2
Cyclobutane	C_4H_8,g	56.1063	27.6	2745.0	2568.9
	C_4H_8,l*		3.7	2721.1	2545.0
Cyclopentane	C_5H_{10},g	70.1329	− 77.1	3319.6	3099.5
	C_5H_{10},l*		− 105.8	3290.9	3070.8
Ethene (ethylene)	C_2H_4,g	28.0532	52.50	1411.2	1323.11
Propene (Propylene)	C_3H_6,g	42.0797	20.00	2058.0	1926.0
	C_3H_6,l*		3.96	2042.0	1909.9
1-Butene	C_4H_8,g	56.1063	− 0.54	2716.8	2540.8
	C_4H_8,l*		− 21.4	2696.0	2519.9
cis-2-Butene	C_4H_8,g	56.1063	− 7.40	2710.0	2533.9
	C_4H_8,l*		− 29.9	2687.5	2511.4
trans-2-Butene	C_4H_8,g	56.1063	− 11.00	2706.4	2530.3
	C_4H_8,l		− 33.00	2684.4	2508.3
2-Methylpropene	C_4H_8,g	56.1063	− 17.1	2700.3	2524.2
(iso-butene)	C_4H_8,l*		− 38.2	2679.2	2503.1
Propadiene (allene)	C_3H_4,g	40.0638	190.92	1944.35	1856.32
1,2-Butadiene	C_4H_6,g	54.0904	162.26	2593.79	2461.74
	C_4H_6,l		138.99	2569.52	2437.51
1,3-Butadiene	C_4H_6,g	54.0904	109.24	2541.74	2409.69
	C_4H_6,l		87.19	2520.11	2388.06
Dimethyl ether	C_2H_6O,g	46.0684	− 184.0	1460.47	1328.42
	C_2H_6O,l*		− 203.5	1440.97	1309.17
Methyl ethyl ether	C_3H_8O,g	60.0950	− 216.4	2107.40	1931.38
	C_3H_8O,l		− 240.7	2083.63	1907.49
Diethyl ether	$C_4H_{10}O$,g	74.1216	− 252.0	2751.06	2530.99
	$C_4H_{10}O$,l		− 279.2	2723.57	2503.50
Ethylene oxide	C_2H_4O,g	44.0526	− 52.63	1306.04	1218.00
Propylene oxide	C_3H_6O,g	58.0791	− 92.76	1945.27	1813.22
	C_3H_6O,l		− 120.8	1917.36	1785.31
Methanal (formaldehyde)	CH_2O,g	30.0260	− 108.6	563.46	519.44
Ethanal	C_2H_4O,g	44.0526	− 166.1	1192.65	1104.62
(acetaldehyde)	C_2H_4O,l		− 192.2	1166.48	1078.46
1-Propanal	C_3H_6O,g	58.0791	− 186.3	1847.40	1715.36
(n-propanaldehyde)	C_3H_6O,l		− 216.2	1817.74	1685.69
Ketene (ethenone)	C_2H_2O,g	42.0367	− 47.7	1011.69	967.76
Diketen	$C_4H_4O_2$,g	84.0734	− 190.2	1955.5	1867.48

The header spans: kJ/mol at 298.15 K (25°C) and 1 bar

(Contd.)

Table AIV.2 (Contd.)

Substance	Formula and state	Molar mass kg/kmol	ΔH_f°	$-\Delta H_c^\circ$ Gross	$-\Delta H_c^\circ$ Net
2-Propanone	C_3H_6O,g	58.0791	− 215.7	1821.30	1689.25
(acetone)	C_3H_6O,l		− 247.3	1791.21	1659.17
Methanoic acid	CH_2O_2,g	46.0254	− 378.8	300.79	257.61
(formic acid)	CH_2O_2,l		− 424.8	254.64	211.46
Ethanoic acid	$C_2H_4O_2$,g	60.0520	− 432.7	924.50	836.21
(acetic acid)	$C_2H_4O_2$,l		− 484.2	874.46	786.42
n-Propanoic acid	$C_3H_6O_2$,g	74.0785	− 452.8		
(propionic acid)	$C_3H_6O_2$,l		− 507.8	1527.08	1395.03
n-Butanoic acid	$C_4H_8O_2$,g	88.1051	− 473.6		
(butyric acid)	$C_4H_8O_2$,l		− 531.6	2182.37	2006.23
Ethanoic (acetic)	$C_4H_6O_3$,g	102.0886	− 432.25	1813.89	1723.68
anhydride	$C_4H_6O_3$,l		− 624.5	1807.45	1675.40
Methyl methanoate	$C_2H_4O_2$,g	60.0520	− 352.4	1008.76	920.90
(methyl formate)	$C_2H_4O_2$,l		− 381.1	980.73	892.45
Ethyl ethanoate	$C_4H_8O_2$,g	88.1051	− 444.5	2265.64	2089.49
(ethyl acetate)	$C_4H_8O_2$,l		− 480.0	2230.91	2054.76
α-Oxalic acid	$C_2H_2O_4$,g	90.0349	− 732.0		
	$C_2H_2O_4$,c		− 829.9	244.76	200.83
Ethyne (acetylene)	C_2H_2,g	26.0373	228.2	1310.1	1257.0
	C_2H_2,l*			1072.9	1028.8
Propyne	C_3H_4,g	40.0638	184.51	1936.7	1848.7
(methyl acetylene)	C_3H_4,l*			1752.2	1664.2
1-Butyne	C_4H_6,g	54.0904	165.23	2596.7	2464.7
(ethyl acetylene)	C_4H_6,l*		141.4	2572.9	2440.9
2-Butyne	C_4H_6,g	54.0904	145.09	2577.4	2445.4
(dimethyl acetylene)	C_4H_6,l*		119.3	2550.8	2418.8
Benzene	C_6H_6,g	78.118	82.93	3301.5	3169.4
	C_6H_6,l		49.08	3267.6	3135.6
Methylbenzene	C_7H_8,g	92.1384	50.117	3948.1	3772.0
(toluene)	C_7H_8,l		12.18	3910.1	3734.0
Styrene	C_8H_8,g	104.1491	148.30	4439.7	4263.66
(phenyl ethane)	C_8H_8,l		103.80	4395.2	4219.16
Ethylbenzene	C_8H_{10},g	106.165	29.92	4607.1	4387.1
	C_8H_{10},l		− 12.34	4564.9	4344.8
1,2-dimethylbenzene	C_8H_{10},g	106.165	19.08	4596.3	4376.2
(o-xylene)	C_8H_{10},l		− 24.35	4552.9	4332.8
1,3-Dimethylbenzene	C_8H_{10},g	106.165	17.32	4594.5	4374.5
(m-xylene)	C_8H_{10},l		− 25.35	4551.9	4331.8
1,4-Dimethylbenzene	C_8H_{10},g	106.165	18.03	4595.3	4375.2
(p-xylene)	C_8H_{10},l		− 24.35	4552.9	4332.8
Methanol	CH_4O,g	32.0419	− 200.94	764.08	676.05
(methyl alcohol)	CH_4O,l		− 239.2	726.13	638.10

(Contd.)

Table AIV.2 (Contd.)

Substance	Formula and state	Molar mass kg/kmol	ΔH_f°	$-\Delta H_c^\circ$ Gross	$-\Delta H_c^\circ$ Net
Ethanol	C_2H_6O,g	46.0684	− 234.95	1410.09	1278.04
(ethyl alcohol)	C_2H_6O,l		− 277.2	1364.54	1235.49
1-Propanol	C_3H_8O,g	60.0950	− 255.20	2067.44	1891.42
(n-propyl alcohol)	C_3H_8O,l		− 304.2	2028.19	1843.81
2-Propanol	C_3H_8O,g	60.0950	− 272.70	2051.42	1875.39
(iso-propyl alcohol)	C_3H_8O,l		318.1	2005.98	1829.96
1-Butanol	$C_4H_{10}O$,g	74.1216	− 274.60	2728.51	2508.43
(n-butyl alcohol)	$C_4H_{10}O$,l		− 327.3	2676.09	2456.01
1-Pentanol	$C_5H_{12}O$,g	88.1482	− 295.6	3381.51	3117.46
(amyl alcohol)	$C_5H_{12}O$,l		− 358.2	3324.61	3060.51
1,2-Ethanediol	$C_2H_6O_2$,g	62.0678	− 389.0		
(ethylene glycol)	$C_2H_6O_2$,l		− 455.7	1189.64	1057.59
Benzoic acid	$C_7H_6O_2$,g	122.1213	− 290.20	3318.37	3186.33
	$C_7H_6O_2$,c		− 385.4	3226.95	3094.90
Phenol	C_6H_6O,g	94.1112	− 96.15	3122.39	2990.35
	C_6H_6O,c		− 165.1	3053.25	2921.48
2-Methylphenol	C_7H_8O,g	108.1378	− 128.57	3769.45	3593.39
(o-cresol)	C_7H_8O,c		− 204.6	3693.43	3517.36
3-Methylphenol	C_7H_8O,g	108.1378	− 132.3	3765.98	3589.91
(m-cresol)	C_7H_8O,c		− 193.8	3704.26	3528.20
4-Methylphenol	C_7H_8O,g	108.1378	− 125.35	3772.71	3596.73
(p-cresol)	C_7H_8O,c		− 199.3	3698.70	3522.64
Carbon tetrafluoride	CF_4,g	88.0043	− 933.5		
(tetrafluoromethane)					
Biphenyl	$C_{12}H_{10}$,g	154.2078	182.09	6333.36	6113.28
	$C_{12}H_{10}$,c		100.49	6251.77	6031.70
Naphthalene	$C_{10}H_8$,g	128.1705	150.96	5229.62	5053.56
	$C_{10}H_8$,c		78.53	5156.95	4980.88
Carbon tetrachloride	CCl_4,g	153.8227	− 95.81	290.79	290.79
(tetrachloromethane)	CCl_4,l		− 135.5	258.07	258.07
Chloromethane	CH_3Cl,g	50.4875	− 81.96	741.40	675.38
(methyl chloride)					
Dichloromethane	CH_2Cl_2,g	84.9326	− 95.40	586.89	542.87
(methylene dichloride)	CH_2Cl_2,l		− 121.5	557.89	513.88
Trichloromethane	$CHCl_3$,g	119.3776	− 102.936	433.30	411.29
(chloroform)	$CHCl_3$,l		− 134.6	401.96	379.95
Chloroethane	C_2H_5Cl,g	64.5141	− 112.26	1394.95	1284.91
(ethyl chloride)					
Fluorotrichloromethane	$CFCl_3$,g	137.3681	− 283.7		
	$CFCl_3$,l		− 301.5		
Difluorodichloro-methane	CF_2Cl_2,g	120.9135	− 490.8		
Trifluorochloro-methane	CF_3Cl,g	104.4589	− 704.2		

(Contd.)

Table AIV.2 (Contd.)

Substance	Formula and state	Molar mass kg/kmol	ΔH_f°	$-\Delta H_c^{\circ}$ Gross	Net
Carbon disulphide	CS_2,g	76.141	117.07	1104.53	1104.53
	CS_2,l			1076.88	1076.88
Aminomethane	CH_5N,g	31.0571	− 22.53	1085.12	975.08
(methylamine)	CH_5N,l		− 47.27	1060.64	950.60
Aminoethane	C_2H_7N,g	45.0837	− 47.47	1741.38	1587.37
(ethyl amine)	C_2H_7N,l		− 74.13	1713.31	1559.29
Aminobenzene	C_6H_7N,g	93.1265	− 87.46	3448.33	3294.27
(aniline)	C_6H_7N,l		31.1	3392.55	3238.50
Hydrogen cyanide	HCN,g	27.0253	130.12	671.53	649.36
	HCN,l		108.9	645.30	623.29
Cyanamide	CH_2N_2,c	42.04	58.99	738.48	694.13
Ammonium cyanide	CH_4N_2,c	44.0559	0.42	965.58	877.55
Acetonitrile	C_2H_3N,g	41.0519	66.63	1303.73	1237.63
	C_2H_3N,l		51.46	1267.33	1201.23
Acrylonitrile	C_3H_3N,g	53.0626	180.6	1794.10	1693.26
	C_3H_3N,l		150.21	1759.37	1727.99
Pyridine	C_5H_5N,g	79.0999	140.37	2822.28	2712.24
	C_5H_5N,l		99.96	2782.07	2672.07
Ammonium bicarbonate	CH_5O_3,N,c	79.0553	− 849.35	258.57	148.53
Urea	CH_4ON_2,c	60.0553	− 333.51	632.20	544.17

@ g : Gaseous state

  1 : Liquid state

  c : Crystalline (solid) state

* at saturation pressure

REFERENCES

1. Reproduced with permission from TRC Thermodynamic Tables–Hydrocarbons and Non-Hydrocarbons, Thermodynamics Research Center, Texas A & M University, College Station TX 77843-3111, USA, 1993.
2. Selected Heats of Formation of Inorganic Compounds are reproduced from "NBS Tables of Chemical Thermodynamic Properties", *J. Phys. Chem. Ref. Data*, Vol. 11, Suppl. 2, 1982.
3. Reproduced with permission from "Enthalpy of Formation for 700 Major Organic Compounds", Yaws, C. L. and Chiang, P. Y., *Chem. Engng.*, Sept. 26, 1988, p. 81–88.

Index